# APPLIED PHARMACOKINETICS
## Principles of Therapeutic Drug Monitoring

# APPLIED PHARMACOKINETICS

Principles of Therapeutic Drug Monitoring

# APPLIED PHARMACOKINETICS

## Principles of Therapeutic Drug Monitoring

Edited by

**William E. Evans,** Pharm.D.
Director, Clinical Pharmacokinetics Laboratory
and Clinical Division of Pharmacy
St. Jude Children's Research Hospital
   and
Associate Professor of Clinical Pharmacy
Department of Pharmacy Practice
University of Tennessee
Center for the Health Sciences
Memphis

**Jerome J. Schentag,** Pharm.D.
Assistant Director, Clinical Pharmacokinetics Laboratory
Millard Fillmore Hospital
   and
Assistant Professor of Pharmaceutics and Pharmacy
State University of New York at Buffalo
Buffalo

**William J. Jusko,** Ph.D.
Director, Clinical Pharmacokinetics Laboratory
Millard Fillmore Hospital
   and
Professor of Pharmaceutics
State University of New York at Buffalo
Buffalo

Applied Therapeutics, Inc.
San Francisco

Applied Therapeutics, Inc.
P.O. Box 31-747
San Francisco, CA 94131

Library of Congress catalog card number 80-53408
ISBN 0-915486-03-2

Published December 1980
First Printing

# Preface

*Applied Pharmacokinetics: Principles of Therapeutic Drug Monitoring* is intended as an authoritative source of the objective criteria and systematic approaches necessary for rational application of pharmacokinetics in clinical practice. Previous texts have dealt mainly with the mathematical basis of pharmacokinetics and not with the principles governing its translation into improved patient care. The appropriate clinical application of pharmacokinetic data requires not only an understanding of the mathematical basis for pharmacokinetic manipulations of drug therapy, but also a comprehension of the relation of drug concentrations in biologic fluids (or tissue) to therapeutic or toxic effects, and of the influence of disease states, concurrent drug therapy and other clinical variables on drug disposition.

The scope of this first edition is limited to those drugs which are commonly monitored by pharmacokinetic methods and have a pharmacodynamic data base large enough to warrant critical review. For each drug, the authors examine the current basis and accepted criteria for application of pharmacokinetic principles in therapeutic drug monitoring. These guidelines are assessed for their accuracy and completeness, and critiqued against future research needs to better define their adequacy. In instances where a consensus does not exist, a primary chapter and one or more "counterpoint" chapters are included to reflect the current positions of several investigators. This format was adopted to compensate for the evolving data base from which pharmacokinetic approaches are being formulated, and thereby provides the reader with a broader representation of the present state-of-the-art.

The ultimate goal of this book is to improve patient care by improving the quality and application of pharmacokinetic principles in clinical practice. By providing a comprehensive and rigorous examination of the published literature, in the context of their own clinical and research experience, the authors have produced an authoritative reference source. If this text can serve as a resource for those involved in pharmacokinetic practice, education and research, and as a starting point for further refinement of our current approaches to applied pharmacokinetics, it will fulfill our intentions.

v

We wish to thank our contributors for their meticulous writing and unceasing cooperation in meeting the many demands required for timely publication of their work. We especially thank Dr. Brian Katcher for his editorial assistance, which was of paramount importance in the development of this first edition.

William E. Evans
Jerome J. Schentag
William J. Jusko

# Contributors

**Amdi Amdisen, M.D.**
Assistant Research Director, Psychopharmacology Research Unit, Department of Psychiatry, Aarhus University, Risskov, Denmark. (Lithium)

**C. Lindsay DeVane, Pharm.D.**
Clinical Pharmacokinetics Laboratory, Millard Fillmore Hospital; Department of Pharmaceutics, State University of New York at Buffalo, Buffalo, NY. (Tricyclic Antidepressants)

**Sydney H. Dromgoole, Ph.D.**
Research Rheumotologist, Department of Medicine, School of Medicine, University of California at Los Angeles, Los Angeles, CA. (Salicylates)

**William E. Evans, Pharm.D.**
Director, Clinical Pharmacokinetics Laboratory and Clinical Division of Pharmacy, St. Jude Children's Research Hospital; Associate Professor of Clinical Pharmacy, Department of Pharmacy Practice, University of Tennessee, Center for the Health Sciences, Memphis, TN. (Methotrexate)

**Margaret A. French, Pharm.D.**
Department of Pharmacy Services, Hartford Hospital, Hartford, CT; Assistant Clinical Professor, School of Pharmacy, University of Connecticut, Storrs, CT. (Cephalosporins)

**Daniel E. Furst, M.D.**
Assistant Professor of Medicine, Department of Medicine, School of Medicine, University of California at Los Angeles, Los Angeles, CA. (Salicylates)

**Thomas P. Gibson, M.D.**
Associate Professor of Medicine, Section of Nephrology/Hypertension, Department of Medicine, Veterans Administration Lakeside Medical Center; Northwestern University Medical School and Northwestern Memorial Hospital, Chicago, IL. (Influence of Renal Disease on Pharmacokinetics)

**Laurence Green, Pharm.D.**
Clinical Pharmacokinetics Laboratory of the Buffalo General Hospital; Department of Pharmaceutics, School of Pharmacy, State University of New York at Buffalo, Buffalo, NY. (Lidocaine Counterpoint)

**Leslie Hendeles, Pharm.D.**
Associate Professor, College of Pharmacy, University of Florida, J. Hillis Miller Health Center, Gainesville, FL. (Theophylline)

**Donald M. Hilligoss, Pharm.D.**
Director of Pharmacokinetic Services, West Virginia University Medical Center, Charleston Division, Charleston, WV. (Neonatal Pharmacokinetics)

**J. Edward Jackson, M.D.**
Division of Clinical Pharmacology, Department of Medicine, University of Arizona, Tucson, AR. (Theophylline Counterpoint)

**George Johnson, Ph.D.**
Associate Professor of Pathology, Director, Clinical Pharmacology and Toxicology Laboratories, University of Iowa, Iowa City, IA. (Theophylline)

**William J. Jusko, Ph.D.**
Director, Clinical Pharmacokinetics Laboratory, Millard Fillmore Hospital; Professor of Pharmaceutics, State University of New York at Buffalo, Buffalo, NY. (Guidelines for Collection and Pharmacokinetic Analysis of Drug Disposition Data)

**Kim L. Kelly, Pharm.D.**
Associate Professor of Clinical Pharmacy, Schools of Pharmacy and Medicine, University of Missouri-Kansas City; Docent Clinical Pharmacist, Truman Medical Center, Kansas City, MO. (Heparin)

**Philip Keys, Pharm.D.**
Assistant Director, Department of Pharmacy, Mercy Hospital, Pittsburgh, PA. (Digoxin)

**David Lalka, Ph.D.**
Clinical Pharmacokinetics Laboratory of the Buffalo General Hospital; Assistant Professor of Pharmaceutics, School of Pharmacy, State University of New York at Buffalo, Buffalo, NY. (Lidocaine Counterpoint)

**Gerhard Levy, Pharm.D.**
Distinguished Professor of Pharmaceutics, School of Pharmacy, State University of New York at Buffalo, Buffalo, NY. (Applied Pharmacokinetics—A Prospectus)

**John J. Lima, Pharm.D.**
Assistant Professor, College of Pharmacy, The Ohio State University, Columbus, OH. (Procainamide)

**Thomas M. Ludden, Ph.D.**
Associate Professor, College of Pharmacy, University of Texas at Austin; Department of Pharmacology, University of Texas Health Sciences Center at San Antonio, San Antonio, TX. (Clinical Pharmacokinetics Consultation Services and Phenytoin Counterpoint)

**Antoinette Mangione, Pharm.D.**
Clinical Pharmacokinetics Laboratory, Millard Fillmore Hospital; Assistant Professor of Pharmacy, State University of New York at Buffalo, Buffalo, NY. (Theophylline Counterpoint)

**Charles Nightingale, Ph.D.**
Director, Department of Pharmacy Services, Hartford Hospital, Hartford, CT; Associate Research Professor, School of Pharmacy, University of Connecticut, Storrs, CT. (Cephalosporins)

**J. Robert Powell, Pharm.D.**
Associate Professor of Clinical Pharmacy, School of Pharmacy, University of North Carolina, Chapel Hill, NC. (Theophylline Counterpoint)

**Richard Quintiliani, M.D.**
Director, Division of Infectious Diseases, Hartford Hospital, Hartford, CT; Associate Professor of Medicine, University of Connecticut, School of Medicine, Farmington, CT. (Cephalosporins)

**John H. Rodman, Pharm.D.**
Associate Professor of Clinical Pharmacy, School of Pharmacy, University of Southern California, Los Angeles, CA. (Lidocaine)

**Philip A. Routledge, M.D.**
Research Assistant Professor of Medicine, Division of Clinical Pharmacology, Duke University Medical Center, Durham, NC. (Propanolol)

**Jerome J. Schentag, Pharm.D.**
Assistant Director, Clinical Pharmacokinetics Laboratory, Millard Fillmore Hospital; Assistant Professor of Pharmaceutics and Pharmacy, State University of New York at Buffalo, Buffalo, NY. (Aminoglycosides)

**David G. Shand, M.B., Ph.D.**
Professor of Pharmacology and Medicine, Division of Clinical Pharmacology, Duke University Medical Center, Durham, NC. (Propranolol)

**Thomas N. Tozer, Ph.D.**
Associate Professor of Pharmacy and Pharmaceutical Chemistry, Department of Pharmacy, School of Pharmacy, University of California San Francisco, San Francisco, CA. (Phenytoin)

**Clarence T. Ueda, Pharm.D., Ph.D.**
Director of Clinical Pharmacokinetics Cardiovascular Center, University of Nebraska Medical Center; Associate Professor and Chairman, Department of Pharmaceutics, College of Pharmacy, University of Nebraska, Omaha, NE. (Quinidine)

**Miles Weinberger, M.D.**
Associate Professor, Pediatrics & Pharmacology, Chairman of the Pediatric Allergy and Pulmonary Division, Department of Pediatrics, University of Iowa, Iowa City, IA. (Theophylline)

**Michael E. Winter, Pharm.D.**
Director, Clinical Pharmacokinetics Consultation Services; Associate Clinical Professor, Division of Clinical Pharmacy, School of Pharmacy, University of California San Francisco, San Francisco, CA. (Phenytoin)

**Grant R. Wilkinson, Ph.D.**
Professor of Pharmacology, Department of Pharmacology, Vanderbilt University, Nashville, TN. (Influence of Liver Disease on Pharmacokinetics)

**Milford G. Wyman, M.D.**
Department of Cardiology, San Pedro and Peninsula Hospital, San Pedro, CA. (Lidocaine Counterpoint)

**Darwin E. Zaske, Pharm.D.**
Associate Professor, College of Pharmacy and School of Medicine, University of Minnesota; Director of Pharmaceutical Services, St. Paul-Ramsey Medical Center, St. Paul, MN. (Counterpoint on Aminoglycosides and Counterpoint on Clinical Pharmacokinetics Consultation Services)

# Contents

# 1

# Applied Pharmacokinetics— A Prospectus

## Gerhard Levy, Pharm. D.

During the last twenty years enormous advances have been made in the development of sensitive and specific methods for the determination of drug and drug metabolite concentrations in biologic fluids, in the mathematical description of the changes of these concentrations as a function of time after drug administration, and in the use of mathematical formulations to predict the concentration-time profiles of drugs during chronic drug administration from knowledge obtained in single dose studies. It has also been established that the intensity of the pharmacologic effects of many drugs is related to their concentration and/or to the concentration of their metabolite(s) in plasma. This has led to the determination of usual therapeutic plasma concentration ranges of such drugs and to an awareness that these concentration ranges can serve as an intermediate therapeutic target for the individualization of drug dosage.

Many genetic characteristics and environmental factors, including diet and concomitant use of other drugs, and pathophysiologic variables such as age, gender, disease and pregnancy can affect the disposition of drugs and therefore can modify the relationship between dose and the drug concentration versus time profile in plasma and tissues. The dose-concentration relationship is also affected by incomplete absorption of the drug due to inadequate bioavailability of a particular dosage form, presystemic biotransformation of certain drugs administered by routes other than intravenous, and possible malabsorption secondary to pathologic conditions affecting the gastrointestinal tract. Another very important problem is poor compliance, either by the patient or by the hospital personnel responsible for drug administration to patients. For all these reasons, there is usually a much better relationship between drug concentration in plasma and the intensity of pharmacologic effects than there is between dose (or dosing rate) and these effects.

Individual adjustment of drug dosage on the basis of a targeted drug concentration in plasma may prevent or minimize adverse effects due to inadvertent overdosage and it may facilitate therapy, particularly in the case of drugs used to prevent periodic pathologic episodes such as epileptic seizures, by providing an alternative to the titration of dosage on the basis of therapeutic response or toxic effects. Moreover, therapeutic response is often difficult to assess in individual patients, particularly when the condition of the patient is unstable. Individualization of drug dosage based on therapeutic response becomes even more difficult if the patient receives several drugs with similar indications.

These considerations have led to the extensive use of therapeutic drug concentration monitoring and to an almost explosive proliferation of drug assay laboratories in recent years. This has been a mixed blessing for patients, their physicians, and for those who must bear the financial burden of this new component of health care. In many settings, therapeutic drug concentration monitoring consists of simply determining the concentration of a drug in plasma from a randomly collected blood sample and reporting the resulting "number" to the attending physician. Such random assays, without reference to the time interval between the last dose and the collection of the blood sample and without considering the duration of drug therapy in relation to the time required to reach steady state conditions, are uninterpretable at best and seriously misleading at worst. Other confounding factors may be interactions of the drug in plasma with the syringe or evacuated container used to collect the blood, administration of heparin shortly before collection of the blood sample (and consequent displacement of certain drugs from plasma proteins), assay interferences by other drugs or by drug metabolites, and lack of assay accuracy or precision. The turn-around time of an assay may be too long for the results to be helpful; assay results may not be charted; or appropriate action may not be taken when it is indicated by the reported drug concentration. Various studies of therapeutic drug concentration monitoring have revealed an enormous waste of resources for the reasons cited. Unless these deplorable practices are promptly reduced to a minimum, the disciplines of clinical pharmacokinetics, clinical pharmacy and clinical pharmacology may suffer a serious loss of credibility even if the poor practices described here are attributable to others.

The application of clinical pharmacokinetic principles to the individualization and optimization of drug dosing regimens is a rational process. It begins with a clear formulation of the therapeutic problem (Why does this patient not respond to a population-average drug dosing regimen? What is the most appropriate drug dosing regimen for this elderly patient with renal failure?), leading to a provisional decision (the dosage adjustment to be made or the initial dosage regimen to be used), followed by an assessment of the outcome of that decision (drug concentration in plasma and therapeutic response). If necessary, the drug regimen must be modified or other actions must be taken. This rational process usually requires a review of the patient's chart (for drug history and pathophysiologic information), an understanding of what the therapist wishes to accomplish, and adequate knowledge of the clinical pharmacokinetic characteristics of the drug.

It should be obvious therefore that the drug assay is only a small, albeit important part of the rational application of clinical pharmacokinetics to drug therapy. More important is the professional competence of the individual who has to determine when, what and how to monitor, and who must interpret the results and recommend appropriate action to the physician responsible for the patient's therapeutic management. This book is devoted to that individual—the clinical pharmacokineticist—and to those pharmacists and physicians who share our view that drug dosage must be individualized and that this should be done, whenever possible, by objective means. The initial chapters of the book are directed to the presentation of general principles and strategies of clinical pharmacokinetics and to a general consideration of the roles of certain pathophysiologic and environmental variables in pharmacokinetics. The following chapters are detailed expositions of the clinically important information required for therapeutic concentration monitoring of specific drugs: the kinetics of their absorption, distribution, metabolism and excretion; the usual therapeutic concentration range, as well as the relationships between concentration and pharmacologic effects and (if known) factors affecting these relationships; the application of the available information concerning the pharmacokinetic characteristics of the drug to the individualization of therapy; available analytical methods, including the advantages and shortcomings of different methods; and an outline of a rational approach to the optimization of drug dosage, including the design of the initial regimen and subsequent adjustments of dosage. This arrangement of the individual chapters epitomizes what I have tried to stress in these introductory paragraphs: there is a huge difference between determining a "blood level" and applying the wealth of our knowledge of the clinical pharmacokinetics of many important drugs to the effective therapeutic management of individual patients. All those whose efforts are devoted, directly or indirectly, to the latter purpose owe a debt of gratitude to the editors of and contributors to *Applied Pharmacokinetics*.

# 2

# Clinical Pharmacokinetics Consultation Services

Thomas M. Ludden, Ph.D.

## Introduction

Within the last ten years the direct application of pharmacokinetic principles to optimization of individual dosage regimens (1-4) has become an important aspect of clinical pharmacy and clinical pharmacology practices. Initial regimens of antiarrhythmics, aminoglycoside antibiotics, cardiac glycosides, theophylline and lithium are now frequently determined by referring to various tables, nomograms, or equations relating pharmacokinetic behavior to physiologic and pathophysiologic characteristics of the patient. Although the predictive use of pharmacokinetics is far from perfect, this approach is obviously an improvement over the past when most patients received a "usual" dose regardless of their individual characteristics. Still, many patients are treated without the benefit of a rationally designed initial dosage regimen.

An even more important application of pharmacokinetic principles is related to the therapeutic monitoring of serum or saliva drug levels (5-9). In the past, dosage regimens were frequently optimized by increasing the dose to the point of toxicity, then decreasing it slightly. For many drugs this method of titration has been replaced by the monitoring of drug levels. The accurate pharmacokinetic and pharmacodynamic interpretation of drug level data is essential for the correct use of this information in evaluating the efficacy or potential toxicity of a particular regimen and as a guide for making appropriate dosage adjustments. For example, a digoxin level obtained within six hours of the dose may be elevated merely because digoxin undergoes a rather slow distribution. A phenytoin level drawn ten days after initiating or changing the dosage regimen may not be indicative of the eventual steady-state level. Incorrect pharmacokinetic or phar-

4

macodynamic interpretation of drug level data may actually be detrimental to the patient.

There also appears to be significant misuse of serum level data. A recent study of changes in digoxin and digitoxin dosage regimens following determination of serum levels (10) demonstrated that no change in regimen was made in 36% of the cases in which there was rational indication for an increase or decrease in dosage. The same study also pointed out that 49% of the digoxin and digitoxin levels ordered were not indicated. Other studies (11,12) have found similar results. There appears to be a real need for improved utilization of drug level monitoring and the resulting data.

One means for providing better initial regimens and appropriate use of drug levels is a Clinical Pharmacokinetics Consultation Service (CPCS) (13). The CPCS can design rational initial regimens, screen requests for drug level determinations, interpret the levels once they are available, and make appropriate recommendations for dosage regimen adjustment based upon the drug level data and the physiologic and pathophysiologic characteristics of the patient. Of course, such a service could be a part of a broader Drug Information, Clinical Pharmacology and/or Clinical Pharmacy Consultation Service, provided the individuals responsible for the service possess adequate knowledge of clinical pharmacokinetics. A CPCS has been quite successful as a joint effort of the Clinical Pharmacy, Clinical Pharmacology, and Clinical Pathology Programs at the University of Texas Health Science Center at San Antonio (12).

This chapter will examine various aspects of the development and operation of a CPCS. Discussions concerning the scope of service, expertise of the consultants, evaluation of data, preparation of the consult, reimbursement and liability are included.

## Initiation of a Clinical Pharmacokinetics Consultation Service

The development of a consult service must be in keeping with the needs of the particular clinical environment for which it is intended. A pilot study involving only a few drugs and a defined patient population should be carried out to confirm the perceived need for the service and to identify potential problems.

Many factors can be used to document the benefits of the CPCS. These include incidence of toxicity, time required for optimization of therapy, rehospitalization for further dosage adjustment, emergency room visits, etc. The result of such a pilot study should be compared to similar data collected for a similar patient population who did not receive the service. It may be possible to express the overall results in terms of a cost-benefit analysis (14). Publication of well designed and executed studies demonstrating the economic benefits of clinical pharmacokinetics (15) are needed to convince health care administrators of their beneficial effect.

The logistics for requesting consults, collecting blood, saliva, or urine samples, transporting samples to the laboratory, obtaining the analytical results, and placing the written consult in the patient's chart will vary from institution to institution. Standard, efficient mechanisms for transfer of information and samples must be established and maintained.

In developing a consult service it is optimal to have requests for drug levels screened before they are actually obtained. This alone should prove to be a savings for the patient. However, proper screening of levels requires knowledge of the patient's data base and the intent of the requesting clinician and therefore involves a significant commitment of time and manpower. Alternately, a training program for physicians, nurses, and laboratory personnel involved with drug level monitoring can be developed. Such a program would deal with indications for levels and their appropriate drawing and timing.

In many situations the clinical pharmacokinetic consultant is a clinical pharmacist or clinical pharmacologist intimately involved with patient care. A patient's physician can then merely notify the pharmacokinetics consultant that an initial regimen or a serum level determination is desired, leaving the details to the consultant. In addition, the clinical pharmacist or clinical pharmacologist may receive a request for a consult of a broader nature which requires a drug level determination for an appropriate recommendation to be given. Since questions of a pharmacokinetic nature can arise at any time, use of a mobile paging system is a convenient way to request consults. However, in a newly initiated service, sitting back and waiting for only solicited consults will not quickly illustrate the contributions that can be made. By working with the analytical laboratory it may be possible to identify certain drug levels whose interpretation is not obvious. Then a brief discussion of the drug level with the clinician may stimulate his interest in requesting consults in the future.

If the results of a pilot study or of the developmental phase of a CPCS are indicative of benefit, then it may be possible to require that a pharmacokinetic consult accompany each drug level determination. In this case the laboratory could notify the CPCS that a level has been requested and that a consult is needed.

Specimen collection can usually be the responsibility of the nursing staff or laboratory personnel, but the consultant must assure himself that samples are obtained, timed and processed correctly and with due consideration for drug stability. The analytical results should be obtained directly from the laboratory. This provides an opportunity for the consultant and the clinical chemist to discuss any problems relative to that day's assays.

After the consult is prepared the consultant should see that it is placed in the patient's chart. In addition, the consultant should verbally discuss the recommendations with the patient's physician. Written consults are easily overlooked in a crowded chart.

The individual attempting to initiate a CPCS must demonstrate its role in patient care and develop an efficient system for its day-to-day operation. Sufficient manpower must be available to appropriately staff the CPCS and ensure continuous, dependable service. Cumbersome logistics or inconsistent availability of qualified consultants will threaten the success of the service.

## Scope of Service

The scope of services provided by a CPCS may vary considerably among institutions, based upon the results of the pilot study referred to previously. In certain cases the consultation service may be restricted to a particular patient population because of manpower limitations or because of the recognition of a special need in a particular group of patients (i.e., neurology or cardiology patients). Likewise, the nature of the services provided may be quite different. The CPCS may be involved with design of initial dosage regimens based upon the physiologic and pathophysiologic characteristics of the patient, using data in the literature relating drug kinetics to these characteristics. On the other hand, many clinicians prefer to design initial regimens, but will seek assistance when it is necessary to evaluate or optimize a patient's current therapy with the aid of drug levels.

There are two ways a consult regarding drug level determinations can be provided. In one case, there is only an interpretation of the serum or saliva drug level. Questions answered by such a consult usually include: "Is the level drawn at an appropriate time? Is it within the usual therapeutic range when such factors as plasma protein binding are considered? Is the drug level likely to be at steady-state or is there a possibility of a continued increase or decrease in concentration? If the level is significantly different from that which was expected based upon dose and/or response, what are the most probable factors (i.e., bioavailability, non-compliance, idiosyncrasy, inaccurate assay results, etc.) responsible for the difference?" While the importance of the above considerations should not be minimized, a more complete consult will contain a recommendation regarding the design of the dosage regimen. This must be worded in an appropriate manner reflecting the scientific basis for the recommendation but also indicating that therapeutic monitoring must be continued. Only individuals capable of evaluating the patient's *entire* clinical data base should make recommendations for dosage regimen alterations. Changes in regimen should never be recommended solely on the basis of a serum drug level. The patient's physiologic and pathophysiologic characteristics as well as concurrent drug administration (including nicotine, alcohol, etc.) must be carefully considered.

Besides consulting on drug levels, the CPCS can serve as a screen for the appropriateness of levels before they are drawn and assayed, as mentioned previously.

In certain situations the kinetic behavior of a drug permits the relatively easy determination of one or more pharmacokinetic parameters for a given patient (i.e., gentamicin or theophylline half-life or digoxin renal clearance). Such determinations usually require a minimum of extra samples. The use of individual gentamicin half-lives for dosage regimen design has been shown to be cost-effective in burn patients when compared to a control period during which pharmacokinetics was not carefully considered (15). In a few cases the CPCS may be asked to perform a detailed evaluation of the absorption, distribution or elimination of a drug to determine the cause of an abnormally high or low level and to rule out compliance as a complicating factor. Such evaluations usually require increased sampling and/or measurement of plasma or urine metabolites. These requests occur infrequently since, in most cases, they are difficult to justify on a cost-benefit basis.

When consulting on drug level data, the CPCS must be limited to those drugs for which there are accurate analytical procedures available in the institution. While the availability of a Clinical Pharmacokinetics Service *Laboratory* is certainly advantageous, it is in no way a requirement if the Clinical Pathology Laboratory provides reliable drug assays with the required turn-around time. The development of radioimmunoassay and the Enzyme-Multiplied Immunotest (EMIT®) has brought reliable clinical drug assays within the financial reach of most laboratories. The recent development of fully automated EMIT®-type systems has made therapeutic monitoring of drug levels even more practical from an analytic point of view.

The greatest advantage in having a Clinical Pharmacokinetics Service Laboratory is the capability of doing free drug levels using appropriate ultrafiltration or equilibrium dialysis techniques. While saliva assays can be useful as a general guide to free drug concentration in plasma, they tend to be inferior to more direct techniques when it comes to quantitation. Few Clinical Pathology Laboratories have the ability to determine free drug concentrations.

## Expertise Required

The knowledge base required to provide pharmacokinetic consults includes several components. The consultant must possess a clear understanding of the basic concepts of pharmacokinetics. This usually requires a graduate level pharmacokinetics course or its equivalent. The text by Gibaldi and Perrier (16) is an excellent guide to the basic concepts of classical pharmacokinetics. Other sources include books by Wagner (17,18) and Ritschel (19) and the review by Levy and Gibaldi (20). The basic concepts of physiologic pharmacokinetics as related to elimination of drug by the liver are discussed by Wilkinson and Shand (21) and Nies, Shand, and Wilkinson (22). While an understanding of the conceptual basis for pharmacokinetics is extremely important to rationally apply pharmacokinetic principles to clinical problems, it is equally important as a basis for the critical evaluation of current and future literature concerning applied biopharmaceutics and pharmacokinetics. Such evaluation and assimilation of new pharmacokinetics information is essential for continued competence.

Besides a thorough knowledge of pharmacokinetics, the individual responsible for consulting on initial dosage regimens, serum drug levels, and alterations in regimens must have a background in pathophysiology and pharmacotherapeutics. The clinical pharmacologist obviously has these other qualifications. Also, many clinical pharmacists, besides being trained in pharmacotherapeutics, have received appropriate instruction in pathophysiology (23), frequently from a medical school faculty. It is obvious that the clinical pharmacokinetics consultant must be able to understand the interplay between physiology, pathophysiology and drug absorption and disposition. Although this text represents a serious effort to bring together this type of information into a single reference source, the individual without in depth training in pathophysiology may find it difficult to properly relate the contribution of pharmacokinetics to the overall treatment of the patient. Although certain individuals who have not had formal training in one or more of the above areas may develop competence in preparing pharmacokinetic consults, they are likely to be the exception.

Besides the acquisition of an appropriate data base in the fields of physiology, pathophysiology and therapeutics and pharmacokinetics, it is of utmost importance that the consultant go through a residency or fellowship period during which his ability to intermix clinical judgement and scientific facts is under the scrutiny of a competent practitioner. The individual who tries to develop his own expertise usually is deprived of this controlled practical learning experience and may be unnecessarily exposing physicians and patients alike to poor advice.

Besides competence in the areas mentioned above, the individual providing interpretations of drug levels or consults based on drug levels must be aware of proper collection and handling procedures for specific drugs in biological fluids and have an appreciation for the potential errors that can occur in a given analytical procedure. The clinical pharmacokinetics consultant must assure himself of the specificity, accuracy and precision of the analytical procedures involved (24–26).

Clinical pharmacy practitioners competent in clinical pharmacokinetics are growing in number. Certain clinical pharmacy programs across the country can now provide excellent training in clinical pharmacokinetics at the graduate or post-graduate (fellowship or residency) level (27). In addition, more and more clinical pharmacology programs have access to expertise in pharmacokinetics.

## Patient Data Base Acquisition

In preparing a pharmacokinetics consult, the consultant must first collect and organize the patient's data base. This includes a drug history (including alcohol, nicotine, and caffeine) with particular emphasis on recent dosing of the drug being consulted upon. One must have an accurate record of all doses within the last three to four drug half-lives before the level was obtained in order to provide a meaningful pharmacokinetic interpretation or consult.

The dosing of drugs other than the one being consulted upon may also be quite important. For example, antacids given simultaneously with digoxin may decrease the bioavailability of digoxin (28), quinidine may cause an increase in digoxin serum levels (29) and salicylates may change the free to total ratio for serum phenytoin (30). Changes in regimens of drugs that influence drug absorption, distribution, metabolism or excretion may have a pronounced effect upon a drug level.

If a patient is seen in an ambulatory setting or has just recently been admitted to the hospital, it is necessary to get much of the drug history from the patient himself. A good deal of interviewing skill is required at this point if the data collected are expected to be accurate. Even if the patient has been hospitalized for considerable time, it is still quite useful to check the nurses' medication record against the patient's own recollections. Charting of a dose occasionally does not correspond to drug administration.

Another component of an individual's data base is his pertinent physiologic characteristics. Important physiologic factors include such things as age, weight (including lean body weight), sex, body surface area and pregnancy. Correct design of dosage regimens and interpretation of serum levels are dependent upon a knowledge of these characteristics.

The consultant must make note of all pathophysiologic findings. Drug kinetics can be influenced by numerous disease processes as illustrated throughout this text. Also, the practical aspects of dosage form selection and therapeutic monitoring may be significantly influenced by such things as neurological disease (i.e., organic brain syndrome). The pathophysiologic data base should contain as much pertinent, quantitative information as is available. A mere list of disease states provides little information of value to the pharmacokineticist. On the other hand, measurements such as serum creatinines, prothrombin times, serum albumins, etc. may be quite useful in a quantitative or semi-quantitative manner. Of course, such measurements must be up to date to be of value. It is important to make note of the past time course of the physiologic or pathophysiologic characteristics. "Has there been a recent history of weight loss? Is his renal function stable?" The answers to these and similar questions may have a significant influence on the final consult. Much of the patient's physiologic and pathophysiologic data base is available in the chart. Additional information required may be obtained from the patient's physician or directly by the consultant, depending of course upon the consultant's clinical capabilities.

The final portion of the patient's data base is comprised of all available drug level information, both current and previous. Too often only the current drug level information is considered by the clinician. A major advantage of providing a pharmacokinetics consult is that the consultant is sensitized to the importance of serial drug levels in characterizing the handling of a particular drug by an individual patient. Patients frequently require repeated monitoring of serum drug levels for the establishment and maintenance of optimum individual regimens. The pharmacokinetics consultant should be capable of extracting the maximum amount of information from such data.

Serum levels of drugs other than the one being consulted upon may also provide important clues for correct interpretation and dosage regimen design. For example, phenytoin pharmacokinetic parameters have been shown to be related to serum phenobarbital levels resulting from primidone administration (31).

A significant amount of the clinical pharmacokinetic consultant's time is devoted to collection and verification of the patient's therapeutic, physiologic, pathophysiologic and pharmacokinetic data bases. Only if this information is reliable can accurate interpretations or consults be provided. Hasty or careless collection of data can lead to inaccuracies with subsequent unfortunate consequences for the patient.

## Data Evaluation

The evaluation of the patient's data base may be performed simultaneously with data collection, but it is important to systematically review the case immediately before preparing the consult. A mental checklist (Table 1) is quite helpful.

**Route of Administration and Dosage Form.** The route of administration and dosage form must be considered in respect to the patient's physiologic and pathophysiologic profile in order to arrive at a proper initial or adjusted dosage regimen or to evaluate a current regimen. The pathophysiology of the patient may make one particular route of administration less desirable than another. For example, congestive heart failure may diminish the rate and possibly the extent of absorption of certain drugs (32).

The biopharmaceutic characteristics of the dosage form must also be carefully considered. If a patient receiving quinidine is having arrhythmias just prior to the time for the next dose, then it may be appropriate to use a sustained release preparation.

Consideration of route and dosage form are also important for proper interpretation of serum drug levels. A pre-dose theophylline level must be interpreted differently depending upon whether the patient is on a parenteral or rapidly absorbed preparation in contrast to a slowly absorbed or sustained release product.

TABLE 1. CHECKLIST OF PERTINENT FACTORS TO CONSIDER WHEN PREPARING A CLINICAL PHARMACOKINETIC CONSULT

Route of administration and dosage form
Compliance
Duration of therapy
Time of level relative to dose
Physiologic and pathophysiologic characteristics
Concurrent drug and food intake
Accuracy of drug assay

**Compliance.** Several studies have illustrated the frequency of non-compliance with prescribed regimens in both hospitalized patients and outpatients (33–35). In designing dosage regimens one must keep in mind that the more complex the regimen the less likely the patient will receive the drug as intended (36). Evaluation of compliance is extremely important when interpreting serum drug levels or making recommendations based upon these interpretations. Serious errors in predicting appropriate regimens may arise if the patient suddenly starts taking his drug as prescribed. The determination of compliance by patient, guardian or nurse interviews, "pill" counts, or other means are always prone to errors.

Serum levels themselves are useful in evaluating compliance. A serum level drawn upon admission and followed two or three drug half-lives by a serum level obtained after continuous, enforced drug administration may give an indication of the patient's compliance prior to admission. Of course, any change in pharmacokinetic parameters secondary to changes in pathophysiology, concurrent drug therapy, etc. during this period can also influence the second drug level. As always, all relevant factors must be considered.

In an outpatient, the presence of stable serum drug levels (usually ± 15%) on repeated visits can be considered indicative of *consistent* drug intake. The patient may still be noncompliant, but in a consistent manner. Of course a lack of stable serum drug levels can be explained by a number of intervening factors other than noncompliance. Instructing patients about the necessity of compliance is important, but undiplomatic accusation of noncompliance will alienate the patient and benefits neither him nor the clinician.

**Duration of Therapy.** Accurate knowledge of the duration of therapy is of utmost importance for the correct interpretation of serum drug levels. A serum level assumed to be obtained after attainment of steady-state, but which is actually representative of a nonsteady-state situation, can lead to serious errors in dosing recommendations. In evaluating a particular serum level as an indication of the eventual steady-state value, the half-life of the drug in that specific patient must be considered. For example, a patient with severe renal failure could exhibit a digoxin half-life of four days or longer instead of the usual half-life of two to two and a half days found in most adult patients. Thus the time required to reach 94% of steady-state could be sixteen days in the patient with severe renal failure instead of eight to ten days in the patient with uncompromised renal function.

If an appropriate loading dose is administered, then the time required for the achievement of steady-state may be shortened considerably. Although four drug half-lives of maintenance dosing are still required to achieve 94% of the *change* in serum level, the absolute difference between the level and the eventual steady-state may be quite small after only one or two half-lives. For example, loading and maintenance doses are calculated for a particular drug on the basis of *estimated* volume of distribution and clearance values to achieve and maintain a serum level of 15 µg/ml. The load actually provides a level of 14 µg/ml and the patient's true clearance value is such that the maintenance dose will result in a steady-state value of 16 µg/ml. After one half-life of maintenance dosing the serum level will be 15 µg/ml and after two half-lives 15.5 µg/ml, 94 and 97% of the eventual steady-state level, respectively. However, significant mismatching of loading and maintenance doses can result in significant deviation from steady-state even after two half-lives. For example, let the patient's true volume of distribution be significantly greater than estimated yielding a post-load level of 11 µg/ml, and his clearance be considerably lower than estimated resulting in an eventual steady-state of 17 µg/ml. After one half-life of post-load maintenance dosing the level would be 13 µg/ml and after two half-lives 14.5 µg/ml, 76 and 85% of the eventual steady-state level, respectively. If no load had been given, levels of 8.5 and 12.8 µg/ml (50 and 75% of the eventual steady-state level) would have been achieved after one and two half-lives, respectively, of maintenance dosing. While after one half-life the loading dose produces a level significantly higher than would have been obtained without the load, the difference between the serum levels after two half-lives is much less. In this example, over three half-lives of post-load maintenance dosing would be required to achieve 94% of steady-state. Obviously one cannot assume rapid achievement of steady-state levels just because the patient has received a loading dose.

The evaluation of the fraction of steady-state levels that a given observed serum level represents is even more difficult for drugs that are eliminated by one or more processes which exhibit Michaelis-Menten pharmacokinetic behavior. The time required to achieve a given fraction of steady-state is a function of not only the individual pharmacokinetic parameters but also of the rate of administration (37).

In general, high Vmax values, low Km values and low rates of administration favor a rapid approach to steady-state. However, certain individuals with low Km values who also have low Vmax values may continue to accumulate phenytoin for prolonged periods. In these individuals the dosing rate required to produce a level within the therapeutic range may be only slightly less than the Vmax value (38).

In estimating the fraction of steady-state represented by a particular serum level, it is extremely important to consider the patient's pathophysiology, compliance, and concurrent drug therapy. Factors that change drug bioavailability, distribution, clearance, and compliance will result in nonsteady-state levels even when the overall duration of therapy has been adequate.

For many drugs there is no rationale for performing serum level determinations *only* after achievement of steady-state. Nonsteady-state serum levels, if properly interpreted, can provide useful dosing information as well as help to decrease the incidence of toxicity.

**Time of Level Relative to Dose.** Knowledge of the time of a drug level relative to the last dose is critical for the proper interpretation of drug levels. Most drugs exhibit significant distribution phases after intravenous administration. During this phase there may be poor correlation of drug levels with pharmacologic effect as well as high inter-and intrasubject variability in the levels. Several drugs such as digoxin and lithium have significant distribution phases even after oral administration. Serum levels, in most cases, should be obtained after this phase is complete. Failure to recognize that a serum level was obtained during the distribution phase can easily lead to misinterpretation of the drug level and erroneous recommendations based upon that interpretation.

It has become common practice to use pre-dose serum levels for therapeutic monitoring. Estimation of peak and mean levels from predose levels is not a problem if levels do not fluctuate greatly over a dosing interval and half-life values are reasonably predictable. On the other hand, a pre-dose serum level of a drug such as theophylline which exhibits a wide range of half-life values may be difficult to use as an indicator of peak or mean levels. For example, a pre-dose theophylline level of 8 µg/ml in a patient receiving uncoated aminophylline tablets might indicate an approximate peak level (usually about one hour post-dose or five hours prior to the pre-dose level) of 32, 16 or 11 µg/ ml depending upon whether the half-life for theophylline was 2.5, 5 or 10 hours. Therefore, both peak and pre-dose levels should be obtained in such cases. The time to draw the blood sample for a peak level will vary, depending upon the drug, dosage form, and patient pathophysiology.

Careful attention should be directed to levels obtained during dosage regimens based on irregular dosing intervals. If the regimen is designed to avoid dosing during the hours of sleep, the peak and pre-dose levels will be low in the morning and progressively increase throughout the day. It may not be possible to accurately predict the overall daily serum level-time profile from serum levels obtained for one dosing interval during the day.

**Physiologic and Pathophysiologic Characteristics of the Pa-**

**tient.** The physiologic and pathophysiologic characteristics of the patient must be carefully evaluated to assess what influence these factors may have or will have on the pharmacokinetic behavior of the drug(s) of interest. In certain cases, quantitative data exist which permit estimation of pharmacokinetic parameters from these characteristics—for example, the calculation of digoxin clearance from creatinine clearance, age and body surface area.

In other cases, the best one can do is a qualitative or semi-quantitative estimate. For example, severe hepatic disease decreases the metabolism of various drugs but even semi-quantitative estimation of the magnitude of impairment has been possible in only a few instances (22).

Patient characteristics must be kept in mind throughout the evaluation of the remainder of the data base. Failure to appreciate or understand the effects of physiologic and pathophysiologic factors on the pharmacokinetic and pharmacodynamic behavior of drugs will lead to incorrect interpretations of serum drug levels and inappropriate recommendations.

**Concurrent Drug and Food Intake.** Concurrent drug and food intake, including alcohol, caffeine and tobacco, must be carefully evaluated to assess the potential effects of this intake on the pharmacokinetic behavior of the drug being consulted upon. Such interactions can be classified on the basis of the pharmacokinetic process involved, i.e., absorption, distribution or elimination (39).

Drug interactions at the level of absorption frequently occur because of physiochemical interactions between two or more drugs or with food stuffs (39). Other interactions involving absorption include the effects of food and other drugs on gastric emptying, gastrointestinal motility and blood flow (39–41). The rate and/or extent of absorption may be altered. Changes in the rate of absorption may alter the time of peak serum levels and change the degree of fluctuation of serum levels during a dosing interval but will usually not change the extent to which drug reaches the systemic circulation and, therefore, will not alter mean steady-state levels. An increase in extent of absorption will usually result in higher serum levels. If the first pass effect for a drug is saturable, then either an increased rate or extent of absorption may decrease the first-pass effect and increased serum levels can result (42).

Drug interactions limited to displacement from plasma binding sites will usually require consideration of chronic dosage adjustments only if the drug is highly but loosely bound in blood, its clearance is flow dependent, and it is given parenterally (21). In other situations involving drug displacement in plasma, any rise in the free drug concentration is likely to be transient. On the other hand, consideration of the fractional binding of drug in serum is important when comparing an observed serum level with a usual therapeutic range. Published therapeutic ranges for drugs are almost always based on total levels observed in patients with fairly normal binding. Therefore, one must adjust the usual therapeutic range to reflect the same fractional binding that is estimated for the patient's level. For example, valproic acid has been shown to alter the *in vivo* plasma binding of phenytoin (43). Therefore, depending upon valproate dosage or levels, one might estimate the fraction of phenytoin free in a given patient's plasma to be 24% instead of the usual 14%. The therapeutic range in terms of total levels for this patient could be considered to be about 6 to 12 μg/ml instead of 10 to 20 μg/ml. More quantitative information concerning the *in vivo* displacement of drugs from plasma binding sites is required before such estimates can be made accurately. For certain drugs, measurement of saliva levels provides a practical method for estimating the free drug concentration in plasma (9). More quantitative results are obtained if equilibrium dialysis or ultrafiltration techniques are used. These later procedures can be tedious and expensive and should probably be reserved for select cases.

Drug interactions involving changes in drug binding in tissue may produce significant changes in drug distribution throughout the body, but unless there is a concurrent change in free drug clearance, as occurs in the digoxin-quinidine interaction (29), the dosing rate may only have to be altered temporarily.

The order of addition may be quite important for drug interactions limited to displacement of drug from inactive tissue sites back into the circulation, where the drug is not only available for producing a pharmacological effect but also for elimination. For example, if drug A displaces drug B from tissue sites, then starting drug B after drug A is at steady-state will not usually require an adjustment in dosage of drug B. On the other hand, if drug B is first dosed to steady-state and drug A is then added, drug B will be displaced into the circulation and a finite time will be required for elimination of this excess drug before the previous steady-state serum level is reestablished. In either case a shorter half-life for drug B will result. This, of course, has implications regarding the time required to achieve steady-state and the fluctuations in serum levels during a dosing interval. If there is a simultaneous decrease in both volume of distribution and clearance, then a significant and sustained increase in serum levels may occur, as is the apparent case for the digoxin-quinidine interaction. If changes in volume of distribution and clearance are of about the same proportion and in the same direction, there may be little change in drug half-life.

The effects of concurrent intake of stimulators or inhibitors of drug elimination including food, environmental contaminants and other drugs must be considered when designing an initial dosage regimen, evaluating a current regimen with serum levels or recommending an adjustment in regimen based upon serum levels. Changes in drug clearance secondary to these factors will, of course, alter steady-state drug levels. For example, patients receiving the enzyme inducer rifampin may require larger than usual doses of certain drugs that are eliminated primarily by hepatic microsomal oxidation. Likewise, administration of an inducer or inhibitor may significantly affect how close an observed serum level is to the eventual steady-state value because of alterations in drug half-life. Likewise, a change in the intake of the inducer or inhibitor may cause a previous steady-state level of the drug in question to change. The rate at which the new steady-state is approached will be a function of the new half-life. In fact, new, reasonably constant, clearance and half-life values for the drug may not be established for some time since the change in metabolism or active transport produced by an inducer or inhibitor will have its own time course. In other words, the clearance and half-life values may change progressively during the onset or alteration in inducer or inhibitor effect.

Obviously, careful consideration of concurrent drug therapy and food intake is an extremely important step in designing or evaluating a dosage regimen or interpreting a serum level.

**Accuracy of Drug Assay.** Evaluation of an analytical procedure requires that the technician performing the assay be blinded to the evaluation (26). This is commonly done by sending known samples, usually weighed-in standards, to the laboratory just as if they were from a patient. This should always be done in cooperation with the director of the hospital laboratory providing the assay. If possible, a control sample from a pool of actual patients' samples should also be used for assay evaluation. Such a sample will contain metabolites as well as parent drug and will serve as a guide to assay specificity. This is particularly useful for evaluating immunoassays in which antibody specificity may vary from lot to lot. Of course, the "true" concentration of drug in such a sample must be determined independently by one or more very specific techniques, the best being gas-liquid or high pressure-liquid chromatography combined with mass-spectrometry.

Lack of assay specificity secondary to concurrent drug therapy is always a potential problem. The mere addition of a potentially interfering drug to blank serum followed by analysis does not take into consideration the possibility that a metabolite of the potentially interfering drug could be the cause of the problem. This question concerning interference can only be adequately answered by assaying serum from patients receiving normal or high doses of the potentially interfering drug but not receiving the drug whose assay is in question. An estimate of the precision of an assay can be obtained by sending two or more identical samples for analysis. This can be easily done by splitting a patient's sample and sending them to the lab as different specimens. Of course, this tells one nothing about assay specificity. If the consultant feels that there is an analytical problem of any type, then he should work with the laboratory personnel to find the source of the problem and correct it.

The accuracy of a given assay result depends upon both the precision and specificity of the assay. Providing accurate drug assays at reasonable cost and with minimal delay continues to challenge the clinical chemist. Recent advances in automated immunoassays are a big step in the right direction, although the expense is still high.

## Preparing the Consult

In general, the consult should be written very concisely but without omitting pertinent information. Of course, the need for proper spelling and grammar is basic to good written communication. There are an endless number of formats that can be used for the consult, but most pharmacokinetic consults must have at least two of the following components.

**Statement of the Problem.** This will include a concise summary of the relevant physiologic (age, height, weight, sex, etc.) and pathophysiologic characteristics (past and present disease states, relevant laboratory data, vital signs, EKG's etc.). A brief drug history should be included, emphasizing the drug being consulted upon, any concurrent drugs that would have an influence on the consult and an assessment of the patient's past and projected future compliance. At this point, a summary of previous serum level data, if available, should be presented. Finally, the reason for the consult should be stated.

**Interpretation of Drug Level Data.** If the consult involves the interpretation of new drug level data, then the level(s) should be clearly presented as to concentration, actual time drawn and time of draw relative to the last dose. Any uncertainty about this data should be stated. A statement of the "usual" therapeutic range should be given and how this level is related to that range in light of the patient's data base, i.e., if the fraction of drug free in plasma is likely to be high, then the possible discrepancy between the "usual" therapeutic range and the patient's therapeutic range must be presented. Next, the consult should provide an assessment of the patient's observed level in comparison to published data in a population of patients similar to the individual being consulted upon. This type of comparison is valuable in detecting an atypical patient or situation. For example, an observed digoxin level of 0.6 ng/ml when the expected level is (based on age, sex, body surface area or weight, and renal, hepatic, and cardiovascular function, etc.) 1.8 ng/ml should stimulate further assessment of compliance and consideration of an individual bioavailability problem. On the other hand, agreement between observed and expected levels may be only fortuitous and secondary to compensating deviations in drug absorption, distribution and elimination.

This section of the consult should also include an assessment of the fraction of steady-state that a given level represents based upon consideration of both the patient's characteristics and the actual level observed. If a patient's characteristics indicate a pre-dose theophylline level of 7 to 10 µg/ml would be expected, then an observed level of 15 µg/ml would strongly suggest that this patient's theophylline half-life could be longer than predicted from his characteristics. This potentially longer half-life should be considered in the evaluation of steady-state.

**Recommendation and Rationale.** Recommendations for dosage regimens based upon previously published or current individual data should be clearly stated as to dose size, dosage form, and dosing interval. The method for determining the regimen should be referenced or described. Appropriate times for obtaining subsequent drug levels should be noted. A range of serum level values expected at these times should be provided. If the pathophysiologic characteristics of the patient are likely to change, then a recommendation for appropriate monitoring of these characteristics, i.e., creatinine clearance, should be made.

This section should always include the rationale for the recommended regimen and subsequent drug levels but need not be overly mathematical unless the requesting clinician so desires. If significant mathematical manipulations are required for either interpretation or recommendations, these should be outlined as briefly and clearly as possible.

Recommendations for dosage regimens must *never* be based upon serum level data alone unless other monitoring parameters are unobtainable. The patient who exhibits adequate response but has a serum level below the usual therapeutic range may have little to gain and much to lose from a higher serum level. However, a major problem is the assessment of adequate response, particularly as regards prophylactic therapy such as with anticonvulsants and antiarrhythmics. Does the patient with a steady-state phenytoin level below the usual therapeutic range but who has not had a seizure in three weeks require an increase in dose? Many neurologists would agree that an increase in phenytoin levels to within the usual therapeutic range would be desirable in this case. On the other hand, if the patient had been seizure free for six months, then there would be little apparent indication for increasing the level. The question becomes "If a seizure has not occurred in a certain length of time, what is the probability that the patient will have a seizure in the future at the same serum level of drug?" A similar problem occurs in deciding whether or not to lower a serum level that is above the usual therapeutic range when there is no evidence of toxicity. One must balance the possibilities that the patient is truly "resistant" to the toxic effects and, therefore, less likely to exhibit toxicity even at a later time, against the fact that for any given individual the higher the dose the greater the frequency of dose-related toxic effects. Levels greater than 10 to 15% above the usual therapeutic range should probably not be maintained unless such levels are clinically justified.

Frequently it is necessary to place dosage regimen recommendations on a contingency basis. For example: "If additional therapeutic effect is desired, an increase in theophylline (sustained-release) dosage to 500 mg every twelve hours would be expected to produce new steady-state serum levels of about 14–18 $\mu$g/ml." Or, "If it is decided to reduce serum levels to within the usual therapeutic range, then a phenytoin (Dilantin®) dosage of 360 mg daily would be an appropriate trial regimen. Skipping one day of therapy before starting the new regimen will facilitate the decline in levels." In a way, this appears to be avoiding the responsibility of making a decision. However, in many cases it is absolutely necessary to defer the decision to the patient's clinician since he may be in the best position to make such a decision. On other occasions, the clinician may clearly prefer that he receive a direct recommendation. However, the clinical pharmacokinetics consultant should never make a recommendation concerning a case that he feels is beyond his expertise. In certain situations a joint consult involving another specialist such as a cardiologist or neurologist may be indicated. On occasion it may be necessary to confer with an analytical or clinical chemist or a more theoretically oriented pharmacokineticist.

## Reimbursement

Reimbursement for consults may take many forms. In government institutions such as Veterans Administration Hospitals the preparation of clinical pharmacokinetic consults may be a designated duty for a clinical pharmacist or be recognized as a clinical contribution from a clinical pharmacologist. In health science centers and university hospitals, where patient fees are frequently returned to the particular department for disbursement in the form of salary supplementation and secretarial and research support, the benefits of a consult service may be indirect. In such an environment it is convenient to route the consults through the Department of Medicine just as many medical subspecialties do. If consults are not performed under the auspices of a recognized medical or surgical department, it may be necessary to negotiate with third-party payment contractors such as Blue Cross/Blue Shield for appropriate reimbursement. This would also be true in the private sector where clinical pharmacokinetics consults could be provided through the hospital pharmacy service, provided the individuals involved were properly trained and could be certified in an appropriate manner. One can even project into the future and visualize a private pharmacy practice in which the monitoring of drug levels is performed simultaneously with the refilling of prescriptions for certain chronic medications. Of course, before third-party payers or patients will provide remuneration to pharmacists for such a non-dispensing function, cost-benefit analysis must be carried out to document the practical benefits of clinical pharmacokinetics (44).

## Liability

The individual preparing a consult concerning patient care must assume moral and legal responsibility for the accuracy and validity of information and/or recommendations provided. It is unthinkable that incorrect information would be provided purposefully, but this is essentially the case if an individual grossly oversteps his capabilities to provide a consult. One must not view a consult as merely information for the patient's physician, but must keep in mind the potential consequences for the patient for whom the consult is written.

Even when care is taken, an error may occur. It is the consultant's responsibility to maintain sufficient liability insurance not only to protect his own financial well being, but that of the patient as well. The physician's liability insurance obviously covers his preparation of consults. However, pharmacy practitioners who undertake the responsibility of providing clinical pharmacokinetic consults must be sure that their professional liability insurance will cover such an activity.

## Summary

The organization and scope of a particular clinical pharmacokinetic consultation service will be determined by the needs of the particular clinical setting, the expertise of the pharmacokinetics consultant, and the analytical capabilities of the clinical pathology or pharmacokinetics laboratory.

Preparation of a clinical pharmacokinetic consult requires careful consideration of the patient's entire clinical data base and a thorough understanding of pharmacokinetics and the influence of physiologic, pathophysiologic and therapeutic factors on pharmacokinetics and pharmacodynamics. In preparing a consult, the consultant assumes moral and legal responsibility for the information and/or recommendations provided.

There are numerous testimonials in the literature describing the presumed benefits of dosage regimen individualization based upon clinical pharmacokinetic principles and/or drug level monitoring. However, few controlled studies have been performed to scientifically document these benefits. Patient (consumer) acceptance of clinical pharmacokinetic consult services will depend upon the perceived benefits in terms of increased quality of care and/or decreased overall health care costs.

## REFERENCES

1. Gibaldi M and Levy G: Pharmacokinetics in clinical practice: 1 Concepts. JAMA 1976; 235:1864–1867.
2. Gibaldi M and Levy G: Pharmacokinetics in clinical practice: 2 Applications. JAMA 1976; 235:1987–1992.
3. Greenblatt DJ and Koch-Weser J: Clinical pharmacokinetics, Part 1. N Engl J Med 1975; 293:702–705.
4. Greenblatt DJ and Koch-Weser J: Clinical pharmacokinetics, Part 2. N Engl J Med 1975; 293:964–970.
5. Koch-Weser J: Serum drug concentrations as therapeutic guides. N Engl J Med 1972; 287:227–231.
6. Koch-Weser J: The serum level approach to individualization of drug dosage. Eur J Clin Pharmacol 1975; 9:1–8.
7. Davies DS and Prichard BNC (Eds): *Biological Effects of Drugs in Relation to Their Plasma Concentrations*, University Park Press, Baltimore, 1973.
8. Richens A and Warrington S: When should plasma drug levels be monitored? Drugs 1979; 17:488–500.
9. Horning MG, Brown L, Nowlin J, Lertiatanangkoon K, Kellaway P, and Zion TE: Use of saliva in therapeutic drug monitoring. Clin Chem 1977; 23:157–164.
10. Slaughter RL, Schneider PJ, and Visconti JA: Appropriateness of the use of serum digoxin and digitoxin assays. Am. J Hosp Pharm 1978; 35:1376–1379.
11. Anderson AC, Hodges GR and Barnes WG: Determination of serum gentamicin sulfate levels. Ordering patterns and use as a guide to therapy. Arch Intern Med 1976; 136:785–787.

12. Taylor JW, McLean AJ, Leonard RG, Ludden TM, Clibon U, duSouich BP, Harris SC, Lalka D, Talbert RL, Vicuna N, Walton CA, and McNay JL: Initial experience of clinical pharmacology and clinical pharmacy interactions in a clinical pharmacokinetics consultation service. J Clin Pharmacol 1979; 1–7.

13. Levy G: An orientation to clinical pharmacokinetics in Levy G (Ed) *Clinical Pharmacokinetics: A Symposium.* American Pharmaceutical Association, Washington, 1974.

14. McGhan WF, Rowland CR and Bootman JL: Cost-benefit and cost-effectiveness: Methodologies for evaluating innovative pharmaceutical services. Am J Hosp Pharm 1978; 35:133–140.

15. Bootman JL, Wertheimer AI, Zaske D, and Rowland C: Individualizing gentamicin dosage regimens in burn patients with gram-negative septicemia: A cost-benefit analysis. J Pharm Sci 1979; 68:267–272.

16. Gibaldi M, and Perrier D: Pharmacokinetics, in Swarbrick J (Ed) *Drugs and the Pharmaceutical Sciences,* Vol. 1, Marcel Dekker, Inc., New York, 1975.

17. Wagner JG: *Biopharmaceutics and Relevant Pharmacokinetics,* Drug Intelligence Publications, Inc., Hamilton, Ill., 1971.

18. Wagner JG: *Fundamentals of Clinical Pharmacokinetics,* Drug Intelligence Publication, Inc., Hamilton, Ill., 1975.

19. Ritschel WA: *Handbook of Basic Pharmacokinetics,* Drug Intelligence Publications, Inc., Hamilton, Ill., 1976.

20. Levy G and Gibaldi M: Pharmacokinetics, in Eichler O, Farah A, Herken H and Welch AD (Eds) *Handbook of Experimental Pharmacology,* Vol. 28, Part 3, Springer Verlag, New York, 1975, pp. 1–34.

21. Wilkinson GR and Shand DG: A physiologic approach to hepatic drug clearance. Clin Pharmacol Ther 1975; 18:377–390.

22. Nies AS, Shand DG and Wilkinson GR: Altered hepatic blood flow and drug disposition. Clin Pharmacokinet 1976; 1:135–155.

23. Bean CL: Definition of clinical pharmacy. Am J Hosp Pharm 1979; 36:744.

24. Pippenger CE, Penry JL, White BG, Daly DD and Buddington R: Interlaboratory variability in determination of plasma antiepileptic drug concentrations. Arch Neurol 1976; 33:351–355.

25. Richens A: Drug level monitoring—quantity and quality. Br J Clin Pharmacol 1978; 5:285–288.

26. McCormick W, Ingelfinger JA, Isakson G and Goldman P: Errors in measuring drug concentrations. N Engl J Med 1978; 299:1118–1121.

27. Levy G: A training program in clinical pharmacokinetics. Drug Intell Clin Pharm 1978; 12:204–209.

28. Braun DD and Juhl RP: Decreased bioavailability of digoxin due to antacids and kaolin-pectin. N Engl J Med 1976; 295:1034–1037.

29. Hager WD, Fenster P, Mayersohn M, Perrier D, Groves P, Marcus FI, Goldman S: Digoxin-quinidine interaction: pharmacokinetic evaluation. N Engl J Med 1979; 300:1238–1241.

30. Fraser DG, Ludden TM, Evens RP, and Sutherland III EW: *In vivo* displacement of phenytoin from plasma proteins with salicylates. Clin Pharmacol Ther 1979; 25:226.

31. Garrettson LK and Gomez M: Phenytoin-primidone interaction. Br J Clin Pharmacol 1977; 4:693–695.

32. Benet LZ, Greither A and Meister W: Gastrointestinal absorption of drugs in patients with cardiac failure, in Benet LZ (Ed), *The Effect of Disease States on Drug Pharmacokinetics,* American Pharmaceutical Association, Washington, 1976.

33. Boyd JR, Covington TR, Stanaszek WF, Coussons RT: Drug defaulting: Determinants of compliance. Am J Hosp Pharm 1974; 31:362–367.
34. Kellaway GSM and McCrae E: Non-compliance and errors of drug administration in patients discharged from acute general medical wards. NZ Med J 1975; 81:508–513.
35. Roth HP and Caron HS: Accuracy of doctors' estimates and patients statements on adherence to a drug regimen. Clin Pharmacol Ther 1978; 23:361–370.
36. Sackett DL and Hayes RB: *Compliance with Therapeutic Regimens,* John Hopkins University Press. Baltimore, 1976, pp32–39.
37. Wagner JG: Time to reach steady-state and prediction of steady-state concentrations of drugs obeying Michaelis-Menten elimination kinetics. J Pharmacokinet Biopharm 1978; 6:209–225.
38. Ludden TM, Allen JP, Schneider LW and Stavehansky SA: Rate of phenytoin accumulation in man: A simulation study. J Pharmacokinet Biopharm 1978; 6:399–415.
39. Kristensen MB: Drug interactions and clinical pharmacokinetics. Clin Pharmacokinet 1976; 1:351–372.
40. Nimmo WS: Drugs, diseases and altered gastric emptying. Clin Pharmacokinet 1976; 1:189–203.
41. McLean AJ, McNamara PJ, duSouich P, Gibaldi M and Lalka D: Food, splanchic blood flow, and bioavailability of drugs subject to first pass metabolism. Clin Pharmacol Ther 1978; 24:5–10.
42. Riegelman S and Rowland M: Effect of route of administration on drug disposition. J Pharmacokinet Biopharm 1973; 1:419–434.
43. Mattson RH, Cramer JA, Williamson PD and Novelly RA: Valproic acid in epilepsy: clinical and pharmacological effects. Ann Neurol 1978; 3:20–25.
44. Soloway AH: Reimbursement for nondispensing services—the critical issue. Am Pharmacy 1979; 19:287.

*Counterpoint Discussion:*

# Clinical Pharmacokinetics Consultation Services

Darwin E. Zaske, Pharm.D.

## Introduction

The need for clinical pharmacokinetic consultations within an institution may be large in relationship to the resources available. An efficient, systematic approach should be developed to provide these pharmacokinetic services. Existing resources should be used to prevent unnecessary cost. This is especially important with capital expenditures such as laboratory instrumentation. In many institutions, the clinical laboratory has the necessary instrumentation for many of the assay methodologies. An efficient clinical pharmacokinetic consulting service also requires cooperation from several different disciplines. Personnel providing the clinical pharmacokinetic consult need to work in a timely and effective manner to be maximally utilized. The following discussion describes the systematic approach used at our institution and suggests responsibilities for various disciplines to optimally provide these services.

## Components of the Clinical Consultant Service

The application of clinical pharmacokinetic principles provides a unique contribution in improving patient treatment. This statement applies to several pharmacologic categories. These services can be systematically provided as part of the institution's clinical pharmacy-pharmacology services. We have subdivided our clinical pharmacokinetic consulting services according to major pharmacologic categories (Figure 1). This enables the clinical pharmacist to develop additional skills, knowledge, and experience in a specific therapeutic area. An individual clinical pharmacist is responsible for one or two pharmacologic groups. He provides clinical consultations in these areas and educational conferences for the medical staff and pharmacy students.

26

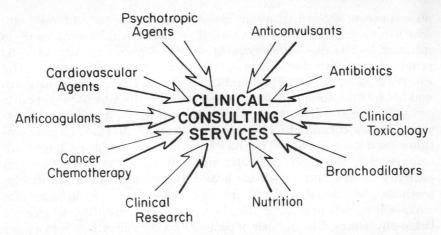

FIGURE 1.   Components of the Clinical Pharmacokinetics Consulting Service

In addition, this is also his/her primary area of clinical research, which further develops the level of practice in that specific area.

Most clinical consulting services provided in acute patient settings are needed on a 24 hour per day, seven day per week schedule. Such continuity allows the medical resident to utilize these services during medical emergencies occurring at night or weekends when the service is often needed the most. This further results in greater utilization throughout the institution, while providing a unique training opportunity for Doctor of Pharmacy residents. The Pharm.D. resident is on call in the institution with a Pharm.D. staff member. Call responsibilities apply to nights and weekends and are shared by members of the staff.

The Pharm.D. staff member provides clinical consulting services primarily in his/her specialization area. The staff member, in turn, is responsible for training his/her colleagues to an acceptable (optimal) level of practice for nights and weekends. Consequently, there needs to be a strong group of clinicians providing 24 hour coverage to optimally provide clinical consultative services in a major institution. The following approach has been used in our hospital to provide these services. This particular model may need to be modified for other institutions.

**Antibiotics.** Individualizing aminoglycoside and vancomycin dosage regimens are primary areas for clinical consultative services with this pharmacologic group. In order to obtain reliable data, it has been necessary in our institution to have the Pharm.D.'s draw serum samples. However, other institutions may have an active phlebotomy team which may provide these services. The pharmacokinetic consult is initiated by the physician's request. Initial dosage regimens may be provided by a member of the clinical pharmacokinetic group. The Pharm.D. determines the optimal times for obtaining serum samples and obtains the samples from the patient. The therapeutic end points are determined collaboratively with the primary physician or infectious disease consultant. The interpretation of the serum concentration time data is conducted by the Pharm.D., and dosage regimens are calculated to achieve therapeutic end points. In our institution, all patients receive aminoglycoside antibiotics by individualized dosage methods. Additional patients are also referred by physicians from outside hospitals and the Pharm.D. provides consultative service for these physicians. The number of patients on the consulting service for aminoglycosides varies but is generally between 20 and 30 patients at any particular time. These patients are followed frequently throughout the course of therapy to monitor renal function and obtain peak and trough serum concentrations to further evaluate the dosage regimen.

**Anticonvulsants.** The services of this unit are provided by the Pharm.D. staff for ambulatory and hospitalized patients. This service provides dosage adjustments for the anticonvulsants, determines kinetic parameters for anticonvulsants in selected patients, monitors clinical efficacy and safety, and provides assessments of patient compliance. The clinical summary of serum concentrations combined with known dosage regimens are used to assist the consultant in evaluating patient compliance in this clinic.

**Cardiovascular Agents.** This consulting service assists medical internists, surgeons, and cardiologists in determining optimal dosage regimens for the dysrhythmics and digitalis glycosides given to hospitalized and ambulatory patients. These services are provided upon physician request. Initial dosage estimates are obtained from renal and cardiac function parameters such as serum creatinine or cardiac output. In selected patients, the dosage regimens are further individualized by the use of serum levels and determination of kinetic parameters.

**Anticoagulants.** Warfarin and heparin are the two major anticoagulants for which pharmacokinetic principles can be utilized to improve patient treatment. Both drugs are particularly difficult for clinicians to use empirically and achieve desired end points. Complications of concern can occur if dosage regimens are not optimal. Individualized approaches are available for both anticoagulants to assist the clinician in rapidly and safely achieving desired end points.

**Bronchodilators.** Theophylline is the major drug in this category. The application of pharmacokinetic principles has clearly made this drug a safe agent in comparison with earlier experiences. A large number of serum theophylline concentrations are measured weekly in our institution. However, most levels are interpreted and necessary dosage adjustments determined by the primary care physician. With more difficult patients, the primary care physician or pulmonary internist requests consultation from one of the clinical pharmacists for further assistance in dosage adjustments.

**Clinical Toxicology.** Clinical consulting services are provided by the department as part of the clinical toxicology treatment team. This treatment team is composed of medical internists, pathologists, neurologists, pediatricians, surgeons, psychiatrists, and clinical pharmacists. The Pharm.D.'s provide information related to toxicologic and pharmacologic aspects of the ingested agent. Suggested treatment modalities are also provided upon request by the physician. The application of clinical pharmacokinetic principles may provide useful information to the clinician in anticipating future or further complications from severe drug ingestions.

**Psychotropic.** Therapeutic end points have been proposed as guidelines to ensure maximal efficacy and safety for several psychotropic drugs. Some data suggest the existence of a "therapeutic window," further justifying the measurement of serum concentrations to individualize dosage regimens for these agents. At our institution, pharmacokinetic principles are being applied to achieve optimal dosage regimens for these agents and this application will likely increase in the near future.

**Cancer Chemotherapy.** The number of patients followed by our oncology service is limited. Within the local medical community, most oncology patients are referred to a separate cancer chemotherapy referral center. Consequently, our staff has little involvement in this area except for consultation with oncologists in local hospitals. However, the pharmacokinetic principles of selected antineoplastic agents should generally be applied in patient care settings to improve the safety and efficacy of these drugs.

**Clinical Research.** The clinical consulting services provide an initial data base for conducting further research in pharmacokinetics. The clinical research conducted from this data base can be multidirectional and may include assessment of pharmacokinetic principles in a large number of patients, relate pharmacologic outcome with pharmacokinetic data, and evaluate the benefit of these services. This component of the department's services necessitates an individual with skills and experience in research design, statistical analysis, pharmacology, and pharmacokinetics. The clinical research needs to be integrated with the components of the clinical consulting service. Consequently, the clinical pharmacist providing clinical services in a particular area also conducts clinical research related to that area.

## Multidisciplinary Approach

Several disciplines need to cooperate effectively to provide clinical pharmacokinetic services in an efficient manner (Figure 2). The total clinical pharmacokinetic service involves a primary care physician, a medical consultant, nursing department, clinical laboratory, and a clinical pharmacokinetic consultant. Within a particular institution, specific departments may have unique resources which may influence service responsibilities. In some institutions, the laboratory component may be part of the clinical pharmacokinetic service. The nursing staff is directly responsible for drug administration in most institutions. Depending upon the complexity of the patient's condition, the primary care physician may elect to consult initially with another medical specialty such as neurology, infectious disease, or pediatrics. In this instance, the clinical pharmacokinetic consultant may interface with either the primary care physician or the medical consultant.

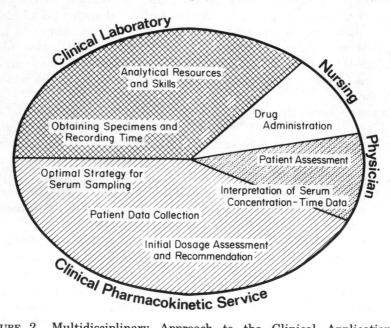

FIGURE 2. Multidisciplinary Approach to the Clinical Application of Pharmacokinetics

An effective clinical pharmacokinetic consultant service requires a multidisciplinary approach. The primary care physician makes decisions regarding the patient's diagnosis and ultimate treatment. The nursing staff is responsible for timely drug administration and adequate records of drug administration. The medical technologist provides timely assays which are sensitive and precise. The clinical pharmacokinetic consultant provides initial estimates of dose requirements, determines an optimal schedule for obtaining specimens for drug analysis, interprets concentration time data, calculates a patient's individual dosage requirement to achieve desired therapeutic end points, and evaluates response to treatment and suggests necessary dosage adjustments or laboratory tests. The pharmacokinetic consultant needs an effective line of communication between the primary physician, nurse and laboratory technologist. Information must be integrated to formulate a suggested treatment for the primary physician. The primary care physician determines the ultimate treatment course, while obtaining essential information from the clinical pharmacokinetic consultant.

## The Clinical Pharmacokinetic Consultant

The consultant in pharmacokinetics must have experience and skills in pathophysiology, clinical pharmacology, and pharmacokinetic principles to make appropriate decisions regarding dosage regimens. In addition, tactful and effective communication skills are essential for any consultant and the clinical pharmacokinetic consultant is no exception. The professional providing consultation services must work effectively with the variety of personalities encountered in the healthcare setting. Additionally, the consultant must recognize that his recommendations are *only* recommendations with which the primary physician may or may not fully agree or fully implement.

# 3

# Influence of Renal Disease on Pharmacokinetics

Thomas P. Gibson, M.D.

## Introduction

Renal failure is commonly thought to have its sole effect on the renal elimination of drugs. As will become apparent, renal failure has a variety of influences on drug kinetics, such as reducing nonrenal (presumably hepatic) drug elimination, protein binding, and volume of distribution of some drugs. Renal failure reduces the bioavailability of some drugs while increasing that of others. For drugs not dependent upon renal function for elimination, renal failure can lead to the accumulation of toxic metabolites that are normally of no concern.

Knowledge of the effects of renal failure on pharmacokinetics is of value in the rational treatment of patients. The most obvious example is the fact that digoxin doses must be reduced as renal failure develops. In this chapter the known influences of renal failure, defined for practical purposes as a glomerular filtration rate (GFR) of 10 ml/min or less, on drug elimination, accumulation, absorption and distribution will be discussed. The effects of the artificial kidney on pharmacokinetics will also be explored. General principles will be given using specific drugs as examples.

## Estimation of Glomerular Filtration Rate

The glomerular filtration rate is a measure of one discrete renal function, namely, the capacity of the kidneys to excrete the waste products of metabolism, such as creatinine and urea. For drugs such as digoxin, gentamicin and N-acetylprocainamide, elimination depends almost entirely upon the kidneys, and an accurate estimate of the glomerular filtration rate is an absolute requirement for rational drug therapy.

The measurement of GFR is based upon the concept of clearance, which relates the quantitative urinary excretion of a substance per unit time to the volume of plasma that, if cleared completely of the same substance, would yield a quantity equivalent to that in the urine. The clearance of any substance that is freely filtered at the glomerulus and is neither reabsorbed, secreted, synthesized, nor metabolized by the kidney is equal to the glomerular filtration rate. The glomerular filtration rate, usually expressed in ml per minute, is calculated as follows:

$$GFR_x = \frac{U_x(V_u)}{P_x} \qquad \text{(Eq. 1)}$$

where x is the substance cleared, U and P are the urinary and plasma concentrations of x given as mg/ml and $V_u$ is urine flow in ml/min. Although inulin fulfills all criteria as the ideal measure of glomerular filtration rate, it does not share with creatinine the important features of convenience, low cost, and widespread availability.

Creatinine, an endogenous product of muscle metabolism (1), is released from muscle at a relatively constant rate (2) so that the plasma creatinine concentration remains stable with time. Unlike inulin, urinary creatinine excretion exceeds the amount filtered by about 10% because of renal tubular secretion. Creatinine is not reabsorbed. However, the usual methods of serum creatinine determination detect noncreatinine chromogens present in the plasma but not in the urine. The net result is that creatinine clearance ($Cl_{cr}$) is slightly less than inulin clearance ($Cl_{in}$); the difference is not clinically important, however.

Normally, the $Cl_{cr}$ is derived from a 24 hour urine collection. The normal 24 hour creatinine excretion is 20 to 25 mg per kg of body weight in males and 15 to 20 mg per kg of body weight in females. Values substantially less than these often indicate incomplete urine collections, which can lead to serious underestimation of the $Cl_{cr}$. The normal glomerular filtration rate in young men averages about 125 ml/min per 1.73 m$^2$ and that in women, about 115 ml/min per 1.73 m$^2$ (3). The $Cl_{cr}$ begins to fall in middle age, even in the absence of underlying renal disease so that at age 60 the $Cl_{cr}$ is about 70% of that in normal young adults.

The normal serum creatinine concentration ($C_{cr}$) varies from 0.6 to 1.0 mg per 100 ml (mg/dl) in females and from 0.8 to 1.3 mg/dl in males. This value remains constant unless there is a change in rate of production or a reduction in the $Cl_{cr}$. Since the $Cl_{cr}$ is dependent upon muscle mass (4), which can vary widely from individual to individual and decreases in the elderly, a normal or nearly normal $C_{cr}$ cannot be directly equated with normal renal function until the $C_{cr}$ is matched with the $Cl_{cr}$ for both. Thereafter, the $C_{cr}$ varies indirectly with the $Cl_{cr}$, such that a twofold increase in the $C_{cr}$ indicates a 50% reduction in the $Cl_{cr}$.

During periods of rapidly declining renal function, as seen in acute tubular necrosis, the plasma creatinine concentration may increase by 1 mg/dl/day and may take as many as seven days to reach a new steady state even if there is not further change in the glomerular filtration rate. In such circumstances it is still possible to estimate the glomerular filtration rate, but the value so determined will be of little use unless a new steady state of renal function has been achieved. More importantly, during these times the $C_{cr}$ bears little relationship to the glomerular filtration rate and will not be a reliable index of glomerular filtration until renal function has stabilized.

Although the serum urea nitrogen concentration is often used to assess glomerular filtration, such a use should be discouraged. Urea once filtered is reabsorbed (4), the extent depending on the rate of urine flow, so that in congestive heart failure and dehydration, the ratio of the serum urea nitrogen to creatinine is greater than the normal 10:1 (5). Urea production by the liver is not constant, as it decreases with severe hepatic disease and increases with a high protein diet, gastrointestinal bleeding, and hypercatabolic states. Therefore, changes in the serum urea nitrogen level do not necessarily reflect changes in renal function, and the serum urea nitrogen value should not be used as a guide to drug dose adjustment in renal disease (5).

## Influence of Renal Disease on Drug Elimination

The overall elimination rate (K) for any drug is the sum of the renal ($k_e$) and nonrenal or metabolic ($k_f$) rate constants:

$$K = k_e + k_f \tag{Eq. 2}$$

For most drugs, K is linearly related to some function (X) of $Cl_{cr}$ such that:

$$K = (X)Cl_{cr} + k_f \tag{Eq. 3}$$

Plotting K on the right ordinate and $k_f$ on the left ordinate versus $XCl_{cr}$ on Cartesian coordinates, the Dettli nomogram (6) is constructed (Figure 1).

Three classes of drugs exist: (A) drugs dependent entirely upon renal function for elimination, (B) drugs dependent entirely upon

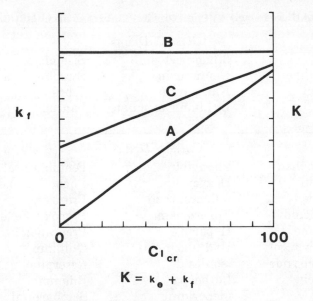

FIGURE 1.   The Dettli Nomogram

hepatic or other nonrenal routes of elimination, and (C) drugs that depend on both renal and nonrenal routes of elimination. The elimination of class B drugs is unaltered by renal disease and no change in the therapeutic regimen is required unless active metabolites are formed that behave as class A or C drugs. Representative drugs from each class are given in Table 1. Using the Dettli nomogram, K for any drug and any $Cl_{cr}$ can be calculated if $k_e$ and $k_f$ are known. If $k_f$ in renal failure has not been established, it can be calculated from data from normals as:

$$k_f = K(1-f) \qquad \text{(Eq. 4)}$$

where f is the fraction of the systemically available drug ultimately excreted unchanged in the urine.

The major caveat of the Dettli nomogram is that renal disease does not alter drug metabolism. However, the metabolism of procainamide (7) and possibly other drugs acetylated by polymorphic N-acetyltransferase is reduced in renal failure. Therefore, an *a priori* estimate of $k_f$ is impossible. Secondly, the Dettli approach assumes that metabolites of class B and C drugs are either inactive or nontoxic. Again with procainamide, N-acetylprocainamide, the major metabolite of procainamide and a potent antiarrhythmic agent itself (8), is a class A drug

TABLE 1. EXAMPLES OF CLASS A, B, AND C DRUGS

### Class A Drugs

| | | |
|---|---|---|
| Amikacin | 5-fluorocytosine | Sisomicin |
| Cephaloridine | Gentamicin | Streptomycin |
| Cephalexin | Kanamycin | Tobramycin |
| Cefazolin | Lithium Carbonate | Vancomycin |
| Colistin | | |

### Class B Drugs

| | | |
|---|---|---|
| Acetaminophen | Phenytoin | Pentobarbital |
| Adriamycin | Doxycycline | Phenothiazines |
| All steroids | 5-fluorouracil | Prazosin |
| Trihexyphenidyl | Flurazepam | Propoxyphene |
| Azathioprine | Heparin | Propranolol |
| Chloramphenicol | Hydralazine | Quinidine |
| Chlordiazepoxide | Isoniazid | Reserpine |
| Clindamycin | Levodopa | Rifampin |
| Clonidine | Meperidine | Secobarbital |
| Codeine | Minoxidil | Theophylline |
| Cyclophosphamide | Morphine | Tricyclic |
| Cytosine Arabinoside | Naloxone | Antidepressants |
| Diazepam | Nitroprusside | Vincristine |
| Digitoxin | Pentazocine | Warfarin |

### Class C Drugs

| | | |
|---|---|---|
| Ampicillin | Digoxin | Methyldopa |
| Carbenicillin | Ethambutol | Nafcillin |
| Cephalothin | Guanethidine | Oxacillin |
| Cloxacillin | Lincomycin | Penicillin G |
| Diazoxide | Methicillin | Phenobarbital |
| Dicloxacillin | Methotrexate | Procainamide |

and accumulates in renal failure (9). Drugs with these characteristics are best avoided in renal failure, unless the capability of quantitating the parent drug and important metabolites exists. Finally, this approach is only valid for steady-state renal function.

## Drug Dosing in Renal Failure

In the absence of a loading dose, the time necessary for the serum concentration of any drug to reach steady-state is solely dependent upon half-life. As a rule of thumb, 90% of the final steady-state value is reached after 3.3 half lives. For drugs such as digoxin, with half-lives as long as 5 to 6 days in renal failure, 90% of steady state with daily oral doses would be reached in 17 to 20 days. If a more rapid achievement of steady state is required, then a loading dose must be given. For most drugs the loading dose in renal failure is the same as in normals. The loading dose (LD) can be calculated if the desired average plasma drug concentration ($\overline{C}$), the volume of distribution of the drug (V), and patient weight (kg), are known:

$$LD = \overline{C} \cdot V \cdot kg \qquad \text{(Eq. 5)}$$

V must be given in terms of L/kg, as reporting V as L serves no useful purpose and should be avoided. Obviously the LD varies with body weight so that there is no universal LD in adults. Likewise, if V in renal failure is different from V in normals, LD will change. An important example is digoxin. The V for digoxin may be reduced from 25 to 50% in renal failure (10,11) as compared to normals and may be due, in part, to the accumulation of immunoreactive digoxin metabolites (12). Therefore, the LD for digoxin should be reduced in renal failure. This is true for end stage renal failure. It is not known at what level of renal function the V for digoxin, or $k_f$ for procainamide begin to change.

Once the loading dose has been established, the maintenance dose (MD) necessary to maintain $\overline{C}$ can be calculated as:

$$MD = \overline{C} \cdot V \cdot K \cdot \tau \qquad \text{(Eq. 6)}$$

where $\tau$ is the dosing interval. Both equations 5 and 6 assume that the dose is given intravenously and is, therefore, completely available. If the dose is given orally and if the absolute bioavailability (F) is less than 1, the LD and MD are

$$F \cdot LD = \overline{C} \cdot V \cdot kg \qquad \text{(Eq. 7)}$$

and
$$F \cdot MD = \overline{C} \cdot V \cdot K \cdot \tau \qquad \text{(Eq. 8)}$$

Therefore, by knowing F, V, and K, the average plasma concentration of any drug can be estimated for any patient. The average plasma concentration is directly related to dose and indirectly related to V, K, and $\tau$. Only the dose and the dosing interval are under physician control. To achieve the same $\overline{C}$ in renal failure patients as in normals, the dose can be kept constant and $\tau$ changed, or $\tau$ kept constant and the dose altered.

If it is desirable to maintain the dose constant, the new dosing interval for renal failure ($\tau^*$) is calculated as

$$\tau^* = \tau \cdot (K/K^*) \tag{Eq. 9}$$

where $K^*$ is the elimination rate constant in renal failure. If a constant dosing interval is desired, the reduction in dose necessary to maintain a constant $\overline{C}$ is:

$$MD^* = MD \cdot (K^*/K) \tag{Eq. 10}$$

where $MD^*$ is the maintenance dose in renal failure.

While both of these methods will give the same $\overline{C}$, they have vastly different effects on the maximum $(C\infty)_{max}$ and minimum $(C\infty)_{min}$ drug concentrations at steady-state (Figure 2). As shown in the following equations, $(C\infty)_{max}$ and $(C\infty)_{min}$ are a function of $MD^*$, V, and $\tau$, and K.

$$(C\infty)_{max} = \frac{MD^*}{V} \left( \frac{1}{1 - e^{-k\tau}} \right) \tag{Eq. 11}$$

and

$$(C\infty)_{min} = \frac{MD^*}{V} \left( \frac{1}{1 - e^{-k\tau}} \right) e^{-k\tau} \tag{Eq. 12}$$

If the dose is kept constant and $\tau$ increased, wide fluctuations in drug concentration will be expected as shown in panel A of Figure 2. If line A in Figure 2 represents the toxic threshold, then the patient could potentially suffer toxic effects for a considerable period of time. Likewise, if line B is the minimum effective concentration, the patient will be undertreated for some time before the next dose. In panel B, the dose has been reduced and $\tau$ increased. If the proper loading dose has been given, the serum concentrations will fluctuate within the therapeutic range but $\overline{C}$ will be the same as in panel A. For drugs with half-lives greater than one day, this method of dosage adjustment is probably the best.

If no loading dose is given, the amount of accumulation of drug at steady-state, when compared to the first dose, is given by the accumulation factor (R), where

$$R = \frac{1}{1 - e^{-k\tau}} \tag{Eq. 13}$$

The information needed to effectively use the above equations, namely V and K, is generally available as mean values obtained from studies on small numbers of patients. There is no assurance that any given patient will conform to those values. Optimal use of these equations can only occur if the predictions are checked against actual drug

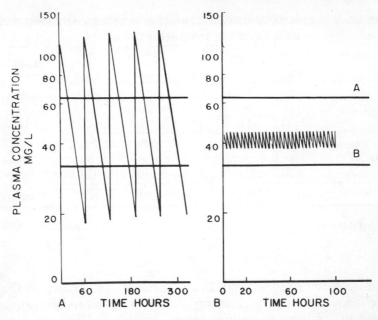

FIGURE 2. Plasma concentrations of a hypothetical drug in an anephric. Panel A—Dosage identical to that in normal renal function but dosing interval is increased. Panel B—Proper loading dose has been given. Maintenance dose has been reduced but dosing interval is the same as in normal renal function. Line A represents toxic threshold, line B minimum effective concentration.

concentrations, preferably with an analysis turnaround time less than one dosing interval. With drug concentration feedback, the prescribed doses can be iteratively changed until the desired results are achieved.

## Influence of Renal Failure on Drug Absorption

The whole area of drug bioavailability in renal failure has been sadly neglected. In general it has been assumed that drug absorption is unimpaired if, after a given oral dose, the drug concentrations in renal failure are the same, or nearly the same, as in normals. This totally neglects the fact that if V is reduced in renal failure, drug concentrations could be similar to those in normals even if availability is substantially reduced. The bioavailability of a given drug formulation is best determined by comparing its plasma concentration versus time curve with that of a reference standard. The best comparison is made with the curve obtained after intravenous administration, since bioavailability by this route is complete. Bioavailability deter-

TABLE 2.    ABSOLUTE BIOAVAILABILITY OF D-XYLOSE IN NORMALS
AND PATIENTS WITH RENAL FAILURE

|  | Vd (l/kg) | t½ ——— | t½$_a$ (Min) | Time to Peak ——— | Peak Height (mg/l) | Absolute Bioavailability |
|---|---|---|---|---|---|---|
| Normals (n = 11) | 0.22 ± 0.05 | 75 ± 11 | 29 ± 14 | 71 ± 15 | 0.53 ± 0.10 | 69.4 ± 13.5 |
| Renal Failure (n = 9) | 0.30 ± 0.80 | 388 ± 137 | 64 ± 62 | 166 ± 82 | 0.48 ± 0.19 | 46.6 ± 12.8 |
| P | <0.01 | <0.01 | <0.01 | <0.01 | ND | <0.01 |

ND = not different

mined by comparison with an intravenous dose is known as the absolute bioavailability. Information about the absolute bioavailability of most drugs in renal failure is not available. However, absolute bioavailability of furosemide (13), D-xylose (14) and pindolol (15) have been reported to be diminished in renal failure.

A comparison of factors relevant to the estimation of the absolute bioavailability of D-xylose in subjects with normal renal function and in renal failure patients requiring maintenance dialysis is given in Table 2. Notice that absolute bioavailability is decreased and V is increased in patients as compared to normals while the peak concentrations are not significantly different.

The peak concentration $(C_1)_{max}$ of a drug after a single dose is given by:

$$(C_1)_{max} = \frac{MD \cdot F \left[ \dfrac{k_a}{K} \right]^{K/(K-k_a)}}{V}$$

(Eq. 14)

$(C_1)_{max}$ is therefore mainly dependent upon the ratio of the rate of absorption $(k_a)$ and K. In the case of D-xylose, K is reduced much more than $k_a$ so that even though F is decreased and V increased, the expected peak concentration in renal failure after a 25 gm oral dose is 0.46 µg/ml compared to 0.49 µg/ml in normals. Therefore, similar peak concentrations do not indicate similar absolute bioavailability. Similarly, extremely disparate peak concentration values do not necessarily indicate poor availability but only slowed absorption. Slow-release medications would be a case in point. Likewise, the time $(t_{max})$ to peak concentration is dependent upon $k_a$ and K:

$$t_{max} = \frac{2.30}{k_a - K} \cdot \log \frac{k_a}{K}$$

(Eq. 15)

While the systemic availability of some drugs may be reduced in renal failure, it has been suggested that the first pass metabolism of some drugs like propranolol (16) and d-propoxyphene (17) may be reduced in renal disease. However, it has been reported that the absolute bioavailability of propranolol in renal failure patients is identical to that in age matched controls (18). On the other hand, animal experiments with d-propoxyphene suggest that the first pass metabolism of this drug is reduced in renal failure (personal communication, G. Levy).

## Effect of Changes in Protein Binding on Pharmacokinetics in Renal Failure

The plasma protein binding of many drugs, especially acidic compounds, is impaired in renal failure (19). The protein binding of some basic drugs, on the other hand, may be increased (20). However, the important change is the reduction in binding. As has been shown with phenytoin, a reduction in protein binding leads to a larger apparent volume of distribution and a greater total body clearance than observed in patients with normal renal function (21). Thus, renal disease can alter the pharmacokinetics of drugs eliminated by nonrenal (metabolic) mechanisms.

This alteration in pharmacokinetics secondary to changes in protein binding does not necessarily indicate that the metabolism of these drugs has been enhanced. Based upon the following assumptions, (a) the kinetics of elimination are apparent first order, (b) the driving force of each elimination process is the concentration of free drug, (c) elimination is not limited or measurably influenced by organ perfusion rate, the total body clearance $(Cl_B)$ of an extensively bound and completely metabolized drug is directly proportional to the free fraction (f) (22), so that

$$Cl_B = Cl_H \cdot f$$

(Eq. 16)

Therefore, $Cl_B$ is linearly related to f. For such drugs, an increase in $Cl_B$ does not necessarily indicate a change in metabolism but only a change in protein binding.

The pharmacologic effect of any drug is presumed to be related to f. An increase in f will theoretically cause an increase in the intensity of the initial pharmacologic response, but the duration of the response may be altered (Figure 3). However, the average concentration of free drug at steady-state will be unchanged if the dose and dosing interval are unchanged:

$$f \cdot \overline{C} = \frac{F \cdot MD}{Cl_H \cdot \tau}$$

(Eq. 17)

Since changes in f will increase V and decrease half-life, the maximum and minimum concentrations (Equations 11 and 12) will increase and decrease respectively (Figure 3), if $\tau$ remains constant.

The net result is that (a) the therapeutic concentration of total drug in the plasma will be reduced, (b) the time to reach steady-state conditions by infusion or repetitive dosing at a fixed interval will be decreased and (c) the fluctuation of drug concentration between doses will increase. Wide fluctuations in drug concentrations in these circumstances can be minimized by decreasing the dosing interval with little or no change in the total daily dose.

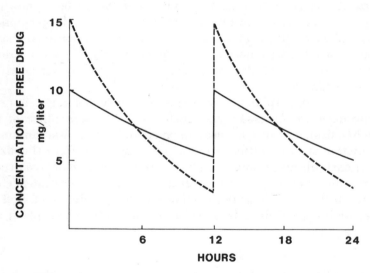

FIGURE 3. Effect of a change in the free fraction of drug in plasma (f) on the time course of free drug concentrations in plasma at steady state when a 100 mg/kg dose of a drug is given intravenously every 12 hours. Key: continuous line, apparent volume of distribution (V) = 0.2 liter/kg, half-life (t½) = 12 hours and f = 0.01; and interrupted line, t increased to 0.03, V increased to 0.25 liter/kg, and t½ decreased, therefore, to 5 hours. (From Levy, J. Pharm. Sci. 1976; 65:1264–1265, with permission.)

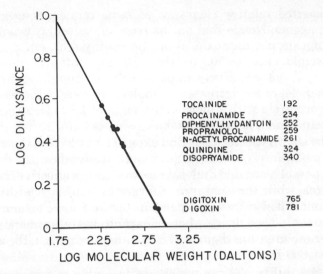

FIGURE 4. Effect of increasing molecular weight on relative hemodialysis clearance of antiarrhythmic agents.

As stated above, changes in elimination half-life can be caused by alterations in drug protein binding. Half-life ($t\frac{1}{2}$) is not a primary pharmacokinetic parameter, but is directly dependent upon V and indirectly dependent upon total body clearance ($Cl_B$):

$$t\frac{1}{2} = \frac{0.693 \cdot V}{Cl_B} \qquad \text{(Eq. 18)}$$

Therefore, $t\frac{1}{2}$ could remain the same if both V and $Cl_B$ doubled. Since $Cl_B$ is the fundamental expression of overall drug elimination, it is obvious that in such a situation the identical $t\frac{1}{2}$ would belie the fact that important changes in drug metabolism and distribution had occurred.

### Effect of Hemodialysis on Pharmacokinetics

The specific properties of a drug that are of importance in predicting the efficacy of conventional hemodialysis are molecular weight or, more properly, molecular volume; water solubility; protein binding; inherent plasma clearance; and dialyzer clearance.

**Molecular Weight.** Hemodialysis membranes can be considered to have discrete pores through which solutes diffuse. These pores can be thought of as cylinders of uniform diameter that perforate the membrane. Because of this, as the molecular weight of a solute increases, diffusiveness through a given membrane decreases. Figure 4 is a plot of the expected relative clearance of some commonly used antiarrhythmic agents. Notice that on the basis of molecular weight alone, neither digoxin nor digitoxin would be readily dialyzable. Once molecular weight exceeds 500 daltons (D), conventional hemodialysis probably will not effectively remove a drug. Therefore, for a given membrane, clearance decreases as molecular weight increases. As a result, vancomycin with a molecular weight of 1,800 D, although only 10% protein bound, is not dialyzable.

It can be shown theoretically and experimentally that the clearance of small molecules (i.e., less than 500 D) is significantly dependent upon the flow of blood and dialysate as well as the effective membrane surface area, while the clearance of larger molecules is, within limits, independent of flow rates and dependent upon effective membrane area (23). Commonly used drugs whose clearance would primarily depend on membrane area are digoxin (781 D), digitoxin (764 D), and vancomycin (1,800 D).

**Water Solubility.** Solutes which are insoluble in water cannot be expected to move from the blood into the aqueous dialysate. The most obvious example is glutethimide. This compound has a molecular weight of 217 D but is insoluble in water. Although there are conflicting reports (24,25), it is apparent that conventional hemodialysis does not substantially increase glutethimide elimination. Another example is phenytoin, which is sparingly soluble in water at pH 7.4.

**Protein Binding.** The driving force in conventional hemodialysis is the concentration gradient of unbound, ultrafilterable solute, between plasma water and dialysate. Therefore, as protein binding increases, clearance decreases. Propranolol, molecular weight 259 D, is 90% to 94% bound and is essentially nondialyzable. Similarly, the protein binding of the semisynthetic penicillins, cloxacillin, dicloxacillin, nafcillin, and oxacillin is greater than 90% and they are therefore not dialyzable.

**Total Body Clearance.** The purpose of hemodialysis is to substantially increase the total body clearance ($Cl_B$) of a drug so as to reduce its half-life. If, during hemodialysis, there are no changes in the inherent metabolic clearance, $Cl_B$, a new $Cl_B$, ($Cl_{BD}$), is established such that:

$$Cl_{BD} = Cl_B + Cl_D \qquad \text{(Eq. 19)}$$

where $Cl_D$ is the dialyzer clearance.

$Cl_D$ must significantly add to $Cl_B$ before dialysis will effectively increase overall solute removal. Levy (26) has suggested that $Cl_D$ must increase $Cl_B$ by 30% to be considered a useful therapeutic adjunct. Therefore, to predict the effectiveness of hemodialysis, accurate estimates of $Cl_B$ and $Cl_D$ are needed.

For any given dialyzer, solute, and blood flow, $Cl_D$ will be constant, but as the weight of the patient increases, the effect of $Cl_D$ on $Cl_B$ will decrease. Therefore extrapolation of results from pediatric patients or small individuals to the patient population as a whole may not be possible. Only if V, $Cl_D$, and patient weight are known, can the effect of dialysis on $t\frac{1}{2}$ be determined.

**Dialyzer Clearance.** The general equation used clinically to calculate solute removal during hemodialysis is

$$Cl_D = \frac{Q(C_A - C_V)}{C_A} \qquad \text{(Eq. 20)}$$

where Q is the flow of blood through the kidney, $C_A$ is the concentration of test substance going into the artificial kidney (arterial side), and $C_V$ is the concentration of the substance leaving the kidney (venous side). Plasma or whole blood clearance can be calculated from

$$Cl_p = \frac{Q_p(C_{Ap} - C_{Vp})}{C_{Ap}} \qquad \text{(Eq. 21)}$$

$$Cl_b = \frac{Q_b(C_{Ap} - C_{Vb})}{C_{Ab}} \qquad \text{(Eq. 22)}$$

where p and b are plasma and blood, respectively. Finally, clearance can be calculated as

$$Cl_x = \frac{Q_b(C_{Ap} - C_{Vp})}{C_{Ap}} \qquad \text{(Eq. 23)}$$

where x is combined.

Calculations of clearance using Equation 23 assume that blood water flow rate through the dialyzer is equal to whole blood flow rate; solute concentration equilibrium, if any, exists between plasma and red cell water along the length of the dialyzer; and there is an absence of significant binding by plasma and red cell proteins. Unfortunately, concentration equilibrium between red cells and plasma may not exist along the length of the dialyzer, hemoglobin binding of solute is known to occur, and blood water flow rate is not equal to whole blood flow rate.

Equations 20 to 23 depend upon an accurate estimation of blood flow. Blood flow is normally determined by pump revolutions/minute or bubble transit time. Gotch has examined both methods (27). The use of calibrated pumps can be accurate if done carefully, but in the clinical setting errors of $\pm 30\%$ to $40\%$ may be encountered. For the bubble transit time, if it is assumed that the flow of the bubble is equal to the flow of blood, there will be a systematic overestimation of $Q_b$ by about 7% at a flow of 100 ml/min, increasing to 16% at a flow of 400 ml/min (27).

Solute concentrations are generally determined in plasma. For solutes transported only in plasma water, such measurements reflect the actual amount in the blood. For substances that are present in red cells and equilibrate with plasma, plasma concentrations underestimate the amount in whole blood and use of Equation 21 may underestimate the amount of solute removal. For drugs present only in plasma, use of Equation 23 will overestimate solute removal by a factor equal to one minus the hematocrit (Hct). On the other hand, if a drug is transported not only by plasma but also by formed elements, $Cl_p$ may underestimate the effective clearance if the drug in the formed elements is available for removal. While $Cl_b$ would therefore appear to be the method of choice to calculate clearance, this is usually not possible since drug concentrations are not generally measured in whole blood. Furthermore, $Cl_b$ is calculated using an entirely different data source (whole blood) than is $Cl_B$ and therefore is not directly comparable to $Cl_B$. Under conditions of ultrafiltration, where movement of plasma water from blood to dialysate occurs, unless the solute moves at the same rate it will become concentrated in the venous sample and clearance will be underestimated as a result of the apparent increase in $C_{Vp}$. If fluid is being administered via the extracorporeal circuit, the solute concentration in V may be diluted and clearance will be overestimated.

In these circumstances, simultaneous measurement of arterial and venous hematocrit or plasma protein concentration will allow for a partial correction of the venous level. An approximation of the venous concentration had ultrafiltration not taken place would be

$$C_{Vp} \text{ actual} = C_{Vp} \text{ observed } [1 - (C_{V\,prot} - C_{A\,prot})/C_{V\,prot}] \qquad \text{(Eq. 24)}$$

where $C_{V\,prot}$ and $C_{A\,prot}$ are venous and arterial protein concentrations respectively. Substituting hematocrit for protein concentration, the same would be true.

Equations 20 to 23 are applicable to those situations where solute does not accumulate in the dialysate. Some clinical centers occasionally use dialysis systems in which the removed substances accumulate in the bath so that the concentration gradient is constantly decreasing. In these situations, removal of solute is expressed as dialysance (D) as shown in Equation 25, where $C_B$ is the concentration of the solute in the dialysis bath.

$$D = \frac{Q(C_A - C_V)}{C_A - C_B} \qquad \text{(Eq. 25)}$$

All the above methods of clearance calculations depend upon the accuracy of measurement of arterial, venous, and bath concentrations of the solute, the accuracy of measurement of whole blood flow, and the assumption of concentration independence of clearance. If a solute is dialyzable, it will be present in the dialysate. If the total amount of solute present in the used dialysate can be determined, clearance can be calculated as:

$$Cl_R = \frac{R}{AUC_0^t} \qquad \text{(Eq. 26)}$$

where R is total amount of solute recovered in dialysate and t is length of dialysis. This method of clearance calculation is independent of blood flow and unaffected by ultrafiltration. If the partition coefficient of the solute between plasma and red cells is known, the product of the partition coefficient and plasma level will give the whole blood level, and whole blood clearance can be determined. For solutes present in plasma and red cell water, plasma clearance calculated by Equation 26 may exceed actual plasma or whole blood flow if the solute is removed from the red cell. Since the amount of drug present in the dialysate, R, is that which is actually removed and is independent of blood flow, this method of clearance calculation should be the standard against which all other methods of clearance are compared.

*Types of Dialyzers.* Besides protein binding and molecular size, $Cl_D$ is obviously dependent upon the type of artificial kidney used. In general, $Cl_D$ increases as surface area (Table 3) and membrane porosity increase (28). Most membranes available today are cuprophan or cellulose, which are similar in porosity. Besides the type of membrane used, the construction of the dialyzer is also important. Different types of membrane supports are used; by impinging on the membrane during ultrafiltration, these can decrease effective surface area. Therefore, dialyzers constructed by different manufacturers but having the same membrane and surface area may not have the same clearance values for a given solute (28).

*In vitro* studies are often undertaken to determine which dialyzer is best for a given solute. Since many of these studies are carried out with the solute dissolved in water, application of the results to the clinical situation requires correction for protein binding and, if the solute is present only in plasma, for the hematocrit. *In vivo* clearance can be estimated from

$$C_{in\ vivo} = C_{in\ vitro} \cdot (\%\ free) \cdot (1 - Hct) \qquad \text{(Eq. 27)}$$

Renal failure may significantly decrease the protein binding of some substances. Therefore, drugs given to patients with renal failure and diminished protein binding may be less efficiently dialyzed than the

TABLE 3.  *In Vitro Dialysis Studies*

| Dialyzer | Surface area (m²) | Membrane thickness (μ) | Clearance (ml/min ± SE) | | | | |
| --- | --- | --- | --- | --- | --- | --- | --- |
| | | | Urea 60** | Procainamide 219** | Phenobarbital 232** | N-acetyl procainamide 261** | Quinidine 324** |
| Dow Model 5 | 2.5 | 30 | 171 ± 3.9 | 114.6 ± 2.4 | 101.6 ± 2.0 | 89.9 ± 2.3 | 70.1 ± 0.6 |
| Dow Model 4 | 1.3 | 30 | 141.9 ± 1.6 | 79.9 ± 5.0 | 97.7 ± 4.4 | 55.3 ± 2.0 | 48.3 ± 0.3 |
| Gambro 17 | 1.02 | 17 | 67.7 ± 2.5 | 50.8 ± 4.7 | 45.6 ± 2.4 | 33.3 ± 4.7 | 39.3 ± 1.3 |
| Gambro 13.5 | 1.02 | 13.5 | 116.9 ± 4.1 | 75.5 ± 0.2 | 74.0 ± 1.5 | | 47.9 ± 0.6 |
| EX 29 | 1.4 | 18 | 155.1 ± 2.8 | 81.4 ± 0.8 | 72.9 ± 9.2 | 78.0 ± 1.6 | 67.6 ± 0.5 |
| EX 25 | 1.0 | 18 | 137.3 ± 1.3 | 71.6 ± 1.4 | 58.3 ± 7.2 | 62.6 ± 1.9 | 57.3 ± 0.8 |
| EX 23 | 0.84 | 18 | 116.6 ± 3.2 | 50.4 ± 3.1 | 47.8 ± 5.4 | 50.4 ± 2.7 | 47.0 ± 1.0 |
| EX 55 | 1.3 | 18 | 82.2 ± 1.3 | 51.8 ± 2.8 | 40.5 ± 4.4 | 53.9 ± 1.3 | 51.6 ± 0.6 |
| Ultra-flow II | 1.9 | 17 | 147.7 ± 0.4 | 78.5 ± 5.4 | 48.3 ± 3.4 | 63.8 ± 2.6 | 46.6 ± 1.3 |
| Ultra-flow 145 | 1.5 | 25 | 132.9 ± 0.5 | 63.4 ± 7.8 | 33.2 ± 6.4 | 50.4 ± 2.6 | 38.3 ± 0.7 |
| Vivacell | 0.5 | 10 | 78.5 ± 5.6 | 37.1 ± 7.0 | 74.5 ± 4.3*** | 27.8 ± 2.2 | 36.0 ± 1.3 |
| XAD-4 650 g | 750/g | NA | 20.6 ± 0.6 | Flow rate | Flow rate | Flow rate | Flow rate |

NA = not applicable
*Q = 200 ml/min
**Molecular weights of test substances
***Results using Vivacell with 1.0 m² surface area

same drug given to normal subjects who are overdosed or patients who may have a higher degree of protein binding. Drugs that are almost entirely confined to the plasma may be better removed in renal failure patients than in normals because, by virtue of their anemia, the plasma flow will be greater in renal failure patients at any given whole blood flow. Patients with polycystic kidneys may be an exception, since they are often not as anemic as the usual dialysis patient.

*Multicompartment Pharmacokinetics.* Equation 19 most properly applies when drug kinetics can be described using a one-compartment model, which assumes that any changes that occur in plasma drug concentration instantaneously and quantitatively reflect changes occurring in tissue drug concentrations. The kinetics of distribution and elimination of most antibiotics can be adequately described with this model. However, many drugs require multiexponential equations to describe the serum level versus time course after intravenous injection, indicating distribution into some tissue(s) other than plasma.

An example of a three-compartment model is given in Figure 5 where $V_c$ is the central (plasma) compartment and $V_f$ and $V_s$ are the fast and slowly equilibrating peripheral compartments. $Cl_f$ and $Cl_s$ represent the rate at which the drug leaves and enters the fast (f) and slow (s) equilibrating compartments from the central compartment. $Cl_T$ is the same as $Cl_B$ in a one-compartment model.

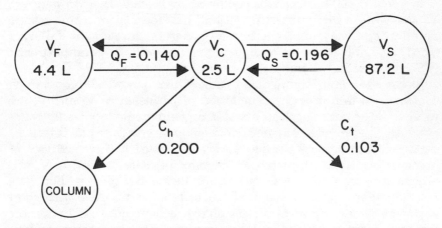

FIGURE 5. Multicompartmental model used to analyze the pharmacokinetics of digoxin in dogs. $Q_F$, $Q_S$, $C_h$, and $C_t$ are the same as $Cl_F$, $Cl_S$, $Cl_H$, and $Cl_B$ respectively. From Gibson (29) with permission.

For drugs with multicompartmental pharmacokinetics, the rate of movement of drug to and from the central compartment not only determines rate decline of serum levels during the distribution phase, but also the effect of dialysis on the serum levels and total body burden (29). One consequence of multicompartmental distribution kinetics is that rebound of plasma levels can be expected after dialysis if the rate of solute removal from plasma exceeds the rate of movement of solute from peripheral compartments into plasma. In Figure 6 and Table 4, a computer simulation of the effect of changing the rate of movement of drug from the peripheral compartments to the central (plasma) compartment is shown, using data for digoxin kinetics in dogs (30).

In panel A, Figure 6, $Cl_s$ has been increased ten-fold over that observed experimentally. With perfusion there is a linear and concordant fall in digoxin levels in all compartments, much as in a one-compartment model. Although serum levels of digoxin only fall from 18.5 to 9.5 ng/ml, 777.2 μg of digoxin are removed (Table 4). The postperfusion rebound is 90% complete within three minutes and levels in $V_c$ re-equilibrated at 10.3 ng/ml.

In panel B, Figure 6, the results are shown with the value of $Q_s$ found experimentally. With hemoperfusion there is a curvilinear decline in serum levels to 6.8 ng/ml. Digoxin concentration in $V_s$ and $V_f$ lag behind that in $V_c$ and only 581.9 μg of digoxin are removed. Seventy-five minutes are required postperfusion before the system has reached 90% of equilibration.

In panel C, $Cl_s$ has been slowed by a factor of 10. Digoxin levels in $V_c$ and $V_f$ fall rapidly to 1.6 ng/ml and hemoperfusion in this setting appears to be very effective. However, digoxin levels in $V_s$ fall very slowly and only 204.8 μg of digoxin are removed. Re-equilibration is 90% complete in 705 minutes.

As can be seen in Figure 6 and Table 4, the amount of digoxin in $V_s$ continues to fall after the completion of perfusion as $V_c$ and $V_f$ are refilled. If the pharmacologic effect of digoxin or any other drug takes place in $V_s$, the adverse effect of those drugs with rapid intercompartmental clearances can be rapidly decreased by hemodialysis or hemoperfusion. As $Cl_s$ decreases, changes in concentration in $V_c$ will become greater with dialysis or hemoperfusion, but there will be little net reduction in pharmacologic effects or total body burden with short perfusion times. However, if the pharmacologic effect is in $V_c$, the toxicity of drugs with slow intercompartmental clearances will be rapidly reversed, only to return as this compartment is refilled from $V_s$.

It is important to point out that if only the changes in serum drug concentration during dialysis are followed, the results shown in panel

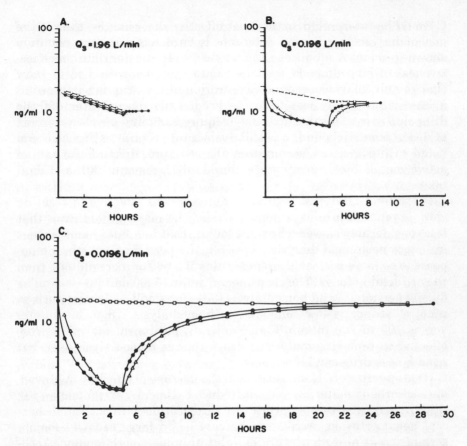

FIGURE 6. Effect of altering $Q_S$ (identical to $Cl_S$) on digoxin concentrations in $V_C$ (o), $V_F$ (Δ), and $V_S$ (□) during and after hemoperfusion. From Gibson (29) with permission.

TABLE 4. CHANGES IN COMPARTMENT CONTENT OF DIGOXIN WITH ALTERATIONS OF $Cl_S$

| $Cl_S$ | Fast | Intermediate | Slow |
|---|---|---|---|
| Amount removed (μg) | 777.2 | 518.9 | 204.8 |
| Amount in $V_C$ (μg) | 46.5 | 46.5 | 46.5 |
| Start | | | |
| Lowest Point | 23.8 | 17.0 | 4.0 |
| Re-equilibrium | 25.8 | 32.5 | 40.5 |
| Amount in $V_S$ (μg) | 1621.7 | 1621.7 | 1621.7 |
| Start | | | |
| End | 904.7 | 1182.6 | 1533.6 |
| Re-equilibration | 901.4 | 1140.8 | 1433.5 |
| Time to 90% re-equilibration (minutes) | 3 | 75 | 705 |

51

C would be interpreted as the most effective dialysis. However, if the goal of dialysis is reduction in total body burden of drug, the situation shown in panel A produces the best result. To substantiate the effectiveness of hemodialysis, sufficient data must be presented to show that the postdialysis serum concentration of the drug is sustained at a level significantly less than the predialysis concentration. If the drug slowly equilibrates, this may require sampling over a very long period of time. Rebound in postdialysis solute concentration has been noted with potassium, serum urea nitrogen, procainamide (9) and its active metabolite N-acetylprocainamide (31), digoxin (30), and digitoxin (32).

**Peritoneal Dialysis.** Peritoneal dialysis is as effective in treating chronic renal failure as is hemodialysis. The major difference is that it is considerably slower. The same factors that influence hemodialysis influence peritoneal dialysis. However, the peritoneal membrane appears to be more permeable to molecules of 5,000 or more daltons than the artificial kidneys. The clearance of inulin (5200 daltons) is similar during peritoneal and hemodialysis (33). For small molecules such as urea, clearance is low compared to hemodialysis, 18 to 30 ml/min versus 100 to 200 ml/min (34). Similarly, peritoneal dialysis is less effective in removing dialyzable drugs than is hemodialysis (35), but nonetheless drug can be removed.

**Hemoperfusion.** Hemoperfusion, the passage of blood through various adsorbent materials, was introduced clinically by Yatzidis (36), who treated two cases of barbiturate intoxication with activated charcoal hemoperfusion. Activated charcoal has a large capacity for absorbing creatinine, barbiturates, glutethimide, methaqualone, ethchlorvynol, and other drugs, but no affinity for urea, electrolytes, and cannot remove water. Also clinically available is Amberlite XAD-4, a synthetic copolymer of styrene and divinylbenzene with affinity for lipophilic molecules such as barbiturates, glutethimide, digoxin, meprobamate, tricyclic antidepressants, quinidine, phenytoin, procainamide, N-acetylprocainamide, and lidocaine. However, XAD-4 has no affinity for urea, creatinine, or water. Regardless of the type of adsorbent used, hemoperfusion has several advantages over hemodialysis in the treatment of drug intoxication.

The physical properties of drugs that restrict the effectiveness of hemodialysis, namely, water solubility, plasma protein binding, and molecular weight, do not appear to limit the effectiveness of hemoperfusion. For example, hemoperfusion with either XAD-4 or activated charcoal removes glutethimide (37), which is 50% bound. Phenobarbital, whose binding varies from 20% to 60% depending on plasma concentration, is rapidly removed (38). With hemoperfusion, the rate limiting factors appear to be affinity of the solute for the adsorbent, rate of movement of solute from tissues to the blood compartment (see above), and capacity of the adsorbent for the solute. Since each molecule of adsorbed solute occupies a binding site on the column, columns of either type will become saturated and may require periodic replacement if hemoperfusion is to be carried out for a prolonged period of time. The principles outlined in the preceding sections apply to hemoperfusion.

**Estimation of Amount of Drug Removed during Dialysis.** If a drug is dialyzable, and if it is necessary to maintain a fairly constant serum concentration, replacement of the drug removed will be required. Several methods can be used. If the same dialyzer is used from treatment to treatment and if the length of dialysis is the same, the amount of drug recovered in the bath can be quantitated and replaced. The plasma clearance of the drug can be determined from Equation 21, and the amount of drug removed from the plasma estimated from the following equation:

$$R_{predicted} = (\overline{Cl}_p)(t)(C_{A\ midpoint}) \tag{Eq. 28}$$

where $R_{predicted}$ is the predicted amount to be recovered and $\overline{Cl}_p$ is the mean plasma clearance. If the drug is removed only from plasma, Equation 28 should give a good estimate of the amount to be replaced. If the drug is removed from red cells and plasma, Equation 28 will underestimate the amount to be replaced. Again, the most accurate estimates will be based on $Cl_R$. Removal of drug from red cells has been documented for procainamide, N-acetylprocainamide, and digoxin (hemoperfusion). Finally, if $Cl_D$ is known, the fraction of the total body burden of drug present at the beginning of dialysis can be estimated as

$$FR = 1 - e^{-kt} \tag{Eq. 29}$$

where k here is $Cl_{BD}/V$ and t is the length of dialysis. The total body burden (BB) of drug at the start of dialysis is

$$BB = C_S \cdot V \tag{Eq. 30}$$

where $C_s$ is the predialysis concentration of the drug in serum or plasma.

Estimation of total amount of drug removed using these formulae assumes that dialysis or hemoperfusion does not alter those physiological parameters such as cardiac output, peripheral resistance, and regional blood flow to either drug storage depots (i.e. skeletal muscle and fat) or to excretory organs such as liver and, in the case of overdoses in otherwise healthy individuals, to the kidneys. Computer predictions of the amount of digoxin and digitoxin removed during canine hemoperfusion have consistently exceeded R. Similarly during conventional hemodialysis, less N-acetylprocainamide was recovered in the bath than was predicted. By decreasing $Cl_s$ during hemoperfusion, the computer prediction and R came into agreement (31). This suggests that hemodialysis and hemoperfusion may limit their own efficacy, by causing hemodynamic changes that retard intercompartmental clearance.

Given the vagaries of half-life, protein binding, dialyzers, methods of calculating dialyzer clearance and possible effects of dialysis or hemoperfusion on intercompartmental clearance, it should be appreciated that all the methods of calculations are only estimates. The adequacy of these methods can be best ascertained by the periodic measurement of drug concentration. As a rule of thumb, it is best to measure drug levels immediately prior (trough level) to the next scheduled dose. By that time, absorption of the drug should be complete and blood concentrations fairly constant. Under such circumstances, if the measured concentration is too high or too low, the dose can be decreased or increased. It should be emphasized that serum drug concentrations measured in the immediate postdialysis period may not accurately reflect the total body burden unless the postdialysis re-equilibration is complete.

## REFERENCES

1. Block K, Schoenheimer R: Studies in protein metabolism XI. The metabolic relation of creatine and creatinine studied with isotopic nitrogen. J Biol Chem 1939; 131:111–119.
2. Bleiler RE, Schedl HP: Creatinine excretion: variability and relationships to diet and body size. J Lab Clin Med 1962; 59:945–955.
3. Renkin EM, Robinson RR: Glomerular filtration. N Engl J Med 1974; 290:785–792.
4. Kassirer JP: Clinical evaluation of kidney function-glomerular function. N Engl J Med 1971; 285:385–389.
5. Dossetor JB: Creatininemia versus uremia. The relative significance of blood urea nitrogen and serum creatinine concentrations in azotemia. Ann Intern Med 1966; 65:1287–1299.
6. Dettli L: Drug dosage in renal disease. Clin Pharmacokinet 1976; 1:126–134.
7. Gibson TP, Atkinson AJ Jr, Matusik E, Nelson E, Briggs WA: Kinetics of procainamide and N-acetylprocainamide in renal failure. Kidney Intl 1977; 12:422–429.
8. Letora JJL, Atkinson AJ, Jr, Kushner W, Nevin MJ, Lee W-K, Jones C, Schmid FR: Long-term antiarrhythmic therapy with N-acetylprocainamide. Clin Pharmacol Ther 1979; 25:273–282.
9. Gibson TP, Matusik EJ, Briggs WA: N-acetylprocainamide levels in patients with end stage renal failure. Clin Pharmacol Ther 1976; 19:206–212.

10. Reuning RH, Sams RA, Notari RE: Role of pharmacokinetics in drug dosage adjustment: apparent volume of distribution of digoxin. J Clin Pharmacol 1973; 13:127–141.
11. Koup JR, Jusko WJ, Elwood CM, Kohli RK: Digoxin pharmacokinetics: role of renal failure in dosage regimen design. Clin Pharmacol Ther 1975; 18:9–21.
12. Gibson TP, Nelson HA: The question of cumulation of digoxin metabolites in renal failure. Clin Pharmacol Ther 1980; 27:219–223.
13. Tilstone WJ, Fine A: Furosemide kinetics in renal failure. Clin Pharmacol Ther 1978; 23:644–650.
14. Craig R, Gibson TP, Murphy P, Quintanilla A: Reduced metabolism and intestinal absorption of D-xylose in renal failure. Amer Soc Neph 1978; 11:14A.
15. Chau NP, Weiss YA, Safar ME, Lavene DE, Georges DR, Milliez PL: Pindolol availability in hypertensive patients with normal and impaired renal function. Clin Pharmacol Ther 1977; 22:505–510.
16. Branchetti G, Graziani G, Brancaccio D, Morganti A, Leonetti G, Manfrin M, Sega R, Gomeni R, Ponticelli C, Morselli PL: Pharmacokinetics and effects of propranolol in terminal uraemic patients and patients undergoing regular dialysis treatment. Clin Pharmacokinet 1976; 1:373–384.
17. Gibson TP, Giacomini KM, Briggs WA, Whitman W, Levy G: Pharmacokinetics of d-propoxyphene in anephric patients. Clin Pharmacol Ther 1977; 21:103.
18. Wood AJJ, Vestal RE, Spannath C, Stone WJ, Wilkinson GR, Shand DG: Propranolol disposition in renal failure. Clin Res 1979; 27:239A.
19. Reidenberg MM: The binding of drugs to plasma proteins from patients with poor renal function. Clin Pharmacokinet 1976; 1:121–125.
20. Belpaire FM, Bogaert MG, Mussche MM: Influence of acute renal failure on the protein binding of drugs in animals and man. Eur J Clin Pharmacol 1977; 11:27–32.
21. Odar-Cederlof I, Borga O: Kinetics of diphenylhydantoin in uraemic patients: consequences of decreased protein binding. Eur J Clin Pharmacol 1974; 7:31–37.
22. Levy G: Clinical implications of interindividual differences in plasma protein binding of drugs and endogenous substances. In: Benet LZ, ed. *The Effect of Disease States on Drug Pharmacokinetics*. American Pharmaceutical Association, Washington DC 1976; 137–151.
23. Babb AL, Popovich RP, Christopher TG, Scribner BH: The genesis of the square meter-hour hypothesis. Trans Amer Soc Artif Intern Organs 1971; 17:81–91.
24. Maher JF, Schreiner GE, Westervelt FB: Acute glutethimide intoxication I. Clinical experience (twenty-two patients) compared to acute barbiturate intoxication (sixty-three patients). Amer J Med 1962; 33:70–82.
25. Chazan JA, Cohen JJ: Clinical spectrum of glutethimide intoxication. JAMA 1969; 208:837–839.
26. Levy G: Pharmacokinetics in renal disease. Amer J Med 1977; 62:461–465.
27. Gotch FA: Hemodialysis: technical and kinetic considerations. In: Brenner BM, Rector FC Jr, eds. *The Kidney*. WB Saunders, Philadelphia 1976; 1672–1704.
28. Gibson TP, Matusik E, Nelson LD, Briggs WA: Artificial kidneys and clearance calculations. Clin Pharmacol Ther 1976; 20:720–726.
29. Gibson TP, Atkinson AJ Jr: Effect of changes in intercompartmental rate constants on drug removal during hemoperfusion. J Pharm Sci 1978; 67:1178–1179.
30. Gibson TP, Lucas SV, Nelson HA, Atkinson AJ Jr, Okita GI, Ivanovich P: Hemoperfusion removal of digoxin from dogs. J Lab Clin Med 1978; 91:673–682.

31. Stec GP, Atkinson AJ Jr, Nevin MJ, Theuot J-P, Ruo TI, Gibson TP, Ivanovich P, del Greco F: N-acetylprocainamide pharmacokinetics in functionally anephric patients before and after perturbation by hemodialysis. Clin Pharmacol Ther (In press)
32. Shah G, Nelson HA, Atkinson AJ Jr, Okita GT, Ivanovich P, Gibson TP: Effect of hemoperfusion on the pharmacokinetics of digitoxin in dogs. J Lab Clin Med 1979; 93:370–380.
33. Nolph KD, Ghods AJ, Brown P, Van Stone J, Miller FN, Wiegman DL, Harris PD: Peritoneal dialysis efficiency. Dial Transpl 1977; 6:52–56.
34. Nolph KD: Peritoneal clearances. J Lab Clin Med 1979; 94:519–525.
35. Regeur L, Colding H, Jensen H, Kampmann JP: Pharmacokinetics of amakacin during hemodialysis and peritoneal dialysis. Antimicrob Agents Chemother 1977; 11:214–218.
36. Yatsidis H: Treatment of severe barbiturate poisoning. Lancet 1965; 2:216–217.
37. Rosenbaum JL, Kramer MS, Raja R: Resin hemoperfusion for acute drug intoxication. Arch Intern Med 1976; 136:263–266.
38. Vale JA, Rees AJ, Widdop B, Goulding R: Use of charcoal haemoperfusion in the management of severely poisoned patients. Br Med J 1975; 1:5–9.

# 4

# Influence of Liver Disease on Pharmacokinetics

Grant R. Wilkinson, Ph.D.

## Introduction

The central role of the liver in drug elimination leads logically to the question of altered disposition and effects in patients with impaired hepatic function. Early studies in this area provided a confused and conflicting picture, especially when contrasted to the analogous situation of renal failure. Several reasons were suggested to account for this situation (1), but even when appropriately designed and interpreted investigations were subsequently performed, they only confirmed that generalizations are extremely difficult. Consequently, the practitioner is still in the quandary of recognizing that drug use in a patient with liver disease may require more than the usual caution; however, there are few reliable aids available to improve the predictability of the clinical response. Accordingly, this chapter will focus on generally applicable principles rather than a collation of the increasingly large descriptive data base, for which there are several recent reviews (1–5). Also, information on specific drugs is presented in other chapters of this book.

## Patient Factors

While the term "liver disease" connotes a well defined and circumscribed disease state, in reality it consists of an assortment of acute and chronic inflammatory, degenerative and/or neoplastic insults to the hepatobiliary system. There may be disturbances in organ structure and architecture as well as altered hemodynamics. Moreover, the assessment of functional abnormality varies widely within any diag-

57

nosed condition because many of the clinical and laboratory criteria for determining the stage and severity are relatively crude. As a result, patients with liver disease exhibit considerable heterogeneity of hepatic function, including drug metabolism and biliary excretion.

The problem is further compounded by dysfunction in other organs or when other disease states are present along with liver disease, such as the hepato-renal syndrome. Additionally, patients may have an altered nutritional status, either self-generated (alcoholic cirrhosis) or imposed by therapeutic considerations (protein restriction). While specific information is lacking for such patients, the effect of diet upon drug metabolism is generally well recognized (6). Finally, it is not unusual for patients with liver disease, in contrast to subjects in controlled clinical studies, to be receiving multiple drugs which may interact, either pharmacokinetically or pharmacodynamically. These interactions add further to the underlying interpatient variability due to genetic, age and environmental factors. As a result of all these factors, drug distribution and elimination in patients with liver disease shows pronounced variability.

## Pharmacokinetic Factors

The effects of liver disease on drug disposition may be manifested as changes in any of the common descriptive pharmacokinetic parameters for total drug, namely systemic clearance ($Cl_S$), volume of distribution (Vd), disposition half-live(s) ($t\frac{1}{2}$) and systemic bioavailability. Since the drugs of most concern are extensively metabolized by the liver, systemic clearance generally reflects hepatic clearance ($Cl_H$). In evaluating such changes it is critical to understand the fundamental inter-relationship between the various terms and also their physiological determinants. Often, apparently paradoxical and confusing situations may be explained by such knowledge.

In considering a drug eliminated only by the liver, systemic clearance is controlled by the three determinants of hepatic removal (7): (a) the ability of the elimination process to irreversibly remove drug from liver water, termed intrinsic free clearance ($Cl'_{int}$), (b) the fraction of drug unbound in the blood ($f_B$), and (c) the rate of drug delivery to the organ as controlled by liver blood flow (Q). A quantitative inter-relationship between these determinants is provided by the "venous equilibration" perfusion model (7–9) as shown in Equation 1.

$$Cl_H = Q \cdot \frac{f_B \, Cl'_{int}}{Q + f_B \, Cl'_{int}}$$

(Eq. 1)

This relationship can be used to explain differences in drug disposition when the various determinants are modified (7). When intrinsic total clearance ($f_B Cl_{int}$) is small compared to liver blood flow, hepatic clearance largely reflects intrinsic clearance, and a change in either binding or drug metabolizing/excretion activity will have a greater effect on organ clearance than changes in liver blood flow. In contrast, when $Q << f_B Cl_{int}$ hepatic clearance is predominantly controlled by liver blood flow, and it is sensitive to changes in this determinant and less sensitive to alterations in binding or intrinsic free clearance.

The volume of distribution subsequent to tissue pseudo-equilibrium may also be explained in physiological terms (Equation 2):

$$Vd = V_B + V_T \frac{f_B}{f_T} \qquad \text{(Eq. 2)}$$

where $V_B$ is the blood volume, $V_T$ is the volume of other body tissues and $f_B$ and $f_T$ are the fractions of unbound drug in blood and tissue, respectively (7,10). Consequently, as the unbound fraction in the blood increases there is an approximately proportional change in the volume of distribution of total drug, especially for drugs with a large Vd (i.e., small $f_T$). Conversely, the distribution volume in terms of unbound drug ($Vd/f_B$) remains essentially constant, except for drugs with a relatively small Vd where an increase in $f_B$ leads to a reduction in this particular distribution volume. Drug distribution may also be altered by tissue binding. When both $f_B$ and $f_T$ change, the resulting alteration is a balance of the two changes, including the possibility of offsetting perturbations leading to no alteration in Vd (11).

Systemic (hepatic) clearance and distribution volume interact to produce the empirical pharmacokinetic parameter, elimination half-life ($t\frac{1}{2}$), according to Equation 3:

$$t\frac{1}{2} = \frac{0.693 Vd}{Cl_S} \qquad \text{(Eq. 3)}$$

Substitution of Equations 1 and 2 into Equation 3 indicates that half-life is affected in a complex fashion when either drug binding, intrinsic free clearance or liver blood flow are altered (7). Such changes are all potentially possible as a result of liver disease and consequently the interpretation of any alteration in elimination half-life is fraught with difficulties. Assessment of changes in clearance and distribution, along with knowledge of the unbound fraction, is far more valuable.

## Intrinsic Free Clearance Changes in Liver Disease

For drugs which are metabolized and enter the liver parenchymal cells by rapid passive diffusion, intrinsic free clearance may be conceptualized as the clearance of the unbound drug from intracellular water. In cases where another step is rate-limiting (e.g., uptake, biliary secretion), $Cl'_{int}$ reflects the process with respect to unbound drug. Intuitively, it would be expected that any liver dysfunction with respect to drug handling would be reflected in this parameter. However, direct assessment of any such impairment in hepatic disposition of drugs is difficult and most evidence is inferential.

Under first-order conditions, $Cl'_{int}$ is equivalent to the ratio of the overall Michaelis-Menten parameters, Vmax and Km, for the removal process (12). Therefore, it might be expected that assessment of the *in vitro* metabolizing capacity of a liver biopsy would provide a useful indicator of overall drug metabolizing ability. Limited studies to date have not, however, been encouraging. Only in severe cases of hepatitis and cirrhosis is oxidative microsomal drug metabolizing activity significantly decreased (13–15), and yet *in vivo* drug clearance is often impaired in patients with much less extensive disease. Measurement of the terminal component of the electron transport chain system, cytochrome P-450, has been similarly disappointing. While a good relationship exists between its biopsy concentration and histological damage, the correlation with antipyrine elimination in a population of alcoholics with a wide-spectrum of liver disease was poor (16). Major problems with such an approach are the assumption of homogeneity of liver structure, which is not likely in severe cirrhosis, and the difficulty of assessing functional liver mass in order to determine total metabolizing activity. Liver enlargement is quite common in liver diseased patients. In mild cases of fatty liver, such hepatomegaly may actually compensate for the decreased enzyme content, but in more severe situations the metabolic impairment appears to dominate (17). Overall, it appears that drug clearance by the diseased liver depends on factors other than the level of drug metabolizing enzyme activity *per se*.

For drugs with a small intrinsic total clearance relative to total liver blood flow ($f_B Cl'_{int} < Q/4$), hepatic clearance is essentially independent of flow and reflects drug metabolizing activity (7–9). When corrected for drug binding in the blood (i.e., hepatic clearance of unbound drug), this parameter is a good estimate of $Cl'_{int}$. Such information exists for a number of drugs in a variety of different liver diseases.

By far the most widely investigated drug is antipyrine, predominantly because it is almost totally metabolized, essentially unbound in plasma, distributed in body water and behaves similarly after both oral and intravenous administration. Its elimination is, therefore, a good indicator of hepatic drug metabolism alone, and it may well become the standard correlative measure of this activity. Following the initial investigation of Branch et al (18), many other investigators have demonstrated impaired clearance in patients with cirrhosis, based on either serum/plasma (19–23) or salivary pharmacokinetics (24). Similarly, the free (25) and total (25,26) clearance of theophylline in cirrhotics, and the free clearance of amobarbital (27) in patients with chronic liver disease and low serum albumin ($< 3.5$ mg/100 ml) are reduced compared to normal subjects. The mean clearance of diazepam from plasma in alcoholic cirrhotics is almost half of that in age-matched controls (28,29). Since plasma binding is also reduced, an even greater impairment in $Cl'_{int}$ is inferred (28,29). A similar situation apparently exists with chlordiazepoxide (30) and diazepam's major metabolite, N-desmethyldiazepam (31). In contrast, the clearance of unbound lorazepam is not affected in cirrhosis, even though the handling of antipyrine and chlordiazepoxide in the same patients is impaired (32). The clearance of oxazepam is similarly unaffected in cirrhosis (33). There is, therefore, good evidence that chronic liver disease, such as cirrhosis, leads to an impairment in the intrinsic ability of the hepatocyte to metabolize drugs. However, it is apparent that in addition to considerable inter-patient variability, all drugs are not equally affected (i.e., there is selective impairment of different routes of metabolism to the effects of a given degree of liver dysfunction).

The differential sensitivity is even more readily apparent in acute viral hepatitis. Plasma clearances of unbound phenytoin (34), tolbutamide (35), warfarin (36), oxazepam (33) and lorazepam (32) are not significantly different from appropriately matched normal subjects. More important, perhaps, is that clearance does not usually change during progression of the disease state to recovery. On the other hand, the clearance of antipyrine (37), diazepam (28), chlordiazepoxide (30) and hexobarbital (38) are impaired in viral hepatitis; although, in general the extent of dysfunction is less than that observed in cirrhosis.

If drug metabolism is impaired in liver disease, it would be expected that alternative pathways of elimination would play a more significant role and thereby alter the quantitative elimination profile. In fact, this information is probably the best *in vivo* evidence of altered metabolizing ability. However, few investigators have explored this approach. The percentage of amylobarbital excreted as the 3-hydroxy metabolite is significantly reduced in chronically diseased patients (27) as is the fraction of hexobarbital eliminated as 3'-ketohexobarbital in patients with viral hepatitis (38). On the other hand, total excretion of the 4-hydroxy metabolite of phenobarbital is reduced in cirrhosis but not acute viral hepatitis (39). The 24 hr urinary excretion of the 4-hydroxy metabolite of antipyrine is reduced in patients with a variety of different types of liver disease and the excretion rate is highly correlated with the clearance of the parent drug (22). Consistent with the hypothesis of selective impairment of different metabolic pathways, the urinary excretion of lidocaine and three of its metabolites were unequally affected in a patient with chronic active hepatitis (40).

In summary, it appears that the intrinsic free clearance of drugs is impaired in patients with liver disease, but there is considerable variability in the extent. In part this may be explained by differences in the type and severity of the disease under consideration. In addition, it is becoming increasingly apparent that for any given degree of dysfunction the metabolism of all drugs is not equally affected, even though a common major biotransformation, such as oxidation, appears to be involved. Some pathways, such as glucuronidation of the benzodiazepines (and other drugs?) appear to be less sensitive to pathological changes than other pathways.

### Plasma and Tissue Binding

Since the liver is the major organ for the synthesis of albumin and other circulating macromolecules to which drugs bind reversibly, it would be expected that hepatic dysfunction would lead to alterations in the unbound fraction present in the plasma ($f_P$) and, therefore, in the blood ($f_B$), where $f_B = f_P/B/P$ and B/P is the blood/plasma concentration ratio. *In vitro* studies are supportive of this concept. For example, the plasma from cirrhotic patients binds a number of drugs, including diazepam (28,41), chlordiazepoxide (30), lorazepam (32), amylobarbitone (27), morphine (42), phenytoin (42,43), phenylbutazone (44), propranolol (51,52), tolbutamide (41), quinidine (43) and thiopental (45), to a lesser extent than normal plasma. Similarly, there is an increase in the unbound fraction of chlordiazepoxide (30), lorazepam (32), tolbutamide (35) and phenytoin (34) in acute viral hepatitis. While reduced levels of binding protein (e.g., albumin) especially in cirrhosis, may account for these changes, a role for qualitative differences in the binding protein(s) cannot be excluded. Additionally, it is possible that the accumulation of endogenous binding inhibitors such as bilirubin may also be involved.

The critically important question is how do such alterations in binding affect the drug's pharmacokinetics *in vivo?* In general, the major concern is for situations where the unbound fraction increases significantly, which is essentially limited to drugs which are less than

10% free. When the extent of binding is below about 90%, pharmacokinetic parameters for total drug tend to be relatively insensitive to the limited pathophysiological changes in binding (46).

Equation 1 indicates that plasma binding only restricts hepatic clearance when a drug's intrinsic free clearance is small relative to liver blood flow. In the reverse situation, the removal process is sufficiently efficient to strip drug from its plasma binding sites during passage through the liver and so, binding is not limiting (7,9). For drugs with restrictive plasma binding (e.g., diazepam (28), chlordiazepoxide (30), and tolbutamide (35)), the increased unbound fraction in liver disease compensates for the decrease in $Cl'_{int}$, and the impairment of hepatic clearance of total drug is an underestimate of the hepatocellular dysfunction. In fact, with tolbutamide the relative change in binding in acute viral hepatitis is larger than the change in $Cl'_{int}$. This results in greater total hepatic clearance and a shorter half-life in such patients than when they have recovered and are disease-free (35)! Accordingly, it is important in patients with liver disease to consider the clearance of both total and unbound drug, especially in chronic dosing situations (47).

Perturbations in binding may also affect drug distribution. An increase in the unbound fraction would be expected to lead to an increase in the total volume of distribution (Equation 2), while the unbound volume ($Vd/f_p$) should remain essentially constant, providing Vd is reasonably large and tissue binding ($f_T$) is not altered (7,11). Such observations have been made with diazepam (28), chlordiazepoxide (30), lorazepam (32), lidocaine (48), pancuronium (49), valproic acid (30), theophylline (25,26), and propranolol (51,52) in cirrhosis; and chlordiazepoxide (30) and lidocaine (53) in acute viral hepatitis. With lorazepam there is no significant impairment of unbound or total plasma clearance in cirrhosis (32). Consequently, the increase in Vd leads to a prolongation in the elimination half-life; a similar situation occurs with chloramphenicol (54). These are vivid examples of the limitations of half-life in assessing the body's ability to metabolize a drug, and the difficulty in interpreting a prolonged half-life in patients with liver disease. In certain cases the expected increase in Vd has not been observed or conflicting data exist. This probably arises because of the small magnitude of the predicted change coupled with the inherent error of estimation and the variance of the study population. Alternatively, it is possible that the extent of tissue binding is altered along with plasma binding changes. This mechanism has been suggested to account for the unchanged distribution of tolbutamide in acute viral hepatitis (11,35). In some instances the presence of ascitic fluid has also been found to alter drug distribution (50,55).

It is clear that changes in drug binding in the plasma (and possibly extravascular tissue) produced by liver disease can have a significant effect on a drug's pharmacokinetics. Moreover, the changes in binding may vary from a few percent to several-fold, dependent on the drug, disease state and individual patient. Although most analytical methodologies determine total drug levels and their time course, it is often critical to interpret these findings in terms of simultaneous estimates of unbound drug, which is generally considered to be the pharmacologically active moiety.

## Liver Blood Flow

In subjects with normal liver function, hepatic clearance of a drug may be limited completely or partly by its rate of delivery to the organ (7–9). This occurs when intrinsic total clearance is larger than liver blood flow (Equation 1). Accordingly, hepatic clearance is sensitive to changes in flow and such drugs are often used to measure liver blood flow. Therefore, the alterations in hepatic hemodynamics occurring in liver disease would be expected to lead to changes in the hepatic elimination of highly extracted drugs. Generally, it is considered that total liver blood flow is somewhat decreased in chronic liver disease (56), while it is unchanged or even slightly elevated in acute viral hepatitis (57–59). It is probable, therefore, that the impaired hepatic clearance of lidocaine (48) and propranolol (51,52,60) in cirrhotics involves a component related to the decreased drug delivery rate. The major problem in assessing the relative contributions of altered blood flow and intrinsic free clearance in impaired hepatic elimination is the present impossibility of routinely estimating functional rather than total liver blood flow (i.e., that blood supply perfusing metabolically active liver cells). Extra-hepatic, intra-hepatic and surgical shunts are frequently present, especially in chronic liver disease, permiting drugs to bypass functioning liver cells. For example, up to 70% of mesenteric and 100% of splenic blood flow may undergo extra-hepatic shunting in alcoholic liver diseases (61–63) and intra-hepatic anastomosis has been reported to range from 3 to 66% (64,65). Furthermore, it must be recognized that with a reduction in intrinsic free clearance the dependency of hepatic clearance on liver blood flow also decreases. Consequently, the altered hemodynamics present in liver disease may not be as pronounced with respect to overall hepatic clearance as might be expected by direct extrapolation from a normal physiological standpoint (52,60).

## Route of Administration

In contrast to other common routes of administration, the oral route does not deliver drug directly into the systemic circulation following absorption. Instead, the blood supply from the upper and middle gastro-intestinal tract flows to the liver via the portal system. As a consequence, drug is exposed to this eliminating organ prior to reaching the systemic circulation, yielding the so-called "first-pass effect." The fraction of the absorbed dose (F) which escapes this pre-systemic elimination is related to the hepatic extraction ratio (E), the parenthetic term in Equation 1, and the fraction of the mesenteric blood flow passing through the functional liver • ($f_H$)

$$F = 1\text{-}f_H E = \frac{Q + f_B Cl'_{int}(1\text{-}f_H)}{Q + f_B Cl'_{int}} \qquad\qquad \text{(Eq. 4)}$$

Thus, when the liver is normally efficient at removing drug (i.e. high extraction/intrinsic total clearance), only a small fraction of drug reaches the circulation and *vice-versa* for a poorly cleared drug. Also, for any degree of reduction in intrinsic total clearance, the effect on the absorbed fraction is greater the higher the initial value of this parameter. The presence of extra- and intra-hepatic shunts will also increase the fraction of the absorbed dose which reaches the systemic circulation, and again the greater the hepatic extraction ratio the larger this effect (66).

Separation of the relative contribution of each of these mechanisms to any increase in bioavailability of drug in liver disease is not presently possible. However, the existence of the overall phenomenon has been clearly demonstrated in cirrhotics receiving meperidine (67), pentazocine (67), salicylamide (67), propranolol (52) and chlormethiazole (68). Increases in the absorbed fraction may be substantial, approaching three-fold for pentazocine and ten-fold for chlormethiazole.

It is readily apparent that oral administration of drugs to patients with liver disease leads to an increased amount of drug reaching the circulation, from which it is eliminated less efficiently (i.e., oral dosing accentuates the effects of impaired hepatic elimination). Importantly, these effects are multiplicative, and the higher the normal hepatic clearance, the greater the enhancement.

## Specific Liver Diseases

While the category of liver disease encompasses a variety of specific pathophysiologies of varying severity, certain broad points of importance may be made with regard to hepatic drug elimination.

**Chronic Liver Disease.** Fibrosis and cirrhosis occur as the end result of liver cell necrosis and inflammation, and may be caused by viral hepatitis, alcohol abuse and biliary obstruction. Various degrees of hepatic dysfunction are usually present. In general, concomitant alterations in all aspects of hepatic drug disposition are present to a greater extent in chronic liver disease than in other forms of hepatic dysfunction. Moreover, the more severe the disease the greater the alterations. Most studies have investigated cirrhosis of alcoholic etiology, but chronic active hepatitis and other types of cirrhosis appear to have a similar spectrum and range of dysfunction. Such patients, especially those with end-stage disease also develop related clinical problems which further complicate drug therapy. Examples include renal dysfunction and a propensity to develop encephalopathy, especially following sedative-hypnotic drug administration.

**Acute Hepatitis.** Although drugs, alcohol and infections may all cause hepatitis, drug disposition in acute viral hepatitis is the most extensively studied. The degree of mean changes in drug disposition is often less than that observed in cirrhosis, but considerable variability is exhibited. In certain cases no impairment of hepatic elimination or distribution may be present. As the disease resolves and the patient recovers, drug disposition tends to return towards normal. However, a lag period of possibly many weeks relative to the normalization of the conventional biochemical liver function tests is often apparent, as has been noted with diazepam (28) and hexobarbital (38). However, one series of studies with antipyrine demonstrated normalization of drug metabolizing activity prior to normalization of liver function tests (37).

**Cholestasis.** There have been few studies of the effects of either intra- or extra-hepatic cholestasis on drug disposition, despite the role of biliary excretion in the hepatic elimination of several drugs. However, the limited studies with antipyrine (69,70), aminopyrine (71), meprobamate (72) and pentobarbital (72) have found only small changes in elimination due to cholestasis. Similarly, surgical relief of extra-hepatic obstruction has had only a small and variable effect (69,70). In contrast, the half-life of tolbutamide is almost halved in patients with gallstones (72), possibly because of the increase in unbound fraction in the plasma secondary to elevated bilirubin levels.

**Hepatic Neoplastic Disease.** Only the disposition of model compounds in patients with hepatic cancer has been investigated, and then only to a limited extent. As a group, such patients exhibit an impaired ability to metabolize antipyrine (73) and aminopyrine (74), although marked variability is present. These differences appear to be the result of the type of neoplasm, primary versus metastatic, the size of the malignancy and the presence of associated parenchymal disease (73). In addition, an altered capacity to metabolize drugs may result from chemotherapy and radiation treatment (75).

**Drug-Induced Hepatotoxicity.** A variety of drugs may induce liver damage, although in general drug-induced hepatic dysfunction is not severe enough to significantly affect drug elimination and it is usually rapidly reversible. However, hepatic injury caused by acute exposure to a large dose of a hepatotoxin may produce a completely different picture. For example, acute centrilobular necrosis following acetaminophen overdose not only reduces elimination of the causative agent (76,77) but also significantly impairs the metabolism of other drugs (77,78). If the patient recovers, impairment generally reverses over a period of several weeks (77). In contrast to other types of liver disease, the extent of impairment is well related to the extent of hepatic damage as assessed by conventional liver function tests (76). Clinical case reports would suggest that other overdosages, especially of sedative-hypnotic drugs (77), also affect to a variable extent the liver's ability to eliminate drugs, but few studies have been made.

## Clinical Considerations

In general, the study of drug disposition and effects in liver disease has been directed towards identification and quantification of changes relative to the normal individual. Presumably, it was hoped that such information would have direct relevance to the clinical situation. Unfortunately, such application has had only very limited success.

A major problem is caused by the scientific methodological approach that has been taken. Patients are generally selected to exclude as many potentially confounding factors as possible, such as other drug administration, diet, age-matching and homogeneity of the disease state, a far cry from the typical clinical situation. Also, drug administration is usually limited to a single dose, frequently by the intravenous route, and often not all of the critical pharmacokinetic parameters are estimated. The more common clinical situation of multiple dosing, especially by the oral route, is handled by theoretical extrapolation rather than empirical evaluation. While this may be satisfactory for unchanged drug, it is of little value when pharmacologically active metabolites are formed, the disposition of which may also be affected by the liver disease. For example, the elimination of desmethyl diazepam, a major psychopharmacologically active metabolite of diazepam, is impaired in a manner similar to the parent drug in chronic liver disease. This impairment of metabolite clearance in turn affects the clearance of diazepam in a different fashion than in normals following chronic dosing (31). Finally, the major thrust has been directed towards alterations in pharmacokinetics. While this is an important consideration, it neglects the pharmacodynamic aspects of drug responsiveness.

**Altered Drug Responsiveness.** The clinical application of pharmacokinetics assumes that differences in drug disposition are largely responsible for interpatient variability in drug responsiveness (i.e., receptor sensitivity is reasonably uniform). However, it must be recognized that liver disease may alter a drug's pharmacodynamics in addition to changing its pharmacokinetics. Furthermore, the pharmacodynamic changes may be more critical in drug therapy than the pharmacokinetic ones. Of special concern is the apparent increase in cerebral "sensitivity" to CNS active drugs in chronic liver disease. Thus, significantly less diazepam is required to produce a given degree of sedation in such patients relative to normals (79), and alterations in drug-related electroencephalographic patterns have also been noted in liver disease patients receiving morphine (80), chlorpromazine (81,82), diazepam (79) and tranylcypromine (83). Clinically, it is also well recognized that sedatives, tranquillizers and analgesics are a major precipitating factor in hepatic encephalopathy (84). While the precise contributions of altered pharmacokinetics and pharmacodynamics are not absolutely clear, there seems to be little doubt that these alterations in responsiveness involve a change in "receptor sensitivity." Another area for concern is where drug action is directly dependent upon liver function, for example, anticoagulant therapy. Even when impairment in drug disposition is not apparent, perturbations in coagulation factors may be present, yielding an unexpectedly pronounced pharmacologic effect following warfarin administration (36). Unfortunately, in such cases clinical assessment of the patient is of little value in predicting the altered responsiveness.

**Predictive Tests of Altered Disposition.** Because there is so much inter-subject variability in pharmacokinetic changes produced by any type of liver disease, it would be of great clinical value to have a predictive test(s) indicative of the degree of impairment in an individual patient. This could then be used in a manner analogous to creatinine clearance in renal dysfunction. Ideally, knowledge of a drug's systemic clearance in terms of both total and unbound forms, elimination half-life, bioavailability and distribution volume(s) would permit rational pharmacokinetic therapy.

Since biochemical liver function tests evaluate the effects of hepatic disease on organ function, one of which is drug metabolism, some correlation might be expected. However, the conventional tests such as SGOT, SGPT, serum levels of bilirubin, gamma glutamyl transpeptidase, albumin, and prothrombin index lack discrimination and have not proven to be consistently reliable correlative indicators. The best findings have been in chronic liver disease where a serum albumin level below 3.0 to 3.5 mg/dl and/or impaired prothrombin activity ($<$ 80% normal) is frequently indicative of impaired drug elimination (18,19,21,26,27,51). This is not too surprising since these two measurements are indices of general hepatic protein systhesis and simply classify the severity of the disease. Certainly no useful continuous correlative relationships have been found.

The lack of success of conventional biochemical function tests as correlative predictors of drug metabolism has led to investigation of specific marker substrates for drug metabolism. Compounds examined include antipyrine (21,52,85,86), galactose (19,20,22,23), indocyanine green (21,53), $^{14}$C-aminopyrine (85,87–90), $^{14}$C-diazepam (85), $^{14}$C-galactose (91) and $^{14}$C-phenacetin (92). The latter radiolabeled drugs have the advantage that the $^{14}CO_2$ formed via drug metabolism and subsequently excreted in the expired air is a non-invasive measurement of hepatic function. Two aspects of such marker compounds need to be considered; how sensitive are they in detecting impaired hepatic drug elimination and how accurately do they predict the altered disposition of other drugs?

With the exception of one study (90), the general trend of available information is that direct determination of a specific aspect of hepatic drug elimination provides an assessment of this capability which is superior to any biochemical function test. As such, these tests could well complement the conventional tests which measure different activities of the liver. Possibly because of their simplicity and non-invasive nature, the breath tests using $^{14}$C-labelled drug will prove to be more advantageous than other approaches. However, further studies are required to determine the merits and limitations of the various specific compounds previously used on an empirical basis (89).

A number of statistically significant correlations have been found between hepatic elimination of various compounds in patients with liver disease and normal subjects, irrespective of the rate-limiting step of the process. For example, the half-lives of antipyrine, lidocaine or acetaminophen were always associated with a corresponding impairment of the other drugs (86); the clearances of propranolol, indocyanine green and antipyrine (51), and diazepam, indocyanine green, aminopyrine and antipyrine were significantly correlated (85). Similarly, antipyrine clearance was linearly related to the galactose elimination rate (19,22) in patients with various types of liver disease.

Unfortunately, there was considerable scatter of individual data about the statistically significant correlation curves. Thus, for individual patients the degree of predictability was quite low, and it appears that this approach will not lead to any clinically useful indicator, given the present state of knowledge.

**Guidelines for Drug Use.** An increased understanding of the interaction of the various biological factors which determine drug disposition has led to a better appreciation of the complex fashion in which liver disease produces changes in pharmacokinetics. The effects of liver disease are not limited to altered hepatic metabolism/excretion; changes in plasma binding, liver blood flow, tissue distribution and altered receptor responsiveness may also occur. However, this knowledge is currently of little practical value in the clinical use of a particular drug in an individual patient with a specific liver dysfunction. Marked inter-patient variability in the perturbations is present and available diagnostic tools are of essentially no value in predicting an individual's overall responsiveness.

Given these constraints, how should essential drugs be used in patients with liver disease? It is important to recognize that even when severe liver dysfunction is present, the resulting mean alterations in drug disposition are usually no greater than two- to threefold. Certain individuals may, however, exhibit greater changes. For many drugs, the inter-subject variability in normal individuals is much greater than this. Accordingly, the need to specifically modify a dosage regimen solely on the basis of a potential impairment in hepatic elimination and/or distribution is somewhat questionable. Sensitivity to the possibility of an enhanced response and cautious empiricism would still appear to be the most appropriate approach; with greater caution being used when active or severe dysfunction is present. Plasma level monitoring along with plasma binding determinations may be helpful, but there is no substitute for dosage adjustment according to the patient's response. Wherever possible, the use of drugs which are eliminated by extra-hepatic routes or known to be unaffected by liver disease is preferred. Furthermore, it is better to administer a drug which is pharmacologically effective *per se*, rather one which is dependent upon hepatic activation. Finally, drugs which are known to produce hepatotoxicity should be avoided unless absolutely essential; when they are necessary, then aggressive monitoring of liver function and clinical response would be mandatory.

Such platitudes may be frustrating to the practitioner, especially if an overestimation of the utility of clinical pharmacokinetics is presented. Hopefully, future studies will permit a less empiric approach, but until that time cautious individualization of therapy based primarily upon clinical responsiveness is the best possible guideline.

# REFERENCES

1. Wilkinson GR and Schenker S: Drug disposition and liver disease. Drug Metab Rev 1975; 4:139—175.
2. Hoyumpa AM, Branch RA and Schenker S: The disposition and effects of sedatives and analgesics in liver disease. Ann Rev Med 1978; 29:205—218.
3. Roberts RK, Desmond PV and Schenker S: Drug prescribing in hepatobiliary disease. Drugs 1979; 17:198—212.
4. Bond WS: Clinical relevance of the effect of hepatic disease on drug disposition. Amer J Hosp Pharm 1978; 35:406—414.
5. Klotz U: Influence of liver disease on the elimination of drugs. Europ J Drug Metab Pharmacokin 1976; 1:129–140.
6. Kappas A, Alvares AP, Anderson KE, Garland WA, Pantuck EJ and Conney AH: The regulation of human drug metabolism by nutritional factors, in Ullrich V et al eds *Microsomes and Drug Oxidation,* Pergamon Press, New York 1977; 703–708.
7. Wilkinson GR and Shand DG: A physiological approach to hepatic drug clearance. Clin Pharmacol Therap 1975; 18:377–390.
8. Rowland M, Benet LZ and Graham GG: Clearance concepts in pharmacokinetics. J Pharmacokin Biopharm 1973; 1:123–136.
9. Pang KS and Rowland M: Hepatic clearance of drugs. I. Theoretical considerations of a "well-stirred" model and a "parallel tube" model. Influence of hepatic blood flow, plasma and blood cell binding and the hepatocellular enzymatic activity on hepatic drug clearance. J Pharmacokin Biopharm 1977; 5:625–653.
10. Gillette JR: Factors affecting drug metabolism. Ann NY Acad Sci 1971; 179:43–66.
11. Gibaldi M and McNamara PJ: Apparent volumes of distribution and drug binding to plasma proteins and tissues. Europ J Clin Pharmacol 1978; 13:373–378.
12. Rane A, Wilkinson GR and Shand DG: Prediction of hepatic extraction ratio from *in vitro* measurements of intrinsic clearance. J Pharmacol Exptl Therap 1977; 200:420–424.
13. Schoene B, Fleischman RA, Remmer H and van Oldershausen HF: Determination of drug metabolizing enzymes in needle biopsies of human liver. Europ J Clin Pharmacol 1972; 4:65–73.
14. Doshi J, Luisada-Opper A and Leevy CM: Microsomal pentobarbital hydroxylase activity in acute viral hepatitis. Proc Soc Exp Biol Med 1972; 140:492–495.
15. Gold MS and Ziegler DM: Dimethylaniline N-oxidase and aminopyrine N-demethylase activities of human liver tissue. Xenobiotica 1973; 3:179–189.
16. Sotaniemi EA, Ahlqvist J, Pelkonen RO, Pirttiaho H and Luoma PV: Histological changes in liver and indices of drug metabolism in alcoholics. Europ J Clin Pharmacol 1977; 11:295–303.
17. Pirttiaho HI, Sotaniemi EA, Ahlqvist J, Pitkänen U and Pelkonen RO: Liver size and indices of drug metabolism in alcoholics. Europ J Clin Pharmacol 1978; 13:61–67.
18. Branch RA, Herbert CM and Read AE: Determinants of serum antipyrine half-lives in patients with liver disease. Gut 1973; 14:569–573.
19. Andreasen PB, Ranek L, Statland BE and Tygstrup N: Clearance of antipyrine-dependence of quantitative liver function. Europ J Clin Invest 1974; 4:129–134.
20. Andreasen PB and Ranek L: Liver failure and drug metabolism. Scand J Gastroenterol 1975; 10:293–297.
21. Branch RA, James JA and Read AE: The clearance of antipyrine and indocyanine green in normal subjects and in patients with chronic liver disease. Clin Pharmacol Therap 1976; 20:81–89.
22. Andreasen PB and Griesen G: Phenazone metabolism in patients with liver disease. Europ J Clin Invest 1976; 6:21–26.

23. Griesen G and Andreasen PB: Two compartment analysis of plasma elimination of phenazone in normals and in patients with cirrhosis of the liver. Acta Pharmacol Toxicol 1976; 38:49–58.

24. Harman AW, Penhall RK, Priestly BG, Frewin DB, Phillips PJ and Clarkson AR: Salivary antipyrine kinetics in hepatic and renal disease and in patients on anticonvulsant therapy. Aust N Z J Med 1977; 7:385–390.

25. Magione A, Imhoff TE, Lee RV, Shum LY and Jusko WJ: Pharmacokinetics of theophylline in hepatic disease. Chest 1978; 73:616–622.

26. Piafsky KM, Sitar DS, Rangno RE and Ogilvie RI: Theophylline disposition in patients with hepatic cirrhosis. New Engl J Med 1977; 296:1495–1497.

27. Mawer GE, Miller NE and Turnberg LA: Metabolism of amylobarbitone in patients with chronic liver disease. Br J Pharmac 1972; 44:549–560.

28. Klotz U, Avant GR, Hoyumpa A, Schenker S and Wilkinson GR: The effects of age and liver disease on the disposition and elimination of diazepam in adult man. J Clin Invest 1975; 55:347–359.

29. Andreasen PB, Hendel J, Griesen G and Hvidberg EF: Pharmacokinetics of diazepam in disordered liver function. Europ J Clin Pharmacol 1976; 10:115–120.

30. Roberts RK, Wilkinson GR, Branch RA and Schenker S: Effects of age and parenchymal liver disease on the disposition and elimination of chlordiazepoxide (Librium). Gastroenterol 1978; 75:479–485.

31. Klotz U, Antonin KH, Brügel H and Bieck PR: Disposition of diazepam and its major metabolite desmethyldiazepam in patients with liver disease. Clin Pharmacol Therap 1977; 21:430–436.

32. Kraus JW, Desmond PV, Marshall JP, Johnson RF, Schenker S and Wilkinson GR: Effects of aging and liver disease on disposition of lorazepam. Clin Pharmacol Therap 1978; 24:411–419.

33. Shull HJ, Wilkinson GR, Johnson R and Schenker S: Normal disposition of oxazepam in acute viral hepatitis and cirrhosis. Ann Intern Med 1976; 84:420–425.

34. Blaschke TF, Meffin PJ, Melmon KL and Rowland M: Influence of acute viral hepatitis on phenytoin kinetics and protein binding. Clin Pharmacol Therap 1975; 17:685–691.

35. Williams RL, Blaschke TF, Meffin PJ, Melmon KL and Rowland M: Influence of acute viral hepatitis on disposition and plasma binding of tolbutamide. Clin Pharmacol Therap 1977; 21:301–309.

36. Williams RL, Schary WL, Blaschke TF, Meffin PJ, Melmon KL and Rowland M: Influence of acute viral hepatitis on disposition and pharmacologic effect of warfarin. Clin Pharmacol Therap 1976; 20:90–97.

37. Burnett DA, Barak AJ, Tuma DJ and Sorrell MF: Altered elimination of antipyrine in patients with acute viral hepatitis. Gut 1976; 17:341–344.

38. Breimer DD, Zilly W and Richter E: Pharmacokinetics of hexobarbital in acute hepatitis and after apparent recovery. Clin Pharmacol Therap 1975; 18:433–440.

39. Alvin J, McHorse T, Hoyumpa A, Bush MT and Schenker S: The effect of liver disease in man on the disposition of phenobarbital. J Pharmacol Exptl Therap 1975; 192:224–235.

40. Adjepon-Yamoah KK, Nimmo J and Prescott LF: Gross impairment of hepatic drug metabolism in a patient with chronic liver disease. Br Med J 1974; 4:387–388.

41. Thiessen JJ, Sellers EM, Denbeigh P and Dolman L: Plasma protein binding of diazepam and tolbutamide in chronic alcoholics. J Clin Pharmacol 1976; 16:345–351.

42. Olsen GD, Bennett WM and Porter GA: Morphine and phenytoin binding to plasma proteins in renal and hepatic failure. Clin Pharmacol Therap 1975; 17:677–684.

43. Affrime M and Reidenberg MM: The protein binding of some drugs in plasma from patients with alcoholic liver disease. Europ J Clin Pharmacol 1975; 8:267–269.
44. Wallace S and Brodie MJ: Decreased drug binding in serum from patients with chronic hepatic disease. Europ J Clin Pharmacol 1976; 9:429–432.
45. Ghoneim MM and Pandya H: Plasma protein binding of thiopental in patients with impaired renal or hepatic function. Anesthesiol 1975; 42:545–549.
46. Blaschke TF: Protein binding and kinetics of drugs in liver disease. Clin Pharmacokin 1977; 2:32–44.
47. Rowland M, Blaschke TF, Meffin PJ and Williams RL: Pharmacokinetics in disease states modifying hepatic and metabolic function, in Benet LZ, ed *Effect of Disease States on Drug Pharmacokinetics*. Amer Pharm Assoc Washington DC 1976; 53–75.
48. Thomson PD, Melmon KL, Richardson JA, Cohn K, Steinbrunn W, Cudihee R and Rowland M: Lidocaine pharmacokinetics in advanced heart failure, liver disease and renal failure in humans. Ann Intern Med 1973; 78:499–508.
49. Duvaldestin P, Agoston S, Henzel D, Kerstein UW and Desmonts JM: Pancuronium pharmacokinetics in patients with liver cirrhosis. Br J Anaesth 1978; 50:1131–1136.
50. Klotz U, Rapp T and Müller WA: Disposition of valproic acid in patients with liver disease. Europ J Clin Pharmacol 1978; 13:55–60.
51. Branch RA, James J and Read AE: A study of factors influencing drug disposition in chronic liver disease using the model drug (+) propranolol. Brit J Clin Pharmacol 1976; 3:243–249.
52. Wood AJJ, Kornhauser DM, Wilkinson GR, Shand DG and Branch RA: The influence of cirrhosis on steady-state blood concentrations of unbound propranolol after oral administration. Clin Pharmacokin 1978; 3:478–487.
53. Williams RL, Blaschke TF, Meffin PJ, Melmon KL and Rowland M: Influence of viral hepatitis on the disposition of two compounds with high hepatic clearance: lidocaine and indocyanine green. Clin Pharmacol Therap 1976; 20:290–299.
54. Azzollini F, Gazzaniga A, Lodola E and Natangelo R: Elimination of chloramphenicol and thiamphenicol in subjects with cirrhosis of the liver. Internat J Clin Pharmacol 1972; 6:130–134.
55. Lewis GP and Jusko WJ: Pharmacokinetics of ampicillin in cirrhosis. Clin Pharmacol Therap 1975; 18:475–484.
56. Branch RA and Shand DG: Propranolol disposition in chronic liver disease: A physiological approach. Clin Pharmacokin 1976; 1:264–279.
57. Preisig R, Rankin JG, Sweeting J and Bradley S: Hepatic hemodynamics during viral hepatitis in man. Circulation 1966; 34:188–197.
58. Lundbergh P: Hepatic circulation during and after infectious hepatitis. Scand J Infect Dis 1974; 6:297–304.
59. Lundbergh P and Strandell T: Changes in hepatic circulation at rest, during and after exercise in young males with infectious hepatitis compared with controls. Acta Med Scand 1974; 196:315–325.
60. Pessayre D, Lebrec D, Descatoire V, Peignoux M and Benhamou JP: Mechanism for reduced drug clearance in patients with cirrhosis. Gastroenterol 1978; 74:566–571.
61. Groszmann R, Kotelanski B, Cohn JN and Khatri IM: Quantitation of portasystemic shunting from the splenic and mesenteric beds in alcoholic liver disease. Amer J Med 1972; 53:715–722.
62. Lebrec D, Kotelanski B and Cohn JN: Splanchnic hemodynamics in cirrhotic patients with esophageal varices and gastrointestinal bleeding. Gastroenterol 1976; 70:1108–1111.

63. Huet PM, Marleau D, Lavoie P and Viallet A: Extraction of [125]I-albumin microaggregates from portal blood; an index of functional blood supply in cirrhotics. Gastroenterol 1976; 70:74—81.

64. Gross G and Perrier CV: Intra-hepatic portasystemic shunting in cirrhotic patients. New Engl J Med 1975; 293:1046.

65. Groszmann RJ, Kravetz D and Paryzow: Arteriovenous (AV) shunting in the liver. Gastroenterol 1976; 70: 983.

66. Gugler R, Lain P and Azarnoff DL: Effect of portacaval shunt on the disposition of drugs with and without first-pass effect. J Pharmacol Exptl Therap 1975; 195:416–423.

67. Neal EA, Meffin PJ, Gregory PB and Blaschke TF: Enhanced bioavailability and decreased clearance of analgesics in patients with cirrhosis. Gastroenterol. 1979; 77:96–102.

68. Pentikäinen PJ, Neuvonen PJ, Tarpila S and Syvälahti E: Effect of cirrhosis of the liver on the pharmacokinetics of chlormethiazole. Brit J Med 1978; 2:861–863.

69. Elfström J and Lindgren S: Disappearance of phenazone from plasma in patients with obstructive jaundice. Europ J Clin Pharmacol 1974; 7:467—471.

70. Hepner GW and Vesell ES: Normal antipyrine metabolism in patients with cholesterol cholelithiasis. Evidence that the disease is not due to generalized hepatic microsomal dysfunction. Amer J Digest Dis 1975; 20:9–12.

71. Hepner GW and Vesell ES: Aminopyrine metabolism in the presence of hyperbilirubinemia due to cholestasis or hepatocellular disease. Combined use of laboratory tests to study disease-induced alterations in drug disposition. Clin Pharmacol Therap 1977; 21:620–626.

72. Carulli N, Manenti F, de Leon P, Ferrari A, Salvioli G and Gallo M: Alteration of drug metabolism during cholestasis in man. Europ J Clin Invest 1975; 5:455–462.

73. Sotaniemi EA, Pelkonen RO, Mokka RE, Huttunen R and Viljakainen E: Impairment of drug metabolism in patients with liver cancer. Europ J Clin Invest 1977; 7:269–274.

74. Hepner GW, Uhlin SR, Lipton A, Harvey HA and Rohrer V: Abnormal aminopyrine metabolism in patients with hepatic neoplasm; detection by breath test. J Amer Med Assoc 1976; 236:1587–1590.

75. Warren RD and Bender RA: Drug interactions with antineoplastic agents. Cancer Treat Reports 1977; 61:1231–1241.

76. Prescott LF, Roscoe P, Wright N and Brown SS: Plasma paracetamol half-life and hepatic necrosis in patients with paracetamol overdosage. Lancet 1971; 1:519–522.

77. Forrest JAH, Roscoe P, Prescott LF and Stevenson IH: Abnormal drug metabolism after barbiturate and paracetamol overdose. Brit Med J 1974; 4:499–502.

78. Prescott LF and Stevenson IH: Liver disease and drug metabolism in man. in Proceedings, Fifth International Congress in Pharmacology, San Francisco 1972; 3:182–190.

79. Branch RA, Morgan MH, James J and Read AE: Intravenous administration of diazepam in patients with chronic liver disease. Gut 1976; 17:975–983.

80. Laidlaw J, Read AE and Sherlock S: Morphine tolerance in hepatic cirrhosis. Gastroenterol 1961; 40:389–396.

81. Read AE, Laidlaw J and McCarthy CF: Effects of chlorpromazine in patients with hepatic disease. Brit Med J 1969; 3:497–499.

82. Maxwell JD, Carrella M, Parkes JD, Williams R, Mould GP and Curry SH: Plasma disappearance and cerebral effects of chlorpromazine in cirrhosis. Clin Sci 1972; 43:143–151.

83. Morgan MH and Read AE: Antidepressants and liver disease. Gut 1972; 13:697–701.

84. Fessel JM and Conn HO: An analysis of the causes and prevention of hepatic coma. Gastroenterol 1972; 62:191.

85. Hepner GW, Vesell ES, Lipton A, Harvey HA, Wilkinson GR and Schenker S: Disposition of aminopyrine, antipyrine, diazepam and indocyanine green in patients with liver disease or on anticonvulsant therapy: Diazepam breath test and correlations in drug elimination. J Lab Clin Med 1977; 90:440–456.

86. Forrest JAH, Finlayson NDC, Adjepon-Yamoah KK and Prescott LF: Antipyrine, paracetamol and lignocaine elimination in chronic liver disease. Brit Med J 1977; 1:1384–1387.

87. Hepner GW and Vesell ES: Quantitative assessment of hepatic function by breath analysis after oral administration of [14]C-aminopyrine. Ann Intern Med 1975; 83:632–638.

88. Bircher J, Küpfer A, Gilakov I and Preisig R: Aminopyrine demethylation measured by breath analysis in cirrhosis. Clin Pharmacol Therap 1976; 20:484–492.

89. Galizzi J, Long RG, Billing BH and Sherlock S: Assessment of the [14]C-aminopyrine breath test in liver disease. Gut 1978; 19:40–45.

90. Noordhoek J, Dees J, Savenije-Chapel EM and Wilson JHP: Output of [14]CO$_2$ in breath after oral administration of [14]C-methyl aminopyrine in hepatitis, cirrhosis and hepatic bilharziasis: Its relationship to aminopyrine pharmacokinetics. Europ J Clin Pharmacol 1978; 13:223–229.

91. Shreeve WW, Shoop JD, Ott DG and McInteer BB: Test for alcoholic cirrhosis by conversion of [14]C- or [13]C- galactose to expired CO$_2$. Gastroenterol 1976; 71:98–101.

92. Breen KJ, Desmond PV, Bury R, Calder I and Mashford ML: A [14]C-phenacetin breath test in the assessment of hepatic function. Gastroenterol 1977; 72:1033.

# 5

# Neonatal Pharmacokinetics

Donald M. Hilligoss, Pharm.D.

## Introduction

The study of neonatal pharmacokinetics has undergone considerable growth in the last ten years. Continual advancement in neonatal and perinatal medicine has created both the need and the opportunity to study drug disposition in these patients who may weigh less than one kilogram.

There are numerous potential benefits to be obtained from the study of neonatal pharmacokinetics. First, and foremost, is the elimination of the "therapeutic orphan" concept. While this term was originally applied to the entire pediatric patient population, it most appropriately describes the neonatal patient of today. It is unfortunate that in this patient population with higher mortality and morbidity rates than any other age group, the least amount of basic information is available.

The primary reason for this knowledge deficit is the inability to directly extrapolate data gathered from older patients to neonates. The potential hazards of this approach have been well documented. For example, utilization of chloramphenicol at doses well tolerated in older pediatric patients causes the potentially lethal "gray baby" syndrome in patients less than two or three months of age. Consequently, it is necessary to study neonates as a separate and unique entity, taking nothing for granted that has been learned from the study of older patients.

While extrapolation of data gathered from older patients to the neonate may be of questionable value, it is gradually becoming apparent that "reverse extrapolation" of information gained from neonatal studies may be of use in other patient groups. Despite the widespread use of aminoglycoside antibiotics in intensive care nurseries, there are no well documented instances of neonatal nephrotoxicity. Adult aminoglycoside nephrotoxicity has been reported to occur in 3 to 25% of patients, dependent on the criteria used to define toxicity. Recent studies have utilized a two-compartment pharmacokinetic model to characterize the disposition of aminoglycosides in adults (1,2). In this model the presence of aminoglycosides persisting in serum long after the cessation of therapy is represented as the washout from a peripheral tissue compartment. Adult aminoglycoside nephrotoxicity has been shown to be related to both peripheral compartment accumulation and the individual patient's inherent sensitivity to these tissue concentrations (3). Neonatal peripheral tissue compartment parameters for gentamicin closely resemble those of adults with similar renal function (4). This dissimilarity in incidence of adult versus neonatal nephrotoxicity in conjunction with the similarity of the two groups tissue compartment parameters implies different inherent tissue sensitivity and may lead to a better understanding of renal toxicity in older patients. A systematic comparison of other aspects of aminoglycoside disposition in adults versus neonates could potentially yield useful information.

Because of their relationship to other patients, neonates may serve as a baseline "control group" in the study of developmental factors that cause changes in drug disposition. Multiple variant analysis of factors such as congestive heart failure, use of potential enzyme inducers, obesity, smoking history and previous use of methylxanthines can account for approximately one-half of the variability of theophylline disposition in adults (5). The remaining variability is thought to be related to genetic predisposition, unknown environmental factors and normal interpatient differences. The variance in neonatal theophylline clearances has recently been shown to be significantly lower than that of older children or adults (6). It now appears that much of the previously unaccounted for variance in adults may appear within the first year of life. Detailed study of patients within this particular age group may eventually yield information that will be of predictive value in adults. Without a neonatal baseline, it would be difficult to isolate the particular time in life when this variance first appears, or to differentiate it from genetic variation present at birth.

While neonatal studies have been, and will continue to be, of considerable direct and indirect value, they do pose certain unique problems. All patients share the common potential for normal interpatient variation and pathological alteration of pharmacokinetic parameters. In addition, neonates are physiologically more dynamic than any other patient population. Changing gastric acidity and motility, hepatic and renal function, protein binding, and total body water and its distribution may all result in alterations in patterns of drug disposition.

No other patient group exhibits these rapid rates of change as a part of their normal physiology. To compensate for increasing clearances, a two week old infant requires a 50% higher dose of aminoglycoside antibiotics on a milligram per kilogram basis than a one week old patient. One of the most interesting areas of pharmacokinetic research today is the characterization and quantification of the many changes occurring within the neonatal period.

Due to limitations in sample volume, neonatal studies often require more sophisticated assay technology than is initially developed for investigations in older patients. Microassay techniques are necessary in studies that require multiple serum samples to be obtained over a short period of time from patients who may have a total blood volume of less than 100 ml. Despite these difficulties, this area of research will continue to grow rapidly, since the potentials for benefit, both directly to the neonatal patient population and indirectly to older patients, certainly outweigh the special problems encountered.

## Absorption

The two primary determinants of gastrointestinal absorption are pH-dependent passive diffusion and gastric emptying time. These two physiological processes differ markedly in neonates when compared to values found in older children and adults. Both processes also undergo considerable change during the neonatal period due to continuous maturation.

Gastric contents at birth are relatively neutral, with pH ranges of 6 to 8. This neutrality is primarily due to the presence of residual, alkaline amniotic fluid which is regularly swallowed during intrauterine life. Products of cesarean-section deliveries that have not undergone gastric compression from the birth process have significantly higher gastric pH's due to the presence of even greater amounts of amniotic fluid (7). Gastric pH rapidly falls to ranges of 1 to 3 within the first 24 hours of life due to passage of alkaline amniotic fluid and production of gastric acid. Mean acid output after betazole stimulation has been quantified in mEq/10 kg/hr as 0.15 at birth, 0.31 at one month of age and 1.22 in three month old babies (8). In comparison, adults and young children produce approximately 2 mEq/10 kg/hr of gastric acid in response to histamine stimulation. This reduced output of titratable acidity in the newborn is related to both volume and concentration of gastric secretions. Frequent feedings with milk or formula may also increase gastric pH.

Studies utilizing feedings that contain radioisotopes have measured gastric emptying times in newborns at one to ten weeks of age. Gastric radioactivity declined in a monoexponential pattern, with a "half-life" (mean ± SD) of 87 ± 29 minutes (9). Comparable studies in normal adults have revealed similar exponential patterns, but with a mean "half-life" of 65 minutes.

These differences in gastric pH and emptying time could have varied and opposite effects on gastrointestinal absorption. Acid labile drugs could have greater bioavailability in neonates secondary to the reduction in gastric acidity. Drugs that are only partially absorbed in adults may undergo more extensive absorption in neonates due to prolonged contact time with gastrointestinal mucosa secondary to the slower gastric emptying times and sporadic peristalsis. Weakly acidic compounds would exist in their ionized form to a greater extent in the neonatal gastric environment, which should cause a reduction in pH-dependent passive diffusion. The opposite would be true for basic drugs. Due to these varied effects, it is apparent that oral bioavailability must be assessed separately for each drug used in neonates. It is impossible to accurately predict the net effect these variables could have on any particular compound.

Penicillin (10), ampicillin (11) and nafcillin (12) have been reported to achieve higher serum concentrations in newborns than in older children and adults after oral administration of similar dosages. These higher concentrations have been attributed to an enhanced bioavailability in newborns, secondary to reduced gastric acidity (13, 14, 15). There is little doubt that newborns do have significantly higher serum concentrations after an orally administered dose of these acid labile penicillins when compared to older children and adults. However, the serum concentration and $AUC_T$ resulting from an oral dose of a drug that confers upon the body the characteristics of a one-compartment model are affected not only by bioavailability but also by the apparent volume of distribution and elimination rate constant, i.e.,

$$AUC_T = \frac{FD}{VK} \qquad \text{(Eq. 1)}$$

where $AUC_T$ is the total area under the drug concentration in plasma versus time curve, F is fraction of the dose which is available, D is the dose, V is the apparent volume of distribution and K the elimination rate constant.

From this relationship, it is apparent that one may not attribute higher serum concentrations of penicillins in newborns entirely to increased bioavailability (F). Smaller elimination rate constants in neonates could easily account for the higher serum concentrations. To definitively quantitate bioavailability in newborns it is necessary to compare intravenous versus oral data obtained in the same neonates within a short period of time. Whether or not the absolute bioavailability of these penicillins differ significantly in newborns as compared to older patients is a matter requiring further investigation.

Phenobarbital has been used extensively in newborns as an anticonvulsant and for the treatment of hyperbilirubinemia. Both the rate and extent of oral absorption are less than that obtained following intramuscular administration to newborns (16). While definitive $AUC_T$'s or excretion data are not easily obtained in the clinical environment due to the extremely long half-life of phenobarbital in neonates, e.g., 59 to 182 hours, the available data indicate that phenobarbital may well be less bioavailable in newborns than the 70 to 90% reported in adults. Considering phenobarbital's pKa of 7.23, this could be the result of a reduction in pH-dependent passive diffusion due to elevated neonatal gastric pH.

There appears to be no appreciable difference between neonates and older patients in regards to gastrointestinal absorption of digoxin. All digoxin orally administered to neonates is in the pediatric elixir form, the most bioavailable of the oral dosage preparations. The bioavailability of orally administered digoxin pediatric elixir (Lanoxin®) in neonates has been estimated as 72 ± 13% (mean ± SD) following comparison of intravenous versus oral 8-hour AUC's (17). This is in close agreement with bioavailability estimates for the same preparation when given to adults (18).

One clinically significant occurrence of reduced neonatal drug absorption has been studied. Premature infants are born with low serum levels of vitamin E (d-alpha tocopherol) (19). These low stores of vitamin E, in conjunction with the use of formulas which contain greater amounts of polyunsaturated fatty acids than breast milk, will lead to the development of a vitamin E-dependent hemolytic anemia. Supplementation with fat-soluble d-alpha tocopherol results in little change in serum tocopherol concentrations or objective measures of RBC fragility. This lack of bioavailability may be attributed to premature neonates' impaired ability to synthesize bile salts and pancreatic enzymes (20). While the absorption of water soluble d-alpha tocopherol polyethylene glycol 1,000 succinate is generally greater in these newborns, some investigators have advocated the use of intramuscular vitamin E in order to avoid the unpredictable gastrointestinal absorption (21). Progressive improvement in the absorption of vitamin E is seen as the chronological equivalent of full term gestational age is approached (22).

In general, neonatal gastrointestinal absorption of drugs appears to be clinically adequate in most cases. Since bioavailability studies require a comparison of the preparation under investigation versus a standard (i.e., intravenous administration or an oral preparation of known bioavailability), extreme care must be taken in the design and interpretation of this kind of study in neonates. Rapidly changing patterns of metabolism and excretion can affect both serum concentration versus time profiles and excretion data. Frequent emesis after feedings and nasogastric suctioning prior to feedings for the prevention of gastric distention can also significantly alter data obtained in the intensive care nursery environment.

## Distribution

The pattern of distribution of a drug is determined by the physicochemical properties of the drug itself (i.e., partition coefficient and pKa), in conjunction with physiological factors unique to the individual patient. While the physiochemical properties of the drug are constant, variations in the physiological determinants (i.e., total body water and its distribution, amount of adipose tissue, amount of drug-binding proteins in serum, affinity of the protein for the drug, and presence of pathophysiological conditions and/or compounds that modify the drug-protein interaction), can significantly alter the specific pattern of distribution from one individual to another. Differences in neonatal drug distribution, as compared to older patients, are to be expected when one considers the dissimilarity between the physiological determinants of these two patient groups.

Total body water (TBW) of full term neonates has been estimated to be 78% of body weight. While this is considerably higher than the 60% estimates for adults, it is lower than the 94% and 85% determinations for fetuses and premature neonates, respectively (23). In general, TBW decreases rapidly during intrauterine life, followed by a more gradual decline throughout childhood.

Concurrent with the reduction of TBW during development is a changing pattern of distribution between the intracellular water (ICW) and extracellular water (ECW) compartments. Neonatal ICW comprises only 43% of TBW with the remaining 57% found in the ECW compartment. Adult ICW accounts for 68% of TBW with only 32% remaining as ECW. This shift of water into the intracellular compartment in conjunction with the decrease in TBW results in ECW accounting for 44% of neonatal body weight as compared to only 19% in adults. It is interesting to note the similarity of these data with the central compartment volumes of 0.48 L/kg and 0.20 L/kg recently reported for gentamicin in neonates and adults with decreased glomerular filtration rates (4). The proportion of body weight accounted for by ICW is more constant with 34% and 41% for neonates and adults, respectively.

Due to the low content of water in adipose tissue, an inverse relationship exists between TBW and amount of fat tissue in the body. The percentage of body weight accounted for by adipose tissue increases rapidly from approximately 0.5% at five months gestation to 12% at full term (24). Increasing presence of fatty breast tissue is actually one of the parameters that are assessed in estimating gestational age (25).

While the 12% fat of full term neonates is similar to that found in athletic individuals, it is substantially less than the fat of an average adult. Due to this reduction in body lipid content, one would anticipate smaller volumes of distribution in neonates for highly lipid soluble drugs if all other variables affecting distribution were equal. In accord with this, the neonatal volume of distribution for diazepam of 1.40 to 1.82 L/kg is smaller than adult values of 2.20 to 2.60 L/kg (13). This smaller volume of distribution is of even greater significance when the protein binding properties of diazepam are considered. The adult values of 94 to 98% bound are greater than the 84% bound reported for neonates (13). This reduction of percent bound to plasma protein should potentially increase diazepam's volume of distribution in neonates. Consequently, the total effect of the differences in body lipid content may be even greater than would be indicated by direct comparison of the volume of distribution values.

The reversible association of plasma proteins with drugs can be mathematically described by the law of mass action. In this relationship, both drug and protein concentration, together with the association constant, determine the specific amount of bound and unbound drug. Most frequently, neonatal data are reported as percent bound or unbound and compared to adult data. While this may be of some clinical value over a limited concentration range, it does not differentiate between changes due to amount of protein or different association constants.

Assuming all else to be equal, drug protein binding would be less in neonates due to the amount of plasma proteins available for drug-protein association. Adult serum usually contains (mean $\pm$ SD) 4.5 $\pm$ 0.4 gm/dl albumin and 7.2 $\pm$ 0.6 gm/dl total protein. Neonatal serum contains approximately 80% as much protein as that of an adult, or 3.7 $\pm$ 0.2 gm/dl albumin (26). The above example of reduced neonatal plasma protein binding of diazepam may be primarily due to lower protein concentrations. The association constant ($K = 4 \times 10^5$

$M^{-1}$ of diazepam to newborn serum has been reported as the same as adult serum (27).

Many drugs bind to a lesser degree with neonatal plasma proteins, irrespective of the quantitative effect of lower protein concentration. Ampicillin (9.5 − 11.9 μg/ml) is 19.3 to 24.2% bound to adult plasma protein. Neonatal plasma proteins bind only 7.6 to 12.1% of ampicillin over the same concentration range of drug (26). Adjustment for the quantitative effect of lower neonatal protein concentrations does not account for the observed degree of reduced binding. Either inherent differences in neonatal plasma proteins or the presence of an endogenous competitor (i.e., bilirubin, free fatty acids or lipids), reduces the affinity for ampicillin.

Of considerable concern to the clinician is the potential of drug competition with bilirubin for neonatal albumin sites. If a drug significantly displaces bilirubin from albumin, the threat of central nervous system damage secondary to kernicterus is increased. Cord serum albumin binds bilirubin ($K = 5.2 \times 10^7 M^{-1}$) with greater affinity than adult albumin ($K = 2.4 \times 10^7 M^{-1}$) (27). Since most drugs have an association constant of $10^4$ or $10^5$, a molar concentration of drug 100 to 1000 times greater than bilirubin would be necessary for displacement by direct competition. Unfortunately, drug-induced alterations in albumin structure may adversely affect bilirubin-albumin binding in neonates. Consequently, direct comparisons of association constants derived *in vitro* do not adequately assess the potential risk. The ability of sulfisoxazole to displace bilirubin from neonatal serum proteins and cause an increased mortality rate due to kernicterus has been well documented (28,29).

With the association constant of neonatal albumin for bilirubin usually being 100 to 1000 times greater than albumin-drug constants, the potential for bilirubin-induced drug displacement exists. Phenytoin binding to albumin has been studied in adults, normal infants and hyperbilirubinemic infants (30). Unbound phenytoin (mean ± SD) in normal infants was 10.6 ± 1.4% as compared with adult values of 7.4 ± 0.7%. This difference can be primarily accounted for by lower neonatal albumin concentrations (3.5 ± 0.4 gm/dl). Hyperbilirubinemic infants (total bilirubin 4.5 ± 0.5 mg/dl, conjugated bilirubin ≤ 1.9 mg/dl) had unbound phenytoin values of 15.5 ± 3.3% with albumin concentrations of 3.8 ± 0.5 gm/dl. At a bilirubin concentration of 20 mg/dl, the unbound fraction of phenytoin was twice as high as in plasma from normal infants. Consequently, one must consider the potential for larger volumes of distribution in hyperbilirubinemic infants for those drugs that may be displaced by bilirubin.

In general, the majority of differences in physiological determinants of drug distribution between adults and neonates tends to favor larger volumes of distribution in the neonates. Larger amounts of TBW with a greater proportion in the ECW compartment, a reduced quantity of plasma proteins available for drug protein binding, a potential for reduction in the affinity of the available protein for drug binding and the presence of compounds, e.g., bilirubin, free fatty acids or lipids, that could further impair drug-protein binding would all tend to increase apparent volumes of distribution for many drugs in neonates. Conversely, the smaller proportion of body lipid tissue in neonates could reduce the apparent volume of distribution for highly lipid soluble drugs, e.g., diazepam, if all other factors were constant. Obviously, these are only general guidelines.

**Metabolism**

For many drugs, the major factor which limits the duration of pharmacological activity is metabolism to less active metabolites. Lipid solubility is necessary for membrane permeability and the attainment of adequate concentrations at specific sites of action to elicit the desired response. Metabolism, usually occurring within the hepatic endoplasmic reticulum, reduces lipid solubility and increases water solubility. Excretion may then occur directly or after conjugation to further enhance water solubility.

The hepatic microsomal enzyme systems can catalyze many drug metabolizing reactions. The major components of these distinct systems are NADPH, NADPH-cytochrome C reductase, cytochrome P-450 and NADPH-cytochrome P-450 reductase. The involved reactions are mainly oxidative, but also include some reductive reactions and numerous conjugations with sulfate, glucuronic acid, acetyl groups or amino acids such as glutathione, cysteine or glycine. A drug often undergoes two or three such reactions before elimination from the body.

Hepatic metabolic activity is generally lower in neonates than it is in adults. During intrauterine existence, a neonate's hepatic enzyme systems are challenged by a comparatively small number of substrates requiring detoxification. The maternal hepatic system is primarily responsible for insuring that potentially toxic substances do not accumulate to harmful concentrations. It is not surprising that these relatively untried biochemical systems are not operating at peak efficiency shortly after birth.

Characterization of the rate of development of neonatal hepatic metabolic activity can be most useful. Toxicity such as the "gray baby" syndrome of the late 1950's can be prevented. Dosages may be increased as metabolic capacity increases, in order to maintain therapeutic serum concentrations. Unfortunately, specific hepatic metabolic processes mature at different rates, making overall characterization particularly difficult when a drug undergoes more than one reaction.

The ability to form conjugates with sulfate appears to be relatively mature at birth (31). While the overall elimination of acetaminophen is slower in 2 to 3-day-old newborns than adults, with average half-lives of 3.5 hours and 2.0 hours respectively, the rate of formation of sulfate conjugates is actually greater in newborns (32). Rate constants for neonatal sulfate conjugation are (M ± SD) $0.099 \pm 0.030$ hr$^{-1}$, compared to adult ranges reported previously as 0.059 to 0.093 hr$^{-1}$. The higher rate of sulfate conjugation may be partially compensatory for the lower neonatal capacity for glucuronide conjugation also reported.

The disposition of para-aminobenzoic acid (PABA) has been studied in premature infants (2 to 6-days-old), full term infants (3 to 5-days-old), infants (5 to 8-weeks-old) and children (8 to 11-years-old) (33). Overall disposition of PABA was slowest in the newborns (t½ = 1.6 hours). Urinary metabolite studies revealed that the primary deficiency in neonatal metabolism of PABA was an inability to conjugate PABA with glycine to form para-amino hippuric acid (PAH). The percentage of total dose excreted as PAH increased from a mean of 12.5% for premature newborns to 26.8% for full term neonates. The 8-week-old infant excreted 39.4% of the PABA dose as PAH, which was still lower than the 45 to 50% found in older children and adults. The older children excreted only 16% of the total dose of PABA as acetyl-PABA. This acetylated metabolite accounted for 35% of the dose in the infants (5 to 8-weeks-old) but only 25% in neonates (2 to 6-days-old). Therefore, it appears that the ability to acetylate PABA increases for at least the first four to six weeks of life. This rate of increase is relatively greater than the maturing glycine conjugation process, which has not reached adult levels at eight weeks of age.

The ability of neonates to conjugate drugs with glucuronic acid has been studied due to the role this process plays in the etiology of neonatal hyperbilirubinemia. *In vitro* studies measuring the extent of 4-methyl-umbelliferone glucuronidation have shown little increase in conjugating ability for the first ten days of life (34). Thereafter, the rate increases to approach adult values at 50 to 70 days of age. In accord with this, "physiological jaundice" in newborns usually ceases to be a problem after the first few days of life (35).

Conjugation with amino acids (i.e., glutathione, cysteine and glycine) may be one of the latest metabolic pathways to mature. In the previously cited study of para-aminobenzoic acid metabolism, the ability to conjugate PABA with glycine was apparently approaching, but still less than, adult values at eight weeks of age. Amino acid conjugation has been noted to mature at approximately three months of age (31). Converse to this, other investigators have concluded that the prolonged retention of sulfobromophthalein (BSP) in 2 to 9-day-old neonates was due to insufficient transport or secretion into the bile rather than impaired conjugating ability (36).

In general, the enzymatic conjugation reactions of the liver may follow a sequence of maturation similar to development in phylogenesis (31). As noted above, sulfation and acetylation capacities appear to be well developed at birth or mature rapidly within the first weeks of life. Conjugation with glucuronic and amino acids matures later. Primitive animals detoxify by sulfation and acetylation while other reactions are representative of more differentiated species.

Caution must be exercised in drawing conclusions concerning a general class of enzymatic reactions from data obtained after a study of only one substrate. Subtle differences in substrate structure could significantly alter metabolic rates. Secondly, age-related changes in enzymes could make them more available to a particular substrate at different points of maturity. Changes in Michaelis-Menten constants have indicated that hepatic bilirubin transferase exists in different forms during development of animals (37).

Previous exposure to a drug, either intrauterine or postnatal, can affect neonatal metabolism. Since hepatic enzyme systems are already present even in intrauterine life, but have lower specific activities than adults, neonates may be more susceptible to enzyme induction than older patients. The half-life of diazepam has been reported to be 40 to 100 hours in premature newborns and 20 to 45 hours in full term newborns (13). Both patient groups have significantly longer half-lives than the 15 to 25 hour range reported for adults. This slower disposition rate is due to reduced demethylation and hydroxylation in the newborn. Intrauterine or postnatal exposure to phenobarbital significantly reduces the apparent plasma half-life of diazepam in newborns to 12 to 16 hours. This reduction in half-life is concurrent with a preferential increase in hydroxylating activities, resulting in an increase in urinary hydroxylated derivatives.

The disposition of phenobarbital in neonates has been characterized with an exponentially increasing elimination rate term (38). Half-lives decreased from 115 hours after one week to 67 hours after four weeks of therapy. The increases in clearance were thought to be related to changing turnover rates of neonatal drug metabolizing enzymes in response to substrate exposure.

Characterization of neonates' ability to metabolize drugs will continue to be a challenging area. Varying maturation rates for different metabolic pathways, potential enzyme-substrate specificity changes during development, and the effect of intrauterine or postnatal exposure to drugs which may increase their own rate of metabolism as well as that of other substances will make this a rewarding area both clinically and academically.

## Renal Excretion

The final elimination of a drug is often via renal excretion. Hydrophilic compounds are excreted directly, while lipophilic compounds are generally excreted after metabolism to more hydrophilic metabolites. Consequently, pathophysiological changes in renal function can significantly alter the excretion rate of drugs and/or their metabolites.

Net renal excretion of drugs is influenced by one or more of three mechanisms: glomerular filtration, tubular secretion, tubular reabsorption. These three processes undergo considerable development and maturation during early postnatal life. Comparison of initial and developmental renal function with that of adults allows one to anticipate that significant differences will be found between urinary excretion patterns in neonates and older patients.

Glomerular filtration rate (GFR) is considerably less in neonates than it is in adults. Inulin clearance, considered to be an indicator of GFR, has been measured in infants 12 hours to 25 days of age (39). Clearances in the first four days of life average (M $\pm$ SD) 10.8 $\pm$ 1.0 ml/min/m$^2$ and increase about twofold by 14 days of age. This inital rapid rate of increase does not continue, since adult values of 70 ml/min/m$^2$ are not reached until approximately one year of age (40). This increase in GFR during the first year of life is mediated via changes in arterial blood pressure, renal vascular resistance, permeability of the glomerulus and the surface area available for filtration.

Tubular secretion is an active, energy-requiring process for transport of drug from the peritubular capillary into the lumen of the renal tubule. Active tubular secretion would therefore increase net renal excretion of a drug in addition to GFR. Two independent transport systems exist, one for weak organic acids and one for weak organic bases. Drugs that are excreted by tubular secretion may also competitively inhibit the renal tubular excretion of endogenous metabolic products.

Compounds undergoing tubular secretion are limited by a transport maximum (Tm). Measurement of the Tm for various substances has

TABLE 1. PHYSIOLOGIC DIFFERENCES BETWEEN NEONATES AND ADULTS THAT COULD ALTER PHARMACOKINETIC PARAMETERS

|  | Neonate | Adult | Reference |
|---|---|---|---|
| Gastric Acid Output (mEq/10kg/hr) | 0.15 | 2 | 8 |
| Gastric Emptying Time (Minutes) | 87 | 65 | 9 |
| Total Body Water (Percent of Body Weight) | 78 | 60 | 23 |
| Extracellular Water (Percent of Body Weight) | 44 | 19 | 23 |
| Intracellular Water (Percent of Body Weight) | 34 | 41 | 23 |
| Adipose Tissue (Percent of Body Weight) | 12 | 12–25 | 24 |
| Serum Albumin (gm/dl) | 3.7 | 4.5 | 26 |
| Glomerular Filtration Rate (ml/min/m$^2$) | 11 | 70 | 39 |

been utilized as an index of tubular function. The Tm of para-aminohippuric acid (PAH) has been found to be lower in newborns than adults (41). However, direct comparison of Tm values for neonates and adults may be an inadequate assessment of tubular function alone, since Tm has been found to be directly related to GFR, (i.e., as GFR increases, Tm increases) (42). In view of the rapidly increasing GFR shortly after birth, it is difficult to quantitate the specific effect that immature tubular secretion might have on the renal excretion of drugs.

Tubular reabsorption of most drugs is a passive, concentration-dependent process by which a compound passes from the renal tubular lumen, through peritubular cells and back into the systemic vascular system via capillaries. As such, this process would reduce net renal excretion. The rate of reabsorption is pH-dependent, since a compound must exist in its nonionized, lipophilic form in order to pass through the lipid peritubular cell membranes.

It is highly probable that adults and neonates have different rates of tubular reabsorption. The lower neonatal GFR and the potentially higher systemic concentrations of parent compounds secondary to slower metabolism could both reduce the concentration gradient necessary for reabsorption. Differences in urinary pH between neonates and adults would alter the proportion of nonionized drug available for reabsorption, depending on whether the compound was weakly basic or acidic (43,44).

In general, renal excretion of drugs is less in early postnatal life compared to older patients. Much of this initial reduction in renal excretion may be accounted for by the significantly lower neonatal GFR. Also, the rapid maturation in GFR in the first weeks of life would be expected to result in similar increases in drug clearance for those agents that are eliminated primarily by renal filtration. In accord with this, standard references recommend that the doses of ampicillin, carbenicillin, penicillin G, ticarcillin, methicillin, gentamicin, kanamycin, and tobramycin should all be significantly increased after the first week of life (45,46).

## Surface Area Versus Body Weight Perspective

Age-related variability in the ratio of body surface area to body weight has been recognized for some time (47). The average 70 kg adult of 1.73 m$^2$ has a ratio of approximately 40 kg/m$^2$. A typical intensive care nursery patient weighing 1.5 kg with a surface area of 0.13 m$^2$ has a ratio of 11.5 kg/m$^2$. This three-fold difference in the weight/surface area ratio between neonates and adults is due to their relative sizes.

Surface area (SA) increases as the square of linear measure while volume, or weight, increases as the cube of linear measure. Consequently, as linear measure increases, or growth occurs, there is a greater increase in weight relative to surface area. This relationship of surface area to weight can be approximated by the simple exponential function,

$$SA = K \cdot W^{2/3} \qquad \text{(Eq. 2)}$$

where SA is surface area in square meters, W is weight in kilograms, and K is a constant (48).

When dosing patients within a relatively small size range, there is no particular advantage to calculations based on surface area as compared to weight. As with any exponential function, the relationship of surface area to weight is relatively constant and linear over a short segment of the independent variable. However, when an attempt is made to standardize dosage recommendations over a broad range of age and size, the surface area perspective is considerably less variable.

We recently reported the two-compartment pharmacokinetic parameters for gentamicin in neonates given 5.0 ± 0.3 mg/kg/day and adults given 2.4 ± 0.8 mg/kg/day (4). The two patient groups were considered to be well matched for renal function on the basis of body surface area. While the dosing regimens were significantly (p<0.001) different based on body weight, this difference was no longer apparent when dosages were adjusted for surface area, with neonates receiving 65 ± 9 mg/m$^2$/day and adults 84 ± 32 mg/m$^2$/day. Adjustment of the pharmacokinetic parameters for surface area also resulted in similarities between neonates and adults that were not apparent from a body weight perspective.

The characterization of the developmental changes in neonatal pharmacokinetics is of particular value. Clinicians may then antici-pate what adjustment in dosing regimens may be appropriate as ther-apy is initiated in or continues through various maturational stages. In a study of the effect of maturational factors on neonatal theophyl-line clearances, the correlation coefficients were consistently higher when clearances were adjusted for surface area rather than weight (6). Rubner's surface area law of 1883 states that in resting, warm-blooded animals, heat loss is the same per square meter of body surface area over a 24-hour period regardless of the size of the animal. Close correlation also exists between surface area and a large number of physiologic processes, such as cardiac output, blood volume, glomer-ular filtration, body organ growth and development, and minute vol-ume of respiration (47). This suggests that pharmacokinetic parame-ters adjusted for surface area may be more appropriate than the usual weight adjustment when studying factors that may affect neonatal drug disposition. This is particularly important for comparisons with older children and adults. Since the ratio of body weight to surface area varies directly with linear dimensions, relationships are dra-matically altered when comparisons are made with other patient groups on a surface area rather than weight basis.

No simple, accurate method exists for obtaining a direct determi-nation of surface area in man. Most estimates are obtained from formulas relating area to height and weight or from tables and nom-ograms derived from these formulas (49). The formula of Dubois and Dubois and nomograms derived from it are probably the most common methods for estimating surface area (50). The formula,

$$A = W^{0.425} \cdot H^{0.725} \cdot 71.84 \qquad \text{(Eq. 3)}$$

where A equals surface area in square centimeters, W equals weight in kilograms and H equals height in centimeters, has been meticu-lously validated in adults. Unfortunately, only one child was included in the subjects whose measured surface areas were used to derive the formula. This method has subsequently been shown to underestimate surface area as values fall below 0.7 $m^2$, with the disparity being greatest in the neonate (7.96%) (51). Consequently, the formula of Haycock, et al,

$$SA = W^{0.5378} \cdot H^{0.3964} \cdot 0.024265 \qquad \text{(Eq. 4)}$$

where SA equals surface area in square meters, W is weight in kilo-grams, and H is height in centimeters, appears to presently be the most appropriate method of estimating neonatal body surface area (51).

## Potential Sources of Error in Neonatal Pharmacokinetic Studies

While all pharmacokinetic studies conducted in the clinical environment are susceptible to a certain degree of error, the uniqueness of the neonate has induced an unacceptable amount of variability in data from some studies. Fortunately, if an investigator is aware of these potential sources of error, they are often avoidable.

After an initial, brief period of weight loss, most patients in an intensive care nursery begin to gain weight at the rate of 1–2% a day if an adequate caloric intake can be maintained. Virtually all drugs are ordered initially as a specific amount in relation to body weight (i.e., theophylline 2 mg/kg every twelve hours would result in a 1.5 kg patient being administered 3 mg of theophylline every twelve hours). It is not customary to routinely increase the administered dose as the patient's weight increases. Consequently, twenty days after therapy is initiated this theoretical patient may now weigh 2.0 kg but still be receiving 3 mg of theophylline or 1.5 mg/kg every twelve hours. Pharmacokinetic calculations based on measured serum concentrations at this time and the original dose of 2 mg/kg would result in clearance and apparent volume of distribution values that would be 33% artifactually high. Failure to account for the neonate's ability to gain weight faster than any other type of patient has resulted in the introduction of significant error in some studies.

Studies utilizing oral medications in neonates are prone to potential sources of error not encountered when parenteral preparations are used. A common problem among premature neonates is their inability to tolerate oral feedings. In attempting to overcome this problem, intensive care nursery patients are often fed small volumes frequently (i.e., every 2 to 3 hours). Since regurgitation is very common after feeding, these patients with prolonged gastric emptying times may lose significant amounts of oral medications via this route. The practice of nasogastric suctioning prior to feedings to prevent gastric distention is another potential source of loss for medication given orally. While this source of error is difficult to quantitatively correct, an investigator can check for its presence by assaying emesis and nasogastric suctioning fluid for drug content.

Many neonatal studies have utilized pharmacokinetic equations that require the attainment of steady-state conditions in order to be valid. Neonates have significantly longer half-lives for virtually all drugs and, consequently, require constant rate dosing for a much longer period to attain steady-state. We have found that patients who were assumed to be at steady-state often were not. When using steady-state equations, data variability has been significantly reduced by eliminating from analysis any patient whose consecutive "trough" concentrations varied by more than the expected assay variability. Close inspection of nursing notes invariably revealed the reason for lack of a steady-state condition (i.e., a missed or held dose). While these points may seem so basic as to preclude their enumeration, we have found them useful in reducing data variability.

## Conclusion

The field of neonatal pharmacokinetics is presently at its introductory stages and will continue to be so for quite some time. In this respect it shares a common characteristic with the patients about which it is concerned. Further study in this area will be of considerable direct benefit to neonatal patients. Of even greater potential value will be the indirect benefit to older patient groups. As we study what we were at our common beginning it is very likely we will better understand ourselves as we are today.

## REFERENCES

1. Schentag JJ, Jusko WJ, Vance JW, Cumbo TJ, Abrutyn E, DeLattre M, Gerbracht LM: Gentamicin disposition and tissue accumulation on multiple dosing. J Pharmacokinetics Biopharm 1977; 5:559–577.
2. Schentag JJ, Lasezkay G, Cumbo TJ, Plaut ME, Jusko WJ: Accumulation pharmacokinetics of tobramycin. Antimicrob Agents and Chemother 1978; 13:649–656.
3. Schentag JJ, Plaut ME, Cerra FB, Wels PB, Walczak P, Buckley RJ: Aminoglycoside nephrotoxicity in critically ill surgical patients. J Surg Res 1979; 26:270–279.
4. Haughey DB, Hilligoss DM, Grassi A, Schentag JJ: Two-compartment gentamicin pharmacokinetics in premature neonates: a comparison to adults with decreased glomerular filtration rates. J Pediatr 1980; 96:325–330.
5. Jusko WJ, Gardner MJ, Mangione A, Schentag JJ, Koup JR, Vance JW: Surveillance of factors affecting theophylline clearances: Age, tobacco, marihuana, cirrhosis, congestive heart failure, obesity, oral contraceptive, benzodiazepines, barbiturates and ethanol. J Pharm Sci 1979 (in press).
6. Hilligoss DM, Jusko WJ, Koup JR, Giacoia G: Factors affecting theophylline pharmacokinetics in premature infants with apnea. Devel Pharmacol Ther 1980; 1:6–15.
7. Avery GB, Randolph JG, Weaver T: Gastric acidity in the first day of life. Pediatrics 1966; 37:1005–1007.
8. Agunod M, Yamaguchi N, Lopez R, Luhby AL, Glass GBJ: Correlative study of hydrochloric acid, pepsin, and intrinsic factor secretion in newborns and infants. Am J Dig Dis 1969; 14:400–414.
9. Signer E, Fridrich R: Gastric emptying in newborns and young infants. Acta Paediatr Scand 1975; 64:525–530.

10. Huang NN, High RN: Comparison of serum levels following the administration of oral and parenteral preparations of penicillin to infants and children of various age groups. J Pediatr 1953; 42:657–668.
11. Silverio J, Poole JW: Serum concentrations of ampicillin in newborn infants after oral administration. Pediatrics 1973; 51:578–580.
12. O'Connor WJ, Warren GH, Edrada LS, Mandala PS, Roseman SB: Serum concentrations of sodium nafcillin in infants during the perinatal period. Antimicrob Agts Chemother 1965; 220–222.
13. Morselli PL: Clinical pharmacokinetics in neonates. Clin Pharmacokin 1976; 1:81–98.
14. Mirkin BL: Drug disposition and therapy in the developing human being. Pediatr Ann 1976; September: 542–557.
15. Cupit GC, Serrano VA: Concepts in pediatric pharmacotherapy I. J Cont Educ Pharmacy 1979; Jan-March: 55–67.
16. Jalling B: Plasma concentrations of phenobarbital in the treatment of seizures in newborns. Acta Paediatr Scand 1975; 64:514–524.
17. Wettrel G, Anderson KE: Absorption of digoxin in infants. Eur J Clin Pharmacol 1975; 9:49–55.
18. Greenblatt DJ, Duhme DW, Koch-Weser J, Smith TW: Evaluation of digoxin bioavailability in single-dose studies. N Engl J Med 1973; 289:651–654.
19. Gross S, Melhorn DK: Vitamin E-dependent anemia in the premature infant. I. Effects of large doses of medicinal iron. J Pediatr 1971; 79:569–580.
20. Gross S, Melhorn DK: Vitamin E-dependent anemia in the premature infant. III. Comparative hemoglobin, vitamin E and erythrocyte phospholipid responses following absorption of either water-soluble or fat-soluble d-alpha tocopheryl. J Pediatr 1974; 85:753–759.
21. Graeber JE, Williams ML, Oski FA: The use of intramuscular vitamin E in the premature infant. J Pediatr 1977; 90:282–284.
22. Melhorn DK, Gross S: Vitamin E-dependent anemia in the premature infant. II. Relationships between gestational age and absorption of vitamin E. J Pediatr 1971; 79:581–588.
23. Friis-Hansen B: Body water compartments in children: changes during growth and related changes in body composition. Pediatrics 1961; 28:169–181.
24. Widdowson EM, Spray CM: Chemical development in utero. Arch Dis Child 1951; 26:205–214.
25. Dubowitz L, Dubowitz V, Goldberg C: Clinical assessment of gestational age in the newborn infant. J Pediatr 1970; 77:1–10.
26. Ehrnebo M, Agurell S, Jalling B, Boreus LO: Age differences in drug binding by plasma proteins: studies on human foetuses, neonates and adults. Eur J Clin Pharmacol 1971; 3:189–193.
27. Krasner K, Yaffe SJ: Drug-protein binding in the neonate. In: Morselli PL, Garrattini S, Sereni F, eds. *Basic Therapeutic Aspects of Perinatal Pharmacology.* New York: Raven Press 1975:356–366.
28. Silverman WA, Anderson DH, Blanc WA, Crozier DN: A difference in mortality rate and incidence of kernicterus among premature infants allotted to two prophylactic antibacterial regimens. Pediatrics 1956; 18:614–624.
29. Odell GB: The dissociation of bilirubin from albumin and its clinical implications. J Pediatr 1959; 55:268–279.
30. Rane A, Lunde PKM, Jalling B, Yaffe SJ, Sjoqvist F: Plasma protein binding of diphenylhydantoin in normal and hyperbilirubinemic infants. J Pediatr 1971; 78:877–882.

31. Gladtke E, Heimann G: The rate of development of elimination functions in kidney and liver of young infants. In: Morselli PL, Garattini S, Sereni F, eds. *Basic and Therapeutic Aspects of Perinatal Pharmacology.* New York: Raven Press, 1975; 393–403.

32. Levy G, Khanna NN, Soda DM, Tsuzuki O, Stern L: Pharmacokinetics of acetaminophen in the human neonate: formation of acetaminophen glucuronide and sulfate in relation to plasma bilirubin concentration and d-glucaric acid excretion. Pediatrics 1975; 55:818–825.

33. Vest MF, Salzberg R: Conjugation reactions in the newborn infant: the metabolism of para-aminobenzoic acid. Arch Dis Child 1965; 40:97–105.

34. Di Toro R, Lupi L, Ansanelli V: Glucuronation of the liver in premature babies. Nature 1968; 219:265–267.

35. Odell GB, Poland RL, Ostrea EM: Neonatal hyperbilirubinemia. In: Klaus MH, Fanaroff AA, eds. *Care of the High-Risk Neonate.* Philadelphia: W.B. Saunders, 1973; 183–204.

36. Vest MF: Conjugation of sulfobromphthalein in newborn infants and children. J Clin Invest 1962; 41:1013–1020.

37. Krasner J: Postnatal developmental changes in hepatic bilirubin UDP-glucuronyl transferase. Biol Neonate 1973; 23:381.

38. Pitlick W, Painter M, Pippenger C: Phenobarbital pharmacokinetics in neonates. Clin Pharmacol Ther 1978; 23:346–350.

39. Guignard JP, Torrado A, Da Cunha O, Gautier E: Glomerular filtration rate in the first three weeks of life. J Pediatr 1975; 87:268–272.

40. Loggie JMH, Kleinman LI, Van Maanen EF: Renal function and diuretic therapy in infants and children. Part I. J Pediatr 1975; 86:485–496.

41. Tudvad F, Vesterdal J: The maximal tubular transfer of glucose and para-aminohippurate in premature infants. Acta Paediatr Scand 1953; 42:337.

42. Deetjen P, Sonnenberg H: Der tubulare transport von PAH. Microperfusions versuche um einzelnephron der rattenniere in situ. Pfluegers Arch 1965; 285:35.

43. Braunlich H: Kidney development: drug elimination mechanisms. In: Morselli PL, ed. *Drug Disposition During Development.* New York: Spectrum Publications, 1977; 89–100.

44. Edelmann CM Jr, Spitzer A: The maturing kidney: a modern view of well-balanced infants with imbalanced nephrons. J Pediatr 1969; 75:509–519

45. Schuberth KC, Fitelli BJ, ed. *The Harriet Lane Handbook.* Chicago: Year Book Medical Publishers, Inc., 1978:115–159.

46. Nelson JD. *Pocketbook of Pediatric Antimicrobial Therapy.* Philadelphia: JB Lippincott Company, 1975.

47. Shirkey HC. Dosage (posology). In: Shirkey HC, ed. *Pediatric Therapy,* 5th edition. St. Louis: The C.V. Mosby Company, 1975; 19–33.

48. Meeh K: Oberflachenmessungen des menschlichen Korpers. Z Biol 1879; 15:425–458.

49. Gehan EA, George SL: Estimation of human body surface area from height and weight. Cancer Chemother Rep 1970; 54:225–235.

50. Dubois D, Dubois EF: A formula to estimate the approximate surface area if height and weight be known. Arch Intern Med 1916; 17:863–871.

51. Haycock GB, Chir B, Schwartz GJ, Wisotsky DH: Geometric method for measuring body surface area: A height-weight formula validated in infants, children, and adults. J Pediatr 1978; 93:62–66.

# 6

# Theophylline

Leslie Hendeles, Pharm.D.
Miles Weinberger, M.D.
George Johnson, Ph.D.

## INTRODUCTION/BACKGROUND

For nearly six decades, theophylline has been prescribed as a bronchodilator, cardiotonic, diuretic, and respiratory stimulant. During this time, however, its use has also been associated with reports of serious toxicity. Recent definition of its pharmacodynamics and pharmacokinetics and the availability of clinically useful drug assays have improved both the safety and efficacy of this drug for acute bronchodilator therapy, treatment of apneic spells in the premature neonate and as a major prophylactic agent in the management of chronic asthmatic symptoms. Specifically, benefit and risk of adverse effects have been demonstrated to relate directly to serum concentration, which is itself a function not only of the dose but also the elimination characteristics of the drug in the individual patient. With the development of new formulations of oral preparations that allow controlled delivery into the gut, theophylline has evolved as a highly effective and very convenient means for maintaining around the clock stabilization of the hyperreactive airways that characterize asthma. It also has been of value in the treatment of Cheyne-Stokes respirations and as an adjunct in the treatment of acute pulmonary edema.

Chemically, theophylline is a dimethylated xanthine similar in structure to caffeine and theobromine which are commonly found in coffee, tea, cola beverages, and chocolate (Figure 1). Dyphylline is the only other xanthine marketed in the United States as a bronchodilator. It is a 7-dihydroxypropyl derivative of theophylline (Figure 2). *In vitro,* the dose response relationship for dyphylline suggests a degree of potency only one tenth that of theophylline (Figure 3). In a clinical study, 1,000 mg of dyphylline demonstrated only one half the bronchodilator effect of a 400 mg dose of theophylline (1). Smaller doses

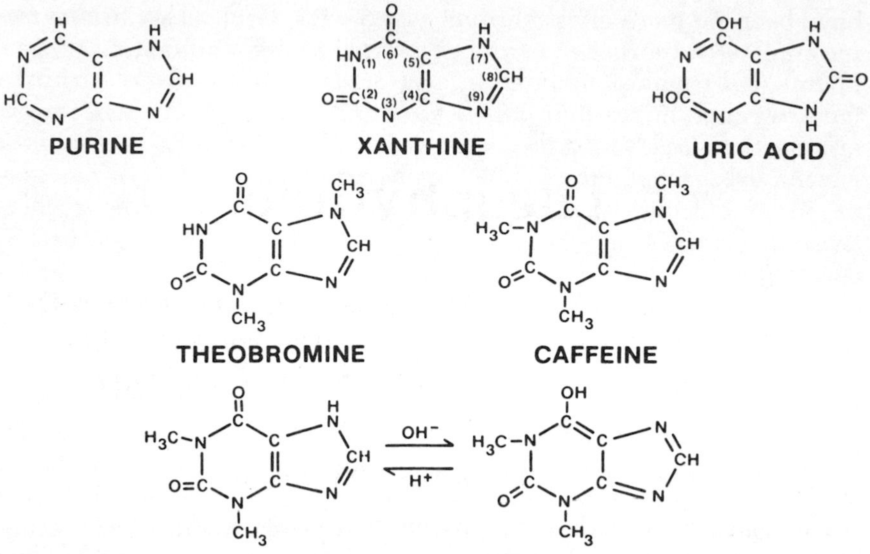

FIGURE 1. Chemical structure of endogenous and dietary xanthines including theophylline (tautomeric shift illustrated).

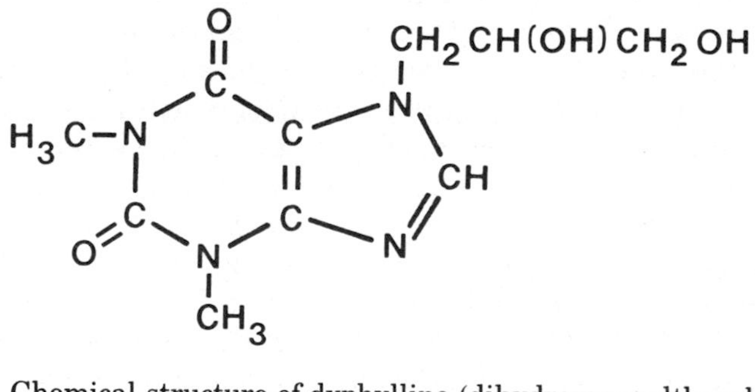

FIGURE 2. Chemical structure of dyphylline (dihydroxpropyltheophylline).

96

have been no more effective than placebo (2). Oral formulations are incompletely absorbed (3,4) and exceedingly rapid elimination (t½ = 2 hours) (3–5) makes maintenance of serum concentration within a narrow range impossible unless the drug is given every four hours around the clock. Outside the United States other "untheophylline" xanthine bronchodilators have been marketed (proxyphylline, acephylline), but offer the same disadvantages (4,6). As a consequence, these derivatives have no role in the contemporary management of asthma.

In contrast to the above stable derivatives, theophylline salts readily dissociate, and at physiologic pH exist only as mixtures with the various bases (ethylenediamine, calcium salicylate, sodium glycinate, and choline). While at high pH a salt may be formed as a result of a tautomeric shift in a hydrogen ion (Figure 1), theophylline is a weak base at physiologic pH and incapable of the implied union. Therefore, there is no rationale for most of the formulations that include added substances with claims of increased solubility or absorption.

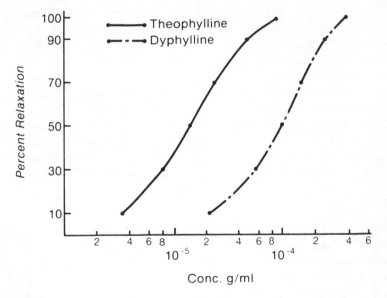

FIGURE 3. *In vitro* dose response relationships for theophylline and dyphylline using human tracheal strips. Dyphylline required 10 times the concentration (one log) of theophylline to produce 50% relaxation (adapted from Svedmyr[6]).

## Absorption

Theophylline is rapidly, consistently and completely absorbed from liquids and plain tablets (Figure 4). Neither the presence of alcohol in solution nor micronized crystals in tablet formulations speeds up absorption to a clinically important degree (7,8). Absorption of theophylline from formulations that decrease the rate of dissolution in the stomach is delayed or slowed. Enteric-coated tablets (9) and some slow-release formulations are erratically and incompletely absorbed (10–13). However, bioavailable slow-release products offer therapeutic advantages for children and other fast metabolizers of theophylline. In these patients, fluctuations in serum concentration between doses of rapidly absorbed products are excessive, even with unrealistically short dosing intervals (Figure 5). Slow-release formulations allow longer dosing intervals with less variation in serum concentrations (14,15).

Absorption from rectal solutions appears to be equivalent to oral theophylline (16,17), but rectal suppositories have repeatedly been associated with slow and erratic absorption (9,16,18). Since oral theophylline is rapidly and completely absorbed (19), the only indication for a rectal solution is the inability of the patient to take oral medication, e.g., in the presence of vomiting from causes other than theophylline toxicity or when fasting before surgery. There is *no* indication for rectal suppositories.

Parenteral theophylline must be given intravenously. The maximal solubility of theophylline in water at a physiologic pH (about 2 mg/ml) is such that precipitation of theophylline will occur in the tissue when the 20 mg/ml intravenous preparation (pH greater than 9.5) is injected intramuscularly. As a consequence, this route of administration is painful and absorption from the site of injection is delayed (9).

## Distribution

Following either intravenous administration or absorption from the gastrointestinal tract, theophylline distributes rapidly into peripheral tissues other than fat. The overall apparent volume of distribution at steady state averages 0.45 L/kg with a range of 0.3 to 0.7 L/kg (20,21) in all ages except neonates, where the weight-adjusted volume of distribution is slightly larger (22). Factors that affect the clearance of theophylline do not, in general, affect the volume of distribution.

Since only 60% of the drug in serum is bound to protein, small changes in the degree of binding do not have a significant effect upon the concentration of free theophylline. In premature neonates (22), and in the presence of acidemia (23), protein binding is reduced.

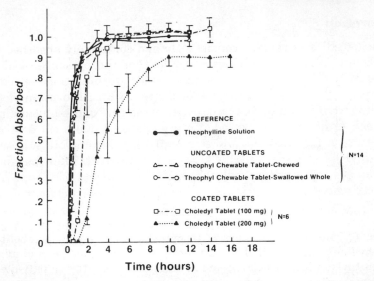

FIGURE 4. Absorption of a theophylline solution, uncoated, and coated tablets. When chewed, the chewable tablet was not significantly different in rate of absorption from the solution and was absorbed slower only during the first half-hour when swallowed whole. Absorption of the coated tablets was delayed.[10] (Reproduced by permission of the New England Journal of Medicine.)

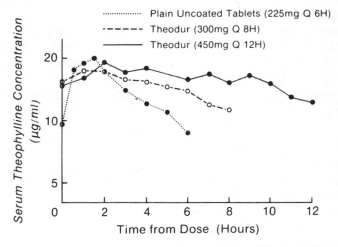

FIGURE 5. Serum concentrations in a 12-year-old boy, who rapidly metabolized theophylline, during a typical dosing interval while receiving plain uncoated tablets every six hours and Theodur at eight and twelve hour intervals. The large fluctuation in serum concentrations during the six hourly regimen was reduced by the slow-release formulation which also permitted an interval between doses that was compatible with a normal life style.[15]

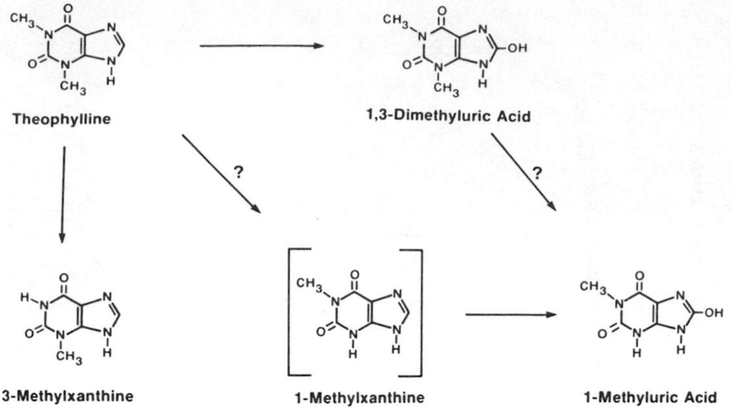

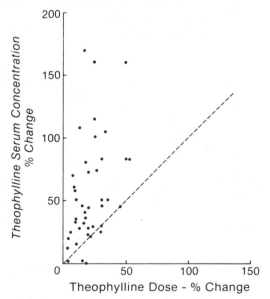

FIGURE 6.   Metabolic pathways of theophylline. The major metabolite for theophylline is the dimethylated uric acid. A variable fraction is eliminated as 3-methylxanthine which appears in decreased quantities in patients who are slow metabolizers. It is not known whether the 1-methyluric acid results directly from demethylation of the dimethyluric acid or oxidation of an intermediate compound, 1-methylxanthine (adapted from Jenne et al[28]).

FIGURE 7.   Relationship between changes in serum concentration and change in dose among 42 patients who had at least two serum concentration measurements at different doses of the same product (from 200 charts reviewed). In 30 of these children, the percent change in serum concentration was 50% greater than the percent change in dose ($\Delta\%$ concentration $\div$ $\Delta\%$ dose $\geq 1.5$). Thus dose dependent kinetics occurred in at least 15% of the 200 children examined.[35]

Therefore the concentration of free drug is greater. Since the assay procedures measure total bound and unbound drug, higher serum concentrations should probably be avoided in these patients.

Theophylline does not appear to concentrate in any tissue and thus any binding that may occur appears to be readily reversible. The rate of distribution into and out of peripheral compartments is rapid. Although it enters the cerebral spinal fluid, neither the rate of equilibration with blood nor the serum to spinal fluid concentration ratio have been defined. Theophylline crosses the placenta and produces a serum concentration in neonatal cord blood equal to the maternal serum concentration (24). The concentration of theophylline in breast milk (25) and saliva (26) is less than in serum. Over 95% of the theophylline found in saliva is unbound (free) drug.

## Metabolism

Theophylline is metabolized in the liver to relatively inactive metabolites via multiple parallel pathways by both first-order and capacity-limited kinetic processes. Less than 10% of the drug is excreted in the urine unchanged (27,28). The remainder is metabolized, apparently in the liver, to uric acid derivatives by oxidation in the 8 position, and to 3-methylxanthine by 1-demethylation (Figure 6). In the neonate, theophylline is metabolized in part to caffeine (29-31). Conversely, theophylline is a minor metabolite of caffeine, even in adults (32). The proportion of theophylline eliminated as 3-methylxanthine is lower in patients who are slower metabolizers (28). It also appears that the enzyme involved in the metabolism of theophylline to 3-methylxanthine is present in sufficiently limited quantities that capacity-limited kinetics occur in the presence of dietary methylxanthines (33). This has been shown to have clinical relevance (34,35) in that changes in dosage frequently result in disproportionately large changes in serum concentration (Figure 7). Changes in theophylline clearance at different serum concentrations have been documented in both children (36) and adults (37).

## Elimination

In 1972, Jenne et al first described the relationship between interpatient variation in theophylline elimination rate, dosage requirements and serum concentration (34). A fixed dose of oral medication administered continuously to a group of asthmatic adults resulted in a wide range of serum concentrations. When dosage was adjusted to maintain serum concentrations within the 10 to 20 $\mu$g/ml range, requirements varied from 400 to 2000 mg/day. A similar variability in rate of elimination has been demonstrated among children where the

## TABLE 1  FACTORS ASSOCIATED WITH VARIATION IN THEOPHYLLINE ELIMINATION

| Factors | Age Mean ± S.D. (years) | No. of Patients | Clearance Mean ± S.D. (ml/min/kg) | Half-Life Mean ± S.D. (hours) | Authors | Reference |
|---|---|---|---|---|---|---|
| *AGE* | | | | | | |
| Premature Neonates with Apnea | 7.5 ± 4.4 days | 6 | 0.29 ± 0.1 | 30 ± 6.5 | Aranda et al, 1976 | 22 |
|  | 41 ± 12 days | 8 | 0.64 ± 0.3 | 20 ± 5.3 | Giacoia et al, 1976 | 105 |
| Infants under 6 mos. | 12 ± 4 weeks | 8 | Incomplete data | 14 ± 4 | Nassif et al, 1979 | 40 |
|  | 18 ± 2 weeks | 3 | 0.8 ± 0.1 | 6.9 ± 1 | Rosen et al, 1979 | 106 |
| 6 to 11 mos. | 34 ± 10 weeks | 4 | 2.0 ± 0.5 | 4.6 ± 1.2 | Rosen et al, 1979 | 106 |
|  | 34 ± 7 weeks | 5 | Incomplete data | 3.7 ± 1 | Simons and Simons, 1978 | 107 |
| Young children 1–4 years | 2.5 ± 0.9 | 10 | 1.7 ± 0.6 | 3.4 ± 1.1 | Loughnan et al, 1976 | 108 |
| Older children 4–12 years | 9.4 ± 3 | 17 | 1.5 ± 0.4 | Not measured* | Ginchansky and Weinberger, 1977 | 38 |
| 13–15 years | 14 ± 0.8 | 6 | 0.8 ± 0.2 | Not measured | Ginchansky and Weinberger, 1977 | 38 |
| 6–17 years | 10.7 ± 2.6 | 30 | 1.4 ± 0.6 | 3.7 ± 1.1 | Ellis et al, 1976 | 109 |
| Adults —otherwise healthy nonsmoking asthmatics | 31 ± 10 | 16 | 0.65 ± 0.19 | 8.7 ± 2.2 | Hendeles et al, 1978 | 21 |

| | | | | | | |
|---|---|---|---|---|---|---|
| —healthy non-smoking volunteers | 22–35[a] | 19 | 0.86 ± 0.35 | 8.1 ± 2.4 | Jusko et al, 1978 | 53 |
| —healthy non-smoking volunteers | 20–32 (25.5)[b] | 15 | 0.67 ± 0.13 | 8.2 ± 1.2 | Powell et al, 1977 | 52 |
| Elderly —nonsmokers with normal cardiac, liver and renal function | 67 ± 5.7 | 9 | 0.59 ± 0.07 | 7.4 ± 1.1 | Nielsen-Kudsk et al, 1978 | 110 |
| *ABNORMAL PHYSIOLOGY* Fever —associated with acute viral upper respiratory tract illness | 9–15[a] | 6 (During illness) | Not measured | 7.0 ± 3.0 | Chang et al, 1978 | 49 |
| | | (1 month later) | Not measured | 4.1 ± 2.4 | | |
| Cor pulmonale | 64[c] | 8 | 0.48 ± 0.2 | Not measured | Vicuna et al, 1979 | 45 |
| Acute pulmonary edema | 71 ± 10 | 9 | 0.33 (0.067–2.35)[d] | 19(3.1–82)[d] | Piafsky et al, 1977 | 43 |
| Hepatic cirrhosis | 52 ± 8.2 | 9 | 0.43 (0.13–3.3)[d] | 14.1(7.1–59.1)[d] | Piafsky et al, 1977 | 41 |
| | 56 ± 4 | 8 | 0.21 (0.1–0.6)[d] | 32(10.4–56)[d] | Mangione et al, 1978 | 42 |

103

TABLE 1   FACTORS ASSOCIATED WITH VARIATION IN THEOPHYLLINE ELIMINATION—CONT.

| Factors | Age Mean ± S.D. (years) | No. of Patients | Clearance Mean ± S.D. (ml/min/kg) | Half-Life Mean ± S.D. (hours) | Authors | Reference |
|---|---|---|---|---|---|---|
| *SMOKING HISTORY* | | | | | | |
| Marijuana alone | 20–25[a] | 7 | 1.2 ± 0.5 | 4.3 ± 1.2 | Jusko et al, 1978 | 53 |
| Marijuana and cigarettes | 19–27[a] | 7 | 1.5 ± 0.4 | 4.3 ± 1 | Jusko et al, 1978 | 53 |
| Cigarettes | 33[c] | 10 | Not measured | 4.1 ± 1 | Jenne et al 1975 | 50 |
| Cigarettes (heavy smokers) | 22–31(27)[b] | 7 | 1.05 ± 0.32 | 5.4 ± 1 | Powell et al, 1977 | 52 |
| Ex-cigarette smokers (for at least 2 years) | 22–39(28)[b] | 6 | 0.85 ± 0.2 | 6.4 ± 1 | Powell et al, 1977 | 52 |
| *CONCURRENT DRUGS* | | | | | | |
| Triacetyloleandomycin (TAO) | 39 ± 15 | 8 (Before) / 8 (After) | 0.70 ± 0.14 / 0.34 ± 0.05 | Not measured / Not measured | Weinberger et al, 1977 | 56 |
| Erythromycin base | 23 ± 2.2 | (Before) / (After) 6 | 0.82 ± 0.17 / 0.60 ± 0.11 | 6.7 ± 1.9 / 8.3 ± 1.8 | Wing et al, 1980 | 58 |
| Phenobarbital | 23–32(27)[b] | (Before) / (After 1 mo.) | 0.75 ± 0.35 / 1.0 ± 0.5 | Not measured / Not measured | Landay et al, 1978 | 55 |

## ABERRANT DIETS

| | | | | | | |
|---|---|---|---|---|---|---|
| Low carbohydrate—high protein | 22–29[a] | 6 (Before) | e | 8.1 ± 2.4 | Kappas et al, 1976 | 111 |
| | | (After 2 wks.) | | 5.2 ± 1 | | |
| Charcoal-broiled beef | 22–32[a] | 8 (Before) | e | 6.0 ± 1 | Kappas et al, 1978 | 112 |
| | | (After 7 days of Diet) | | 4.7 ± 0.4 | | |

[a] Age range. Individual ages were not reported.
[b] Age range and mean. Standard deviation was not reported.
[c] Mean age. Individual data not reported.
[d] Median and range. Mean and standard deviations were not meaningful because of large range of values.
[e] Calculation on weight basis not reported.

105

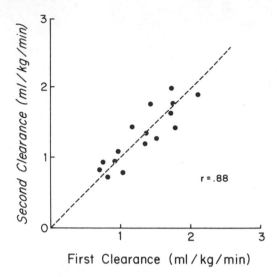

FIGURE 8.   Relationship of clearances among 16 children with chronic asthma performed at two different points in time (mean interval = 5 months). The dotted line represents identity. Clinically important variability of clearance over time was not observed in these patients.[38] (Reproduced by permission of the Journal of Pediatrics.)

dose required to achieve a therapeutic serum concentration ranged from 16 to 40 mg/kg/day in the age group under nine (38).

Since there is a two-fold variation in volume of distribution and an eight-fold difference in the elimination rate, the product of these two pharmacokinetic parameters, total body clearance, most accurately reflects the removal of theophylline from the body. Interpatient variability in clearance appears to be due primarily to differences in the rate of hepatic biotransformation, which changes with age, physiological abnormalities, aberrations in diet, and concurrent drug therapy (Table 1). Under normal circumstances, clearance (38), dosage requirements (39), and serum concentration (34), remain relatively constant over time (Figure 8).

Theophylline clearance and thus dosage requirements are markedly reduced in neonates (22), infants under 6 months of age (40), and in acutely ill adults with hepatic cirrhosis (41,42), cardiac decompensation (43,44), and cor pulmonale (45). Theophylline toxicity as a result of excessive serum concentrations has often been associated with the use of usual dosages in patients with liver failure or cardiac decompensation including cor pulmonale (46–48). In patients with these

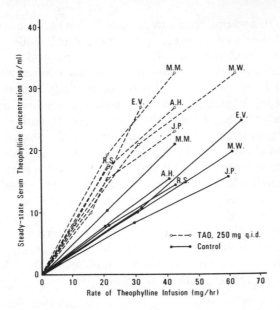

FIGURE 9. Steady-state serum theophylline concentration resulting from continuous intravenous infusion of theophylline at two different doses to six patients while receiving troleandomycin, 250 mg qid, and during the control period when no troleandomycin or related antibiotic was being taken. A 50% reduction in clearance is indicated by the relationship of serum theophylline concentration to dosage; as a result, steady-state serum concentrations were generally twice as high during the period when troleandomycin was being administered as compared with the control period.[56]

concurrent functional abnormalities, theophylline dosage regimens must be markedly reduced in order to prevent toxicity (Table 2).

Sustained fever associated with viral respiratory tract infections has also been associated with reduced theophylline elimination and thus might require a dosage reduction (49). In contrast, cigarette smokers (50–52) and those who use marijuana (53) have rapid average clearance rates which may increase dose requirements. The Boston Collaborative Drug Surveillance Program confirmed that clinical toxicity from theopylline was more frequent in nonsmokers than in cigarette smokers who presumably were receiving similar dosages (54). Anticonvulsant doses of phenobarbital administered for one month also increase theophylline clearance, but the magnitude of this effect is not likely to be clinically important (55).

Troleandomycin (triacetyloleandomycin), a macrolide antibiotic, decreases theopylline clearance 50% in patients with normal liver function (Figure 9) and can result in accumulation of toxic concentrations of theophylline when administered concurrently (56). Pfeiffer et al (57) concluded that the related macrolide antibiotic, erythromycin, had no significant effect on theophylline disposition when administered for 24 hours, although the mean half-life was prolonged and clearance reduced among the nine patients studied. However, the failure to detect a significant difference may have been due to the small study population and a lack of power in the statistical analysis. A subsequent study which examined the effect of seven days of erythromycin demonstrated that theophylline clearance was significantly reduced and half-life prolonged an average of 25% (58). Adverse effects associated with accumulation of excessive serum concentrations of theophylline in children have occurred 36 to 48 hours after concurrent erythromycin was initiated (59). Tetracycline increases the frequency of gastrointestinal side effects when taken concurrently with theophylline (54). Whether this is due to an effect on theophylline clearance or local irritation remains to be defined.

## CONCENTRATION versus RESPONSE and TOXICITY

### Efficacy

The bronchodilator effect of theophylline increases in proportion to the logarithm of the serum concentration (60,61) over a range of 5 to 20 µg/ml (Figure 10). The relationship between serum concentration and therapeutic response has also been demonstrated for exercise-induced bronchospasm, a nearly universal manifestation of asthma (62). Serum concentrations above 10 µg/ml inhibit bronchospasm in response to a standardized treadmill exercise stress, with an even more profound blocking effect occurring at serum concentrations above 15 µg/ml (Figure 11). The effect of theophylline in preventing exercise-induced bronchospasm is maintained with continuous dosing and development of tolerance does not appear to occur (63).

Prevention of the symptoms of chronic asthma is impressive when serum theophylline concentrations are maintained on a continuous around-the-clock basis at levels within the 10 to 20 µg/ml range (64–66). In a double-blind controlled evaluation, theophylline alone, in individualized doses resulting in serum theophylline concentrations between 10 and 20 µg/ml, was associated with much better control of asthma than either placebo or a fixed dose combination of theophylline plus ephedrine which resulted in serum concentrations under 10 µg/ml (Figure 12).

In premature infants, lower serum concentrations in the range of 5 to 10 μg/ml appear to be effective in decreasing the frequency of apneic episodes (67). However, the relationship between serum concentration and efficacy in this situation is unclear since theophylline in neonates is partially converted to caffeine which stimulates the CNS and is effective itself in suppressing apneic spells (68). Thus the relative efficacy and safety of theophylline in comparison with caffeine for this indication awaits further study.

While theophylline is effective in reducing Cheyne-Stokes respirations (69) and may be useful as an adjunct in the treatment of acute pulmonary edema, the relationship of serum concentration and efficacy for these two indications has not been defined.

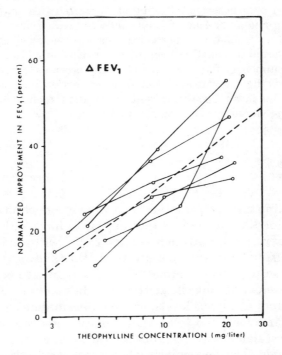

FIGURE 10. Relationship between serum theophylline concentration and the one second forced expiratory volume (FEV$_1$) among nine otherwise healthy asthmatic patients during the recovery phase of an acute exacerbation. Plots for each subject are presented individually (o—o—o), as well as the unweighted least squares regression for the whole group (———).[60] (Reproduced by permission of the New England Journal of Medicine.)

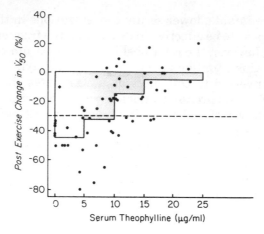

Figure 11. Relationship between serum theophylline concentration and exercise-induced bronchospasm following standardized treadmill exercise performed before and at 2, 4 and 6 hours following 7.5 mg/kg of theophylline administered to 12 children. The shaded area represents mean values for the intervals of serum theophylline concentration. The dotted line indicates 30% decrease in pulmonary function conventionally accepted as clinically important. The $V_{50}$ is the flow rate at 50% of vital capacity during a maximal forced expiration. The mean Spearman rank correlation coefficient was 0.71 (p <0.01).[62] (Reproduced by permission of Pediatrics.)

## Toxicity

Theophylline has the potential for a wide range of adverse effects. Minor caffeine-like side effects that appear to have little direct relationship to serum concentration are associated with rapidly acquired tolerance during long-term therapy. In contrast, adverse effects associated with serum concentrations above 20 μg/ml are persistent and include nausea, vomiting, headache, diarrhea, irritability, insomnia (34,70,71), and, at higher levels, seizures, brain damage, cardiac arrhythmias, and death (46,48). Cardiac arrest and death in adults has also been associated with the administration of a rapid intravenous bolus of theophylline, particularly when injected directly into a central venous catheter (72).

In one of these reports, 75% of patients with serum concentrations over 25 μg/ml experienced adverse effects that were uncommon between 15 and 25 μg/ml and not observed below 15 μg/ml (71).

Deaths have been most frequently reported among small children

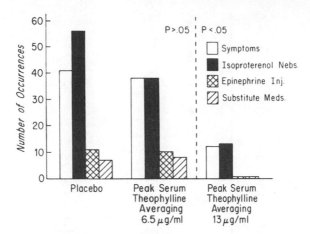

FIGURE 12. Frequency and severity of asthmatic symptoms during one week's treatment with each of placebo, an ephedrine-theophylline combination in conventional doses that resulted in serum theophylline concentrations averaging 6.5 µg/ml, and individualized theophylline doses that resulted in serum theophylline concentrations averaging 13 µg/ml. Asthmatic symptoms during each one-week period were promptly treated when necessary with inhaled isoproterenol; if symptoms were not promptly relieved, epinephrine was administered subcutaneously. If the patient was unresponsive to these measures, known drugs were substituted for the double-blind medications.[64] (Reproduced by permission of the Journal of Pediatrics.)

who have received multiple adult-size doses, commonly administered as suppositories (73). Irritability, vomiting of "coffee-ground" material, and seizures from which the patient did not regain consciousness characterized the common clinical course in such cases. Theophylline-induced seizures were observed in eight adult patients over a period of 10 months at a university hospital with a large and highly competent pulmonary disease service (Figure 13). Four of these patients died. These eight patients generally had considerably higher serum theophylline concentrations (mean 54 µg/ml) than patients with less severe adverse effects (mean 35 µg/ml). Serum concentrations in patients without adverse effects averaged under 20 µg/ml (48). Most noteworthy was the apparent *absence* of adverse effects in seven of the eight patients prior to the seizure. Clearly, minor symptoms of toxicity such as nausea and vomiting cannot be used as a dosing endpoint. If doses likely to attain therapeutic serum concentrations are to be used, *only serum theophylline measurements can reliably forewarn the physician of impending life-threatening toxicity.*

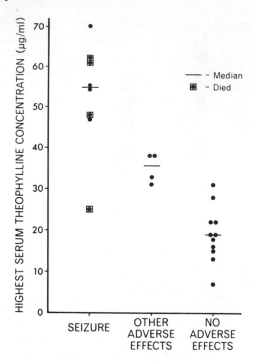

FIGURE 13.   Relationship between serum theophylline concentration and seizures. Eight patients with seizures were identified on the pulmonary service at the University of Colorado Hospitals over a 10 month period; four of them died. Other adverse effects including nausea, vomiting, and headache occurred without seizures at a significantly lower mean serum concentration.[48] (Reproduced by permission of Postgraduate Medicine.)

## CLINICAL APPLICATION OF PHARMACOKINETIC DATA

### Intravenous or Emergency Therapy

**Loading Dose.** The peak serum concentration attained from an initial or loading dose of a drug that has rapid absorption, such as theopylline, is related more to the apparent volume of distribution (V) of the drug (the apparent space into which the drug diffuses), than to its clearance from the body. Since the concentration of a drug (C) attained following rapid absorption is equal to the dose administered (D) divided by the apparent volume of distribution (V),

$$C = \frac{D}{V}$$

(Eq. 1)

each mg/kg (ideal body weight) of theophylline administered in a rapidly absorbed form (i.e., intravenous, oral solution, or rapid dissolution tablet) will result in an average 2 µg/ml increase in the serum theophylline concentration, assuming a volume of distribution of about 0.5 L/kg.

Thus, 7.5 mg/kg administered as a 30 minute intravenous infusion, by an oral or rectal solution, or an uncoated tablet with rapid dissolution characteristics, will result in a peak serum theopylline concentration of approximately 15 µg/ml when administered to patients who have not had recent theophylline-containing medication (19).

When theophylline has been taken prior to the clinical need for a loading dose, estimation of the serum concentration based on the history is unreliable (Figure 14), and an immediate measurement is indicated. The desired loading dose can then be determined as follows:

$$\text{Loading Dose} = (\text{Desired C} - \text{Measured C})\,(\text{V}) \qquad \text{(Eq. 2)}$$

where the mean volume of distribution is estimated to be 0.5 L/kg (74).

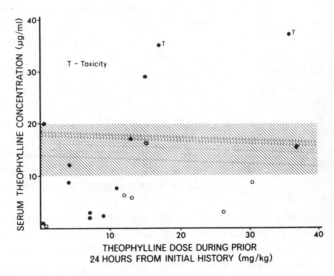

FIGURE 14. Relationship between the measured serum theophylline concentration and the history of theophylline dosage among 19 patients seen at the emergency room of the University of Colorado Medical Center. There was little correlation between history of prior theophylline intake and resultant serum concentrations.[47] (Reproduced by permission of the Journal of the American Medical Association.)

Excessively rapid intravenous administration will result in a transiently higher than predicted serum concentration because of the finite time required for distribution from a central compartment into the whole body theophylline distribution space. On the other hand, delayed gastric emptying, as when oral medication is taken with food in the stomach (75) or antacids (76), might result in a later and somewhat lower peak serum concentration as a result of slower (though equally complete) absorption. Even under ideal circumstances, however, variability will occur in peak serum theophylline concentrations produced by a loading dose, as a function of the intersubject variability in volume of distribution (21). For this reason, the loading dose should aim for a mean serum concentration near the lower end of the therapeutic range, (i.e., 10 to 15 µg/ml). Furthermore, since theophylline does not readily enter adipose tissue, ideal body weight should be used for obese patients.

**Continued Infusions.** The optimal method to maintain serum theophylline concentrations, once a therapeutic level is attained with a loading dose, is by a continuous infusion at a rate that matches the elimination rate at the desired serum concentration (77). Unfortunately, variable plasma clearances among individuals result in a wide range of dosage requirements for continued therapy (47). Mitenko and Ogilvie recommended a constant infusion of approximately 0.75 mg/kg/hr of theophylline (expressed as 0.9 mg/kg/hr of aminophylline) to maintain an average serum concentration of 10 µg/ml (60). While their methodology served as a useful model for determining drug doses, the study population was small and not representative of the patients who require intravenous theophylline. In their study, the average rate of elimination was twice that subsequently found in the nonsmoking adult population. As a consequence, this dosage recommendation resulted in a wide range of serum concentrations which averaged 20 µg/ml (rather than 10 µg/ml) and was associated with frequent toxicity (Figure 15) when administered to critically ill hospitalized adults.

Rates of infusion that will result in an average serum concentration of 10 µg/ml have been derived from mean pharmacokinetic data appropriate for patients of various ages and clinical conditions (Table 2). Adults require, on the average, lower weight-adjusted infusion rates than children. However, the variability in plasma clearance among similar patients is so great that no one constant infusion can reliably yield both optimum benefit and safety. For adults in particular, serum concentrations must be monitored if theophylline is to be continued at full therapeutic doses for more than 12 to 24 hours.

Ideally, the initial infusion rate should be started and serum concentrations at the beginning of the infusion and 4 to 8 hours later

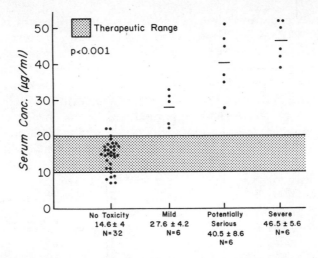

FIGURE 15. Serum theophylline concentrations resulting from intravenous theophylline dosage administered to adults in the medical intensive care unit of the University of Iowa Hospital. Doses averaged 0.7 mg/kg/hr of theophylline (0.9 mg/kg/hr of aminophylline). Using these previously recommended infusion rates, 17 of 49 patients experienced varying degrees of theophylline toxicity as a result of elevated serum concentrations. *Mild* toxicity included nausea, vomiting, headache, insomnia, and nervousness. *Potentially serious* adverse effects included sinus tachycardia with or without symptoms of mild toxicity. *Severe* toxicity included cardiac arrhythmias and seizures. Thus, the relationship between the degree of toxicity and serum theophylline concentration was supported by these data.[46] (Reproduced by permission of Drug Intelligence and Clinical Pharmacy.)

TABLE 2. CONTINUOUS THEOPHYLLINE DOSAGE FOR ACUTELY ILL PATIENTS FOLLOWING AN INITIAL LOADING DOSE

| Patient age/Clinical condition | Infusion rate* (mg/kg/hr) |
| --- | --- |
| Neonates | 0.13 |
| Infants 2–6 months | 0.4 |
| Infants 6–11 months | 0.7 |
| Children 1–9 years of age | 0.8 |
| Children over 9 and otherwise healthy adults who smoke | 0.6 |
| Otherwise healthy non-smoking adults | 0.4 |
| Cardiac decompensation, cor pulmonale, and liver dysfunction | 0.2 |

* These are guidelines for initial infusion rates of theophylline (aminophylline = theophylline/0.80) to achieve a target serum concentration of 10 μg/ml (7.5 μg/ml for neonates). Final dosage requirements may be higher or lower and should be guided by serum theophylline measurement. Use ideal body weight for obese patients.

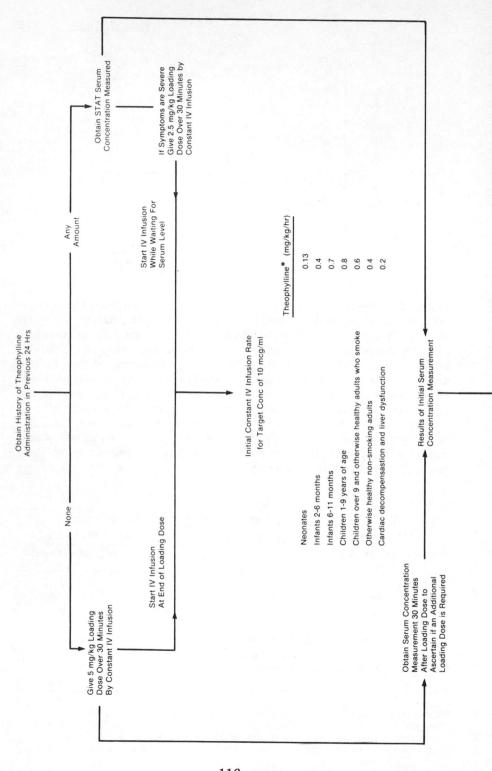

Obtain History of Theophylline
Administration in Previous 24 Hrs

None

Any Amount

Give 5 mg/kg Loading
Dose Over 30 Minutes
By Constant IV Infusion

Start IV Infusion
At End of Loading Dose

Obtain STAT Serum
Concentration Measured

If Symptoms are Severe
Give 2.5 mg/kg Loading
Dose Over 30 Minutes by
Constant IV Infusion

Start IV Infusion
While Waiting For
Serum Level

Initial Constant IV Infusion Rate
for Target Conc of 10 mcg/ml

| | Theophylline* (mg/kg/hr) |
|---|---|
| Neonates | 0.13 |
| Infants 2-6 months | 0.4 |
| Infants 6-11 months | 0.7 |
| Children 1-9 years of age | 0.8 |
| Children over 9 and otherwise healthy adults who smoke | 0.6 |
| Otherwise healthy non-smoking adults | 0.4 |
| Cardiac decompensastion and liver dysfunction | 0.2 |

Obtain Serum Concentration
Measurement 30 Minutes
After Loading Dose to
Ascertain if an Additional
Loading Dose is Required

Results of Initial Serum
Concentration Measurement

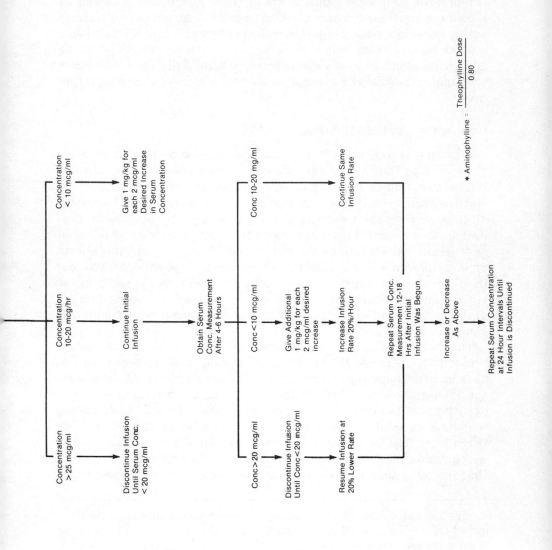

FIGURE 16.   Algorithm for therapy with intravenous theophylline.

117

compared to determine the direction taken by the serum concentration (Figure 16). Empirical adjustments of the infusion rate followed by repeat serum measurements can then maintain serum concentrations within the therapeutic range. Once the appropriate dose is established and the patient's condition improved, subsequent theophylline can be administered orally by dividing the same total daily dose into intervals appropriate for the absorption characteristics of the preparation used.

## Continued Oral Medication

Initiation of oral theophylline therapy may be associated in some patients with mild transient caffeine-like side effects which are unrelated to serum concentration. This problem can often be avoided by starting with a small dose which can be slowly increased, if tolerated, at intervals no shorter than every three days to maximum premeasurement doses (Figure 17). When this dosage schedule is followed and serum concentrations do not exceed 20 μg/ml, adverse effects among children are rare (Table 3). Only about 1% of children and less than 5% of adults appear to have absolute intolerance to the drug at low serum concentrations (78). On the other hand, *transient intolerance is very common when larger initial doses are used without this slow titration procedure.*

The dosage of theophylline required to achieve a serum concentration within the range of 10 to 20 μg/ml during chronic therapy in the absence of confounding factors varies with age (Table 4). At these age-specific weight-adjusted mean dosages, serum concentrations in 50% of patients will be less than 10 μg/ml, while about 10 to 20% of patients will have concentrations over 20 μg/ml and be at risk of toxicity (Figure 18). Therefore, these or higher doses should not be maintained without obtaining a peak serum theophylline measurement to assure that the concentration does not exceed 20 μg/ml. Once the mean age-

---

FIGURE 17. Algorithm for determining optimal theophylline dosage for therapy of chronic asthma. Doses are expressed as 24-hour totals and should be divided to maintain serum theophylline concentrations as stable as possible on an around-the-clock basis. Products with rapid dissolution characteristics require administration at intervals of approximately six hours for most patients, while slow-release products may allow eight or 12 hour dosing intervals depending upon the rate of absorption of the products used.[104] Final dosage adjustment guidelines based upon serum concentration measurement are provided in Table 5. (Reproduced by permission of the American Journal of Diseases of Children.) ⟶

# INITIAL DOSE

# MAXIMUM PRE-MEASUREMENT DOSE

# FINAL DOSE

16 mg/kg/day
(8 mg/kg/day for infants 6-24 weeks)
or
400 mg/day
WHICHEVER IS LESS

*increase dose IF TOLERATED in approximately 25% increments at 3 day intervals to maximum premeasurement dose*

Not to exceed the following:

| Age | Total daily dose (ideal body weight) |
|---|---|
| Infants 6-51 weeks | dose (mg/kg/day) = (0.3) (age in) + 8 weeks |
| Children 1-9 years | 24 mg/kg/day |
| Children 9-12 years | 20 mg/kg/day |
| Adolescents 12-16 years | 18 mg/kg/day |
| Adults | 13 mg/kg/day or 900 mg/day (whichever is less) |

(WARNING:  DO NOT ATTEMPT TO MAINTAIN ANY DOSE THAT IS NOT TOLERATED)

*measure peak serum theophylline i.e. NO missed doses for previous 48 hours: blood drawn at 2 hours after most recent dose for rapid dissolution preparations -- -- 4 hours after sustained release preparations*

Adjust according to Table

*SIMULTANEOUSLY*
Clear non-bronchodilator responsive airway obstruction with short course of high dose prednisone

If final dose not tolerated
and
resulting serum concentration does not exceed 20 µg/ml
and
lower dose doesn't control patient

**Medication tolerated and Disease controlled**

**Medication tolerated but Disease not controlled**

Trial of substitute medication. e.g. cromolyn

Maintain dose until remission suspected (may be months or years), recheck serum concentration at 6 to 12 month intervals If occasional acute exacerbations occur, treat vigorously with additional measures

Add additional measures as indicated

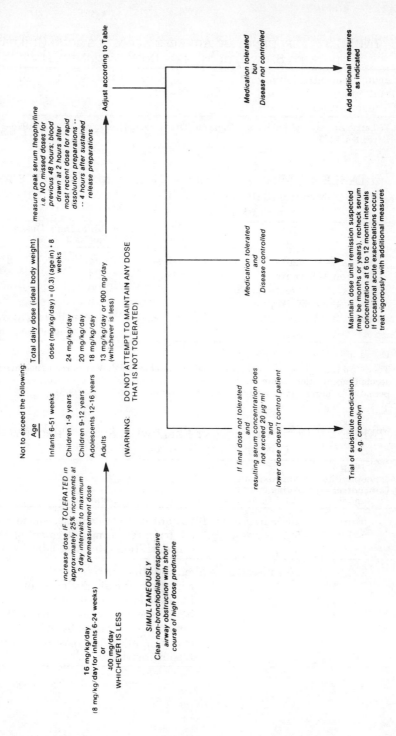

119

TABLE 3. FREQUENCY OF ADVERSE EFFECTS AMONG CHILDREN FOLLOWING SLOW TITRATION OF DOSE OVER NINE DAYS *

| Serum Concentration (µg/ml) | 5–10 | 10.1–15 | 15.1–20 | >20 |
|---|---|---|---|---|
| Total number of patients | 25 | 121 | 120 | 57 |
| Patients with adverse effects (%) | 0 | 1.6 | 2.5 | 26 |

* Pediatric Allergy and Pulmonary Division, The University of Iowa, January 1978– December 1979.

TABLE 4. MEAN AGE-SPECIFIC DOSAGE REQUIREMENTS TO MAINTAIN SERUM THEOPHYLLINE CONCENTRATIONS WITHIN THE 10–20 µg/ml RANGE.[39,40]

| Age | Mean Total Daily Dosage (mg/kg/24 hrs)† |
|---|---|
| Infants 6–51 weeks | dose $= (0.3)$(age in weeks) $+ 8$* |
| Children 1–9 years | 24 |
| 9–12 years | 20 |
| Adolescents 12–16 years | 18 |
| Adults > 16 years | 13 (or 900 mg/day, whichever is *less)* |

† Use ideal body weight for obese patients.

* There is a linear relationship between age (in weeks) and dose required to achieve a serum concentration within the 10–20 µg/ml range among infants after the neonatal period. The formula is based upon data in 39 infants ($r = 0.72$, $p<0.0001$).[40]

TABLE 5. DOSE ADJUSTMENT FOLLOWING SERUM THEOPHYLLINE CONCENTRATION MEASUREMENT [104]

| Peak Theophylline Concentration (µg/ml) | Approximate Adjustment in Total Daily Dose* | Comment |
|---|---|---|
| <5 | 100% increase | If patient is asymptomatic, consider trial |
| 5–7.9 | 50% increase | off drug; repeat measurement of serum concentration after dose adjustment. |
| 8–9.9 | 20% increase | Even if patient is transiently asymptomatic at this level, an increased serum concentration may better prevent symptoms when the airways are stressed by vigorous exertion, allergen exposure, or a viral respiratory infection. |

120

# TABLE 5. DOSE ADJUSTMENT FOLLOWING SERUM THEOPHYLLINE CONCENTRATION MEASUREMENT [104]—CONT.

| Peak Theophylline Concentration (μg/ml) | Approximate Adjustment in Total Daily Dose* | Comment |
|---|---|---|
| 10–13.9 | Cautious 10% increase *if* clinically indicated | If patient is asymptomatic, no increase is necessary; if bronchodilator responsive symptoms persist, increase cautiously as indicated. |
| 14–19.9 | None | If "breakthrough" in asthmatic symptoms occurs at the end of dosing interval, change to slow-release product and repeat serum theophylline measurements. |
| | Occasional intolerance requires a 10% decrease | If side effects occur, decrease total daily dose as indicated. |
| 20–24.9 | 10% decrease | Even if side effects are absent. |
| 25–29.9 | 25% decrease | Even if apparent side effects are absent, omit next dose and decrease total daily dose as indicated; repeat measurement of serum concentration after adjustment. |
| 30–34.9 | 33% decrease | |
| ≥35 | 50% decrease | Omit next two doses, decrease as indicated, and repeat measurement of serum theophylline concentration after adjustment. |

* To avoid toxicity:

(1) Assure that the sample represents a peak concentration obtained at steady state (e.g. no missed or extra doses with close approximation of prescribed dosing intervals during previous 48 hours).

(2) Use a reliable laboratory; if result appears questionable, repeat determination if not initially performed in duplicate.

(3) The increase of 50% or 100% should be made in 25% increments at two-day intervals to further assure safety and tolerance. The serum concentration may increase disproportionate to dosage increase as the therapeutic range is entered.[34,35]

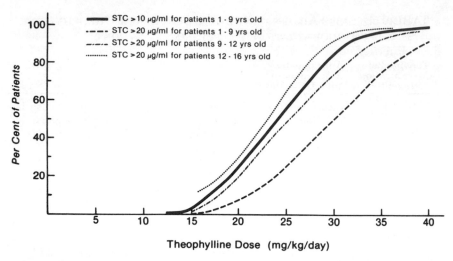

FIGURE 18. Cumulative frequency distribution for theophylline dosage likely to exceed serum concentration (STC) of 10 µg/ml among patients one to nine years of age, for doses likely to result in serum theophylline concentrations greater than 20 µg/ml among the same patients, and for doses likely to result in serum theophylline concentrations in excess of 20 µg/ml among preadolescents and adolescents. Examination of the consequences of a 24 mg/kg/day dosage administered to children under nine years of age illustrates that this "average" or median (50th percentile) dose which would be expected to result in 50% of the children exceeding 10 µg/ml could also result in 20% of the same population of children having serum concentrations over 20 µg/ml. If dosage guidelines are not made age specific and this "average childhood dose" is administered to older children, even greater risk of toxicity would result. For adults, the curve would have shifted even further to the left. These data emphasize the necessity for measurement of serum theophylline in determining optimal safe dosage and provide the basis for appropriate selection of dosages suitable for clinical titration prior to measurement of serum theophylline.[39] (Reproduced by permission of the Journal of Pediatrics.)

specific dosage is reached, subsequent adjustment (if necessary) is made according to the results of a serum concentration measurement (Table 5). It is important that dosage adjustments be made cautiously and in small increments, since dose-dependent elimination kinetics have been documented for theophylline (36) (see section on Metabolism), and a relatively small change in dose might result in a disproportionately larger change in serum concentration (Figure 7). The dose of theophylline must never be doubled at serum concentrations

>5 µg/ml. Dosage should never exceed the average values in Table 4 unless a low serum concentration documents the need for a higher dose. Furthermore, even the average dosages in Table 4 should not be *maintained* without confirmation of their safety by measurement of serum theophylline concentration.

It is important that blood samples obtained for guidance of long-term therapy be collected when steady-state conditions are present. A serum measurement is valid only if no doses have been missed in the previous 48 hours, no extra doses have been taken, the interval between doses has been approximately equal and no erythromycin or other factors that might transiently alter clearance have been present. Dosage adjustment should be guided predominantly by an estimation of the peak serum concentration. Samples should be obtained 2 hours after the dose with solutions and plain uncoated tablets with rapid dissolution characteristics (19), and at 4 hours with slow-release preparations such as Slo-Phyllin Gyrocaps® (10). During therapy with Theodur® or Sustaire®, samples can be obtained 3 to 7 hours after the morning dose to approximate the peak concentration in most patients (15).

Measurement of trough concentrations (obtained at the end of a dosing interval) generally does not provide clinically essential information. Instead, a careful history can guide the dosing interval. For example, increased asthmatic symptoms repeatedly occurring at the end of a dosing interval in a patient with a peak serum concentration within 10 to 20 µg/ml suggest that the trough concentration may be too low. In this situation, symptoms may be eliminated by dividing the same total daily dose into smaller portions and administering them more frequently or by changing the product to a more slowly absorbed formulation (Figure 5). Either strategy should result in approximately the same mean serum concentration but with smaller peak-trough differences and thus greater stability of the airways. The use of a slow-release formulation, however, would be more convenient for the ambulatory patient and less likely to result in a compliance problem.

Following the establishment of a dosage regimen that maintains serum concentrations within the therapeutic range, measurements only need to be obtained yearly, since clearance (38) and thus dosage requirements normally remain stable for extended periods (34,39). In children, however, growth effectively results in decreasing weight-adjusted dosages and repeat measurements of serum theophylline may be needed as frequently as every six months during periods of rapid growth (39). Changes in concurrent drug therapy (i.e., erythromycin), the presence of prolonged fever, or alterations in liver or cardiovascular function may influence drug elimination and warrant measurement of serum concentrations (see section on Elimination). Patients who successfully stop smoking following initiation of theophylline therapy have an increased risk of toxicity if dosage is not modified, since elimination of the drug may subsequently decrease (51,52) and result in increased serum concentrations.

**Measurement of Saliva Concentrations of Theophylline.** The use of saliva to estimate serum theophylline has intrigued a number of investigators (26,79,80). However, subsequent reports indicate that the ratio of saliva to serum concentrations often do not remain constant within the same patient and predictions of serum concentrations are unreliable (81,82). Moreover, the early interest in salivary levels occurred prior to the current micromethodology for drug assays and was also based on the assumption that large numbers of measurements might be required to define kinetic characteristics of individual patients. For clinical purposes, however, relatively few (often only one) serum samples are needed to determine final long-term dosage requirements (83). Even among children, small blood samples by venipuncture are generally well tolerated and within the capability of any clinician competent to manage asthma. There is, therefore, insufficient need to replace the established use of serum levels with estimates based on salivary concentrations which may be unreliable.

**Effect on Other Drugs.** Theophylline appears to decrease phenytoin serum concentrations and thereby may result in decreased seizure control (84). Renal excretion of lithium is significantly increased after a single dose of theophylline (85). This could result in a reduction in lithium's therapeutic effect, although this interaction has not been investigated during chronic administration.

**Management of Theophylline Poisoning.** Ingestion of an oral dose exceeding 10 mg/kg requires prompt emergency treatment with syrup of ipecac, followed by activated charcoal (86) and sodium sulfate after vomiting. Serum concentrations should be measured and all patients with excessive levels monitored in an intensive care unit. Many patients with very high serum theophylline levels survive unscathed. When seizures occur, however, death and permanent brain damage are common sequelae. Charcoal hemoperfusion can rapidly remove theophylline (87,88) and may be clinically indicated when the serum concentration is over 60 µg/ml. Seizures may thereby be prevented by promptly reducing the serum concentration to safe levels. In most cases, however, hemoperfusion has been instituted after the onset of seizures and the clinical outcome has not matched the chemical success of the procedure (89). It is therefore recommended that,

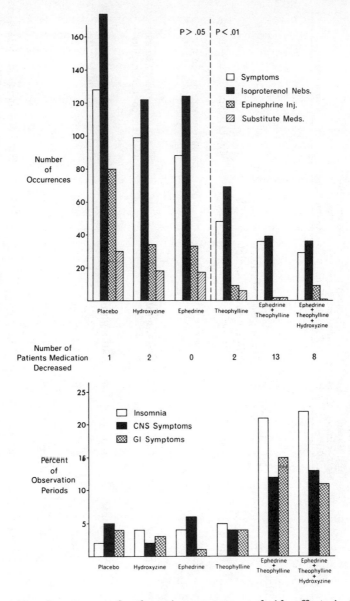

FIGURE 19. Occurrence of asthmatic symptoms and side effects in 23 pediatric patients treated with single drugs and combinations. The combinations contained theophylline, ephedrine, and hydroxyzine in a commercially available fixed-dose ratio of 130:15:10 (Marax). The number of patients who reduced the dose because of adverse effects with each particular medication is given in the space between the diagrams.[65] (Reproduced by permission of Clinical Pharmacology and Therapeutics.)

TABLE 6.  THEOPHYLLINE PRODUCTS WITH DOCUMENTED BIOAVAILABILITY [a]

| Dosage Form And Brand Name | Manufacturer | Dosing Interval (hrs) Children and Rapid Metabolizing Adults | Dosing Interval (hrs) Non-Smoking Adults | Strength (Anhydrous Theophylline) | Measurable Dose Increment[b] (mg) | Comment |
|---|---|---|---|---|---|---|
| Rapidly absorbed products for acute therapy: Plain uncoated tablets | | | | | | |
| Slo-Phyllin | Wm. Rorer | 4–6 | 8 | 100 mg scored tablet 200 mg scored tablet | 50 100 | |
| Theophyl Chewable | Knoll | 4–6 | 8 | 100 mg double scored | 25 | Microencapsulated—must wash down tablet and swallow rapidly to avoid bitter taste |
| Oral liquids (alcohol free) | | | | | | |
| Elixicon Suspension | Berlex | 4–6 | 8 | 20 mg/ml | 10 | Shake vigorously to assure uniform concentration—sugar free. |
| Slo-Phyllin-GG Syrup | Wm. Rorer | 4–6 | 8 | 10 mg/ml | 5 | Contains glyceryl guiacolate which is an inert ingredient. |
| Theolair Syrup | Riker | 4–6 | 8 | 5.3 mg/ml | 2.5 | |
| Rectal Solution Somophyllin[c] | Fisons | 6 | 8 | 48 mg/ml | 16 | |
| Intravenous Solution Aminophylline[c] | Invenex | Constant infusion | | 20 mg/ml | 5 | Rubber stoppered vials avoid glass particles that result from breaking ampules. |

126

Slow-release products for chronic asthma:[d]

| | | | | | | |
|---|---|---|---|---|---|---|
| Slo-Phyllin Gyrocaps | Wm. Rorer | 6–8 | 8–12 | 60 mg capsule 125 mg capsule 250 mg capsule | 30 | Beads can be sprinkled on food for administration to infants and small children. One-half the contents of a 60 mg size capsule can be used for 30 mg doses. |
| Sustaire | Pfizer | 12 | 12 | 100 mg scored tablet 300 mg scored tablet | 50 | Some rapid metabolizers may require 8 hour dosing intervals to avoid breakthrough of symptoms. |
| Theodur | Key | 12 | 12 | 100 mg scored tablet 200 mg scored tablet 300 mg scored tablet | 50 | Some rapid metabolizers may require 8 hour dosing intervals to avoid breakthrough of symptoms. |

[a] Only products with dosage forms that permit incremental dose increases are listed. All prescriptions should state theophylline concentration of the desired product.
[b] Accuracy of measurement decreases below 0.5 ml with suspensions and syrups because of viscosity; smaller amounts cannot be accurately measured. All liquid dosage forms should be measured with a syringe.
[c] On rare occasion, the ethylenediamine compound of aminophylline may cause urticaria or exfoliative dermatitis.
[d] Despite claims of other manufacturers (Theovent, Elixophyllin SR, Quibron-bid, LaBid, etc.), only Sustaire and Theodur have sufficiently slow and complete absorption to allow 12 hour dosing with minimal serum concentration fluctuations in most patients.

when available, the risks of charcoal hemoperfusion be considered at the facility where the patient is being treated. If risks of the procedure are judged not to be excessive, then treatment should be promptly instituted *prior* to obvious clinical toxicity. This is not warranted when the serum concentration is less than 40 µg/ml, since the risk of the procedure probably outweighs the potential benefit. In the range of 40 to 60 µg/ml, the decision to dialyze must be individualized depending on the presence of clinical symptoms such as nausea, vomiting, headache, tachycardia, irritability, confusion, etc. Peritoneal dialysis and other extracorporeal methods of removal are not adequate for the management of theophylline poisoning (89).

**Theophylline Formulations.** The commonly prescribed fixed dose combinations of ephedrine and theophylline with other ingredients (Marax®, Tedral®, etc.) are irrational. Ephedrine adds little benefit to doses of theophylline achieving therapeutic serum concentrations, while the combination of these two drugs produces a synergistic toxicity (Figure 19) (64,65,90).

Rapidly absorbed formulations of theophylline are most appropriate for acute therapy, while slow-release products offer therapeutic advantages for chronic asthma. There are a variety of plain uncoated tablets, capsules, and oral liquids, and a chewable tablet which have equivalent absorption characteristics (Table 6).

A rectal solution is appropriate when the oral route cannot be used. For example, young children tend to vomit medication during acute exacerbations of asthma not severe enough to require hospitalization. This formulation assures rapid absorption of theophylline without the need for parenteral medication. Suppositories, however, are slowly and erratically absorbed, and are therefore contraindicated (9,16,17).

Slow-release formulations have been established as the formulations of choice for management of chronic asthma. While some are incompletely and erratically absorbed, others have reliable absorption characteristics (Table 6). Slo-Phyllin Gyrocaps®, Theodur®, and Sustaire® are particularly useful because they are available in capsule and tablet sizes that allow dosage adjustment in the small increments *essential* for safe and effective use. Slo-Phyllin Gyrocaps® (particularly the 60 mg size capsule) can be administered to small children by sprinkling the beaded contents on a spoonful of soft food which is then followed by a beverage to wash the beads down intact. Theodur® and Sustaire® are the only bioavailable products with sufficiently slow absorption to reliably allow 12 hour dosing intervals. Patients with very large dose requirements as a result of rapid elimination, however, may require eight hour intervals to prevent repeated asthmatic symptoms prior to the next dose.

## ASSAY METHODS

Five different methods of measuring serum theophylline concentrations have been developed and are currently being utilized in clinical laboratories. They differ in sensitivity, specificity, sample size, technical difficulty and amount of technician time required to perform the procedure (Table 7). While the accuracy of these various procedures is similar under experimental conditions, results from clinical laboratories participating in proficiency testing programs have indicated that some methods are more prone to technician error than others (Table 8). For example, the coefficient of variation of 97 laboratories using the enzymatic immunoassay procedure (EMIT) for a 15 μg/ml spiked quality control sample was 11.8% compared to 21% for 41 laboratories using high pressure liquid chromatography (91). Of even greater concern to the clinician using these results to guide dosage adjustments is the precision (day-to-day variation) of the specific laboratory performing the assay. When a pooled serum sample spiked with 15 μg/ml of theophylline was aliquoted and disguised as three different patient specimens and sent through local physicians on separate days to 28 laboratories in Iowa, 15 of them reported values for one or more samples outside an acceptable range of 13 to 18 μg/ml. In contrast, 64 aliquots of this pooled sample measured in the Pediatric Allergy/Pulmonary Research Laboratory of The University of Iowa using the EMIT® enzymatic immunoassay, the most prevalent methodology among both the accurate and inaccurate labs, averaged 15.8 μg/ml and all results were within 13 to 18 μg/ml (92). Therefore, it seems essential for one to ascertain in a similar manner if a specific laboratory can be relied upon to provide accurate results before using this information to guide dosage adjustments in patients.

**UV Spectrophotometric Assay.** Schack and Waxler described the first method of determining theophylline concentration in biological fluids. The procedure consisted of extracting the drug from serum with organic solvent and measuring the absorbance of ultraviolet light in a spectrophotometer (93).

Since most laboratories have a spectrophotometer, the method can be implemented without an investment in new equipment. However, it requires a large sample size, a variety of commonly used drugs (i.e., furosemide, aspirin, etc.) interfere with this method producing false results (94), a large amount of technician time is required, and the reproducibility of the results is often poor (Table 8). Therefore, this method should not be relied upon to guide dosage adjustments.

**Gas Liquid Chromotography (GLC).** The poor specificity and large sample size required for the UV spectrophotometric method led

TABLE 7. COMPARISON OF CURRENTLY AVAILABLE METHODS OF MEASURING SERUM THEOPHYLLINE CONCENTRATION

| Analytical Method[a] | Specificity for Theophylline[b] | Sample Volume for Analysis | Sensitivity | Metabolite Analysis | Usage in Clinical Labs[c] | Analyst Skill and Training | Analysis Time[d] | Comments |
|---|---|---|---|---|---|---|---|---|
| Enzyme Immunoassay (EMIT) | 1 | 50 µl or less | 1 | 5 | 59% | average | 0.5 hr (0.8 hr) | Only procedure that has been widely automated with high volume analyzers. |
| Radioimmunoassay (RIA) | 1 | 25 µl | 2 | 5 | 10% | average | 1 hr (1.5 hr) | |
| Liquid Chromatography (HPLC) | 3 | 20–100 µl | 3 | 1 | 24% | above average | 0.8 hr (2.1 hr) | Capable of analyzing polar non-extractable metabolites. Reverse-phase procedure can be easily set up and maintained. |
| Gas Chromatography (GLC) | 2 | 20–50 µl | 4 | 4 | 3% | superior | 1.5 hr (3.0 hr) | Nitrogen-phosphorus detector is necessary for specificity and sensitivity. |
| UV-Spectrophotometry | 5 | 3 ml | 5 | 5 | 4% | average | 0.8 hr (2.5 hr) | Not recommended for use in a hospital environment because of interference from multiple drugs. |

[a] Any laboratory is capable of achieving a day-to-day precision of 10% or less (C.V.) with all of the procedures listed. Differences between the various methods in clinical labs are generally a function of technician error.

[b] Arbitrary Ranking Scale of 1 (Excellent) to 5 (Poor) with a score of 3 being average or nominal.

[c] Data from College of American Pathologists Therapeutic Drug Monitoring Survey (1979, Set 7-D).

[d] Approximate times to analyze one sample, or a ten sample batch (shown in parentheses) and one control. All procedures are assumed to be non-automated.

TABLE 8. PROFICIENCY OF MEASURING SERUM THEOPHYLLINE
CONCENTRATION IN 15 µg/ml QUALITY CONTROL SAMPLES AMONG 197
LABORATORIES PARTICIPATING IN A TESTING PROGRAM CONDUCTED BY
THE CENTER FOR DISEASE CONTROL IN 1978 UNDER THE CLINICAL
LABORATORIES IMPROVEMENT ACT OF 1967 [91]

| | Number of Labs | Mean* (µg/ml) | Standard Deviation (µg/ml) | Coefficient** Variation (%) |
|---|---|---|---|---|
| Enzyme Immunoassay (EMIT) | 97 | 15.3 | 1.8 | 11.3 |
| High Pressure Liquid Chromatography | 41 | 15.4 | 3.2 | 21.0 |
| Ultraviolet Spectroscopy | 33 | 15.6 | 4.2 | 27.0 |
| Gas Chromatography | 14 | 13.8 | 3.4 | 24.6 |
| Radioimmunoassay | 10 | 15.5 | 1.6 | 10.3 |
| Mass Spectroscopy | 2 | 15.5 | 4.9 | 31.6 |

* Spiked samples contained 15 µg/ml.
** The coefficient of variation is the standard deviation divided by the mean.

investigators to develop a GLC method for measuring theophylline
(95). It involves a technically demanding extraction and derivitization
procedure. While it is very specific and requires only a small sample
size, it is a lengthy procedure and has a high potential for errors
unless the analyst is very skilled. As a consequence, few laboratories
currently use this procedure.

**High Pressure Liquid Chromotography (HPLC).** Reverse-phase
liquid chromotography, the most commonly used HPLC method in
clinical laboratories, offers a substantial advantage over GLC since
sample preparation is simple and the procedure requires only 30 to
40 minutes to perform (96). Although theophylline metabolites and
derivatives, such as dyphylline, do not cause interference, a few drugs
when administered in large doses (ampicillin, cephalothin (97), acetazolamide (98), trisulfapyrimidine (99)) may cause falsely elevated
results under some operating conditions.

**Enzyme Immunoassay (EMIT).** The EMIT system of enzyme immunoassay by Syva Corporation (Palo Alto, California) was the first
commercially available method using an antibody inhibition technique to quantify the concentration of theophylline in serum or
plasma. Although introduced onto the marketplace only a few years
ago, it has become the most extensively used theophylline assay (Table
7). It is rapid, specific and requires a small sample size (100,101). In
addition, the same system can be utilized for a variety of other drug
assays including anticonvulsants, aminoglycoside antibiotics, and cardiac antiarrhythmiac drugs. It is also economical, allowing minimal

technician time for *stat* assays, and it can be adapted to automated batch processing procedures which can deal with large numbers of samples rapidly.

**Radioimmunoassay (RIA).** This procedure also utilizes an antibody inhibition technique, but instead of measuring the ability of residual enzyme activity to act on a substrate, it utilizes radioactive tagging as the marker. It also requires only a small sample size, is highly specific, and while somewhat slower than the EMIT system, still is relatively rapid (102). Sample handling is not as simple as with the EMIT system, however, and batch processing has not been automated.

**Fluorescent Immunoassay (Ames).** This variation of the antibody inhibition method for quantitating theophylline uses a fluorescent marker. Information on this method is limited (103). It is purported to use only 2 microliters of serum and takes only 20 minutes for a sample including determination of a standard curve. While equipment costs may be considerably less than other methods, no information is yet available about reagent costs for performing the assay. Its specificity for theophylline may be somewhat less than the other antibody inhibition techniques with a 2 µg/ml false elevation of serum theophylline measurement reported at serum caffeine concentrations of 10 µg/ml. Since it is not yet commercially available, its precision under laboratory conditions cannot be accurately estimated.

## SUMMARY

Theophylline is a potent bronchodilator and respiratory stimulant effective in the treatment of acute and chronic asthma, Cheyne-Stokes respirations, and neonatal apnea. It is also used as an adjunct in the treatment of congestive heart failure and acute pulmonary disease. Benefits and risks from theophylline have been demonstrated to relate directly to serum concentration, which is itself a function of not only dosage but also the elimination characteristics of the drug in an individual patient. When used to treat acute symptoms, an initial loading dose of theophylline based on a mean volume of distribution is required to rapidly obtain maximum bronchodilator effect. Because of large interpatient differences in elimination, infusion rates for continued therapy must be determined empirically by monitoring serum theophylline concentrations at intervals and making subsequent adjustments until a steady state serum concentration is reached within the 10 to 20 µg/ml therapeutic range. Intravenous, oral or rectal solutions, and plain uncoated tablets are appropriate for acute therapy, while reliably absorbed slow-release formulations offer therapeutic advantages for the management of chronic asthma, particularly in children. A dosage for long-term therapy is determined by starting with doses sufficiently low to allow virtually complete acceptance of the medication, followed by gradual increases if tolerated at three day intervals until mean age-specific dosages are reached. Serum theophylline measurement is essential for management of chronic asthma and when rapidly available, it increases the utility of theophylline for acute therapy. Of the various methods available, the Enzyme Immunoassay (EMIT) appears to have distinct advantages for most laboratories with regard to cost, specificity, ease of operations, speed of the assay and potential application of the equipment for assaying drugs other than theophylline.

# REFERENCES

1. Hudson LD, Tyler ML, Petty TL: Oral aminophylline and dihydroxypropyl theophylline in reversible obstructive airway disease: A single dose, double-blind, crossover comparison. Curr Ther Res 1973; 15:367–372.
2. Lindholm B, Helander E: The effect on the pulmonary ventilation of different theophylline derivatives compared to adrenalin and isoprenaline. Acta Allergol 1966; 21:299–306.
3. Gisclon LG, Ayres JW, Ewing GH: Pharmacokinetics of orally administered dyphylline. Am J Hosp Pharm 1979; 36:1179–1184.
4. Zuidema J, Merkus FWHM: Chemical and biopharmaceutical aspects of theophylline and its derivatives. Curr Med Res Op 1979; 6:14–25 (Suppl 6).
5. Simons FER, Simons JK, Bierman CW: The pharmacokinetics of dihydroxypropyl theophylline: A basis for rational therapy. J Allergy Clin Immunol 1975; 56:347–355.
6. Svedmyr N: The role of the theophyllines in asthma therapy. Scand J Resp Dis (Suppl) 1977; 101:125–137.
7. Koysooko R, Ellis EF, Levy G: Effect of ethanol on theophylline absorption in humans. J Pharm Sci 1975; 64:299–301.
8. Apold J, Bakke OM: Is microcrystalline theophylline really better? Lancet 1979; 1:667–668.
9. Waxler, SH, Schack JA: Administration of aminophylline (theophylline ethylenediamine). JAMA 1950; 143:736–739.
10. Weinberger M, Hendeles L, Bighley L: Relationship of product formulation to absorption of oral theophylline. N Engl J Med 1978; 299:852–857.
11. Mitenko PA, Ogilvie RI: Bioavailability and efficacy of a sustained-released theophylline tablet. Clin Pharmacol Ther 1974; 16:720–726.
12. Spangler DL, Kalof DD, Bloom FL, Wittig HJ: Theophylline bioavailability following oral administration of six sustained-release preparations. Ann Allergy 1978; 40:6–11.
13. Bell T, Bigley J: Sustained-released theophylline therapy for chronic childhood asthma. Pediatrics 1978; 62:352–358.
14. Dasta J, Murtallo JM, Altman M: Comparison of standard and sustained-release theophylline tablets in patients with chronic obstructive pulmonary disease. Am J Hosp Pharm 1979; 36:613–617.

15. Weinberger M, Hendeles L, Wong L: Fluctuations in serum theopylline concentration during 8 and 24 hour dosing with a slowly absorbed formulation compared with 6 hour dosing with conventional tablets. J Allergy Clin Immunol 1980; 65:177–178.

16. Ridolfo AS, Kohlstaedt KD: A simplified method for the rectal instillation of theophylline. Am J Med Sci 1959; 237:585–589.

17. Bolme P, Edlund PO, Eriksson M, Paalzow L, Winbladh B: Pharmacokinetics of theophylline in young children with asthma: Comparison of rectal enema and suppositories. Eur J Clin Pharmacol 1979; 16:133–139.

18. Lillehei JP: Aminophylline oral vs. rectal administrations. JAMA 1968; 205:530–533.

19. Hendeles L, Weinberger M, Bighley L: Absolute bioavailability of oral theophylline. Am J Hosp Pharm 1977; 34:525–527.

20. Mitenko PA, Ogilvie RI: Pharmacokinetics of intravenous theophylline. Clin Pharmocol Ther 1973; 14:509–513.

21. Hendeles L, Weinberger M, Bighley L: Disposition of theophylline following a single intravenous aminophylline infusion. Am Rev Resp Dis 1978; 118:97–103.

22. Aranda JV, Sitar DS, Parsons WE, Loughnan PM, Neimo AH: Pharmacokinetic aspects of theophylline in premature newborns. N Engl J Med 1976; 295:413–416.

23. Vallner JJ, Speir WA, Kolbeck RC, Harrison GN, Bransome ED: Effect of pH on the binding of theophylline to serum proteins. Am Rev Respir Dis 1979; 120:83–86.

24. Arwood LL, Dasta JF, Friedman C: Placental tranfer of theophylline: Two case reports. Pediatrics 1979; 63:844–846.

25. Yurchak AM, Jusko WJ: Theophylline secretion into breast milk. Pediatrics 1976; 57:518–520.

26. Koysooko R, Ellis EF, Levy G: Relationship between theophylline concentration in plasma and saliva of man. Clin Pharmacol Ther 1974; 15:454–460.

27. Levy G, Koysooko R: Renal clearance of theophylline in man. J Clin Pharmacol 1976; 13:329–335.

28. Jenne JW, Nagasawa HT, Thompson RD: Relationship of urinary metabolites of theophylline to serum theophylline levels. Clin Pharmacol Ther 1976; 19:375–381.

29. Bory C, Baltassat P, Porthault M, Bethenod M, Frederich A, Aranda J: Metabolism of theophylline to caffeine in premature newborn infants. J Pediatr 1979; 94:988–993.

30. Bada HS, Khanna NN, Somani SM, Tin AA: Interconversion of theophylline and caffeine in newborn infants. J Pediatr 1979; 94:993–995.

31. Boutroy MJ, Vert P, Royer RJ, Monin P, Royer-Morrott MJ: Caffeine, a metabolite of theophylline during the treatment of apnea in the premature infant. J Pediatr 1979; 94:996–998.

32. Midha KK, Sved S, Hossie RD, McGilveray IJ: High performance liquid chromatographic and mass spectrometric identification of dimethylxanthine metabolites of caffeine in human plasma. Biomed Mass Spectrom 1977; 4:172–177.

33. Caldwell J, Lancaster R, Monks TJ, Smith RL: The influence of dietary methylxanthines on the metabolism and pharmacokinetics of intravenously administered theophylline. Br J Clin Pharmacol 1977; 4:637P–638P.

34. Jenne JW, Wyze MS, Rood FS, McDonald FM: Pharmacokinetics of theophylline application to adjustment of the clinical dose of aminophylline. Clin Pharmacol Ther 1972; 13:349–360.

35. Sarrazin E, Hendeles L, Weinberger M, Muir K, Riegelman S: Dose dependent kinetics for theophylline: Observations among ambulatory asthmatic children and a method of dosage adjustment. J Allergy Clin Immunol (Abstract) 1980; 65:177.

36. Weinberger MM, Ginchansky E: Dose-dependent kinetics of theophylline disposition in asthmatic children. J Pediatr 1977; 91:820–824.
37. Shen DD, Fixley M, Azarnoff DL: Theophylline bioavailability following chronic dosing of an elixir and two solid dosage forms. J Pharm. Sci 1978; 67:916–919.
38. Ginchansky E, Weinberger M: Relationship of theophylline clearance to oral dosage in children with chronic asthma. J Pediatr 1977; 91:655–660.
39. Wyatt R, Weinberger M, Hendeles L: Oral theophylline dosage for the management of chronic asthma. J Pediatr 1978; 92:125–130.
40. Nassif EG, Weinberger M, Guiang SF, Jimenez D: Theophylline disposition in infancy. Presented at American Academy of Pediatrics Annual Meeting, San Francisco, 1979.
41. Piafsky KM, Sitar D, Rangno RE, Ogilvie RI: Theophylline disposition in patients with hepatic cirrhosis. N Engl J Med 1977; 296:1495–1497.
42. Mangione A, Imhoff TE, Lee RV, Shum LY, Jusko W: Pharmacokinetics of theophylline in hepatic disease. Chest 1978; 73:616–622.
43. Piafsky KM, Sitar DS, Rangno RE, Ogilvie RI: Theophylline kinetics in acute pulmonary edema. Clin Pharmacol Ther 1977; 21:310–316.
44. Powell JR, Vozeh S, Hopewell P, Costello J, Sheiner LB, Riegelman S: Theophylline disposition in acutely ill hospitalized patients. Am Rev Resp Dis 1978; 118:229–238.
45. Vicuna N, McNay JL, Ludden TM, Schwertner H: Impaired theophylline clearance in patient with cor pulmonale. Br J Clin Pharmacol 1979; 7:33–37.
46. Hendeles L, Bighley L, Richardson RH, Hepler CD, Carmichael J: Frequent toxicity from IV aminophylline infusions in critically ill patients. Drug Intell Clin Pharm 1977; 11:12–18.
47. Weinberger MM, Matthay RA, Ginchansky EJ, Chidsey CA, Petty TL: Intravenous aminophylline dosage. Use of serum theophylline measurement for guidance. JAMA 1976; 235:2110–2113.
48. Zwillich CW, Sutton FD, Neff TA, Cohn WM, Matthay RA, Weinberger MM: Theophylline-induced seizures in adults; Correlation with serum concentrations. Ann Intern Med 1975; 82:784–787.
49. Chang KC, Bell TD, Lauer BA, Chai H: Altered theophylline pharmacokinetics during acute respiratory viral illness. Lancet 1978; 1:1132–1134.
50. Jenne J, Nagasawa H, McMugh R, MacDonald F, Wyse E: Decreased theophylline half-life in cigarette smokers. Life Sci 1975; 17:195–198.
51. Hunt SN, Jusko WJ, Yurchak AM: Effect of smoking on theophylline disposition. Clin Pharmacol Ther 1976; 19:546–551.
52. Powell JR, Thiercelin J, Vozeh S, Sansom L, Riegelman S: The influence of cigarette smoking and sex on theophylline disposition. Am Rev Resp Dis 1977; 116:17–23.
53. Jusko WJ, Schentag JJ, Clark JH, Gardner M, Yurchak AM: Enhanced biotransformation of theophylline in marijuana and tobacco smokers. Clin Pharmacol Ther 1978; 24:406–410.
54. Pfeifer HJ, Greenblatt DJ: Clinical toxicity of theophylline in relation to cigarette smoking. Chest 1978; 73:455–459.
55. Landay RA, Gonzalez MA, Taylor JC: Effect of phenobarbital on theophylline dispositon. J Allergy Clin Immunol 1978; 62:27–29.
56. Weinberger M, Hudgel D, Spector S, Chidsey C: Inhibition of theophylline clearance by troleandomycin. J Allergy Clin Immunol 1977; 59:228–231.
57. Pfeifer HJ, Greenblatt DJ, Friedman P: Effect of three antibiotics on theophylline kinetics. Clin Pharmacol Ther 1979; 26:36–40.
58. Wing D, Prince R, Weinberger M, Hendeles L: The effect of erythromycin on theophylline disposition. Manuscript in preparation.

59. Kozak PP, Cummins LH, Gillman SA: Administration of erythromycin to patients on theophylline. J Allergy Clin Immunol 1977; 16:149–151.
60. Mitenko PA, Ogilvie RI: Rational intravenous doses of theophylline. N Engl J Med 1973; 289:600–603.
61. Levy G, Koysooko R: Pharmacokinetics analysis of the effect of theophylline on pulmonary function in asthmatic children. J Pediatr 1975; 86:789–793.
62. Pollock J, Kiechel F, Cooper D, Weinberger M: Relationship of serum theophylline concentration to inhibition of exercise-induced bronchospasm and comparison with cromolyn. Pediatrics 1977; 60:840–848.
63. Bierman CW, Shapiro GG, Pierson WE: Acute and chronic theophylline therapy in exercise-induced bronchospasm. Pediatrics 1977; 60:845–849.
64. Weinberger MM, Bronsky EA: Evaluation of oral bronchodilator therapy. J Pediatr 1974; 84:421–427.
65. Weinberger MM, Bronsky EA: Interaction of ephedrine and theophylline. Clin Pharmacol Ther 1975; 17:585–592.
66. Hambleton G, Weinberger M, Taylor J, et al: Comparison of cromoglycate (cromolyn) and theophylline in controlling symptoms of chronic asthma. Lancet 1977; 1:381–385.
67. Dietrich BA, Krauss AN, Reidenberg M, Drayer D, Auld P: Alterations in state in apneic pre-term infants receiving theophylline. Clin Pharmacol Ther 1978; 24:474–478.
68. Aranda JV, Gorman W, Bergsteinsson H, Gunn T: Efficacy of caffeine in treatment of apnea in the low-birth-weight infant. J Pediatr 1977; 90:467–472.
69. Dowell AR, Heyman A, Sieker HO, Tripathy MD: Effect of aminophylline on respiratory-center sensitivity in Cheyne-Stokes respiration and in pulmonary emphysema. N Engl J Med 1965; 273:1447–1453.
70. Kordash TR, Van Dellen RG, McCall JT: Theophylline concentrations in asthmatic patients after administration of aminophylline. JAMA 1977; 238:139–141.
71. Jacobs MH, Senior RM, Kessler G: Clinical experience with theophylline: relationship between dosage, serum concentration, and toxicity. JAMA 1976; 235:1983–1986.
72. Camarata SJ, Weil MH, Hanashiro PK, Shubin H: Cardiac arrest in the critically ill: I. A study of predisposing causes in 132 patients. Circulation 1971; 44:688–695.
73. Ellis EF: Theophylline and derivatives. In: Middleton E, Reed CE, Ellis EF, eds. *Allergy Principles and Practice*. St. Louis: CV Mosby Co., 1978:434–453.
74. Floyd RA, Cohen JL: Pharmacokinetics in drug therapy II: Applications of clinical pharmacokinetics in the assessment of theophylline therapy. Am J Hosp Pharm 1977; 34:402–407.
75. Welling PG, Lyons LL, Craig WA, et al: Influence of diet and fluid on bioavailability of theophylline. Clin Pharmacol Ther 1975; 17:475–480.
76. Arnold LA, Spurbeck GH, Shelver WH, Henderson WM: Effect of an antacid on gastrointestinal absorption of theophylline. Am J Hosp Pharm 1979; 36:1059–1062.
77. Mitenko PA, Ogilvie RI: Rapidly achieved plasma concentration plateaus, with observations on theophylline kinetics. Clin Pharmacol Ther 1972; 13:329–335.
78. Weinberger M, Ginchansky E: Theophyllinization of the child with chronic asthma. In Gouveia WA, Tognoni G, Van der Kleign E (eds). *Proceedings of the International Symposium on Clinical Pharmacy and Clinical Pharmacology*. Amsterdam: North-Holland Biomedical Press, 1976.

79. Eney RD, Goldstein EO: Compliance of chronic asthmatics with oral administration of theophylline as measured by serum and salivary levels. Pediatrics 1976; 57:513–517.

80. Galant SP, Gillman SA, Cummins LH, et al: Reliability of salivary theophylline as a guide to plasma theophylline levels. Am J Dis Child 1977; 131:970–972.

81. Hendeles L, Burkey S, Bighley L, Richardson R: Unpredictability of theophylline saliva measurements in COPD. J Allergy Clin Immunol 1977; 60:335–338.

82. Boobis S, Trembath DW: Plasma-saliva ratio of theophylline following oral theophylline derivatives. Br J Clin Pharmacol 1978; 6:456P–457P.

83. Ekwo E, Hendeles L, Mercer B, Weinberger M: The frequency and cost of theophyllic serum concentration measurements during chronic prophylactic therapy of asthma. Manuscript in preparation.

84. Hendeles L, Wyatt R, Weinberger M, Schottelois D, Fincham R: Decreased oral phenytoin absorption following concurrent theophylline administration. J Allergy Clin Immunol 1979; 63:156.

85. Thomsen K, Schou M: Renal lithium excretion in man. J Physiol 1968; 215:823–827.

86. Sintek C, Hendeles L, Weinberger M: Inhibition of theophylline absorption by activated charcoal. J Pediatr 1979; 94:314–316.

87. Ehlers SM, Zaske DE, Sawchuk RJ: Massive theophylline overdose. Rapid elimination by charcoal hemoperfusion. JAMA 1978; 240:474–475.

88. Russo ME: Management of theophylline intoxication with charcoal column hemoperfusion. N Engl J Med 1979; 300:24–26.

89. Weinberger M, Hendeles L: Role of dialysis in the management and prevention of theophylline toxicity. Dev Pharmacol Ther 1979; 1:26–30.

90. Bierman CW, Pierson WE, Shapiro GG: Excercise-induced asthma: Pharmacological assessment of single drugs and drug combination. JAMA 1975; 234:295–298.

91. Center for Disease Control: Proficiency testing summary analysis—Drug Monitoring 1978. Atlanta, GA 30333.

92. Bonham A, Hendeles L, Weinberger M, Vaughan L: Unreliability of serum theophylline measurements in community hospitals and commercial laboratories. Manuscript in preparation.

93. Schack JA, Waxler SH: An ultraviolet spectrophotometric method for the determination of theophylline and theobromine in blood and tissues. J Pharmacol Exp Ther 1949; 97:283–291.

94. Matheson LE, Bighley L, Hendeles L: Drug interference with the Schack and Waxler plasma theophylline assay. Am J Hosp Pharm 1977; 34:496–499.

95. Least CJ, Johnson GF, Solomon HM: Gas-chromatographic micro-scale procedure for theophylline, with use of a nitrogen-sensitive detector. Clin Chem 1976; 22:765–768.

96. Orcutt JJ, Kozak PP, Gillman SA, Cummins LH: Micro-scale method for theophylline in body fluids by reversed-phase high-pressure liquid chromatography. Clin Chem 1977; 23:599.

97. Kelly RC, Prentice DE, Hearne GM: Cephalosporin antibiotics interfere with the analysis for theophylline by high performance liquid chromatography. Clin Chem 1978; 24:838–839.

98. Robinson CA, Dobbs, J: Acetazolamide interference with theophylline analysis by high-performance liquid chromatography. Clin Chem 1978; 24:2208–2211.

99. Bond LW, Thornton DL: Trisulfapyrimidine interference with liquid-chromatrographic analysis for theophylline and dyphylline. Clin Chem 1979; 25:1186–1187.

100. Koup JR, Brodsky B: Comparison of homogeneous enzyme immunoassay and high-pressure liquid chromatography for the determination of theophylline concentration in serum. Am Rev Respir Dis 1978; 117:1135–1138.
101. Chang JY, Bastiani RJ: Performance evaluation of the EMIT theophylline assay. Clinical Study No. 41 Summary Report. Palo Alto, California, Syva Corporation, 1977.
102. Neese Al, Soyka LF: Development of a radioimmunoassay for theophylline. Clin Pharmacol Ther 1977; 21:633–640.
103. Messenger LJ, Li TM, Benovic JL, Burd JF: STAT assay for theophylline concentrations in human serum using a modified substance labeled fluorescent immunoassay. J Allergy Clin Immunol (Abstract) 1980; 65:175.
104. Hendeles L, Weinberger M, Wyatt R: Guide to oral theophylline therapy for the treatment of chronic asthma. Am J Dis Child 1978; 132:876–880.
105. Giacoia G, Jusko WJ, Menke J, Koup JR: Theophylline pharmacokinetics in premature infants with apnea. J Pediatr 1976; 89:829–832.
106. Rosen JP, Danish M, Ragni MC, Saccar CL, Yaffe SJ, Lecks HI: Theophylline pharmacokinetics in the young infant. Pediatrics 1979; 64:248–251.
107. Simons FER, Simons KJ: Pharmacokinetics of theophylline in infancy. J Clin Pharmacol 1978; 18:472–476.
108. Loughnan PM, Sitar DS, Ogilvie RI, Eisen A, Fox Z, Neims AH: Pharmacokinetic analysis of the dispositon of intravenous theophylline in young children. J Pediatr 1976; 88:874–879.
109. Ellis EF, Koysooko R, Levy G: Pharmacokinetics of theophylline in children with asthma. Pediatrics 1976; 58:542–547.
110. Nielsen-Kudsk F, Magnussen I, Jakobsen P: Pharmacokinetics of theophylline in ten elderly patients. Acta Pharmacol Toxicol 1978; 42:226–234.
111. Kappas A, Anderson KE, Conney AH, Alvares AP: Influence of dietary protein and carbohydrate on antipyrine and theophylline metabolism in man. Clin Pharmacol Ther 1976; 20:643–653.
112. Kappas A, Alvares AP, Anderson KE, et al: Effect of charcoal-broiled beef on antipyrine and theophylline metabolism. Clin Pharmacol Ther 1978; 23:445–450.

*Counterpoint Discussion:*

# Theophylline

J. Robert Powell, Pharm.D.
J. Edward Jackson, M.D.

## Introduction

Despite an extensive literature on theophylline, many gaps remain in our understanding of the pharmacokinetics and pharmacodynamics of this important drug. It is admittedly difficult to perform good pharmacologic studies in seriously ill patients, and many subjects are needed so that confounding variables can be isolated. Certain areas, such as drug interactions and dose-dependent kinetics, may lend themselves to simple, but definitive, studies in patients and healthy subjects. Many of the papers reviewed in the preceding chapter suffer from weak study design and analysis, small sample size, and incorrect extrapolation by subsequent authors of the results of a limited study. Multiple-regression analysis of uncontrolled or poor quality data is not an adequate substitute for carefully designed studies in which relevant variables are controlled.

This counterpoint to the preceding chapter will take the form of a critical review of the three areas of theophylline pharmacokinetics that are most important to the clinician: plasma concentration-response relationships, clearance estimates, and dosing recommendations.

## Therapeutic Concentration Range

**Variables Influencing Concentration-Response Relationship.** The theophylline therapeutic plasma concentration range is usually stated to be either 5 to 20 µg/ml or 10 to 20 µg/ml. The therapeutic concentration range concept indicates that within this range there is an optimal probability for achieving the desired clinical response (i.e., relief of symptoms, bronchodilation) and a minimal and acceptable probability of toxicity. Although 5 to 20 µg/ml may be the therapeutic

TABLE 1.  VARIABLES WHICH MAY INFLUENCE THEOPHYLLINE
PLASMA CONCENTRATION-RESPONSE RELATIONSHIP

Principal Diagnosis:
    Asthma (extrinsic vs intrinsic)
    Chronic bronchitis
    Emphysema
    Pulmonary edema
    Apnea in newborn infants
    Bronchopulmonary dysplasia
    Cystic fibrosis

Secondary Diagnosis:
    Respiratory infection
    Cardiac arrhythmias
    Seizure disorders
    Peptic ulcers
    Anxiety

Severity:
    Mechanical ventilation
    Status asthmaticus (hospitalized)
    Chronic perennial asthma (steroid dependent vs not)
    Seasonal asthma

Patient Age and Aging

Concomitant Drugs:
    Sympathomimetic (selective $Beta_2$ vs nonselective)
    Sympatholytic (metoprolol)
    Cromolyn
    Corticosteroid (local vs systemic)
    Caffeine from diet

concentration range for theophylline, this issue is far more complex than has been stated previously, as there are few convincing studies in this area.

Variables which may influence the theophylline plasma concentration-response relationship and the therapeutic range estimation are listed in Table 1. For the conditions listed under principal diagnosis, theophylline is used as a bronchodilator to treat "wheezes" with the exception of pulmonary edema and apnea. Although there are many studies that indicate theophylline is effective in treating acute and chronic asthma (1–9), there is little evidence of efficacy in a significant percentage of patients with chronic bronchitis and emphysema. Even though pulmonary function does improve in some patients with chronic bronchitis or emphysema, recent studies found no improve-

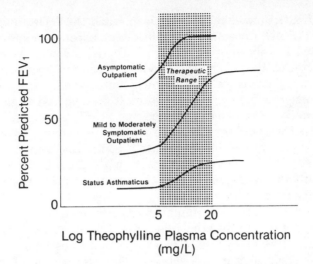

FIGURE 1. A conceptual representation of the theophylline plasma concentration pulmonary function response curves at different stages of asthma severity.

ment in the patients' subjective assessment (10,11). Of twelve patients with cystic fibrosis treated with theophylline, ten showed no improvement or worsening in pulmonary function tests and ten experienced adverse symptoms which were attributed to the drug. This demonstrates an important point in the clinical use of theophylline: The seriously ill patient, in whom the drug has questionable efficacy (e.g., emphysema), is most likely to experience life-threatening theophylline toxicity (seizures, cardiac arrhythmias).

Even considering asthma alone, severity of the disease will have a profound effect on the theophylline plasma concentration-response relationship. Figure 1 is a schematic representation of theophylline plasma concentration-response curves at three different severity stages of asthma. This might very well be the same patient at different times. As asthma worsens, one would expect: (a) the baseline (prior to theophylline) pulmonary function level to decrease, (b) the log-linear slope of the curve to decrease, and (c) the maximum acute response to decrease. In this example, the mild to moderately symptomatic outpatient demonstrates the largest absolute change in pulmonary function with theophylline. This is because the nearly normal asthmatic has little room to improve to achieve normality and the severely obstructed patient will require time to reach the "responsive" phase of asthma (13). The seasonal asthmatic is an excellent example of this time-related intrapatient change in theophylline plasma concentration-response patterns. The theophylline plasma concentration-*toxicity* response relationship may be most important in the severely ill patient, since this type of patient is most predisposed to toxicity due to factors decreasing drug clearance (e.g., CHF, pneumonia) and decreasing the threshold for adverse effects (e.g., acidosis, hypoxia). The seriously ill patient can least tolerate theophylline toxicity.

Drugs administered concomitantly with theophylline certainly change both the therapeutic and toxic concentration-response relationships for theophylline.

The coadministration of sympathomimetic drugs (epinephrine, isoproterenol, ephedrine, isoetharine, metaproterenol, terbutaline, etc.) with theophylline gives rise to two important questions that are not easily answered: (a) Can one achieve a greater degree of bronchodilation with theophylline and a sympathomimetic drug than with either drug alone? (b) At the same degree of bronchodilation and therapeutic response, is there less toxicity from the combined use of theophylline and a sympathomimetic drug than with either agent alone? In answering these questions, in addition to controlling the variables in Table 1, the route of administration (inhalation, oral, intravenous) will influence the pattern of therapeutic and toxic response. At the same degree of bronchodilation, oral or intravenous administration of terbutaline produces more tremor, hypotension, and tachycardia than administration by inhalation (14). Some evidence indicates that the pattern of bronchodilation may also be influenced by the route of administration. Inhalation of salbutamol increases forced expiratory volume at one second ($FEV_1$) much more than forced vital capacity (FVC) whereas, oral salbutamol produces a similar increase in both tests (15). This difference may indicate that systemic administration produces a greater effect on small peripheral airways.

In order to answer the first question, studies would need to be conducted where a dose-response curve achieving maximal bronchodilator response would be constructed for theophylline, a sympathomimetic drug, and a combination. Based on the studies we have reviewed to date (8,16–26), there is no study which fulfills these criteria and, therefore, the first question has not been answered. A well-designed multiple dose study of 54 outpatients treated with oral theophylline, the oral $\beta_2$ sympathomimetic drug, salmefamol, and the combination, indicates the improvement in peak expiratory flow rate from the combination is due to an additive, not synergistic effect (18).

In the emergency treatment of asthma, the combination of intravenous aminophylline and subcutaneous epinephrine offered no advantage over the use of epinephrine alone (26). However, this study did not evaluate the effect of aminophylline alone.

Regarding the second question, data suggest that to achieve the same degree of bronchodilation some patients can tolerate the combination of a $\beta_2$ sympathomimetic drug and theophylline better than either drug alone (21,24,25). The results from these single dose studies need to be confirmed by multiple dose studies of longer duration. However, it seems reasonable to believe that the combination of theophylline with a $\beta_2$ sympathomimetic drug may predispose to tremor. It is not surprising that the combination of theophylline and ephedrine, which have similar toxic effects (insomnia, nervousness, nausea, vomiting), would result in a higher incidence of toxicity and, therefore, a therapeutic disadvantage compared to either drug alone (8).

Other drugs can also modify the concentration-response curve of theophylline. The use of cardioselective $\beta_1$ blocking drugs in patients with cardiac and pulmonary disease (e.g. paroxysmal atrial tachycardia with chronic bronchitis) would be expected to shift the theophylline plasma concentration response curve to the right. In patients with chronic asthma, the combination of theophylline and cromolyn produced more objective and subjective improvement than cromolyn alone (27). The combination was not significantly better than theophylline alone.

Since other methylxanthines (caffeine, theobromine) produce qualitatively the same pharmacologic effects as theophylline, large quantities of these drugs in the diet would increase the apparent sensitivity of a patient to theophylline toxicity. It is not rare to find patients ingesting nearly one gram of caffeine per day from coffee and carbonated beverages in addition to the prescribed theophylline dose. What may be perceived as theophylline intolerance in these patients may be corrected by removing caffeine from the diet. With the recent reports of worsening anxiety and depression in psychiatric patients attributed to caffeine in the diet (28,29), one wonders about the chronic behavioral effects of theophylline, particularly in children, the elderly, and patients with depression and/or anxiety.

Secondary diagnoses may render the patient more susceptible to theophylline toxicity. Because of the known adverse effects of theophylline (tachycardia, seizures, nausea), one might expect patients with cardiac arrhythmias, a seizure disorder, or peptic ulcer to be particularly sensitive to theophylline toxicity. A recent well-conducted study indicates that the $\beta_2$ stimulant, terbutaline, offers no advantage in patients with premature ventricular contractions and, in fact, is worse than theophylline, which was no different from placebo in arrhythmogenicity (30). On the other hand, when compared to several sympathomimetics (ephedrine, epinephrine, isoproterenol, and metaproterenol), aminophylline was the only bronchodilator which significantly increased gastric acid secretion (31). It was concluded that peptic ulcer patients requiring a bronchodilator should either use a sympathomimetic drug or combine theophylline with antacids and/or cimetidine. Although we are not aware of studies documenting clinical experience of seizure patients taking theophylline, the drug is epileptogenic in rats (32). We have had experience with an adult with major motor seizures and asthma who experienced seizures on several hospitalizations for acute asthma. On each occasion the seizure occurred within several hours after receiving an intravenous loading dose which resulted in theophylline levels in the 20 to 25 µg/ml range. When the theophylline level was maintained below 15 µg/ml as an outpatient, seizures were rare. When choosing a bronchodilator for a patient with a seizure disorder, it is probably best to avoid theophylline and ephedrine, and instead use metaproterenol, terbutaline, or isoproterenol which do not distribute significantly into the brain (33, 34).

**Critical Evaluation of the Literature.** In studies relating theophylline plasma concentration to clinical response, desirable characteristics include: (1) a prospective, (2) double-blinded, (3) placebo controlled study design in which neither the patient nor the evaluator knows the theophylline dose or plasma concentration, (4) predetermined, sensitive and valid assessment criteria, (5) an unbiased method for subject selection, (6) accurate description of patient population, (7) characterization of intra- and interpatient variation, and (8) an adequate sample size to safely project to the population of concern. Care should be taken to include, but control, many of the variables in Table 1.

Studies should be conducted in acute, severe, and in chronic, stable obstructive lung disease. In acute, severe disease the plasma concentration-response relationship for theophylline should be studied over a brief time period in an attempt to limit variation in disease severity from influencing results. This type of study might increase the theophylline plasma level until either toxicity occurs or improvement in pulmonary function ceases. Outpatient studies in chronic disease should be conducted over a period of months and should include a variety of objective and subjective measurements much like earlier cromolyn efficacy studies (35,36). Assessment criteria would include home pulmonary function testing several times a day (e.g. Wright Peak Flow Meter), records of doses of aerosol bronchodilator, records of daily patient global self-assessment, and records of the number of days the patient is unable to go to school or work.

There should be appropriate controls. Since pulmonary function tests are effort dependent, a placebo control is necessary when assessing the therapeutic effect of theophylline. It is important to determine if the theophylline plasma level helps distinguish patients who are truly toxic from patients who have symptoms of theophylline toxicity which are due to the patient's disease(s) or drugs other than theophylline. In toxicity studies an appropriate control group would be patients with symptoms of toxicity which do not change when the theophylline dose is decreased or discontinued. The subject's age, type of disease, disease severity, and concomitant drugs are important variables. To avoid bias, toxicity studies should include all patients presenting to a hospital or clinic over a time period and not only those in whom a theophylline level is requested. Similarly, efficacy could be overestimated if patients are selected based upon prior knowledge of an excellent response to bronchodilators.

Sample size should be determined by the ability to measure the response, variability of response, and magnitude of response. Depending on the subject sample and the nature of the study, toxicity studies will require more patients than short-term efficacy studies. Generally we feel that toxicity studies involving fewer than 40 patients and efficacy studies with fewer than 10 patients will be difficult to extrapolate to the general population of patients receiving theophylline. Ideally, repeated measures of efficacy and toxicity in the same subject at the same theophylline level would provide an index of intrasubject variation.

In Table 2 we have summarized several representative studies regarding compliance with the above criteria. Many of the early studies (37,38) are similar to that by Turner-Warwick (1). Based on the clinical judgment of the investigator and some spirometric data, these studies generally concluded that a minimal theophylline plasma concentration of 10 μg/ml was necessary to relieve bronchospasm. Though these studies do not meet many of the above criteria, they are, on the whole, not as inferior to more modern studies as might be expected.

The single dose intravenous aminophylline study conducted by Maselli and associates (4) is well conceived, but the conclusions which can be drawn are restricted for several reasons. The maximum average theophylline plasma concentration achieved was 7 to 8 μg/ml. It is known that improvement in pulmonary function by theophylline may increase to plasma concentrations at least up to 20 $\mu$g/ml. Probably because of this low theophylline level, no toxicity was noted. The study was neither double nor single-blinded. Since $FEV_1$ is effort dependent, it is important that the investigator and patient should not be aware of the treatment. Although a large number of patients was studied (n = 59), only mean $FEV_1$ values were reported and hence there is no index of intersubject or intrasubject variation. Levy and Koysooko used Maselli's data to model the relationship between theophylline plasma concentration and change in $FEV_1$ (39).

The acute intravenous aminophylline study conducted by Mitenko and Ogilvie (4) is an excellent study which provides theophylline plasma concentration-pulmonary function response data over a wide concentration range in nine patients. Unfortunately, subsequent authors referring to this study have extrapolated the results further than the study warrants. The nine patients were at the end of a hospitalization for an exacerbation of asthma. Since the patients were in a period of changing asthma severity, they may not be representative of stable patients of greater or lesser severity. Three aminophylline infusion rates were used. For this type of study it may be better to produce the same theophylline plasma concentrations in all patients and increase the plasma concentration until pulmonary function no longer improves or toxicity occurs or some pre-selected maximum serum concentration is reached. Since the maximum average level achieved in six patients was about 21 $\mu$g/ml, it would be worthwhile to know if further benefit could be achieved by a higher theophylline level in most, some, or no other patients.

Jenne and associates (7) attempted to correlate changes in airway resistance in a single blind study of seven patients who also received a placebo. Patient characteristics were not detailed. In reviewing the data from this study, it is difficult to clearly differentiate and quantitate the effect of theophylline versus placebo. Some patients demonstrated a similar reduction in airway resistance with theophylline and placebo, baseline measurements were not obtained in some cases, the magnitude of change in theophylline level was small in some cases (< 5 $\mu$g/ml), the placebo period was frequently shorter than the theophylline period, and the crossover was not randomized. A separate group of 83 patients on chronic theophylline was evaluated for toxicity in a retrospective chart review conducted by a technologist. Using predetermined criteria, the incidence of definite or possible toxicity was 54% in those patients with plasma theophylline concentrations >20 $\mu$g/ml, 19% in the 10 to 20 $\mu$g/ml range, and 0% in the <10 $\mu$g/ml region. Although the technologist was not aware of the theophylline

TABLE 2.   ANALYSIS OF THEOPHYLLINE PLASMA CONCENTRATION-RESPONSE STUDIES IN PATIENTS WITH AIRWAY OBSTRUCTION

| Study | Type of Study | Prospective | Double Blind | Control | Predetermined Valid Response Criteria | Unbiased Patient Selection | Accurate Sample Description | Adequate Sample Size | Intra-Patient Variation |
|---|---|---|---|---|---|---|---|---|---|
| Turner-Warwick[1] | Ther, C | Yes | No | No | No | Yes | No | Yes | No |
| Maselli et al[3] | Ther, Tox, A | Yes | No | No | Yes | Yes | Yes | Yes | No |
| Levy & Koysooko[39] | | | | | | | | | No |
| Mitenko & Ogilvie[4] | Ther, Tox, A-C | Yes | Single Blind | Yes | Yes | No | Yes | No | No |
| Hendeles et al[40] | Tox, A | Yes | ? | No | Yes | No | No | Yes | No |
| Jacobs et al[41] | Tox, A | No | No | No | No | No | No | Yes | No |
| Jenne et al[7] | Ther, Tox, C | Ther–Yes Tox–No | Single Blind | Ther–Yes Tox–No | Yes | Yes | No | Ther–No Tox–Yes | No |
| Pollock et al[6] | Ther, C | Yes | Yes | Yes | Yes | Yes | Yes | Yes | No |
| Bierman et al[5] | Ther, C | Yes | No | Yes | Yes | Yes | Yes | Yes | Yes |

Type of Study: Ther = Therapeutic Effect
Tox = Toxic Effect
A = Acute, Severe Disease
C = Chronic Disease

plasma concentration, this study suffers from many of the problems of the other cited toxicity studies.

While comparing the efficacy of theophylline to cromolyn in inhibiting exercise-induced bronchospasm in 12 children, Pollock and associates (6) also attempted to obtain a correlation with theophylline serum concentration (see Figure 11 in preceding chapter). This is a particularly well designed study where inhibition of exercise-induced bronchospasm was evaluated at two hour intervals for 6 hours after a single theophylline dose. Although the data presented in the figure suggest a relationship between theophylline serum concentration and inhibition of exercise-induced bronchospasm, it would be helpful to link the data points for each subject. A number of patients with theophylline levels between 5 and 10 µg/ml did not show significant exercise-induced bronchospasm (using the author's criteria). Use of a logarithmic scale for theophylline concentration might produce a more typical dose-response curve. The study does not give an index of interpatient variation in response. Contrary to this study, Bierman and associates (5) were unable to find an association between theophylline plasma concentration and inhibition in exercise-induced bronchospasm. However, there are marked differences in study design.

Hendeles and associates (40) reported a study which is frequently referred to as providing evidence for the theophylline plasma concentration-toxicity response relationship (see Figure 15 from preceding chapter). There is no indication that the physician who evaluated the patient or the chart was unbiased by knowledge of the theophylline level. The patient selection apparently did not include all patients seen during the study period. There is also no indication that the patient was evaluated for toxicity within 1 to 2 hours of the sampling time for the theophylline level. There is no index of patient severity. Since all the patients in the study were receiving intravenous aminophylline, the conclusions may not apply to the outpatient population. Similarly, it is possible that the signs and symptoms attributed to theophylline were due instead to the disease process itself. A patient in respiratory failure may have cardiac arrhythmias from hypoxia, acidosis or other bronchodilators (30). Similarly, patients may be nauseated from illness or from other drugs. Since the mean age was 56 years, many of the patients had chronic obstructive airway disease, and some had congestive heart failure, we wonder how many patients were also taking digoxin. If this drug was present, there is no indication that digitalis toxicity (e.g., nausea, vomiting, PVC's) was absent in this particularly susceptible population. No attempt was made to grade the severity of respiratory failure, liver dysfunction, and cardiac failure. These diseases can make the patient susceptible to or cause the toxic symptoms attributed to theophylline.

A retrospective study that attempts to correlate theophylline serum concentration to toxicity was reported by Jacobs and associates (41). Virtually every criticism of the previously cited study applies to this one. This study goes a step further in that it attempts to determine the incidence of toxicity at various theophylline levels. For a patient to be included in the study, a theophylline level had to be measured. One reason for obtaining a theophylline level is because there is a question of toxicity. It is possible, indeed probable, that many patients receiving theophylline responded well to treatment, had no signs of toxicity, and did not have a theophylline level drawn. If this is true, the toxicity incidences reported would be overestimates because of an incorrect denominator. Just as these studies indicate that the incidence of theophylline toxicity increases at levels greater than 20 μg/ml, another study found the incidence above 20 μg/ml was 11% (2/18) and below 20 μg/ml was 12% (4/33) (42).

There is probably a reasonably good correlation between theophylline plasma concentration and clinical response. However, large, well designed studies are needed to clearly define this relationship.

## Factors Which Affect Clearance

Though theophylline has a low hepatic extraction and clearance (43), most conditions which cause hepatic congestion decrease theophylline clearance. This is particularly important clinically since the indications for use of theophylline are often associated with decreased hepatic perfusion. Tables of dose adjustments for disease states usually represent mean values from small numbers of patients, often based on only a single theophylline level in each patient. Further problems in adjusting individual dosage arise from the spectrum of each disease state (e.g., varying degrees of liver dysfunction), and from physiologic variations which occur as the pathologic state is treated (e.g., diuresis leading to resolution of congestive heart failure). Diseased populations consistently show much greater variation in theophylline metabolism than do normal subjects.

Let us examine several of these states and the data available regarding the effects on theophylline clearance, and consider a practical approach to adjusting individual theophylline dosages.

**Congestive Heart Failure (CHF).** Theophylline has long been recommended in the treatment of congestive heart failure (44,45), and one large study has implicated theophylline as the most frequent cause of fatal drug toxicity in coronary care units (46). Six papers present data on theophylline kinetics in congestive heart failure (40, 47–51), but only a total of 14 patients were carefully studied (47–50).

Piafsky et al (47) studied theophylline kinetics for 24 hours following a single 28 minute infusion in nine patients with acute cardiogenic pulmonary edema. Compared to 19 normals, the volume of distribution at steady state ($V_{ss}$) did not change, but a marked reduction in clearance (41 ml/kg/hr in patients and 62 ml/kg/hr in normals), corresponding to mean elimination half-life of 22.9 and 6.7 hr (both groups included smokers and nonsmokers) was found during pulmonary edema. In addition to the reduced clearance, the patients showed a much greater variation in their elimination of the drug, with elimination half-lives ranging from 3.1 to 82 hr (more than 20-fold), while the normals varied from 3.6 to 12 hr (less than four-fold). Liver functions and clinical appearance did not allow patients with low clearances to be distinguished from patients with higher clearances. Among the nonsmoking patients, however, there was a tendency for those with abnormal liver function tests to have lower clearances. The authors note in their introduction that "there is no clear evidence of the need for theophylline treatment" in acute left ventricular failure.

Powell et al (48) evaluated theophylline pharmacokinetics in a group of acutely ill patients receiving continuous IV infusions of aminophylline. Pharmacokinetic studies were performed during the first 24 hours of hospitalization and immediately prior to ending the infusion (determined by the patient's attending physician) using a modified single dose method (see Figures 2 and 3 for experimental design). All patients had obstructive airways disease. The three patients with CHF as well had signifcantly lower (p<.01) initial clearances (26.6 ml/kg/hr) than patients with uncomplicated asthma or chronic bronchitis (44.5 ml/kg/hr) or normal controls (46.8 ml/kg/hr), though the clearances following improvement were similar (66.4 and 53.4 ml/kg/hr respectively). Volumes of distribution were unchanged. Of particular note here is the marked increase in clearance in all three patients following improvement of their congestive heart failure (statistically significant at p<0.01). This study is limited by the small number of patients with congestive heart failure, making it impossible to correlate initial severity of disease with either initial clearance or degree of improvement, and making extrapolation to all patients with heart failure tentative.

A case report by Jenne et al (47) shows a similar increase in elimination rate following improvement of congestive heart failure. Data are not available to allow volume or clearance calculations, and the

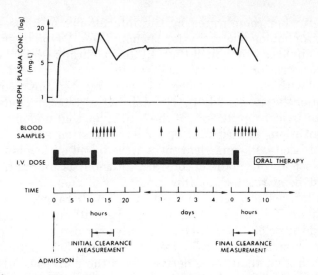

FIGURE 2. Design of study showing relationship of intravenous (I.V.) dose of aminophylline to plasma theophylline (theoph.) concentration, blood sampling times, and clearance determinations. (Reproduced with permission of Am Rev Resp Dis.[48])

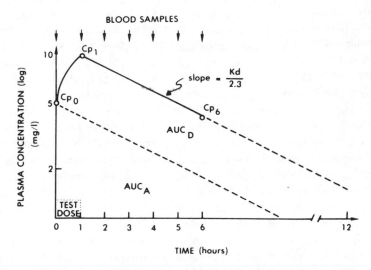

FIGURE 3. Study design for determination of theophylline pharmacokinetic parameters. (Reproduced with permission of Am Rev Resp Dis.[48])

Clearance (Cl) = Dose/$AUC_D$, V = Cl/kd or V = dose/($Cp_1$-$Cp_o$)

151

study is further complicated by the interference of furosemide with the spectrophotometric assay for theophylline. Weinberger et al (50) report a single case in which theophylline clearance (based on steady-state concentration during a constant infusion) rose from 33 to 56.4 ml/kg/hr "with clinical evidence of improvement of the heart failure."

A frequently cited study by Hendeles et al (40) concludes, despite lack of statistical significance at the 0.10 level, that undefined "cardiac decompensation" is a risk factor for accumulation and thus for theophylline toxicity. Plasma clearances were based on levels following a loading dose and 12 hours of constant infusion, assuming that steady-state had been reached at this time. Given that the other studies report half-lives averaging in the 15 to 25 hour range, it is clear that a single point following a 12 hour infusion will not represent steady-state, and thus clearance will be seriously over-estimated. Correspondingly, the plasma clearances and suggested rates for constant infusions are much higher than those derived from the more careful studies of Piafsky (47) and Powell (48) and confirmed by the two case reports cited (49,50).

The recent paper of Vicuna et al (51) involved the study of a large number of patients with the clinical diagnoses of chronic obstructive pulmonary disease (COPD) or chronic obstructive pulmonary disease with cor pulmonale (COPD + CP). Consistent with the preceding studies, the presence of cor pulmonale resulted in decreased theophylline clearance. This study bases its clearance values on single theophylline levels in 36 patients (28 COPD, 8 COPD + CP) "after at least 36 hours of constant infusion." Data from oral dosing are also presented, based on a single trough level in each of 45 patients (39 COPD, 6 COPD + CP) "after at least 48 hours of continuous therapy" on a q 6 hour regimen. Since the mean half-lives in congestive heart failure seem to be about 20 hours (46–50), the subjects with CP were most probably *not* at steady-state. Use of a single level is extremely risky as there is no indication of laboratory error. No comments are made regarding smoking status, liver disease, infection, or severity of pulmonary obstruction. While their data demonstrate a significant decrease in clearance in COPD + CP when compared to COPD alone, the magnitude of this difference cannot be realistically assessed due to the pharmacokinetic methods employed.

Based on the best available data, the aminophylline loading dose should be unchanged (6 mg/kg), and the initial maintenance infusion in congestive heart failure should be about 0.2 mg/kg/hr (i.e., normal doses multiplied by a factor of 0.4). The marked interpatient variability in the presence of cardiac decompensation requires careful clinical and drug level monitoring even during the early phases of the maintenance infusion. Maintenance doses will need to be increased as congestive failure resolves and theophylline clearances return towards normal.

Further studies seeking to explain this gross variation in theophylline metabolism among patients with heart failure are important. These must involve careful pharmacokinetic studies with fairly large numbers of patients, and attempt to identify the most significant markers of altered theophylline kinetics: clinical (e.g., Killip class, hepatomegaly), physiologic (cardiac output, pulmonary capillary wedge pressure, etc.), and biochemical (e.g., liver function abnormalities). The current use of one clearance estimate to determine dosing for all patients with "heart failure" leaves considerable room for improvement.

**Liver Disease.** Three papers address theophylline kinetics in patients with liver disease. Piafsky et al (52) studied theophylline kinetics following a 15 minute intravenous infusion in nine cirrhotics. Theophylline clearance was significantly reduced in the cirrhotics (42 ml/kg/hr) compared to 19 normal subjects (62 ml/kg/hr), corresponding to mean half-lives of 25.6 hours (range 7.1 to 59.1 hr) and 6.7 hours (range 3.6 to 12 hr). $V_{ss}$ appeared to be larger in the cirrhotics, but the difference was not significant at the 0.05 level (0.785 L/kg vs. 0.508 L/kg), and $V_{ss}$ did not correlate with the presence of ascites. The only laboratory test which correlated with reduced theophylline clearance was serum albumin. Marked decreases in theophylline clearance were observed in the three patients with serum albumins of 2.9 gm/dl or less. Binding of theophylline to plasma proteins was reduced in the three subjects in whom it was studied. The diseased subjects exhibited a much greater variability in theophylline metabolism than the normals. Eight patients were smokers (amount unquantified), four were taking spironolactone, one taking multiple anticonvulsants, and one had a history of longterm barbiturate use. Each of these drugs has been implicated in changing the clearance of theophylline or other hepatically metabolized drugs. All subjects had been abstinent from ethanol for at least one week before study, but their drinking habits immediately prior to this were not mentioned. In this patient sample, the effects of smoking will tend to mask the decrease in clearance due to liver disease, and thus the reported clearances may underestimate the reduction in metabolism seen with cirrhosis alone.

Mangione et al (53) investigated the disposition of oral theophylline in eight cirrhotics, 57 young normals, and 25 age-matched controls. The cirrhotics had markedly decreased clearances (18.8 ml/kg/hr) when compared to age-matched controls (53.7 ml/kg/hr) and young normals (63 ml/kg/hr), corresponding to elimination half-lives of 28.8 hours in the cirrhotics and 6 hours in the normals and controls. $V_{ss}$ was slightly increased in the cirrhotics (0.563 L/kg vs. 0.483 L/kg in normals, p <0.01), probably due to decreased protein binding (29% in cirrhotics and 65% in normals, p<0.001). A significant negative correlation was found between theophylline clearance and serum bilirubin, with clearances significantly greater in patients with bilirubin less than 1.5 mg/dl (32.6 ml/kg/hr) compared to those with elevated bilirubin levels (10.5 ml/kg/hr). Again, the patients exhibited much greater variability in theophylline kinetics than did the normal controls. Similar to Piafsky's study (52), most of the cirrhotics were smokers, and many were on multiple medications. This study would be more meaningful if an intravenous theophylline dose had been used, as it was not demonstrated that aminophylline bioavailability is unchanged in cirrhosis. This makes the calculations of $V_{ss}$ particularly suspect. If oral absorption is delayed compared to normals, a falsely elevated elimination half-life may result.

The previously discussed paper by Hendeles and co-workers (40) reported that patients with undefined "liver dysfunction" tended to have lower theophylline clearances than the other patients they studied (p<0.10). However, steady-state concentrations were not documented, and it was *assumed* that the single level after 12 hours of constant infusion represented the steady-state. Since 12 hours is about half of the average half-life reported in the two well-designed investigations of theophylline kinetics in liver disease, drug accumulation was still occurring when the assumed steady-state level was drawn. Therefore, clearance was overestimated.

Seizures have occurred in several cirrhotic patients found to have theophylline levels much higher than would be expected with normal elimination of the drug (7,54).

In view of the reduced clearance of theophylline and the roughly unchanged volume of distribution, patients with cirrhosis should receive the usual loading dose of aminophylline (6 mg/kg), but their maintenance infusion should be about 0.2 mg/kg/hr (i.e., usual doses multiplied by a factor of 0.4). We recommend this rather low figure because most of the patients in the two studies were smokers and because theophylline protein binding is decreased in cirrhotics. Because of decreased protein binding, one might expect both therapeutic and toxic drug effects to occur at lower serum concentrations. Data are not available to allow prediction of dosing requirements in lesser degrees of liver dysfunction (e.g., hepatitis, cholestasis). Further studies are needed to identify the clinical markers for decreased theophylline clearance in patients with liver disease and to determine what, if any, dose adjustments are needed in the presence of other liver disease. Changes in kinetics with improvement in hepatic function also remain unexplored.

**Severe Pulmonary Obstruction.** While a number of papers report or suggest decreased theophylline clearance in patients with severe pulmonary obstruction (7,40,50), only one paper has addressed this issue in an experimental design which allows pulmonary obstruction to be evaluated as an independent variable (48). The methods used by Powell et al (48) to evaluate theophylline kinetics at two points during hospitalization for airway obstruction have been outlined earlier in this critique (see discussion of heart failure). Twenty patients hospitalized with uncomplicated asthma or chronic bronchitis were studied within 24 hours of admission, and 16 of these patients had a second kinetic study during the same hospitalization. Whether the admitting diagnosis was asthma or chronic bronchitis had no effect on theophylline kinetics. However, severe obstruction ($FEV_1 < 1$ liter, or $PEF < 100$ L/min, or $P_{aCO2} > 45$ torr) was associated with a significant ($p < 0.01$) decrease in clearance which averaged 16% (34.4 ml/kg/hr) when compared to patients with mild or moderate obstruction (40.9 ml/kg/hr—both clearance figures for nonsmokers). None of these patients had evidence of congestive heart failure or liver disease. An impressive increase in clearance occurred among the 15 patients whose pulmonary functions improved (initial mean 44.5, final mean 53.4 ml/kg/hr, including both smokers and nonsmokers), while the one patient whose pulmonary function deteriorated showed a decrease in clearance.

This is the only study carefully investigating this problem, and the number of patients with severe obstruction was small. Further investigation to identify those clinical factors which best predict such decreased drug clearance is important, and to be definitive such a study must be prospective, involve a substantial number of patients, control for other variables (e.g., smoking, heart failure, etc.), and involve repeated clearance determinations using meticulous pharmacokinetic methods.

Though the data are limited, it does appear that theophylline dosage should be reduced by about 20% in the presence of severe obstruction, and steady-state plasma levels will be expected to decrease as pulmonary function improves.

**Respiratory Infection.** Powell et al (48) noted that their three patients with pneumonia had markedly reduced theophylline clearances when compared to those with uncomplicated asthma or chronic bronchitis (27.5 vs. 55.2 ml/kg/hr, all patients being smokers). The one patient whose pneumonia resolved had a marked increase in clearance, while the patient who deteriorated had a modest decrease in clearance, and the third patient was lost to follow up. No other authors have reported on pneumonia as a variable in prediction of theophylline clearance.

Several intriguing reports of decreased theophylline clearance during viral upper respiratory infections have appeared recently. Chang and associates (55) studied the kinetics of intravenous theophylline in ten asthmatic children during and one month after febrile upper respiratory infections. In five of the six with seroconversion, theophylline half-lives were markedly prolonged during the febrile period, while the four sero-negative children had no significant change in their theophylline half-lives. This paper reported only elimination half-lives, and used a spectrophotometric analytical method which is subject to interference by other drugs. No data are supplied on the pulmonary status of these patients, so increasing pulmonary obstruction could be involved here. Fleetham et al (56) describe a case in which a mild upper respiratory tract infection caused a marked decrease in theophylline clearance in a healthy volunteer involved in a pharmacokinetic study (32.8 ml/kg/hr while ill and $82.8 \pm 15.4$ ml/kg/hr on three separate determinations while well), as well as a slight decrease in $V_{ss}$ (0.61 L/kg while ill, $0.74 \pm 0.011$ L/kg when well). Renton has suggested that these changes are due to decreased levels of hepatic mixed function oxidases during viral illness, as observed in experimental animals (57).

This area of theophylline kinetics is clearly in flux, and definitive studies have yet to be performed. Given present knowledge, it seems prudent to use a much reduced dose of theophylline (about 40% of the usual maintenance dose) in patients with obstructive lung disease and pneumonia, and to closely monitor both clinical status and drug levels in asthmatics with upper respiratory infections (including rechecking the steady-state level after the infection has resolved).

**Smoking and Other Enzyme Inducers.** Four studies have shown that smoking increases theophylline elimination rates by from 50 to 100% (48,50,59,60). In all studies, the variation in kinetics was greater among the smoking group than among nonsmokers. The time course of this effect is not well defined. Hunt et al (59) noted a decrease in theophylline clearance in three of the four smokers who stopped smoking for three months, with a corresponding increase in elimination half-life, though these changes in the direction of nonsmokers were not statistically significant. The smokers had a slightly, but significantly, larger $V_{ss}$ than nonsmokers, though this is calculated from data following oral dosing, and bioavailability data for their dosage form was not presented.

Powell et al (60) found a significant increase in clearance among 15 nonsmokers when compared to seven heavy smokers (at least 15 cigarettes per day), with six ex-smokers (smoked at least one pack per day for a mean of 3.5 years, but stopped at least two years before the study) falling in between (and being insignificantly different from either smokers or nonsmokers). There were no differences in apparent V. No effect of smoking on $V_{ss}$ was seen in hospitalized patients with asthma or chronic bronchitis (48). Jenne and associates reported that elimination half-life was decreased in smokers (58).

Smoking clearly requires a major adjustment in theophylline dosage. Since about one-third of the American adult population abuses tobacco, the interaction of smoking with theophylline metabolism is undoubtedly one of the most frequently seen drug interactions. Time from onset of smoking to enzyme induction and the time required to return to normality after stopping smoking are not well defined. The minimum number of cigarettes required to cause a change, as well as the relationship between tobacco dose and increased theophylline clearance are also unknown. Data from Piafsky et al (63) suggest that a small amount of tobacco use may not have a sustained effect on theophylline metabolism, as the mean theophylline clearance after an intravenous dose was the same for a group of six nonsmokers and six subjects who smoked less than 10 cigarettes per day and stopped smoking three weeks prior to study. These data are at variance with those reported by Powell et al (60) (see above). As "low tar" cigarettes become increasingly popular, one must wonder if the type of cigarette smoked plays a significant role in determining theophylline clearance. The effects of parental smoking habits on theophylline metabolism in children are also unknown.

In animals, phenobarbital increases theophylline metabolism both *in vivo* and *in vitro*. (61,62). The data on the phenobarbital-theophylline interaction in man are conflicting. Piafsky et al (63) found no significant difference between theophylline disposition before and after two weeks of phenobarbital treatment. Landay and coworkers (64), on the other hand, found a significant increase in clearance following four weeks of phenobarbital treatment, which returned to baseline four weeks after discontinuation of phenobarbital in six normal subjects. Landay states that there is no change in V, though actual data are not presented. The two studies do not present their data in strictly comparable terms, as Piafsky reports clearance in L/kg/hr, while Landay used L/hr/1.73 m², and data on adiposity are not provided. Since Piafsky's study has about one chance in three of missing a 20% change in elimination half-life, it seems likely that there is a small increase in theophylline clearance following chronic phenobarbital treatment.

While very high doses of theophylline (150 mg/kg/day) have been shown to stimulate hepatic theophylline metabolism in experimental animals (61, 62), the significance of dietary methylxanthine intake in man is undefined. Allopurinol has recently been shown to have no effect of theophylline kinetics in man (65). Propranolol decreases theophylline clearance, though these drugs will probably never be used together clinically (66). The mechanisms proposed are reduction in hepatic blood flow (43, 67), and inhibition of microsomal enzymes due to binding of reactive intermediates produced during propranolol metabolism. This latter mechanism has been demonstrated in rats both *in vivo* and *in vitro* (68). Metoprolol causes a smaller decrease in theophylline clearance (66). The effects of other drugs known to interact with microsomal metabolism (e.g., phenytoin, rifampin, steroids) on theophylline kinetics remain to be studied.

Dietary factors causing induction of hepatic microsomal enzymes increase theophylline clearance (69,70). Charcoal-broiled beef at a dose of 14 oz per day for five days caused a 30% increase in theophylline clearance in eight normal volunteers (69). These values returned to pretreatment levels after seven days on the control diet. The same investigators also reported an increase in theophylline clearance in six normal subjects fed a high protein low carbohydrate diet for two weeks, with a return to control values in two weeks (70). It is not known whether this effect is due to the protein itself or to other molecules which are also present in the usual sources of protein.

The effects of xenobiotics on theophylline metabolism are generally poorly characterized, and undoubtedly there are clinically significant interactions awaiting discovery. At present, the theophylline dosage in smokers should be increased to 1.6 times that for nonsmokers, and plasma levels carefully monitored when new drugs are added to a patient's regimen.

**Dose-Dependent Theophylline Clearance.** The possibility that theophylline exhibits dose-dependent clearance is alarming. The available evidence for and against dose-dependent clearance has been reviewed by Lesko (71). The report of a theophylline overdose in a 17-month-old child gives convincing evidence for saturable elimination (72). The breakpoint in the biphasic theophylline elimination curve in this case was in the 20 to 30 µg/ml region. Serum concentrations above this had a 12.6 hour elimination half-life and below this region had a 5.4 hour half-life. The data presented in Figure 7 of the previous chapter are consistent with dose-dependent clearance, but are open to misleading interpretation. It would be useful to plot theophylline dose versus steady-state theophylline serum concentration instead of percent change for these variables. In the original study of this phenomenon by Weinberger and Ginchansky (73), the average initial and final theophylline infusion rates were 0.74 and 1.42 mg/kg/hr. Using the relationship presented in Figure 7 from the previous chapter, dose-dependent clearance might be erroneously expected if the dose was changed from 0.074 to 0.142 mg/kg/hr—ten-fold lower doses. In comparing Figure 7 with a similar curve in Weinberger and Ginchansky's report (73), the point in the curves where nonlinearity begins appear to be different. This may suggest differences in Michaelis-Menten parameters for the two samples. Indeed, there is recent evidence for population differences in theophylline pharmacokinetics in children (74). The clinical significance of these apparently dose-dependent kinetics is unclear. In a figure from Weinberger and Ginchansky's original study showing a curve fitted to their mean data for theophylline elimination, there is a very nearly linear relationship between dose and serum concentration up to a dose of 3 mg/kg/hr, a dose much higher than is generally used in patients (73). Even their curve from a patient with a much lower apparent Km is very close to linear to a dose of about 1.5 mg/kg/hr.

Sophisticated studies on the mechanism and nature of dose-dependent theophylline elimination are needed. Population estimates of Km and Vmax must be determined with an index of inter- and intrasubject variation. Are the Km and Vmax influenced by age, disease, and other drugs (e.g., caffeine)? It is possible that present dosing recommendations and labeling will require changes following answers to these questions.

## A Method For Theophylline Dosing

We can summarize the current data on theophylline kinetics with a simple method for calculating theophylline dosage in various disease states. Rather than memorizing a list of various maintenance dosages, we find it conceptually easier and more satisfying to use a standard maintenance infusion rate for normal adults, and multiply this by correction factors for various disease states to determine the actual infusion rate for any individual patient. This method has the advantage of allowing easy computation of initial dosage rates for patients with multiple disease states, e.g., a smoker with congestive heart failure and pneumonia. In patients previously treated with theophylline products, the best approach is to use the previous kinetic data, with adjustments using the appropriate factors for new disease states.

Because of the tremendous variability in critically ill patients, we have chosen an initial target plasma level of 10 µg/ml, with 95% confidence limits of 4.4 and 22.5 µg/ml, based on the data of Powell et al (48) and in close agreement with that reported by Jusko and co-workers (75). If a higher target were chosen, a substantial amount of toxicity would be expected, as the 95% confidence interval for a target of 12 µg/ml is 5 to 27 µg/ml.

To achieve an average steady state level of 10 µg/ml, an average adult with uncomplicated asthma or chronic bronchitis will require 0.5 mg/kg/hr of aminophylline. The data supporting our recommendations for various disease states have been detailed and critically reviewed earlier in this chapter. Our method for calculating loading and maintenance infusions of aminophylline in adult patients is outlined in Table 3. Because of the marked variation which exists even after correction for these various disease states, careful clinical and drug level monitoring remains very important if toxicity is to be avoided.

TABLE 3.   RECOMMENDATIONS FOR INTRAVENOUS AMINOPHYLLINE
DOSAGE IN ADULTS

---

1. Loading Infusion: 6 mg/kg (at rate no faster than 0.2 mg/kg/min).
   a. If plasma theophylline concentration before loading is estimated to be greater than 0, calculate the reduced loading infusion as

$$\text{LD (mg/kg)} = (10 \text{ µg/ml} - \text{current concentration})/1.6$$

2. Maintenance dose (IV aminophylline)
   Infusion rate (mg/kg/hr) = 0.5 mg/kg/hr × Disease Factor(s)

| Disease State | Factor |
|---|---|
| Nonsmoker | 1.0 |
| Smoker | 1.6 |
| Congestive heart failure | 0.4 |
| Pneumonia | 0.4? |
| Cirrhosis | 0.4 |
| Severe obstruction | 0.8 |

Example: a. 60 kg male smoker with heart failure and moderate COPD:
   Infusion rate = 0.5 mg/kg/hr × 60 kg × 1.6 × 0.4 = 19.2 mg/hr
   b. 75 kg cirrhotic with severe asthma ($P_{aCO2}$ = 50 mm Hg)
   Infusion rate = 0.5 mg/kg/hr × 75 kg × 0.4 × 0.8 = 12 mg/hr

---

In an effort to increase the therapeutic index of theophylline in critically ill patients, Vozeh et al (76) have developed a protocol to estimate individual clearance and perform early dosage adjustments, using the two-point method for rapid estimation of drug clearance of Chiou and coworkers (77). Following an initial loading dose and maintenance infusion adjusted for disease states, plasma theophylline levels were determined at 1 and 5 hours after the infusion began, and total body clearance (TBC) of theophylline calculated as:

$$TBC = \frac{2K_o}{Cp_1 + Cp_2} + \frac{2V\,(Cp_1 - Cp_2)}{(Cp_1 + Cp_2)(t_2 - t_1)}$$

where $Cp_1$ and $Cp_2$ are the plasma concentrations at times $t_1$ and $t_2$ respectively, $K_0$ the infusion rate, and V the apparent volume of distribution (assumed to be 0.5 L/kg by Vozeh et al). (For the derivation of this equation, see reference 77).

If needed, a repeat bolus was given to raise plasma levels to the steady-state target concentration desired by the clinician, and the infusion rate set to equal the calculated TBC. Using this method, all 15 patients had steady-rate theophylline concentrations very close to the desired goal (mean difference from goal ± standard deviation— 0.1 ± 1.58 µg/ml, ranging from −3.4 to +3.0 µg/ml from goal. Use of the standard infusion rates, even though corrected for smoking, heart failure, and liver disease, resulted in a mean prediction error ± standard deviation of 3.8 ± 13.2 µg/ml, with the actual error ranging from −9.4 to +31.5 µg/ml.

While this method appears ideal for optimizing theophylline therapy, it does require an extremely reliable laboratory which is both willing and able to rapidly and reproducibly measure theophylline concentrations 24 hours a day, exact notation of the times when plasma samples are drawn, and infusion of theophylline at a constant and reliable rate.

Both worsening and improving disease states will change theophylline clearance, necessitating re-adjustment of the dosage as the clinical status changes (48,78).

## Conclusion

In conclusion, solid data on which to base clinical decisions regarding theophylline dosing are limited. While the toxic range is fairly well defined, our current notions of the therapeutic concentration range require further study. The efficacy of theophylline in treatment of chronic obstructive pulmonary disease (as opposed to acute asthma) has never been adequately demonstrated, despite the many thousands of courses of aminophyline given each year for this condition.

There are convincing data that doses must be reduced in heart failure, cirrhosis, and severe pulmonary obstruction, and increased for smokers. There are inconclusive, but suggestive, data that upper respiratory infection as well as pneumonia decrease theophylline clearance. Use of an initial maintenance infusion derived from Table 3 will avoid serious toxicity in almost all patients. Still, there is marked interpatient variability, as indicated by the wide confidence intervals of the resulting levels. Further individualization of infusion rates using the method of Chiou et al (76,77) should give excellent control of serum levels and allow maximum therapeutic benefit while minimizing the risk of toxicity. As pulmonary obstruction and heart failure improve, doses will need to be increased to maintain therapeutic effects.

Much research remains to be performed to define theophylline kinetics in varying states of liver disease, in varying degrees of heart failure, and in the presence of respiratory infections, as well as to determine the significance of other drug effects on theophylline elimination, and to determine the significance of alleged dose-dependent kinetics. Particular attention needs to be given to careful studies extending the acute dose-response data to chronic treatment situations, as the present literature has little to offer on this important issue.

Though our focus has been primarily pharmacologic, decisions regarding both efficacy and toxicity in the individual patient are based on clinical evaluation. We strongly concur with the preceding authors that drug levels and pharmacokinetic expertise remain an important aid to, but not a substitute for, careful observation and good clinical judgment.

Supported by research grant 5T32-GMO7533 from the National Institutes of Health, U.S. Public Health Service, Department of Health, Education, and Welfare.

## REFERENCES

1. Turner-Warwick M: Study of theophylline plasma levels after oral administration of new theophylline compounds. Brit Med J 1957; 2:67–69.
2. Pierson WE, Bierman CW, Stamm SJ, Van Arsdel PP: Double-blind trial of aminophylline in status asthmatious. Pediatrics 1971; 48:642–646.
3. Maselli R, Casal G, Ellis EF: Pharmacologic effects of intravenously administered aminophylline in asthmatic children. J Peds 1970; 76:777–782.
4. Mitenko PA and Ogilvie RI: Rational intravenous doses of theophylline. N Engl J Med 1973; 289:600–603.
5. Bierman CW, Shapiro GG, Pierson WE, Dorsett CW: Acute and chronic theophylline therapy in exercise-induced bronchospasm. Pediatrics 1977; 60:845–849.

6. Pollack J, Kieckel F, Cooper D, Weinberger M: Relationship of serum theophylline concentration to inhibition of exercise-induced bronchospasm and comparison with cromolyn. Pediatrics 1977; 60:840–844.
7. Jenne JW, Wyze E, Rood FS, MacDonald FM: Pharmacokinetics of theophylline. Application to adjustment of clinical dose of aminophylline. Clin Pharmacol Ther 1972; 13:349–360.
8. Weinberger MM and Bronsky EA: Evaluation of oral bronchodilator therapy in asthmatic children. J Peds 1974; 84:421–427.
9. Svedmyr K, Mellstrand T, Svedmyr N: A comparison between effects of aminopylline, proxyphylline, and terbutaline in asthma. Scand J Resp Dis 1977; (Suppl. No. 101) 139–146.
10. Alexander MR, Dull WL, Kasik JE: The treatment of chronic obstructive pulmonary disease with oral theophylline: A double-blind controlled study. Clin Pharmacol Ther 1980; (Abstract) 27:243–244.
11. Eaton ML and Niewoehner DE: Efficacy of theophylline in "irreversible" airway obstruction. Clin Pharmacol Ther 1980; (Abstract) 27:251.
12. Shapiro GG, Bamman J, Kanarek P, Bierman CW: The paradoxical effect of adrenergic and methylxanthine drugs in cystic fibrosis. Pediatrics 1976; 58:740–743.
13. Rebuck AS and Read J: Assessment and management of severe asthma. Am J Med 1971; 51:788–798.
14. Thiringer G and Svedmyr N: Comparison of infused and inhaled terbutaline in patients with asthma. Scand J Resp Dis 1977; (Supplement 101) 95–96.
15. Larsson S and Svedmyr N: A comparison of two modes of administering beta$_2$-adrenoceptor stimulants in asthmatics: Tablets and metered aerosol. Scand J Resp Dis 1977; (Supplement 101) 79–83.
16. Hartnett BJS and Marlin GE: Comparison of oral theophylline and salbutamol by inhalation in asthmatic patients. Br J Clin Pharmac 1976; 3:591–594.
17. Svedmyr K, Mellstrand T, Svedmyr N: A comparison between effects of aminophylline, proxyphylline, and terbutaline in asthmatics. Scand J Resp Dis 1977; (Supplement #1) 139–146.
18. Dyson AJ and Campbell IA: Interaction between choline theophyllinate and salmefamol in patients with reversible airways obstruction. Br J Clin Pharmac 1977; 4:677–682.
19. Sims JA, do Pico GA, Reed CE: Bronchodilating effect of oral theophylline-ephedrine combination. J Allergy Clin Immunol 1978; 62:15–21.
20. Campbell IA, Middleton WG, McHardy GJR, Shotter MV, McKenzie R, Kay AB: Interaction between isoprenaline and aminophylline in asthma. Thorax 1977; 32:424–428.
21. Wolfe JD, Tashkin DP, Calvarese B, Simmons M: Bronchodilator effects of terbutaline and aminophylline alone and in combination in asthmatic patients. N Engl J Med 1978; 298:363–367.
22. Marlin GE, Hartnett BJS, Berend N, Hacket NB: Assessment of combined oral theophylline and inhaled β-adrenoceptor against bronchodilator therapy. Br J Clin Pharmac 1978; 5:45–50.
23. Billing B, Dahlqvist R, Garle M, Hornblad Y and Ripe E: Theophylline and terbutaline in asthma. Br J Dis Chest 1979; (Abstract) 73:423.
24. Evans WV and Monie RDH: Aminophylline, salbutamol, and combined intravenous infusions in acute severe asthma. Br J Dis Chest 1979; (Abstract) 73:428.
25. Svedmyr K and Svedmyr N: Combined therapy with theophylline and Beta$_2$-adrenostimulants in asthmatics. Br J Dis Chest 1979; (Abstract) 73:424.
26. Josephson GW, MacKenzie EJ, Lietman PS, Gibson C: Emergency treatment of asthma: A comparison of two treatment regimens. JAMA 1979; 242:639–643.

27. Hambleton G, Weinberger M, Taylor J, Gavanaugh M, Ginchansky E, Godfrey S, Tooley M, Bell T, Greenberg S: Comparison of chromoglycate and theophylline in controlling symptoms of chronic asthma. Lancet 1977; 1:381–385.

28. Greden JF, Fontaine P, Lubetsky M, Chamberlin K: Anxiety and depression associated with caffeinism among psychiatric inpatients. Am J Psychiatry 1978; 135:963–966.

29. DeFreitas B and Schwartz G: Effects of caffeine in chronic psychiatric patients. Am J Psychiatry 1979; 136:1337–1338.

30. Banner AS, Sunderrajan EV, Agarwal MK, Addington WW: Arrhythmogenic effects of orally administered bronchodilators. Arch Intern Med 1979; 139:434–437.

31. Foster LJ, Trudeau WL, Goldman AL: Bronchodilator effects on gastric acid secretion. JAMA 1979; 241:2613–2615.

32. Walker JE, Lewin E, Moffit B: Production of epileptiform discharges by application of agents which increase cyclic AMP levels in rat cortex. Proceedings of the Hans Berger Centennial Symposium, Edinburgh, Scotland, 1973. In Harris P and Maudsley C (Editors): *Epilepsy*, Churchill Livingston, Edinburgh, 1974. pp. 30–36.

33. Axelrod J, Weil-Malherbe H, Tonchick R: The physiologic disposition of $H^3$-epinephrine and its metabolite metanephrine. J Pharmacol Exper Ther 1959; 127:251–256.

34. Bodin NO, Hansson E, Ramsay CH, Ryrfeldt A: The tissue distribution of $^3H$-terbutaline in mice. Acta Physiol Scand 1972; 84:40–47.

35. Smith JM and Devey GF: Clinical trial of disodium cromoglycate in treatment of asthma in children. Brit Med J 1968; 2:340–344.

36. Hyde JS, Isenberg PD, Floro LD: Short and long-term prophylaxis with cromolyn sodium in chronic asthma. Chest 1973; 63:875– 880.

37. Jackson RH, McHenry JI, Moreland FB, Raymer WJ, Etter RL: Clinical evaluation of elixophyllin with correlation of pulmonary function studies and theophylline serum levels in acute and chronic asthmatic patients. Dis Chest 1964; 45:75–85.

38. Schluger J, McGinn JT, Hennessy DJ: Comparative theophylline blood levels following the oral administration of three different theophylline preparations. Amer J Med Sci 1957; 233:296–302.

39. Levy G and Koysooko R: Pharmacokinetic analysis of the effect of theophylline on pulmonary function in asthmatic children. J Ped 1975; 86:789–793.

40. Hendeles L, Bighley L, Richardson RH, Hepler CD, Carmichael J: Frequent toxicity from I.V. aminophylline infusions in critically ill patients. Drug Intell Clin Pharm 1977; 11:12–18.

41. Jacobs MH, Senior RM, Kessler G: Clinical experience with theophylline: Relationships between dosage, serum concentration, and toxicity. JAMA 1976; 235:1983–1986.

42. Kordash TR, Van Dellen RG, McCall JT: Theophylline concentrations in asthmatic patients after administration of aminophylline. JAMA 1977; 238:139–141.

43. Blaschke, TF: Protein binding and kinetics of drugs in liver diseases. Clin Pharmacokinetics 1977; 2:32–44.

44. Spann JF and Hurst JW: Treatment of heart failure, in JW Hurst, RB Logue, RC Schlant and NK Wenger, eds., *The Heart*, 4th ed., McGraw-Hill, New York, 1978. p. 580–586.

45. Braunwald E: Heart failure, in KJ Isselbacher, RD Adams, E Braunwald, RG Petersdorf and JD Wilson, eds. *Harrison's Principles of Internal Medicine,* 9th ed., McGraw-Hill, New York, 1980, p. 1035–1044.

46. Camarata SJ, Weil MH, Hanashiro PK and Shubin H: Cardiac arrest in the critically ill. Circulation 1971; 44:688–695.

47. Piafsky KM, Sitar DS, Rangno RE and Ogilvie RI: Theophylline kinetics in acute pulmonary edema. Clin Pharmacol Ther 1977; 21:310–316.

48. Powell JR, Vozeh S, Hopewell P, Costello J, Sheiner LB, and Riegelman S.: Theophylline disposition in acutely ill hospitalized patients, Am Rev Resp Dis 1978; 118:229–238.

49. Jenne JW, Chick TW, Miller BA, and Strickland RD: Apparent theophylline half-life fluctuations in acute left ventricular failure. Am J Hosp Pharm 1977; 34:408–409.

50. Weinberger MW, Matthay RA, Ginchansky EJ, Chidsey CA and Petty TL: Intravenous aminophylline dosage. JAMA 1976; 235:2110–2113.

51. Vicuna N, McNay JL, Ludden TM and Schwertner H: Impaired theophylline clearance in patients with cor pulmonale. Br J Clin Pharmac 1979; 7:33–37.

52. Piafsky KM, Sitar DS, Rangno RE and Ogilvie RI: Theophylline disposition in patients with hepatic cirrhosis. N Engl J Med 1977; 296:1495–1497.

53. Mangione A, Imhoff TE, Lee RV, Shum LY and Jusko WJ: Pharmacokinetics of theophylline in hepatic disease. Chest 1978; 73:616–622.

54. Zwillich CW, Sutton FD Jr, Neff TA, Cohn WM, Matthay RA and Weinberger MW: Theophylline-induced seizures in adults. Ann Int Med 1975; 82:784–878.

55. Chang KC, Lauer BA, Bell TD and Chai H: Altered theophylline pharmacokinetics during acute respiratory viral illness. Lancet 1978; 1:1132–1133.

56. Fleetham JA, Nakatsu K and Munt PW: Theophylline pharmacokinetics and respiratory infections. Lancet 1978; 2:898.

57. Renton KW: Theophylline pharmacokinetics in in respiratory viral illnesses. Lancet 1978; 2:160–161.

58. Jenne J, Nagasawa H, McHugh R, MacDonald F and Wyse E: Decreased theophylline half-life in cigarette smokers. Life Sci 1975; 17:195–198.

59. Hunt SN, Jusko WJ and Yurchak AM: Effect of smoking on theophylline disposition. Clin Pharmacol Ther 1976; 19:546–551.

60. Powell JR, Thiercelin JF, Vozeh S, Sansom L and Riegelman S: The influence of cigarette smoking and sex on theophylline disposition. Am Rev Resp Dis 1977; 116:17–23.

61. Lohmann SM and Meich RP: Theophylline metabolism by the rat liver microsomal system. J Pharmacol Exp Ther 1976; 196:213–225.

62. Williams JR and Szentivanyi A: Implications of hepatic drug metabolizing activity in the therapy of bronchial asthma. J Allergy Clin Immunol 1975; (Abstract) 55:125.

63. Piafsky KM, Sitar DS, Ogilvie RI: Effect of phenobarbital on the disposition of intravenous theophylline. Clin Pharmacol Ther 1977; 22:336–389.

64. Landay RA, Gonzalez MA, Taylor JC: Effect of phenobarbital on theophylline disposition. J Allergy Clin Immunol 1978; 62:27–29.

65. Vozeh S, Powell JR, Cupit GC, Riegelman S, Sheiner LB: Influence of allopurinol on theophylline disposition in adults. Clin Pharmacol Ther 1980; 27:194–197.

66. Conrad KM, Nyman DW: Influence of metoprolol and propranolol on theophylline elimination. Abstract, World Congress on Clinical Pharmacology and Therapeutics, London, August, 1980.

67. Greenblatt DJ, Franke K, Huffman DH: Impairment of antipyrine clearance in humans by propranolol. Circulation 1978; 57:1161–1164.

68. Pritchard JF, Schneck DW, Hayes AH, Jr: The inhibition of rat hepatic microsomal propranolol metabolism by a covalently bound reactive metabolite. Res Comm Chem Path Pharmacol 1980; 27:211–222.

69. Kappas A, Alvares AP, Anderson KE, Pantuck EJ, Pantuck CB, Chang R, Cooney AH: Effect of charcoal-broiled beef on antipyrine and theophylline metabolism. Clin Pharmacol Ther 1978; 23:445–450.

70. Kappas A, Anderson KE, Conney AH, Alvares AP: Influence of dietary protein and carbohydrate on antipyrine and theophylline metabolism in man. Clin Pharmacol Ther 1977; 20:643–653.

71. Lesko LJ: Dose-dependent elimination kinetics of theophylline. Clin Pharmacokinetics 1979; 4:449–459.
72. Kadlec GJ, Jarboe CH, Pollard SJ, Sublett JL: Acute theophylline intoxication. Biphasic first order elimination kinetics in a child. Ann Allergy 1978; 41:337–339.
73. Weinberger M and Ginchansky E: Dose-dependent kinetics of theophylline disposition in asthmatic children. J Peds 1977; 91:820–824.
74. Bell T, Yaffe S, Lecks H, Danish M, Ragni M, Simon T, Katsampes C: Theophylline pharmacokinetics: Variation between two study populations using oral oxtriphylline syrup. Ann Allergy 1980; 44:67–70.
75. Jusko WJ, Koup JR, Vance JW, Schentag JJ, Kuritzky PM: Intravenous theophylline therapy: Nomogram guidelines. Ann Int Med 1977; 86:400–404.
76. Vozeh S, Kewitz G, Follath F: Accurate prediction of theophylline serum concentrations using a rapid estimation of theophylline clearance. Clin Pharmacol Ther 1980; (Abstract) 27:291.
77. Chiou WL, Gadella MAF, Peng GW: Method for the rapid estimation of the total body drug clearance and adjustment of dosage regimens in patients during a constant-rate intravenous infusion. J Pharm Biopharm 1978; 6:135–151.
78. Vozeh S, Powell JR, Riegelman S, Costello JF, Sheiner LB, Hopewell P: Changes in theophylline clearance during acute illness. JAMA 1978; 240:1882–1884.

*Counterpoint Discussion:*

# Theophylline

## Antoinette Mangione, Pharm.D.

Theophylline is an agent that has fascinated pharmacokineticists for a number of years. Due to this fascination, there is a wealth of literature and viewpoints on the clinical application of the pharmacokinetic data. A review of the excellent theophylline monograph of Dr. Hendeles and co-workers compels this investigator to re-emphasize selected points and offer additional information. All comments will follow the format of the monograph.

### Distribution

Data from Gal et al (1) suggest that theophylline is indeed distributed into body fat. A linear increase in apparent volume of distribution (V) as total body weight (TBW) increases was demonstrated. When V was normalized for body weight, V best correlated with TBW. In obese subjects mean V was 0.77 L/kg using ideal body weight (IBW) vs 0.38 L/kg using TBW. In normal subjects V averaged 0.52 L/kg IBW and 0.48 TBW. Since apparent volume of distribution determines the initial serum concentration following the loading dose, this observation is an important one. The results suggest that a weight approaching that of TBW rather than IBW should be utilized to calculate the loading dose.

A large and variable decrease in the protein binding of theophylline in cirrhotic patients has been observed (29, SD ± 16%) (2). On the average, this results in doubling of the free fraction of theophylline (35 to 71%). As in neonates, the large increase in free fraction is of concern since the quantitative response to a given concentration of theophylline may be increased. It should be noted that selected cirrhotic patients may have a therapeutic response at levels normally considered subtherapeutic.

## Elimination

A study of 200 theophylline patients by Jusko et al (3) examined various factors that may affect theophylline clearance. The relative importance of age, obesity, sex, pregnancy, liver disease, congestive heart failure, and history of use of theophylline, steroids, tobacco, marijuana, caffeine, ethanol, oral contraceptives and various enzyme inducers was examined using the computer program NYBAID (4) which determines the priority, order and combinations of independent variables correlating with body clearance. The factors identified to be of primary importance in determining the clearance of theophylline include smoking (cigarette and marijuana), age, liver and cardiac disease (Figure 1). Population analysis such as this becomes of major importance for maintenance dosing of an agent whose clearance is affected by so many factors.

As previously stated, smoking has clearly been identified in young adults as a major factor affecting theophylline clearance (see monograph). In addition, heavy smoking has also been observed to offset the diminished clearance found in patients greater than 40-years-old with moderate to severe congestive heart failure (3). A question that is still unanswered is the duration of time necessary to dissipate the inducing effect of smoking on theophylline metabolism. Heavy smokers who stopped smoking for at least three months experienced only a small decrease in clearance (5). The mean clearance of subjects who had not smoked for at least two years was noted to lie midway between that of heavy and nonsmokers (6). This suggests that more than three months and perhaps over two years is required to fully negate the effect of cigarette smoking in heavy smokers (generally defined as greater than 15 cigarettes/day). After discontinuation of smoking, careful monitoring is important to help prevent toxicity as clearance decreases.

Diet is another factor that has been observed to affect the elimination of theophylline. While a high protein diet (7) and charcoal-broiled foods (8) increase elimination rate, dietary methylxanthines (primarily caffeine) (9) and a high carbohydrate diet (7) have been found to decrease elimination rate in normal volunteers.

Phenobarbital has been noted to increase the elimination rate of theophylline under clinical conditions (3) and in normal volunteers after four weeks of administration (10). Others found no effect after shorter duration treatment in normal volunteers (11).

Theophylline elimination rate is also increased by hemodialysis. Dialysis clearances of theophylline averaging 32.8 ($\pm$6.3) ml/min (12) and 88.5 ($\pm$9.2) ml/min (13) have been reported. The higher dialysis clearance seen in the later study is ascribed to greater blood flow rate through the dialyzer and different dialysis equipment. These data indicate that hemodialysis may increase theophylline clearance one-half to twofold in normal smoking adults and as much as two to sixfold in patients with cirrhosis or congestive heart failure. Another technique that increases theophylline elimination rate is charcoal hemoperfusion. This technique has successfully been employed in cases of theophylline overdose (14,15).

Total Body Clearance of Theophylline, ml/hr/kg  IBW

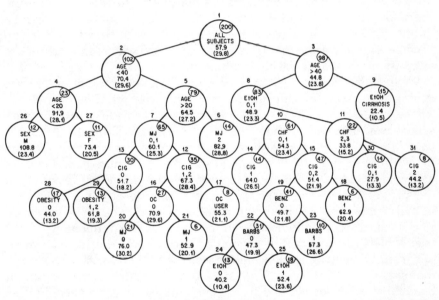

FIGURE 1   Cascade of factors determining theophylline total body clearances. The NYBAID statistical computer program was used to seek the order, priority and combinations of independent variables that correlate with theophylline clearances. The circles list the number of subjects (circled), descriptive factor, group mean and standard deviation (in parentheses).

Description of variables: O = no use; MJ = marijuana, 1 = <1 and 2 = ≥2 joints/week; ETOH = ethanol use, 1 = social drinker; CHF = congestive heart failure, 1 = mild, 2 = moderate, 3 = severe; CIG = cigarette, 1 = <1 and 2 = ≥1 pack/day; OC = oral contraceptives, 1 = user; BENZ = benzodiazepine, 1 = user; BARBS = barbiturate, 1 = user; OBESITY, 1 = 15–55% and 2 = >55% overweight.

## Continued Therapy

It is undisputed that maintenance dosage guidelines are essential for a drug like theophylline. The difficulty lies with simply and rationally applying the wealth of published theophylline pharmacokinetic data to maintenance dosing. A maintenance dose of theophylline can be estimated for various patient groups from the following steady-state pharmacokinetic equation:

$$\frac{\text{Dose}}{\tau} = C_{ss} \times Cl_{B}$$

Where the dose is given at time intervals ($\tau$), $C_{ss}$ is the desired steady-state serum concentration (10 to 12 $\mu$g/ml), and $Cl_{B}$ is the body clearance of theophylline. Using the mean body clearances of theophylline listed by Hendeles et al in Table 1 of the monograph, the average maintenance dose for each group can be calculated. However, this can become a cumbersome and time-consuming procedure. In attempts to simplify maintenance dosing, many guidelines have been proposed.

We have summarized recent recommendations for the maintenance dosing of theophylline in adults (including that of Hendeles et al). These guidelines (Table 1) are intended to achieve a steady-state serum concentration of theophylline of 10 $\mu$g/ml. Table 1 illustrates that in most patient groups a reasonable consensus has been reached for maintenance dosing of theophylline. The patient groups listed in Table 1 include the factors identified by the surveillance study of Jusko et al (3) to be the major factors affecting theophylline clearance, namely smoking, age, liver and cardiac disease. The wide variation in clearance observed in hepatic cirrhosis and acute pulmonary edema (see Table 1, monograph) in particular necessitates the measurement of serum concentration of theophylline. For patients with severe pulmonary edema, Piafsky et al (16) state that a maintenance dose cannot be safely recommended due to the extreme variance in theophylline clearance (0.067 to 2.35 ml/kg/min). The authors suggest that only a loading dose be administered since patients with acute left ventricular failure are often improved clinically within a few hours of initiating treatment.

A point worthy of re-emphasis is the need for rapid analysis and interpretation of theophylline serum concentrations. Unfortunately, in many institutions the capability for measuring serum concentrations of theophylline is limited. In addition, a recent study of serum theophylline assay utilization in a hospitalized population has identified major problems in the use of the assay (Kimelblatt et al, not yet published). First, the timing of the serum sample was not specified in

TABLE 1. A COMPARISON OF VARIOUS MAINTENANCE DOSE RECOMMENDATIONS FOR ADULTS.
(Intended to achieve a theophylline steady-state concentration of 10 μg/ml)

| Patient Group | Further Division | Theophylline mg/kg/hr* | References |
|---|---|---|---|
| Otherwise Healthy Nonsmoking Adults | — | 0.4 | monograph |
| | — | 0.43 | 17 |
| | >20 y.o. | 0.53* | 3 |
| Otherwise Healthy Smoking Adults | | 0.6 | monograph |
| | >10 cig/day × 2 yrs | 0.68 | 17 |
| | 20–40 y.o. >1 pack/day | 0.67* | 3 |
| | 20–40 y.o. marijuana >2 joints/wk | 0.83* | 3 |
| Hepatic Cirrhosis | — | 0.2 | monograph |
| | — | 0.17 | 17 |
| | Serum bilirubin >1.5 mg/dl | 0.14 | 2 |
| | Serum bilirubin <1.5 mg/dl | 0.32 | 2 |
| Congestive Heart Failure | — | 0.2 | monograph |
| | — | 0.17 | 17 |
| | Nonsmokers or < 1 pack/day | 0.28* | 3 |
| | Smokers > 1 pack/day | 0.44* | 3 |
| | Acute Pulmonary Edema | ** | 16 |

*Based on ideal body weight
**Maintenance dose not recommended

45%. Second, 20% of the assays ordered did not reach the chart. The third, and perhaps the most significant problem, lies with inappropriate use of assay results. In 36% of the assays, dosage alterations were not carried out when indicated. The assay results appeared to be ignored. Steps should be undertaken in all institutions to help minimize such problems with theophylline assays.

## Formulations

Since the marketing of sustained release theophylline products with reliable and complete absorption characteristics, these products have generally become the formulation of choice for chronic treatment of rapid theophylline metabolizers. However, the therapeutic advantage of sustained release preparations is likely to be less marked in the older age population, especially nonsmokers and those with organ impairment. Due to prolonged serum t½ in these patients (Table 1, monograph), safe and efficacious serum levels may be maintained with a non-sustained release product given at intervals of eight hours or greater. Thus in slower eliminators of theophylline, uncoated aminophylline may be the formulation of choice for chronic oral treatment since this product can be administered at one-half or less of the expense of sustained release theophylline products.

## REFERENCES

1. Gal P, Jusko WJ, Yurchack AM: Theophylline disposition in obesity. Clin Pharmacol Ther 1978; 23:438–444.
2. Mangione A, Imhoff TE, Lee RV, et al: Pharmacokinetics of theophylline in liver disease. Chest 1978; 73:616–622.
3. Jusko WJ, Gardner MJ, Mangione A, et al: Factors affecting theophylline clearances: Age, tobacco, marijuana, cirrhosis, congestive heart failure, obesity, oral contraceptives, benzodiazepines, barbiturates and ethanol. J Pharm Sci 1979; 68:1358–1366.
4. Sonquist JA, Morgan JN: The detection of interaction effects, monograph No. 35, Survey Research Center, Institute for Social Research, University of Michigan (1964) as program NYBAID by the Computing Center of the State University of New York.
5. Hunt SN, Jusko WJ, Yurchak AM: Effect of smoking on theophylline disposition in man. Clin Pharmacol Ther 1976; 19:546–551.
6. Powell JR, Thiercelin JF, Vozeh S, et al: The influence of cigarette smoking and sex on theophylline disposition. Am Rev Resp Dis 1977; 116:17–23.
7. Kappas A, Anderson KE, Conney AH, et al: Influence of dietary protein and carbohydrate on antipyrine and theophylline metabolism in man. Clin Pharmacol Ther 1977; 20:643–653.
8. Kappas A, Alvares AP, Anderson KE, et al: Effect of charcoal-broiled beef on antipyrine and theophylline metabolism. Clin Pharmacol Ther 1978; 23:445–450.

9. Caldwell J, Lancaster R, Monks J, et al: The influence of dietary methylxanthines on the metabolism and pharmacokinetics of intravenously administered theophylline. Br J Clin Pharmacol 1977; 4:637–638.

10. Landay RA, Gonzalez MA, Taylor JC: Effect of phenobarbital on theophylline disposition. J Allergy Clin Immun 1978; 62:27–29.

11. Piafsky KM, Sitar DS, Ogilvie RI: Effect of phenobarbital on the disposition of intravenous theophylline. Clin Pharmacol Ther 1977; 22:336–339.

12. Levy G, Gibson T, Whitman W, et al: Hemodialysis clearance of theophylline. J Am Med Assoc 1977; 14:1466–1467.

13. Lee C, Marbury T, Perrin J, et al: Hemodialysis of theophylline in uremic patients. J Clin Pharmacol 1979; 19:219–226.

14. Ehlers SM, Zaske DE, Sawchuk RJ: Massive theophylline overdose; Rapid elimination by charcoal hemoperfusion. J Am Med Assoc 1978; 240:474–475.

15. Russo ME: Management of theophylline intoxication with charcoal-column hemoperfusion. N Engl J Med 1979; 300:24–26.

16. Piafsky KM, Sitar DS, Rangno RE, et al: Theophylline kinetics in acute pulmonary edema. Clin Pharmacol Ther 1977; 21:310–316.

17. Powell JR, Vozeh S, Hopewell P, et al: Theophylline disposition in acutely ill hospitalized patients. Am Rev Resp Dis 1978; 118:229–238.

# 7

# Aminoglycosides

Jerome J. Schentag, Pharm.D.

## INTRODUCTION/BACKGROUND

The aminoglycoside antibiotics are frequently chosen drugs in the treatment of life threatening gram negative bacterial infections. These agents are bactericidal *in vitro* and probably *in vivo,* and their activity is often synergistic with that of β-lactam antibiotics (penicillins and cephalosporins). For this reason the combination of aminoglycosides and either β-lactam antibiotics or clindamycin is one of the most frequently used regimens in acutely ill patients.

All aminoglycosides are both oto- and nephrotoxic, and a low margin of safety is their sole disadvantage. Close monitoring is always indicated when seriously ill patients are given aminoglycosides. These antibiotics are among the most frequently selected agents for pharmacokinetic consultation and monitoring (1,2) because of their narrow therapeutic window. Even though pharmacokinetic monitoring of aminoglycosides is widespread, there is a general lack of consensus regarding appropriate criteria for clinical applications. There is no precise definition of the therapeutic peak and trough concentration range for aminoglycosides, which is compounded by the fact that the appropriate pharmacokinetic model is controversial. Finally, although numerous authors recommend therapeutic monitoring because serum levels are not predictable (3,4), other clinical studies challenge the value of serum levels, and point out their inability to avoid drug toxicity (5).

This chapter is written to address these issues, and attempt to lend perspective. It is hoped that the time period between universal availability of blood levels and the eventual optimal use of blood levels can be shortened by this critical review of our current knowledge and our present practices.

Of the several thousand aminoglycoside molecules synthesized in laboratories and by fungi, only three are commonly used in the treatment of human disease. These include gentamicin, tobramycin and amikacin. Netilmicin and perhaps sisomicin may also be introduced within the next two to four years. Most of the following discussion will also be applicable to netilmicin and sisomicin, as it is unlikely that either of these agents will demonstrate major differences in spectrum or toxicity.

Kanamycin and streptomycin are older drugs being used less and less frequently. Their few remaining indications are quite specialized. Kanamycin remains popular in the treatment of infections in neonates. However, bacterial resistance has been increasing, and the future of this indication is unclear. Streptomycin is occasionally employed as an adjunct in the treatment of group D streptococcal endocarditis or tuberculosis, although newer drugs are replacing streptomycin for both of these indications.

## Absorption

Patients must receive aminoglycosides by either the intramuscular or intravenous route, because the drugs are not absorbed from the gastrointestinal tract. The drugs are water soluble, and are completely absorbed from intramuscular injection sites in normal volunteers. Completeness of intramuscular (IM) absorption is seldom a problem in ambulatory patients, but the reliability of IM absorption after repeated injections into the same site might be questioned if peak blood levels are lower than expected. Intramuscular administration is never completely reliable in critically ill patients (52) and is best avoided.

Intravenous infusion is the preferred administration route for most aminoglycosides. The drugs are diluted in 25 to 100 mls of dextrose or saline, and infused over 15 to 60 minutes. Although shorter infusion times invariably result in elevated but transient peaks, this transient peak is of no apparent therapeutic or toxicologic significance, even though it usually exceeds 12 µg/ml.

Because high but transient peaks have little toxicologic significance, aminoglycosides might also be given by rapid intravenous injection (6,7,8), but we point out that this route is not approved in the manufacturer's package insert. Continuous intravenous infusion has also been employed, primarily in critically ill patients with infections complicating malignancy (9,10,11). However, since animal studies provide evidence that continuous infusion is more nephrotoxic than intermittent injection (12), continuous infusion cannot be recommended unless it can be shown more effective in the management of life threatening infections.

Topical use of the systemic aminoglycosides gentamicin, tobramycin or amikacin, should be discouraged because the widespread low level exposure will increase bacterial resistance. Neomycin and kanamycin are given orally for gut sterilization, little absorption occurs, and short term use of this method can be highly successful. Both are also used in the surgical washing of body cavities. Drug absorption during irrigation is appreciable (13,14), and both oto- and nephrotoxicity have resulted from the topical use of neomycin as an irrigant (14,15). Neomycin may shortly be withdrawn due to its toxicity when used as a wound irrigant (Federal Register, July 23, 1979).

## Distribution

Following intravenous administration, the drugs rapidly distribute to highly perfused organs and within extracellular water, and a very rapid distributive phase (half-life: 5 to 15 minutes) can be quantitated. After completion of this early distributive phase, a second phase of serum concentration decline begins. In adults, this second phase half-life is approximately 2.0 hours if renal function is normal, but the second phase half-life increases in proportion to decline in creatinine clearance (CCr). Because of its primary dependence on renal function, the second phase is used both in dosing and therapeutic monitoring. Although a one compartment model is usually chosen, two processes are occurring during this second phase. As serum levels decline, most of the drug is being excreted unchanged by glomerular filtration, while the remainder is being taken up by body tissues (16).

A third phase of serum level decline is first noted 8 to 24 hours after either a single dose or after the final dose in a multiple dose regimen. In all age groups, the half-life of this phase normally exceeds 100 hours (17,18,19,20,21). During the third phase, intracellularly bound aminoglycoside is released and excreted unchanged in urine (17,18,21). Because aminoglycosides are tightly bound intracellularly, and slowly released, and since any circulating drug that is available to the kidney is rapidly excreted, the rate-limiting step in the terminal phase is drug release from tissues.

After dosing, aminoglycosides readily distribute throughout extracellular water. Serum protein binding is low, and ranges 0 to 20% (27,28,29). Aminoglycoside protein binding is affected by ion concentrations, and will be reported as variable until all influencing factors are identified or controlled.

Interstitial fluid concentrations peak about 4 hours after the dose, and are one-fourth to one-half as high as serum (22,23,24). The delayed peak in interstitial fluid is further evidence that the second phase in serum decline is also influenced by distribution.

Most body fluids also have readily measurable concentrations of aminoglycosides. The drugs are measurable in nonobstructed bile (30,31,31), in synovial fluid (33), in renal lymph fluid (34,35), in sputum and bronchial secretions (36,37,38,39), and in pleural fluid. Most of this distribution data has been generated from single dose studies, and it is notable that concentrations at all of these sites will also rise slowly during multiple dosing.

In contrast to most body fluid barriers, aminoglycosides do not pass the blood brain barrier in therapeutically adequate concentrations. To achieve adequate cerebrospinal fluid (CSF) concentrations for the treatment of meningitis, either intralumbar (40) or intraventricular (41) administration must be chosen. Although intraventricular administration yields more reliable CSF concentrations, insertion of another foreign body may occasionally complicate the management of certain patients. Also, neurotoxic side effects can be noted after either route of administration into CSF (42). Unfortunately, there is little information available regarding the CSF aminoglycoside concentrations associated with these adverse effects.

All body tissues bind and accumulate aminoglycosides intracellularly. The early stages of drug uptake primarily consist of binding to cell membranes, rather than intracellular penetration. Aminoglycoside transport into cells is a slower process, and pharmacokinetic and *in vitro* evidence suggests that the half-life of intracellular penetration ranges between 7 and 70 hours (17,25).

The drugs are detectable in all body tissues, and the tissue concentrations of all patients slowly rise with multiple dosing (12,16,18,26). Highly perfused organs such as liver, lung, and kidney usually have concentrations above those in serum, while muscle, fat, and hard bone usually have concentrations lower than serum (16,17,20,62). The highest concentrations in the body are found in the kidneys, except in severe chronic renal failure, where liver or lung will often be higher.

### Excretion

Aminoglycosides are excreted unchanged in urine after glomerular filtration and some tubular reabsorption. There is no evidence that aminoglycosides are metabolized, although metabolism was postulated when early investigators noted intercepts in the relation between CCr and Kel (43), or were unable to recover the entire administered dose in a 24-hour urine (44,45). Complete urine recovery can be accomplished when urine is collected for 20 to 30 *days* (21), and a two compartment model explains the intercept (16). There is no evidence for renal secretion, as probenecid does not alter the renal clearance of aminoglycosides (46).

## Effects of Disease on Normal Pharmacokinetic Parameters

Liver disease has no apparent influence on aminoglycoside serum half-life, probably because the drugs are not metabolized. However, patients with liver disease and ascites may have large fluid compartments and manifest an enlarged central volume of distribution. This may result in a lower initial peak serum concentration. Patients with fever may also have a larger than normal central compartment volume after a single dose (47), but as yet there has been neither a mechanism proposed, nor conclusive evidence to document that distribution volume remains larger with multiple dosing. Hypoxia may prolong serum half-life (48), but may also lower the antibacterial activity (49,50). In some clinical situations, these opposing forces may cancel.

Early investigators suggested a relationship between distribution into red cells and aminoglycoside distribution, based on a correlation between hematocrit and peak serum concentration (51). These findings have not been confirmed in subsequent studies. Also, a thorough study of the relation between distribution and hematocrit must first account for the effects of renal disease, one of which is anemia. Since this has not been accomplished, at present there is little to support a proposed decrease in aminoglycoside dosage to compensate for the effects of anemia.

Obesity may also affect aminoglycoside distribution. Obesity will artificially contract the apparent central volume of distribution (52), because adipose tissue contains less water than lean body mass of equal weight. This effect may be normalized by considering a factor of ideal body weight (IBW) and 40% of actual body weight (ABW) in the calculation of a weight-related central volume of distribution (53). However, there may be some risk associated with this practice, for we have observed at least four obese patients whose initial peak concentrations were very low, suggesting normal partitioning in fat. The peak serum concentrations of these patients were predictable only on the basis of total body mass. For this reason, obese patients who are critically ill should be given loading doses based on actual body weight, to insure adequate blood levels in the first 24 hours.

Altered urine pH may influence both therapeutic effect and nephrotoxicity. In rats, acidic urine both increases the risk of nephrotoxicity (54,57) and decreases the effectiveness of aminoglycosides on bacteria (55). Alkaline urine has precisely the opposite effects on both nephrotoxicity (54) and bactericidal activity (55). Neither of these pH manipulations change aminoglycoside renal excretion to a marked degree (56), although aminoglycoside renal tissue levels tend to increase in acidic urine and decrease in alkaline urine (54).

In addition to the effects of urine pH, changes in urine ion concentrations probably also change both the urine concentration effective on bacteria (55,58) and alter the risk of nephrotoxicity (59). An increased urine sodium concentration will both decrease the tissue accumulation and decrease the severity of nephrotoxicity in rats (59). The protective effects of sodium might occur because aminoglycosides and positively charged sodium ions compete for binding sites on the renal tubular membrane.

Because renal excretion by glomerular filtration is the major elimination route for these drugs, the predominant effect of renal disease is a decrease in drug filtration. The effects of renal disease are predominant, and the correlation between elimination rate constant in serum and creatinine clearance is generally quite reasonable (60). This correlation is the basis for numerous aminoglycoside dosing adjustment nomograms.

In comparison to the effects of renal disease on excretion, the effects of renal disease on aminoglycoside distribution and tissue accumulation are minor. In severe renal impairment, the central compartment volume is about 10% larger (16) and the rate of tissue uptake is somewhat slower (16,17). Renal tissue uptake occurs after the drug is filtered, and although renal uptake generally accounts for 40% of the total body load of aminoglycosides in patients with functional kidneys, patients with severe renal parenchymal disease have renal tissue concentrations which are dramatically reduced (63,64,65). Because chronic renal disease eliminates 40% of the aminoglycoside binding sites, at identical serum levels, individuals with renal impairment have lower aminoglycoside steady state volumes of distribution, lower total body load, and a greater percentage of total body aminoglycoside in skeletal muscle and fat (manuscript in preparation).

## Effects of Dialysis

Hemodialysis is effective in the removal of circulating aminoglycosides, and 4 to 6 hours of hemodialysis can remove as much as half of the drug present in the blood (66). In this setting, hemodialysis will remove an appreciable percentage of total body amount, since the absence of viable kidneys increases the proportion of total body load which is circulating in blood. Appreciable hemodialysis removal has resulted in the recommendation that half the loading dose be administered after 4 to 6 hours of hemodialysis.

Despite the highly effective hemodialysis removal of circulating drug in chronic renal failure, hemodialysis may be markedly less effective in the treatment of aminoglycoside nephrotoxicity. A higher proportion of total body aminoglycoside is sequestered in the tissues of nephrotoxic patients when compared to chronic renal failure patients having nonviable kidneys. In those patients who are nephrotoxic, hemodialysis of the circulating drug removes a much lower proportion of total body load, as most of their drug is tissue bound and inaccessible during hemodialysis. Redistribution from tissues to blood will occur after stopping dialysis, and may return serum concentrations almost to predialysis levels.

Peritoneal dialysis is generally less effective than hemodialysis, removing only about 25% of a dose in 48 to 72 hours (67,68). There are no data available regarding hemoperfusion removal of aminoglycosides.

## Mechanisms of Nephrotoxicity

Aminoglycosides are freely filtered by the glomerular basement membrane, while their nephrotoxic damage is specific to the lining cells of the renal proximal tubule. Decreases in glomerular filtration occur as a protective response to the failure of proximal tubular reabsorptive function, although the precise mechanism remains somewhat controversial (69–76). Regardless of the precise mechanism, changes in glomerular filtration rate (GFR) are a late effect of aminoglycoside proximal tubular damage, and serum creatinine as a marker of GFR is a retrospective marker of aminoglycoside nephrotoxicity (5,77).

Extensive studies of cellular transport mechanisms have provided evidence for a link between normal renal proximal tubular reabsorption of basic amino acids and the damage resulting from normal reabsorption of aminoglycoside antibiotics. After filtration, these drugs are actively reabsorbed from the urine by the brush border membranes of the renal proximal tubule (78,79,80). Aminoglycosides attach to the same negatively charged binding sites on the proximal tubular brush border membrane that attract basic amino acids (65). Most of this reabsorption occurs after filtration, because the 100 to 1 greater surface area of the luminal side is in predominant contact with these drugs as urine is formed. Little if any drug enters the cell by transport from the peritubular capillary. Aminoglycoside transmembrane transport is probably accomplished by the same transport system responsible for the reabsorption of basic amino acids such as lysine. Pinocytosis follows the initial electrophilic binding to the brush border membrane. A lysosomal vacuole is formed at the surface of the cell membrane, and the drug is ingested into the cell (78,79,80). Once inside, initial damage occurs in the lysosome, and results in its disruption (80,81,82,83,84). The aminoglycoside is then released intracellularly and is free to act as an uncoupler of oxidative phosphorylation and inhibit mitochondrial ATP formation (85).

The drug may also directly attack the transport functions of the cell membrane, and directly inhibit membrane Na+/K+ ATPase enzymes (86). Although some of the final stages are not yet precisely characterized, the end result appears to be the inability of the cell to maintain normal Na+/K+ gradients, cellular swelling, and eventual osmotic rupture. The death of significant numbers of proximal tubular lining cells will result in the nephron being unable to carry out its normal reabsorptive functions. This defect in reabsorption is detected by the macula densa, and filtration ceases in the damaged nephron. Serum creatinine begins to rise only when significant numbers of nephrons no longer function, as further outlined below.

## Clinical Presentation of Aminoglycoside Nephrotoxicity

Aminoglycosides are relatively mild nephrotoxic substances, in that they do not produce fulminant acute renal failure within 24 to 48 hours of dosing. Rather, the onset of aminoglycoside related damage is apparent only after 5 to 7 days. Although aminoglycosides might be involved in as much as 25% of the high output renal impairment described in the acute care setting (87), their nephrotoxicity is often mild and generally carries a good prognosis. Damage to renal tubules is nearly always reversible, because the renal proximal tubular lining cells have tremendous regenerative capability. However, it may require 20 to 60 days before complete recovery of baseline renal function, because renal damage is closely associated with both elevated and prolonged aminoglycoside tissue concentrations. In a small percentage of cases, renal insufficiency may first appear only after the final dose of drug.

The diagnosis of aminoglycoside nephrotoxicity, as opposed to other causes of renal failure, is primarily a diagnosis of exclusion, as no aminoglycoside-specific lab tests are available to assess nephrotoxicity. Serum creatinine is essentially a marker of glomerular filtration, and its elevation could result from any extrarenal or renal insults which produce a decline in glomerular filtration rate. Since aminoglycoside induced renal impairment is usually not associated with oliguria until renal failure is advanced, nephrotoxicity may completely escape detection if only urine output is monitored.

There is mounting evidence that aminoglycoside related proximal tubular damage is readily detectable 5 to 10 days prior to the initial rise in serum creatinine (77,88). Tests useful for the detection of renal tubular damage include urinary $\beta_2$microglobulin (89,90), urinary cast excretion (91,92), and urinary enzyme excretion (88,93,94,95). Although they do provide earlier warning, even these nonspecific tests of tubular damage cannot always determine whether the drug or another tubular insult is the specific cause of renal failure. At present, elevated aminoglycoside tissue uptake prior to onset of renal tubular damage is the most specific means of deciding if aminoglycosides are the cause of renal tubular damage (77,100), but these tests are still experimental and limited to research settings.

We attribute clinically apparent renal damage to the aminoglycosides in those patients whose serum creatinine rises after five days of treatment, who are also without apparent clinical renal insults, whose urinalysis reveals increased excretion of granular casts and protein prior to creatinine rise, and only if all of these criteria occur after abnormal tissue accumulation (77). If there are well defined clinical insults also present and the renal insufficiency is nonoliguric and tissue accumulation is not excessive, then tubular injury produced by a combination of aminoglycosides and clinical insults is most likely. Finally, overwhelming septic shock or severe hypotension are sufficient to cause oliguric renal failure, and in most of these patients we do not attribute damage to the drug.

Aminoglycosides should always be discontinued if renal failure occurs and that option is *available,* but the severity of infection may often preclude cessation of treatment. Therefore, it is highly important for the consultant to make some judgment as to the specific cause of nephrotoxicity, because only patients with clearly aminoglycoside-related damage will require cessation of treatment. Our previous studies suggest that only about half of the seriously ill patients with creatinine rise have aminoglycoside nephrotoxicity (77), and aminoglycoside treatment should not always be stopped solely on the basis of creatinine rise in treated patients, unless damage is caused by the aminoglycoside. The patient with oliguric renal insufficiency is not necessarily at greater risk for nephrotoxicity, provided dose adjustments are made to keep serum concentrations "normal". This is because renal accumulation occurs after filtration, and these patients will not accumulate the drug in renal tissue after cessation of glomerular filtration. Thus, even though oliguric renal failure may worsen as a result of progressive disease, many of these patients will recover baseline renal status if infection can be controlled by effective use of aminoglycosides (77).

Rats in renal failure from aminoglycosides also recover baseline renal function, both functionally and histologically. Surprisingly, the rats will recover baseline renal function even when treatment is *continued* (96,97). The observation is provocative, and might be explained by considering the life cycle of individual nephrons. A mature single nephron filters, reabsorbs, then irreversibly binds aminoglycosides inside its proximal tubular lining cells. These cells die, filtration ceases, and the cells disintegrate, forming casts in the urine which contain aminoglycoside and remove the offending drug. Since filtration has now ceased, no drug enters the newly forming proximal cells. Furthermore, the immature and partially functional proximal cells are resistant to the development of new damage (98,99). When the cell is fully mature it once again is sensitive to tubular damage and the process will likely be repeated if exposure continues.

The mechanism proposed might explain most facets of the recovery of renal function with continued therapy. The mechanism also provides some hope that continued treatment in some patients already in renal failure will not prolong the time to recovery. However, these observations were made in rats, and until further tested it remains prudent to discontinue aminoglycosides whenever renal insufficiency develops.

## CONCENTRATION versus RESPONSE and TOXICITY

### Response

The optimum aminoglycoside serum concentrations, and indeed, optimum serum concentrations for any antibiotic, remain obscured by the complexities of the organisms and environment. The problem is at least twofold. It is very difficult to separate the bactericidal effects of the immune system from those of the drugs in the clinical setting, expecially since different organisms have different lethal concentrations. To make matters worse, some bacteria survive in the presence of nearly any drug concentration, because only cells actively engaged in metabolic processes are sensitive, or because drug resistant mutants are part of any bacterial population. The killing of bacteria is a statistical exercise on a population of individual microorganisms, much like the difficulties presented by cancer chemotherapy.

The available literature suggests that aminoglycoside peak concentrations are most useful in the assessment of clinical effect (5). Desired peak concentrations can be roughly estimated as ranging from 4 to 12 µg/ml for gentamicin, tobramycin, netilmicin and sisomicin, and 12 to 36 µg/ml for amikacin. Within these ranges, infection site and host factors must be considered the major variables influencing therapeutic response.

The basis for these therapeutic peak ranges are reports by Noone (106), establishing a peak of 5.0 µg/ml as therapeutic, and 8.0 µg/ml as effective for pneumonias; by Jackson (107), establishing a gentamicin peak of 4.0 μg/ml as therapeutic for pseudomonas; and by Bodey (108), establishing 15.0 μg/ml as an effective amikacin level during constant intravenous infusion. There are no reports in humans correlating trough concentrations with therapeutic response.

## Toxicity

There is controversy whether peak concentrations are useful in the assessment of toxicity. Most studies which quote a toxic peak establish a value above 12 μg/ml for gentamicin or tobramycin and above 35 μg/ml for amikacin. Similar toxic values are stated for both oto- and nephrotoxicity.

Early concentration versus toxicity studies are difficult to interpret, since oto- and nephrotoxicity were correlated with serum peak concentrations measured after serum creatinine was already rising. Since serum creatinine rise is a result of established nephrotoxicity, these studies by definition did not establish serum concentration ranges which produce toxicity. Because of the pronounced delay between actual damage to renal tubules and serum creatinine rise, the important relationship is the correlation between toxicity and the peak concentration *prior* to renal damage, rather than the peak concentration achieved as a result of continued dosing after renal damage is established. To date, there has been no correlation between these early serum peak concentrations and the later development of either oto- (101,102) or nephrotoxicity (100,101,102). Furthermore, it is difficult to conceptualize a direct relationship between peak concentrations in blood and drug toxicity in organs with multicompartment drugs like aminoglycosides. Peak tissue concentrations with these drugs are not achieved for at least 10 days. Since the peak serum concentration occurs days earlier than the peak tissue concentration, it would be more valuable to search for correlation between toxicity and the peak drug concentration in the kidney or ear. This receptor site concentration may be better reflected by the trough concentration rather than the peak (16,21,77), since the trough is a better reflection of post distribution equilibrium between blood and tissue compartments.

Animal studies further support the lack of correlation between aminoglycoside peak concentrations and either oto- or nephrotoxicity. In each of these animal studies, the same total dose is less toxic when given as a single injection versus constant infusion (12) or versus divided doses (103). Although once daily total dose has not yet been attempted in humans, administration of divided doses by IV bolus versus slow infusion has never demonstrated group differences (6,7), which would at least suggest that the high and transient peaks resulting from IV injection present no greater risk of either oto- or nephrotoxicity than peak concentrations which never exceed 12 μg/ml.

Trough concentrations have been associated with nephrotoxicity by many investigators (104,105,118), and the nephrotoxic trough has been quoted between 2.0 and 4.0 μg/ml (5,104,105,118). Much of the same controversy surrounding the ability of peaks to predict nephrotoxicity is applicable to the ability of troughs to predict nephrotoxicity. It might be presumed that, since troughs reflect tissue site concentrations better than peaks, trough concentrations would be more reliable correlates of toxicity. The data of most investigators support this hypothesis (77,100,102,104,105). However, since a change in glomerular filtration is a late effect of aminoglycoside toxicity rather than its cause, trough concentrations, as a marker of glomerular filtration, rise rapidly only after cessation of glomerular filtration (77). Due to their dependency on glomerular filtration, early trough concentrations may not be a reliable means to predict the eventual development of aminoglycoside nephrotoxicity, just as is true with early peaks.

To date, there have been few studies of toxicity correlated with area under the serum concentration vs time curve. Although some recommend it (5), this approach requires more sampling, as well as being equally sensitive to changes in renal function. Thus like peaks and troughs, area methods are often retrospective markers of nephrotoxicity.

## CLINICAL APPLICATION OF PHARMACOKINETIC DATA

### Dosing

Aminoglycosides may produce either dose related or non-dose related nephrotoxicity (77). Optimizing the dose to avoid overdosage can protect patients only against the dose related nephrotoxic damage, while within the optimum serum range, tissue uptake unique to the individual patient determines which patients develop the non-dose related damage. Thus, even though they will not always prevent toxicity, serum levels are valuable tools in the achievement and maintenance of defined therapeutic concentrations, even though factors beyond the control of serum levels may determine renal damage in those patients optimized.

Seriously ill patients require immediate attention and aggressive use of aminoglycosides. A 1.7 to 2.0 mg/kg actual body weight (ABW) gentamicin or tobramycin loading dose should be given intravenously as soon as cultures are taken. The loading dose of amikacin is 7.5 mg/kg ABW. Although some markedly obese patients will have elevated peak concentrations due to loading doses based on ABW rather than IBW, this situation is preferable to the risk of subtherapeutic concentrations in the event distribution volume is a function of ABW. Early in therapy, dosing error on the high side is preferable to the risks of undertreatment, since death from infection presents an immediate risk, while tissue-uptake mediated toxicity requires 5 to 7 days to develop.

Maintenance dosing should be calculated as mg/kg of IBW. Ideal Body Weight may be calculated from height and weight as below (113):

$$\text{IBW Males} = 50 \text{ kg} + 2.3 \text{ kg/inch over } 5' \qquad \text{(Eq. 1)}$$

$$\text{IBW Females} = 45.5 \text{ kg} + 2.3 \text{ kg/inch over } 5' \qquad \text{(Eq. 2)}$$

The goal of maintenance dosing is to replace drug excreted during the dosing interval, and several methods are effective. Ideally, maintenance doses should be given to replace only the drug recovered from urine during the dosing interval, since lower than predicted urine recovery would also identify patients with abnormally high tissue uptake. The practical difficulties associated with obtaining accurate urine collections make this method a poor choice for most hospitals. It is unfortunate that abnormal tissue uptake and lost urine produce the same conclusion, because they are quite difficult to discriminate.

The next best alternative would be dosing based on some estimate of drug filtered by the glomerulus. This would provide no information on tissue accumulation, but at least dosage could be altered if filtration is lower than normal. Creatinine clearance (CCr) is a reasonable estimate of glomerular filtration, and can be used to account for filtered drug. It provides no insight into the amount reabsorbed, and accordingly provides little insight into the risks of nephrotoxicity from accumulation. Nevertheless, CCr should be considered a viable method of clinical dosage adjustment. Creatinine clearance can be predicted from nomograms (110) as accurately as most hospitals can measure it in 24-hour collections (111). The nomogram chosen must include patient's age, sex, and ideal body weight if it is to derive reliable CCr values from serum creatinine.

Once CCr is determined, the nomograms of Hull and Sarubbi (52,112) or Chan (43) will generate appropriate maintenance doses for older seriously ill patients. Some younger patients with normal renal function may not receive adequate dosing from conventional recommendations of 5 mg/kg/day gentamicin and tobramycin or 15 mg/kg/day amikacin. In these patients the monitoring of serum concentrations will disclose the reason for therapeutic failure as underdosing.

An alternative approach to nomograms is individualization of dosage based on derived pharmacokinetic parameters (114,115). This method of dosing adjustment, although requiring more frequent blood level measurements, has particular advantages in younger patients who are often underdosed by conventional recommendations. Underdosing in burn victims or younger patients who are bacteremic may be a result of increased fluid turnover, or disease associated elevations in their creatinine clearances (116,117). More of these infections responded well when aminoglycoside dosages were calculated from their measured serum half-life (116).

In spite of its advantages in younger patients, individualized dosing based on serum half-life and volume of distribution may demonstrate little advantage over traditional CCr and nomogram methods in older patient populations. Standard aminoglycoside doses given to older adults almost always either adequately dose or overdose initially. Patients overdosed and monitored with serum concentrations will be decreased to the therapeutic range after the first trough level is reported as elevated. Measuring one trough takes less time than individualized therapy, and is therefore, more cost effective. Of most importance, once older patients are in the therapeutic range by either of the available dosing techniques, there will be a random occurrence of non-dose related nephro- (and probably oto-) toxicity which cannot easily be avoided by the use of serum concentrations alone. Because of this problem, individualized dosing methods are unlikely to prevent more nephrotoxicity than would appropriate use of nomograms. If less nephrotoxicity is noted when this method is compared with standard dosing, in my view it is because of population differences, or because renal parameters are not being monitored after therapy is individualized. Indeed, a recent report from this group gives little evidence that either blood levels or serum creatinine are monitored after four days treatment (158), providing an alternate explanation for the absence of nephrotoxicity.

Of the two choices in dosing technique, the individualization method of Sawchuk (125,126) has clear advantages in younger critically ill patients because of increased efficacy, although this method has yet to be compared with dosing increases based on serial trough concentration alone. In older patients, where toxicity is a more common problem than therapeutic failure, it appears more cost effective to employ nomograms alone, or combine nomograms with occasional measurement of trough concentrations to achieve the recommended range.

Neither of these methods will protect against nephrotoxicity, although both will lower its incidence. Whenever nephrotoxicity must be avoided in either type of patient, monitoring sensitive indices of renal tubular damage offers the best chance to identify early signs of nephrotoxicity. As a principle of aminoglycoside monitoring, resources and time should be concentrated in the few patients at greatest risk. The critically ill patients who cannot afford the loss of renal function deserve the most intense surveillance, because they may decompensate as a result of even mild renal insufficiency. When renal tubular monitoring is not feasible, the serial use of less sensitive tests such as serum creatinine may be as reliable as aminoglycoside trough concentrations. Although more cost effective than monitoring renal tubular indices, neither creatinine or blood levels can be expected to avoid renal damage in all seriously ill patients.

## Consideration of Pharmacokinetic Modeling in Aminoglycoside Monitoring

Aminoglycoside doses are usually calculated from nomograms based on a one compartment pharmacokinetic model, but at least a two and probably a three compartment model must be employed to accurately describe the serum concentrations of these compounds (16,17,18,19). The normal 8 to 24-hour dosing intervals represent more frequent dosing than the tissue half-life of 100 hours, and because dosing at the usual maintenance intervals is dosing in excess of terminal elimination, a slow accumulation of aminoglycoside must occur. Tissue accumulation is manifested as slowly rising peak and trough serum concentrations in the face of stable creatinine clearances. The tissue accumulation has toxicologic significance, as it includes uptake by both the kidney and inner ear. Individuals vary markedly in rate and extent of tissue uptake. Some patients have high tissue uptake early, and continue until toxicity develops (77,100). In these, toxicity is not related to dose.

Although knowledge of the slow tissue accumulation is important for understanding the course of renal damage during aminoglycoside treatment, the fact that aminoglycosides accumulate in tissues does not mean that doses cannot be adjusted based on the nomograms or individualization methods derived from a one compartment model. These methods are of high value in initiating proper regimens, and reasonably useful in the prediction of blood levels during therapy.

Nevertheless, new understanding of tissue accumulation means that effective serum level monitoring must be based on comparison between measured and model predicted trough concentrations in search for more rapid than normal serum accumulation. If these comparisons are made, it is possible to identify abnormal serum accumulation with either one or two compartment pharmacokinetic models.

TABLE 1. SUMMARY OF REGRESSION EQUATIONS
FOR MAJOR PARAMETERS AND CCR[1]

|  |  | Gentamicin | Tobramycin |
|---|---|---|---|
| $V_c$ (Central)[2] | = | $-.00025$ CCr + .308 | $-.00002$ CCr + .276 |
| $V_{ss}$ (Steady State)[2] | = | .0048 CCr + .60 | .00785 CCr + .744 |
| $K_{12}$ (Central-Tissue)[3] | = | .00023 CCr + .003 | .00019 CCr + .0025 |
| $K_{21}$ (Tissue-Central)[3] | = | .00002 CCr + .0055 | .000021 CCr + .0035 |
| $K_{10}$ (Central-Elim)[3] | = | .0025 CCr | .0027 CCr |

[1] Values for gentamicin and tobramycin were calculated from regressive analysis of 120
patients in each group. All parameters were derived from *nontoxic* patients.
[2] Expressed as L/kg IBW
[3] In units hr$^{-1}$

Since the focus in serum concentration monitoring is serial measurement of trough concentrations to detect patients with an abnormal rate of rise, either model might be employed to predict trough concentrations. The one compartment model will predict steady-state concentrations sooner than will a two compartment model, and accordingly, the amount of trough level deviation between the predicted and measured values of a prenephrotoxic patient will be greater than with a two compartment model.

The advantage of a two compartment model is that this model provides some estimation of average tissue uptake with time on a prospective basis. Parameters of distribution and elimination can be estimated from their relation to renal function, and the regression line equations for model parameter vs CCr are summarized for gentamicin and tobramycin in Table 1. These relationships and knowledge of the patient's CCr allow calculation of average $V_c$, $V_{ss}$, $K_{12}$, $K_{21}$, and $K_{10}$ of each aminoglycoside, for employment in a two compartment model simulation (16). To effectively use these parameters, the clinician only has to compare the rise in two compartment model calculated trough concentrations with the rise in measured values. In this manner, patients with abnormal accumulation may be identified earlier.

This two compartment model approach has been an integral part of our pharmacokinetic consultation service for several years. As an example of the simulation, we have reproduced a completed consult as Figure 1. The solid lines indicate values predicted from the two compartment parameters of Table 1, while closed circles indicate measured serum concentrations. This patient shows deviation in measured trough concentrations from predicted as early as 7/23. In this particular case, we attributed the increase in peak and trough to lab variation in a stable patient and did not alter the dosage. Serum creatinine

Reason for Consultation:

Consultation Note:

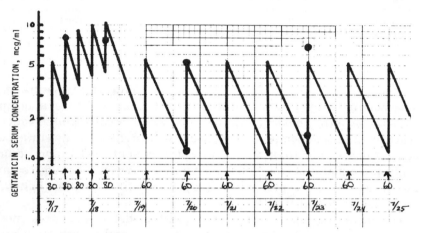

Predicted values indicated by solid lines, measured values indicated by solid circles.

Mr. D. is a 74 yo white male with a history of COPD, chronic UTI and Parkinsonism. He was admitted 7/17/77 with gross hematuria secondary to traumatic catheterization, fever of 104° and BP of 70/0. Keflin (1 gm q 6 h) and Gentamicin (80 mg IV q 8 h) were started because of the possibility of sepsis.

Based on age, sex, weight and serum creatinine 2.5, this patient's calculated creatinine clearance is approx. 28 ml/min.

REC: In view of this patient's renal function, we feel that his Gentamicin should be held for 24 hours then re-started at 60 mg q 24 hrs. This new regimen should provide therapeutic peak levels of over 5 mcg/ml and valleys of 1.1 mcg/ml. We would request weekly weights and serum creatinine determinations QD or QOD. We will follow his blood levels and renal function with you. Thank you for this consult.

Prepared by _____

FORM 4097

FIGURE 1. Completed pharmacokinetic consultation form, illustrating computer predicted peak and trough concentrations (based on two compartment parameters derived from Table 1). The graph shows measured serum concentrations as closed circles, and comparison of measured with the predicted values demonstrates abnormally rapid accumulation at an early stage.

190

began to rise five days later, and declined to baseline ten days after stopping treatment. This case illustrates the particular insensitivity of trough concentrations, even when employed serially.

## Clinical Use of Serum Concentrations

Aminoglycoside serum concentrations can be used to improve the care of treated patients, provided that basic principles of pharmacokinetics and renal physiology are used by those who interpret laboratory results. The success of therapeutic monitoring depends on control of several mechanical details, the first of which is proper timing of blood samples. Trough concentrations should be obtained immediately prior to the dose, as this represents the lowest possible value. Since the trough best represents distribution equilibrium between blood and tissue, trough concentrations are more useful than peaks for prediction of tissue accumulation, and for assessment of the risk of nephrotoxicity.

Peak concentrations should be taken after the rapid distributive phase is completed. One hour after an intramuscular injection, or immediately following intravenous infusions of less than one hour, are optimal for most situations. All drug must have been infused before the peak can be obtained, and the clinician should note the time of blood sampling, as well as its relation to the time after drug infusion was started. In most settings, peak concentrations need be obtained only if there is question of therapeutic failure, as an adequate peak level in a patient with renewed fever might alert the clinician to the development of resistant superinfection, or the presence of undrained abscesses.

In therapeutic monitoring as opposed to initial dosing, there are few indications for repeated peak level determinations. If the initial peak concentrations are accurately measured, in the appropriate range and renal function does not change, the peak will remain relatively constant. One possible exception is repeated intramuscular injections into the same injection site.

Trough concentrations may have a greater role in therapeutic monitoring. Troughs will rise in all patients to some degree because of tissue accumulation. Although patients with more rapid rate of rise are generally at higher risk for the development of nephrotoxicity, a rise in trough concentration must be interpreted in the context of simultaneous predicted values based on accurate assessment of renal function. The most effective early use of aminoglycoside trough concentrations would be to employ them as a marker of renal tissue uptake. Serum trough concentrations rise in two phases in patients who develop nephrotoxicity (77). The first slope correlates with the rate of renal tissue uptake by tubular reabsorption, while the second and more rapid rise occurs in response to cessation of glomerular filtration. Drug reabsorption is the first of several steps leading to cellular damage, and careful surveillance of troughs may lend insight into the rate of drug reabsorption by the proximal tubule. Although in most cases these relationships would argue in favor of serial measurements of trough concentrations, interpretation of changes in troughs is difficult because very large increases in renal tissue concentration are reflected as only minor increases in trough concentration. These minor changes are easily attributed to lab variation or shifts in physiologic status, as happened to our patient in Figure 1. Also, any clinical insult producing a change in GFR will also cause rising troughs. Thus, because of their poor relative sensitivity, trough concentrations face a declining role in the serial monitoring of aminoglycoside nephrotoxicity, especially as the relation between glomerular filtration and trough concentrations is better appreciated.

Finally, a great number of aminoglycoside treated patients do not need intensive blood level monitoring, because risk is low. In my view, serial trough concentrations are not cost justifiable unless patients are both at high risk for toxicity and cannot afford to incur mild renal compromise. Thus, most patients can be monitored with serum creatinine, because even if renal insufficiency develops, it is generally mild and reversible, and of no major concern to relatively healthy individuals. Those that are seriously ill and *do* require intensive monitoring, should have determinations daily or every other day.

## Pharmacologic Effect Monitoring

In any group of 100 appropriately dosed patients, there will be 90 who tolerate the seven to ten day course of therapy without adverse renal or otologic effects. The other 10 of these 100 patients will experience adverse effects, and one to five of these will have severe renal failure or almost complete deafness. These few sensitive patients are clinically indistinguishable from the majority who tolerate the drug without complications. However, because they do exist, and because serial trough concentrations, or rising serum creatinines, or complaints of deafness can only confirm that damage has already occurred, the goal in monitoring aminoglycosides is to develop more sensitive methods of detecting early renal or auditory damage, before damage progresses to severe compromise.

**Ototoxicity.** Proper assessment of hearing requires baseline assessment as well as serial monitoring, because as many as 75% of older adults already have significant high frequency hearing loss at baseline, yet will assert that their hearing is normal (101). Although detectable high frequency hearing loss probably precedes irreversible deafness by many days, audiometric testing is difficult to perform in the environment where most problems occur. Because it requires the cooperation of critically ill patients, monitoring the ear is relatively easy in principle, but practically impossible in critical care practice. Thus, effective pharmacologic monitoring of ototoxicity awaits the development of sensitive tests which do not require patient cooperation.

**Nephrotoxicity.** Monitoring the kidney with pharmacologic tests means serial assessment of proximal tubular function, as this is the site of aminoglycoside damage (77,89). In patients who suffer aminoglycoside nephrotoxicity, a lag time of three to ten days can be demonstrated between initial proximal tubular effects and later rise in serum creatinine (77).

This is adequate time for decisions regarding dose adjustment or alternate therapy. Tests which might have a major role in monitoring proximal tubular effect include urinary excretion of $\beta_2$microglobulin (89,90), urinary enzymes (88,93,94,95), or quantitative cast counts (92). All of these tests share the disadvantage of being nonspecific tests, as their excretion is altered in any proximal tubular insult. However, all proximal tubular tests are at least specific for the site of aminoglycoside damage, while serum aminoglycoside concentrations and serum creatinine measurements (as markers of GFR) completely lack specificity for the proximal tubule. Serum creatinine or blood levels always rise regardless of the cause of GFR decrease.

The other advantages of the proximal tubular tests lie in their greater sensitivity to tubular insults. However, some are more sensitive than others, and rank order from most sensitive to least would include $\beta_2$microglobulin, renal enzymes, protein, and casts, all preceding serum creatinine elevation by at least two days (77). The tubular indices are still under development and testing, and firm criteria for their use in therapeutic decisions are not yet evolved. Renal proximal testing should remain investigational at this time, or be restricted to daily use on 24 hour urines in high risk cases. No single test should be employed as criteria to discontinue treatment, but rather, elevation of proximal tubular indices should prompt use of frequent aminoglycoside blood levels, use of the lowest effective dosage, and a careful search for renal insults concurrent with the aminoglycosides.

## Clinical Considerations in the Use of Aminoglycosides

Early reports of aminoglycoside nephrotoxicity quoted incidences between 2 and 10% (118). Since 1974, the reported incidence has been rising in clinical studies, but paradoxically declining in reports by the aminoglycoside manufacturers. In clinical studies using a serum creatinine rise of $\geq 0.5$ mg/dl as minimum criteria, the reported incidence of renal insufficiency has been as high as 37%. However, studies done in younger patients with good baseline renal function report far lower nephrotoxicity rates than studies done in older patients with baseline renal insufficiency (116). Since dosing recommendations and patterns of use have changed little, undoubtedly the incidence of nephrotoxicity is rising because patients are now more carefully monitored, and because these drugs are finally being studied in the older, more seriously ill patients who most often require them.

We must conclude that between-study differences in side effects are primarily a result of differences between study populations, and directly related to intensity of surveillance. Because of this population dependence, new aminoglycosides must be evaluated in terms of the baseline characteristics of the study population. Conclusions based solely on one population might not apply to another, and untested extrapolations might pose danger to high risk individuals.

Those involved in optimizing aminoglycoside dosage regimens must devote careful attention to concurrent nephrotoxic substances, because many agents can shift the relationship between tissue concentration and toxic effect. The concurrent use of furosemide (119,120), amphotericin B (121), or platinum compounds (122), should provoke extra caution in therapeutic monitoring. Avoidance of dehydration, hypoxia and hyponatremia are prudent measures. Careful attention should also be paid to patients with diabetes.

The role of cephalosporins as concurrent nephrotoxins is controversial. Animal studies usually demonstrate protection from nephrotoxicity (123,124), while clinical anecdotes (125,126,127) and comparative studies (128,129) demonstrate potentiation of nephrotoxicity. The matter cannot be considered resolved by the available clinical studies, because believable controls were not present, even in the clinical trials. A believable control group for comparative studies would be aminoglycoside *alone*, versus aminoglycoside/cephalosporin. Most studies employ control groups receiving carbenicillin or methicillin, which is likely to be protective, since it lowers the incidence of nephrotoxicity to 2–5% (128), compared with the 10–15% usually seen with aminoglycoside alone (134). Until the matter is clarified, the combination of cephalosporins and aminoglycosides should be avoided when it offers no therapeutic advantage over aminoglycosides alone. The controversy will rage until mechanisms of either cephalosporin protection from, or potentiation of nephrotoxicity are understood.

Another problem not yet resolved is the effects of concurrent carbenicillin or ticarcillin on aminoglycoside blood levels. These drugs form an irreversible and inactive complex when mixed and allowed to stand. The reaction is dependent on the molar ratio, time, temperature, and medium (130). The reaction is of most significance in severe renal disease, where it may double the rate of aminoglycoside elimination from serum (131,132). Amikacin is least sensitive to the effects of the penicillins, and should be used whenever patients with renal insufficiency require both drugs. Penicillinase lysis of the penicillin nucleus will slow the reaction, and penicillinase should always be added to blood collection tubes when both drugs are used concurrently.

When evaluating aminoglycosides for their relative antibacterial activity, gentamicin is preferred over tobramycin for serratia sensitive to both drugs, and tobramycin is to be preferred over gentamicin for pseudomonas sensitive to both antibiotics (133). For all other gram negative bacteria sensitive to both aminoglycosides, they are equally effective. Present evidence favors reserving amikacin for resistant organisms, as it is the most effective for multiresistant strains (133), as well as less potent when strains are more sensitive. Under this model, amikacin would be aminoglycoside of first choice in those institutions with a high percentage of resistant bacteria.

Choice between aminoglycosides might also be based on relative toxicity, at least in hospitals where bacteria are sensitive to all aminoglycosides. Amikacin and gentamicin have similar oto- and nephrotoxic potential (134). Netilmicin is clearly less nephrotoxic than gentamicin in animals (135,136), but the results of human clinical trials have thus far not shown significant differences (137,138,139). There are no human data comparing the nephrotoxic potential of netilmicin and tobramycin, while in animals they appear similar. There are many studies comparing the relative nephrotoxic potential of gentamicin and tobramycin. All studies show either no difference, or clear advantage for tobramycin. As the toxicologic data favoring tobramycin over gentamicin continues to accumulate, it can be reasonably stated that the use of tobramycin is preferred over gentamicin, because this aminoglycoside is both less nephrotoxic (77,120, 140,141,142), and less ototoxic (101,143) than gentamicin.

Selection of aminoglycosides and correct usage is a complex process, and there are no standard criteria applicable to all clinical situations. In view of the discussion above, we have outlined our approach to the use of these drugs as an algorithm, which appears as Figure 2. This algorithm, plus the text itself, may be helpful in the decision process.

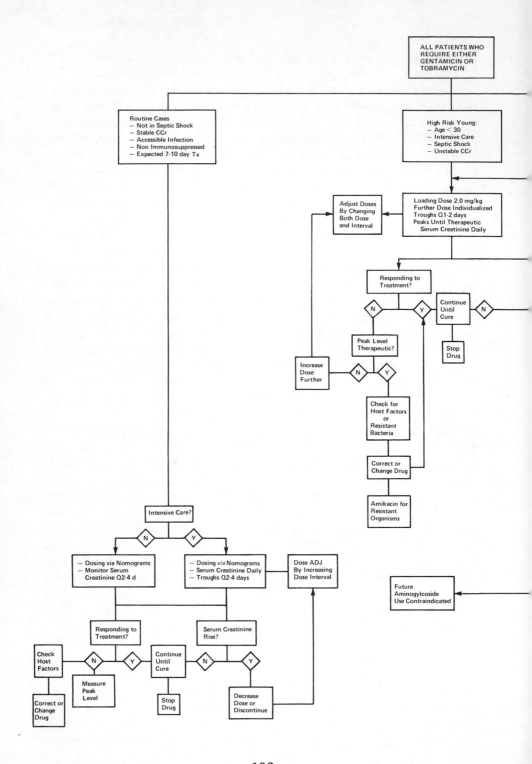

ALL PATIENTS WHO
REQUIRE EITHER
GENTAMICIN OR
TOBRAMYCIN

Routine Cases
— Not in Septic Shock
— Stable CCr
— Accessible Infection
— Non Immunosuppressed
— Expected 7-10 day Tx

High Risk Young:
— Age < 30
— Intensive Care
— Septic Shock
— Unstable CCr

Loading Dose 2.0 mg/kg
Further Dose Individualized
Troughs Q1-2 days
Peaks Until Therapeutic
Serum Creatinine Daily

Adjust Doses
By Changing
Both Dose
and Interval

Responding to
Treatment?

N      Y      Continue
              Until      N
              Cure

              Stop
              Drug

Peak Level
Therapeutic?

Increase
Dose        N      Y
Further

Check for
Host Factors
or
Resistant
Bacteria

Correct or
Change Drug

Amikacin for
Resistant
Organisms

Intensive Care?

N      Y

— Dosing via Nomograms        — Dosing via Nomograms        Dose ADJ
— Monitor Serum               — Serum Creatinine Daily      By Increasing
  Creatinine Q2-4 d           — Troughs Q2-4 days           Dose Interval

Future
Aminogylcoside
Use Contraindicated

Responding to                 Serum Creatinine
Treatment?                    Rise?

Check
Host      N      Y      Continue      N      Y
Factors                 Until
                        Cure

Measure                 Stop         Decrease
Peak                    Drug         Dose or
Level                                Discontinue

Correct or
Change
Drug

196

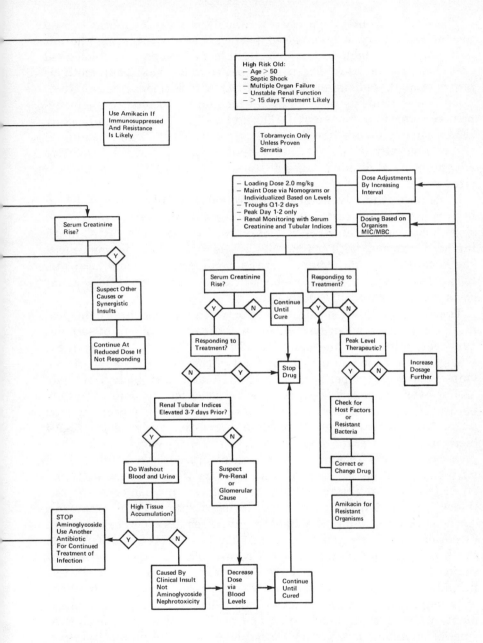

FIGURE 2. Algorithm for the application of pharmacokinetics to aminoglycoside therapy.

## ASSAY METHODS

There are currently a variety of aminoglycoside assay methods, and new ones are frequently proposed, perhaps because all have inherent deficiencies. Available techniques might be divided between biological and chemical methods. The three most common biological methods are microbial, radioimmunoassay (RIA) and radioenzymatic (REA) assay. Two promising new biological techniques include the homogeneous enzyme immunoassay (EMIT), and the fluorescent immunoassay (FIA). High pressure liquid chromatography (HPLC) and gas-liquid chromatography (GLC) are the present chemical methods. Relative advantages and disadvantages of the available methods are summarized in Table 2.

In general, the advantages of microbiological plate assays lie in high volume at low cost, but disadvantages lie in low specificity and slow turnaround. The REA can be viewed as similar to RIA, until further experience with commercial kits is reported. Radioimmunoassay is capable of high volume, and is rapid, sensitive, and accurate. It is not economical for small laboratories, as equipment and reagent costs are high with small daily runs.

There is generally good agreement between the first three biological methods, at least when tests are done on small numbers of samples run over a limited time period (152). However, all three of these biological methods will drift in and out of control over the long term. Our experiences in performing both RIA and microbiological plate assays over the past five years reveal a need for frequent attention, both to insure agreement, and to insure reproducibility over the long term. There is little doubt that these difficulties are widespread. All bioassays measure an endpoint which is a drug effect, rather than measure the precise amount of chemical present. The multitude of variables affecting the intermediate steps between concentration and effect preclude long term stability of results even when constant vigilance is exercised. Thus, their daily use requires both a standard curve and control samples with each run, if results are to be employed in patient care. The newer biological methods, EMIT and FIA, hold much promise as techniques of the future. This is especially true as radioactive waste disposal and exposure grow as a problem worldwide. In addition to the lack of radioactivity exposure, the newer methods offer more stable reagents, they can be done on less expensive equipment, are potentially more rapid, and are at least as specific as RIA. One disadvantage is that they cannot be employed for quantitation of aminoglycoside washout concentrations below 1.0 µg/ml, although modification and adjustment might eventually solve this problem.

TABLE 2. COMPARISON OF THE RELATIVE ADVANTAGES AND DISADVANTAGES OF THE VARIOUS AMINOGLYCOSIDE ASSAY METHODS[*1]

| Analysis Method | Specificity for Aminoglycoside | Limit of Sensitivity (mcg/ml) | Assayable Samples | | | | Minimum Sample Volume Required in microliters | Speed [*2] | | Analysis Cost [*3] | | Preference & Rank [*6] | | | (References) Suppliers |
|---|---|---|---|---|---|---|---|---|---|---|---|---|---|---|---|
| | | | Serum and Urine | Plasma | Tissue Homogenates | Other | | 1–10 Samples | 10–100 Samples | Estimated Reagent and Tech. Costs | Initial Equipment Costs | Small Service | Large Service | Research | |
| I. Microbiological: | | | | | | | | | | | | | | | |
| A. Bacillus subtilis | 4 | 0.5 | [*4] | [*4,*5] | [*4] | [*4] | 10–25 | 2 | 2 | 2 | 2 | 4 | 4 | 1 | (144) |
| B. Multi Resistant Strains | 2 | 0.5 | [*4] | [*4,*5] | [*4] | [*4] | 10–25 | 3 | 3 | 2 | 2 | 2 | 2 | 1 | (145, 146) Monitor Science, New England Nuclear, Diagnostic Products |
| II. Radioimmunoassay (RIA) | 2 | 0.01 | Yes | [*5] | Yes | Yes | 50–100 | 4 | 5 | 4 | 5 | 3 | 3 | 5 | P.O. Biochemicals, Milwaukee (147, 148) |
| III. Radioenzymatic (REA) | 2 | 0.5–1.0 | Yes | [*5] | Yes | Yes | 10 | 4 | 4 | 4 | 4 | 2 | 5 | 4 | |
| IV. Homogeneous Enzyme Immunoassay (EMIT) | 2 | 1.0 | Yes | [*5] | Yes | Yes | 50 | 5 | 4 | 5 | 3 | 4 | 4 | 4 | Syva Corp (155, 156) |
| V. Fluorescent Immunoassay (FIA) | 2 | 1.0 | Yes | [*5] | Yes | Yes | 100 | 5 | 4 | 5 | 3 | 3 | 4 | 4 | Ames, Div. Miles Labs (157) |
| VI. Gas Liquid Chromatography (GLC) | 1 | 0.5 | Yes | [*5] | Yes | Yes | 400 | 4 | 2 | 2 | 4 | 1 | 1 | 2 | (149) |
| VII. High Pressure Liquid Chromatography (HPLC) | 1 | 0.25 | Yes | [*5] | Yes | Yes | 500–1000 | 4 | 2 | 2 | 4 | 1 | 2 | 5 | (150, 151) |

[*1] Arbitrary Ranking Scale of 1 (Excellent) to 5 (Poor) with a score of 3 being average or normal.
[*2] Most Rapid = 5
[*3] Highest Cost = 5
[*4] Requires a standard curve in the fluid to be assayed
[*5] Never used heparinized plasma, because of aminoglycoside inactivation
[*6] Preferred Method = 5

199

The HPLC and GC are most specific and very precise. However, although HPLC and GC are very rapid for one to ten samples, they can be quite slow for larger numbers. Chemical methods such as HPLC and GLC offer the best hope for long term stability in assay results. Unfortunately, these techniques are not yet refined to the point where their full potential is apparent. Problems with day to day variations, or poor sensitivity are not yet solved. In HPLC, both pre and post column derivitization with relatively unstable fluorescence is especially sensitive to daily variation. Thus, these promising techniques require further investigation before their routine service use can be recommended.

It is apparent that routine aminoglycoside assays can be performed after capital expenditures below $1,000, or the chosen assay might be a research procedure requiring as much as $20,000 in equipment alone. Some methods are initially inexpensive, but have the long term disadvantage of high reagent costs, or the requirement for highly trained technical personnel to achieve reproducible results. An important consideration before selection of an assay is available equipment and personnel, as one method or another might be very economical solely on the basis of baseline resources. For example, the RIA has high equipment costs when no equipment is available, but might be a very economical method for the laboratory already equipped with a scintillation counter and having technical staff routinely performing digoxin RIA.

In summary, a person beginning without cash reserves would be advised to begin with a *Bacillus subtilis* microbiologic assay. We would caution this person to frequently assay known controls, and to be aware of all concurrent antibiotics. Penicillins and older cephalosporins can be inactivated with a commercial β-lactamase (153), but tetracyclines, clindamycin, and chloramphenicol will cause assay interference (154). The increasing use of β-lactamase stable cephalosporin derivitives might herald the end of micro assay usefulness, unless more potent β-lactamase enzymes become commercially available.

Startup costs are declining rapidly for the EMIT and FIA techniques, and it may soon reach the point where these assays have startup costs competitive with agar plate assays. Reagent costs remain high however, and daily costs must be considered before adopting these techniques. The attraction of EMIT and FIA extends beyond their use in assay of aminoglycosides, because after an initial purchase of equipment, the technique can be easily used for almost all monitored drugs. Therefore, EMIT and FIA offer multi-drug flexibility for the clinical pharmacokineticist which cannot be matched by RIA, GC, or HPLC. Radioimmunoassay, FIA or EMIT are recommended for established and higher volume services, as it has high volume capabilities, rapid turnaround, and high specificity. High RIA reagent costs can be overcome by batching of samples, while EMIT procedures can be performed on centrifugal analyzers which reduces reagent volumes four-fold. Quality control must be rigid, and good laboratory technique is essential to ensure accurate results over the long term.

## PROSPECTUS

There is a pattern to the clinical use of drug levels in patient monitoring, and this pattern describes the evolving use of aminoglycoside serum levels. Initial therapeutic monitoring closely follows the development of an assay. Early investigators determined the major influences on the half-life, and renal disease was easily identified. Nomograms were created to be used when blood level determinations were unavailable. The nomograms were not perfect substitutes, so the use of blood levels continued to increase. Assay techniques were improved, and problems induced by improper timing in specimen collection were identified and solved. Before long, most clinicians had access to drug concentrations and used them frequently. The literature on the use of blood levels reported increases in efficacy and decreases in toxicity in glowing terms. Then, patients were discovered who did not follow the expected pattern. In the face of appropriate dosing and appropriate levels, some patients experience toxicity or therapeutic failure. The first reports of this phenomenon were dismissed, but when later confirmed, and further supported, a few vocal and influential clinicians stated that blood level determinations should be considered meaningless. Confusion and arguments follow, as some defend present practices, and others voice disbelief. Still others look for mechanisms to explain these exceptions. New information derived from mechanistic research provides perspective, and more appropriate monitoring begins on a limited scale. The newer methods always rely more heavily on observation of the patient for drug effect rather than, or in addition to lab tests. However, these practices are little more than our admission that not all factors affecting blood levels are yet understood.

The pattern above is not unique to aminoglycosides; one only need examine the use of digoxin levels since 1965 to note the precise stages in a similar order. Indeed, medical practice follows a similar and cyclical pattern in the diagnosis and treatment of disease.

New insight into kinetic monitoring of aminoglycosides awaits further research. We have not yet gathered sufficient data to understand our actions, but are beginning to recognize some of the larger pitfalls. It is sufficient for the prudent clinician to examine the present evidence, cautiously apply what is known, question what is not, and be alert for those patients who are the exceptions; for here, careful study will point the way to our future understanding.

Supported in Part by NIGMS grant 20852 from the National Institutes of Health.

## REFERENCES

1. Greenlaw CW, Blough SS, Haughen RK: Aminoglycoside serum assays restricted through a pharmacy program. Am J Hosp Pharm 1979; 36:1080–1083.
2. Bootman JL, Zaske D, Wertheimer Al, et al: Cost of individualizing aminoglycoside dosage regimens. Am J Hosp Pharm 1979; 36:368–370.
3. Barza M, Brown RB, Shen D, Gibaldi M, Weinstein L: Predictability of blood levels of gentamicin in man. J Infect Dis 1975; 132:165–174.
4. Kaye D, Levison ME, Labovitz ED: The unpredictability of serum concentrations of gentamicin: Pharmacokinetics of gentamicin in patients with normal and abnormal renal function. J Infect Dis 1974; 130:150–154.
5. Barza M, Lauermann M: Why monitor serum levels of gentamicin? Clin Pharmacokinetics 1978; 3:202–215.
6. Mendelson J, Portnoy J, Dick V, Black M: Safety of the bolus administration of gentamicin. Antimicrob Agents Chemother 1976; 9:633–638.
7. Korner B: Gentamicin therapy administered by intermittent intravenous injections. Acta Path Microbiol Scand Section B 1973; 81(Suppl)241:15–23.
8. Nielsen AB, Elb S: The use of gentamicin intravenously. Acta Path Microbiol Scand Section B 1973; 81(Suppl)241:23–29.
9. Bodey GP, Chang H-Y, Rodriquez V, Stewart D: Feasibility of administering aminoglycoside antibiotics by continuous intravenous infusion. Antimicrob Agents Chemother 1975; 8:328–333.
10. Keating MJ, Bodey GP, Valdivieso M, Rodriguez V: A randomized trial of three aminoglycosides. Medicine 1979; 58:159–170.
11. Issell BF, Keating MJ, Valdivieso M, Bodey GP: Continuous infusion tobramycin combined with carbenicillin for infections in cancer patients. Am J Med Sci 1979; 277:311–318.
12. Reiner NE, Bloxham DD, Thompson WL: Nephrotoxicity of gentamicin and tobramycin given once daily or continuously in dogs. J Antimicrob Chemother 1978; 4S:85–101.
13. Ericsson CD, Duke JH, Pickering LK: Clinical pharmacology of intravenous and intraperitoneal aminoglycoside antibiotics. Ann Surg 1978; 188:66–70.
14. Weinstein AJ, McHenry MC, Gavan TL: Systemic absorption of neomycin irrigating solution. JAMA 1977; 338:152–152.
15. Masur H, Whelton PK, Whelton A: Neomycin toxicity revisited. Arch Surg 1976; 111:822–825.
16. Schentag JJ, Jusko WJ, Vance JW, et al: Gentamicin disposition and tissue accumulation on multiple dosing. J Pharmacokin Biopharm 1977; 5:559–577.
17. Schentag JJ, Lasezkay G, Plaut ME, Jusko WJ, Cumbo TJ: Comparative tissue accumulation of gentamicin and tobramycin in patients. J Antimicrob Chemother 1978; 4S:23–30.

18. Schentag JJ, Jusko WJ, Plaut ME, Cumbo TJ, Vance JW, Abrutyn E: Tissue persistence of gentamicin in man. JAMA 1977; 238:327–329.
19. Kahlmeter G, Jonsson S, Kamme C: Multiple-compartment pharmacokinetics of tobramycin. J Antimicrob Chemother 1978; 4S:5–11.
20. Fabre J, Rudhardt M, Blanchard P, Regamey C: Persistence of sisomicin and gentamicin in renal cortex and medulla compared with other organs and serum in rats. Kidney Int 1976; 10:444–449.
21. Schentag JJ, Jusko WJ: Renal clearance and tissue accumulation of gentamicin. Clin Pharmacol Ther 1977; 22:364–370.
22. Gerding DN, Hall WH, Schierl EA, Manion RE: Cephalosporin and aminoglycoside concentrations in peritoneal capsular fluid in rabbits. Antimicrob Agents Chemother 1976; 10:902–911.
23. Kozak AJ, Gerding DN, Peterson LR, Hall WH: Gentamicin intravenous infusion rate: Effect on interstitial fluid concentration. Antimicrob Agents Chemother 1977; 12:606–608.
24. Carbon C, Contrepois A, Lamotte-Barrillon S: Comparative distribution of gentamicin, tobramycin, sisomicin netilmicin and amikacin in interstitial fluid in rabbits. Antimicrob Agents Chemother 1978; 13:368–372.
25. Tulkens P, Trouet A: The uptake and intracellular accumulation of aminoglycoside antibiotics in lysosomes of cultured rat fibroblasts. Biochem Pharmacol 1978; 27:415–424.
26. Bergeron MG, Trottier S: Influence of single or multiple doses of gentamicin and netilmicin on their cortical, medullary, and papillary distribution. Antimicrob Agents Chemother 1979; 15:635–641.
27. Gordon RC, Regamey C, Kirby WMM: Serum protein binding of the aminoglycoside antibiotics. Antimicrob Agents Chemother 1972; 2:214–216.
28. Ramirez-Ronda CH, Holmes RK, Sanford JP: Effects of divalent cations on binding of aminoglycoside antibiotics to human serum proteins and to bacteria. Antimicrob Agents Chemother 1975; 7:239–245.
29. Myers DR, DeFehr J, Bennett WM, et al: Gentamicin binding to serum and plasma proteins. Clin Pharmacol Ther 1978; 23:356–360.
30. Mendelson J, Portnoy J, Sigman H: Pharmacology of gentamicin in the biliary tract of humans. Antimicrob Agents Chemother 1973; 4:538–541.
31. Smithivas T, Hyams PJ, Rahal JJ: Gentamicin and ampicillin in human bile. J Infect Dis 1971; 124Suppl:S106–S108.
32. Pitt HA, Roberts RB, Johnson WD: Gentamicin levels in the human biliary tract. J Infect Dis 1973; 127:299–302.
33. March DC, Matthew EB, Persellin RH: Transport of gentamicin into synovial fluid. JAMA 1974; 228:607.
34. DeBroe ME: Antibiotics in renal lymph. Arch Int Pharmacodyn Ther 1973; 201:193–194.
35. Chisholm GD, Calnan JS, Waterworth PM: Distribution of gentamicin in body fluids. Br Med J 1968; 2:22–24.
36. Pennington JE, Reynolds HY: Pharmacokinetics of gentamicin sulfate in bronchial secretions. J Infect Dis 1975; 131:158–162.
37. Pennington JE, Reynolds HY: Concentrations of gentamicin and carbenicillin in bronchial secretions. J Infect Dis 1973; 128:63–68.
38. Wong GA, Peirce TH, Goldstein E, Hoeprich PD: Penetration of antimicrobial agents into bronchial secretions. Am J Med 1975; 59:219–223.
39. Pines A, Raafat H, Plucinski K: Gentamicin and colistin in chronic purulent bronchial infections. Br Med J 1967; 2:543–545.

40. Rahal JJ, Hyams PJ, Simberkoff MS, Rubinstein E: Combined intramuscular and intrathecal gentamicin for gram negative meningitis. NEJM 1974; 290:1394–1398.
41. Kaiser AB, McGee ZA: Aminoglycoside therapy of gram negative meningitis. NEJM 1975; 293:1215–1220.
42. Hollifeld JW, Kaiser AB, McGee ZA: Gram negative bacillary meningitis therapy. JAMA 1976; 236:1264–1266.
43. Chan RA: Gentamicin therapy in renal failure. Ann Int Med 1972; 76:773–778.
44. Simon VK, Mosinger EU, Malerczy V: Pharmacokinetic studies of tobramycin and gentamicin. Antimicrob Agents Chemother 1973; 3:445–450.
45. Gyselynck AM, Forrey A, Cutler R: Pharmacokinetics of gentamicin: Distribution and plasma and renal clearance. J Infect Dis 1971; 124S:S70–S76.
46. Bergan T, Brodwall EK, Westlie L, Oyri A: Renal excretion of gentamicin and effect of probenecid. Acta Path Microbiol Scand Section B 1973; 241:95–98.
47. Pennington JE, Dale DC, Reynolds HY, MacLowry JD: Gentamicin sulfate pharmacokinetics: Lower levels of gentamicin in blood during fever. J Infect Dis 1975; 132:270–275.
48. Mirhij NJ, Roberts RJ, Myers MG: Effects of hypoxemia on aminoglycoside serum pharmacokinetics in animals. Antimicrob Agents Chemother 1978; 14:344–347.
49. Reynolds AV, Hamilton-Miller JMT, Brumfitt W: Diminished effect of gentamicin under anerobic and hypercapnic conditions. Lancet 1976; 1:447–449.
50. Verklin RM, Mandell GL: Alteration of effectivesness of antibiotics by anaerobiosis. J Lab Clin Med 1977; 89:65–71.
51. Riff LJ, Jackson GG: Pharmacology of gentamicin in man. J Infect Dis 1971; 124Suppl:S98–S105.
52. Hull JH, Sarubbi FA: Gentamicin serum concentrations: Pharmacokinetic predictions. Ann Intern Med 1976; 85:183–189.
53. Schwartz SN, Pazin GJ, Lyon JA, Ho M, Pasculle AW: A controlled investigation of the pharmacokinetics of gentamicin and tobramycin in obese subjects. J Infect Dis 1978; 138:499–505.
54. Chiu PJS, Miller GH, Long JF, Waitz JA: Renal uptake and nephrotoxicity of gentamicin during urinary alkalinization in rats. Clin Exp Pharmacol Physiol 1979; 6:317–326.
55. Minuth JN, Musher DM, Thorsteinsson SB: Inhibition of the antibacterial activity of gentamicin by urine. J Infect Dis 1976; 133:14–21.
56. Mariel C, Veisshy P, Pechere JC, et al: Urinary pH and excretion of gentamicin. Br Med J 1972; 2:406.
57. Hsu CH, Kurtz TW, Easterling RE, Weller JM: Potentiation of gentamicin nephrotoxicity by metabolic acidosis. Proc Soc Exp Biol Med 1974; 140:894–897.
58. Gilbert DN, Kutscher E, Ireland P, et al: Effect of the concentrations of magnesium and calcium on the *in-vitro* susceptibility of Pseudomonas aeruginosa to gentamicin. J Infect Dis 1971; 124 Suppl:S37–S44.
59. Bennett WM, Hartnett MN, Gilbert DN, et al: Effect of sodium intake on gentamicin nephrotoxicity in the rat. Proc Soc Exp Biol Med 1976; 151:736–738.
60. Pechere JC, Dugal R: Clinical pharmacokinetics of aminoglycoside antibiotics. Clin Pharmacokin 1979; 4:170–199.
61. Luft FC, Kleit SA: Renal parenchymal accumulation of aminoglycoside antibiotics in rats. J Infect Dis 1974; 130:656–659.
62. Edwards CQ, Smith CR, Baughman KL, Rogers JF, Lietman PS: Concentrations of gentamicin and amikacin in human kidneys. Antimicrob Agents Chemother 1976; 9:925–927.

63. Whelton A, Carter GG, Bryant HH, Fox L, Walker WG: Therapeutic implications of gentamicin accumulation in severely diseased kidneys. Arch Intern Med 1976; 136:172–176.
64. Bennett WM, Hartnett MN, Craven R, et al: Gentamicin concentrations in blood, urine, and renal tissue of patients with end stage renal disease. J Lab Clin Med 1977; 90:389–393.
65. Whelton A, Carter GG, Craig TJ, Bryant HH, Herbst DV, Walker WG: Comparison of the intrarenal disposition of tobramycin and gentamicin: Therapeutic and toxicologic answers. J Antimicrob Chemother 1978; 4S–13–22.
66. Danish M, Schultz R, Jusko WJ: Pharmacokinetics of gentamicin and kanamycin during hemodialysis. Antimicrob Agents Chemother 1974; 6:841–847.
67. Gary NE: Peritoneal clearance and removal of gentamicin. J Infect Dis 1971; 124 Suppl:S96–S97.
68. Jusko WJ, Baliah T, Kim KH, Gerbracht LM, Yaffe S: Pharmacokinetics of gentamicin during peritoneal dialysis in children. Kidney International 1976; 9:430–438.
69. Schnermann J, Levine DZ: Tubular control of glomerular filtration rate in single nephrons. Can J Physiol Pharmcol 1975; 53:325–329.
70. DiBona GF, McDonald FD, Flamenbaum W, Dammin GJ, Oken DE: Maintenance of renal function in salt loaded rats despite severe tubular necrosis induced by $HgCl_2$. Nephron 1971; 8:205–220.
71. Thurau K, Boylan JW: Acute renal success. The unexpected logic of oliguria in acute renal failure. Amer J Med 1976; 61:308–315.
72. Schnermann J, Persson EG, Agerup B: Tubuloglomerular feedback. J Clin Invest 1973; 52:862–869.
73. Sato T, McDowell EM, McNeil JS, Flamenbaum W, Trump BF: Studies on the pathophysiology of acute renal failure. III. A study of the juxtaglomerular apparatus of the rat nephron following administration of mercuric chloride. Virchows Arch B Cell Pathol 1977; 24:279–293.
74. Schnermann J, Stowe N, Yarimiza S, Magnusson M, Tingwald G: Feedback control of glomerular filtration rate in isolated, blood-perfused dog kidneys. Amer J Physiol 1977; 233:F217–F224.
75. Wright FS: Intrarenal regulation of glomerular filtration rate. New Engl J Med 1974; 291:135–141.
76. Thurau KWC, Dahlheim H, Gruner A: Activation of renin in the single juxtoglomerular apparatus by sodium chloride in the tubular fluid at the macula densa. Circulation Res 1972; 30–31 Suppl:II 182–186.
77. Schentag JJ, Plaut ME, Cerra FB, Wels PB, Walczak P, Buckley RJ: Aminoglycoside nephrotoxicity in critically ill surgical patients. J Surg Res 1979; 26:270–279.
78. Silverblatt FJ, Kuehn C: Autoradiography of gentamicin uptake by the rat proximal tubule cell. Kidney International 1979; 15:335–345.
79. Just M, Erdmann G, Habermann E: Renal handling of polybasic drugs. Naunyn-Schmeidebergs Arch Pharmacol 1977; 300:57–66.
80. Just M, Habermann E: Renal handling of polybasic drugs, Part II. Naunyn-Schmeidebergs Arch Pharmacol 1977; 300:67–76.
81. Vera-Roman J, Krishnakantha TP, Cuppage FE: Gentamicin nephrotoxicity in rats, I. Acute biochemical and ultrastructural effects. Lab Invest 1975; 33:412–417.
82. Tulkens P, Aubert-Tulkens G, Van Hoff F, Trouet A: The lysosomal toxicity of aminoglycosides. In: Fillastre JP, ed. Nephrotoxicity. Interaction of drugs with membranes systems mitochondria-lysosomes. New York: Masson, 1978:231–252.

83. Kosek JC, Mazze RI, Cousins MJ: Nephrotoxicity of gentamicin. Lab Invest 1974; 30:48–57.
84. Morin JP, Fresel J, Fillastre JP, Vaillant R: Aminoglycoside actions on rat kidney lysosomes in vivo and in vitro. In: Fillastre JP, ed. Nephrotoxicity. Interaction of drugs with membranes systems mitochondria-lysosomes. New York: Masson, 1978: 253–264.
85. Bendirdjian JP, Foucher B, Fillastre JP: Influence des aminoglycosides sur le metabolisme respiratoire des mitochondries isolees de foie et de rein de rat. In: Fillastre JP, ed. Nephrotoxicity. Interaction of drugs with membranes systems mitochondria-lysosomes. New York: Masson, 1978:315–332.
86. Lietman PS: Aminoglycoside inhibition of a renal sodium-potassium ATP'ase: a possible model for nephrotoxicity. 18th Interscience Con. on Antimicrobial Agents and Chemotherapy, Atlanta, 1978; Abstract #328.
87. Anderson RJ, Linas SL, Berns AS, et al: Nonoliguric acute renal failure. New Engl J Med 1977; 296:1134–1138.
88. Mondorf AW, Breier J, Hendus J, et al: Effect of aminoglycosides on proximal tubule membranes of the human kidney. Europ J Clin Pharmacol 1978; 13:133–142.
89. Schentag JJ, Sutfin TA, Plaut ME, Jusko WJ: Early detection of aminoglycoside nephrotoxicity with urinary beta-2-microglobulin. J Med 1978; 9:201–210.
90. Peterson PA, Ervin PE, Berggard I: Differentiation of glomerular, tubular, and normal proteinuria: Determinations of urinary excretion of $B_2$-microglobulin, albumin, and total protein. J Clin Invest 1969; 48:1189–1198.
91. Schreiner GE: The identification and clinical significance of casts. Arch Intern Med 1957; 99:356–369.
92. Schentag JJ, Gengo FM, Plaut ME, Danner D, Mangione A, Jusko WJ: Urinary casts as an indicator of renal tubular damage in patients receiving aminoglycosides. Antimicrob Agents Chemother 1979; 16:468–474.
93. Mondorf AW, Zegelman M, Klose J, Hendus J, Breier J: Comparative studies on the action of aminoglycosides and cephalosporins on the proximal tubule of the human kidney. J Antimicrob Chemother 1978, 4 Suppl A:53–57.
94. Patel V, Luft FC, Yum MN, et al: Enzymuria in gentamicin induced kidney damage. Antimicrob Agents Chemother 1975; 7:364–369.
95. Stroo WE and Hook JB: Enzymes of renal origin in urine as indicators of nephrotoxicity. Toxicol Appl Pharmacol 1977; 39:423–434.
96. Luft FC, Rankin LI, Sloan RS, Yum MN: Recovery from animoglycoside nephrotoxicity with continued drug administration. Antimicrob Agents Chemother 1978; 14:284–287.
97. Gilbert DN, Houghton DC, Bennett WM, et al: Reversibility of gentamicin nephrotoxicity in rats. Proc Soc Exp Biol Med 1979; 160:99–103.
98. Luft FC, Yum MN, Kleit SA: The effect of concomitant mercuric chloride and gentamicin on kidney function and structure in the rat. J Lab Clin Med 1977; 89:622–631.
99. Hunter WC: Experimental study of acquired resistance of the rabbits renal epithelium to mercuric chloride. Ann Intern Med 1929; 2:796–806.
100. Schentag JJ, Cumbo TJ, Jusko WJ, Plaut ME: Gentamicin tissue accumulation and nephrotoxic reactions. J Am Med Assoc 1978; 240:2067–2069.
101. Fee WE, Vierra V, Lathrop GR: Clinical evaluation of aminoglycoside toxicity: Tobramycin versus gentamicin. A preliminary report. J Antimicrob Chemother 1978; 4S:31–36.

102. Smith CR, Maxwell RR, Edwards CQ, Rogers JF, Lietman PS: Nephrotoxicity induced by gentamicin and amikacin. Johns Hopkins Med J 1978; 142:85–90.
103. Frame PT, Phair JP, Watanakunakorn C, Bannister TW: Pharmacologic factors associated with gentamicin nephrotoxicity in rabbits. J Infect Dis 1977; 135:952–956.
104. Goodman EL, VanGelder J, Holmes R, et al: Prospective comparative study of variable dosage and variable frequency regimens. Antimicrob Agents Chemother 1975; 8:434–438.
105. Dahlgren JG, Anderson ET, Hewitt WL: Gentamicin blood levels; A guide to nephrotoxicity. Antimicrob Agents Chemother 1975; 8:58–62.
106. Noone P, Parsons TMC, Pattison JR, et al: Experience in monitoring gentamicin therapy during treatment of serious gram negative sepsis. Br Med J 1974; 2:477–481.
107. Jackson GG, Riff LJ: Pseudomonas bacteremia: Pharmacologic and other bases for failure of treatment with gentamicin. J Infect Dis 1971; 124 Suppl: S185–S191.
108. Bodey GP, Rodriguez V, Valdivieso M: Amikacin for treatment of infections in patients with malignant diseases. J Infect Dis 1976; 134 Suppl: S421–S426.
109. Kahlmeter G, Hallberg T, Kamme C: Gentamicin and tobramycin in patients with various infections. J Antimicrob Chemother 1978; 4 Suppl A:47–52.
110. Siersbaek-Nielsen K, Molholm Hansen J, Kampmann J, Kristensen M: Rapid evaluation of creatinine clearance. Lancet 1971; 1:1133–1134.
111. Wheeler LA, Sheiner LB: Clinical estimation of creatinine clearance. Am J Clin Pathol 1979; 72:27–31.
112. Sarubbi FA, Hull JH: Amikacin serum concentrations: Predictions of levels and dosage guidelines. Ann Intern Med 1978; 89:612–618.
113. Devine B: Gentamicin therapy. Drug Intell Clin Pharm 1974; 8:650–655.
114. Sawchuk RJ, Zaske DE: Pharmacokinetics of dosing regimens which utilize multiple intravenous infusions: Gentamicin in burn patients. J Pharmacokin Biopharm 1976; 4:183–195.
115. Sawchuk RJ, Zaske DE, Cipolle RJ, Wargin WA: Kinetic model for gentamicin dosing with the use of individual patient parameters. Clin Pharmacol Ther 1977; 21:362–369.
116. Zaske DE, Sawchuk RJ, Gerding DN, Strate RG: Increased dosage requirements of gentamicin in burn patients. J Trauma 1976; 16:824–828.
117. Loirat P, Rohan J, Baillet A, et al: Increased glomerular filtration rate in patients with major burns. N Engl J Med 1978; 299:915–919.
118. Hewitt WL: Gentamicin: Toxicity in perspective. Postgrad Med J 1974; 50S:55–59.
119. Lawson DH, Macadam RF, Singh H, Gavras H, Hartz S, Turnbull D, Linton AL: Effect of furosemide on antibiotic-induced renal damage in rats. J Infect Dis 1972; 126:593–600.
120. Chiu PJS, Long JF: Effects of hydration on gentamicin excretion and renal accumulation in furosemide-treated rats. Antimicrob Agents Chemother 1978; 14:214–217.
121. Churchill DN, Seely J: Nephrotoxicity associated with combined gentamicin-amphotericin B therapy. Nephron 1977; 19:176–181.
122. Gonzales-Vitale JC, Hayes DM, Cvitkovic E, Sternberg S: Acute renal failure after cis-dichlorodiammineplatinum and gentamicin-cephalothin. Cancer Treatment Rep 1978; 62:693–698.
123. Bloch R, Luft FC, Rankin LI, et al: Protection from gentamicin nephrotoxicity by cephalothin and carbenicillin. Antimicrob Agents Chemother 1979; 15:46–49.

124. Dellinger P, Murphy T, Barza M, et al: Effect of cephalothin on renal cortical concentrations of gentamicin in rats. Antimicrob Agents Chemother 1976; 9:587–588.
125. Fillastre JP, Laumonier R, Humbert G, et al: Acute renal failure with combined gentamicin and cephalothin therapy. Br Med J 1973; 2:396–397.
126. Bobrow SN, Jaffe E, Young RD: Anuria and acute tubular necrosis associated with gentamicin and cephalothin. J Am Med Assoc 1972; 222:1546–1547.
127. Cabanillas F, Burgos RC, Rodriguez RC, Baldizon C: Nephrotoxicity of combined cephalothin-gentamicin regimen. Arch Intern Med 1975; 135:850–851.
128. Wade JC, Smith CR, Petty BG, et al: Cephalothin plus an aminoglycoside is more nephrotoxic than methicillin plus an aminoglycoside. Lancet 1978; 2:604–606.
129. Klastersky J, Hensgens C, Debusscher L: Empiric therapy for cancer patients. Antimicrob Agents Chemother 1975; 7:640–645.
130. Riff LJ, Jackson GG: Laboratory and clinical conditions for gentamicin inactivation by carbenicillin. Arch Intern Med 1972; 130:887–891.
131. Davies M, Morgan JR, Anand C: Interactions of carbenicillin and ticarcillin with gentamicin. Antimicrob Agents Chemother 1975; 7:431–434.
132. Ervin FR, Bullock WE, Nuttal CE: Inactivation of gentamicin by penicillins in patients with renal failure. Antimicrob Agents Chemother 1976; 9:1004–1011.
133. Appel GB, Neu HC: Gentamicin in 1978. Ann Intern Med 1978; 89:528–538.
134. Smith CR, Baughman KL, Edwards CQ, Rogers JF, Lietman PS: Controlled comparison of amikacin and gentamicin. N Engl J Med 1977; 296:350–353.
135. Luft FC, Yum MN, Kleit SA: Comparative nephrotoxicities of netilmicin and gentamicin in rats. Antimicrob Agents Chemother 1976; 10:845–849.
136. Ormsby AM, Parker RA, Plamp CE, et al: Comparison of the nephrotoxic potential of gentamicin, tobramycin and netilmicin in the rat. Curr Ther Res 1979; 25:335–343.
137. Panwalker AP, Malow JB, Zimelis VM, Jackson GG: Netilmicin: Clinical efficacy, tolerance and toxicity. Antimicrob Agents Chemother 1978; 13:170–176.
138. Trestman I, Parson J, Santoro J, Goodhart G, Kaye D: Pharmacology and efficacy of netilmicin. Antimicrob Agents Chemother 1978; 13:832–836.
139. Snydman DR, Tally FP, Landesman SH, et al: Netilmicin in gram negative bacterial infections. Antimicrob Agents Chemother 1979; 15:50–54.
140. Gilbert DN, Plamp C, Starr P, Bennett WM, Houghton DC, Porter G: Comparative nephrotoxicity of gentamicin and tobramycin in rats. Antimicrob Agents Chemother 1978; 13:34–40.
141. Smith CR, Lipsky J, Laskin O, Hellman D, Mellits D, Longstreth J, Lietman PS: Double blind comparison of the nephrotoxicity and auditory toxicity of gentamicin and tobramycin. N Engl J Med 1980; 302:1106–1109.
142. Schentag JJ, Plaut ME, Cerra FB: Nephrotoxicity of gentamicin and tobramycin in patients: Pharmacokinetic and clinical studies. Current Chemotherapy and Infectious Disease: Proc. 11th ICC and 19th ICAAC. Ed. Nelson JD and Grassi C, ASM Publications, Washington, DC, 1980; 614–616.
143. Brummett RE, Fox KE, Bendrich TW, Himes DL: Ototoxicity of tobramycin, gentamicin, amikacin and sisomicin in the guinea pig. J Antimicrob Chemother 1978; 4 Suppl:73–83.
144. Winters RE, Litwick KD, Hewitt WL: Relation between dose and levels of gentamicin in blood. J Infect Dis 1971; 124 Suppl: S90–S95.
145. Alcid DV, Seligman SJ: Simplified assay for gentamicin in the presence of other antibiotics. Antimicrob Agents Chemother 1973; 3:559–561.

146. Lund ME, Blazevic DJ, Matsen JM: Rapid gentamicin bioassay using a multiresistant strain of Klebsiella pneumoniae. Antimicrob Agents Chemother 1973; 4:569–573.

147. Smith DH, Van Otto B, Smith AL: A rapid chemical assay for gentamicin. N Engl J Med 1972; 286:583–586.

148. Case RV, Mezei LM: An enzymatic radioassay for gentamicin. Clin Chem 1978; 24:2145–2150.

149. Mayhew JW, Gorbach SL: Assay for gentamicin and tobramycin by Gas-Liquid Chromatography. Antimicrob Agents Chemother 1978; 14:851–855.

150. Anhalt JP, Brown SD: High performance liquid chromatographic assay of aminoglycoside antibiotics. Clin Chem 1978; 24:1940–1947.

151. Maitra SK, Yoshikawa TT, Hansen JL: Gentamicin assay by high performance liquid chromatography. Clin Chem 1977; 23:2275–2278.

152. Stevens P, Young LS, Hewitt WL: Radioimmunoassay, radioenzymatic assay, and microbioassay of gentamicin. J Lab Clin Med 1975; 86:349–359.

153. Waterworth PM: An enzyme preparation inactivating all penicillins and cephalosporins. J Clin Pathol 1973; 26:596–598.

154. Giamarellou H, Zimelis VM, Matulionis DO, Jackson GG: Assay of aminoglycoside antibiotics in clinical specimens. J Infect Dis 1975; 132:399–406.

155. Standefer JC, Saunders GC: Enzyme immunoassay for gentamicin. Clinical Chemistry 1978; 24:1903–1907.

156. Rubenstein KE, Schneider RS, Ullman EF: Homogenous enzyme immunoassay—a new immunochemical technique. Biochem Biophys Res Commun 1972; 42:846–851.

157. Burd JF, Wong RC, Feeney JE, Carrico RJ, Boguslaski RC: Homogenous reactant-labeled fluorescent immunoassay for therapeutic drugs exemplified by gentamicin determination in human serum. Clin Chem 1977; 23:1402–1408.

158. Zaske DE, Cipolle RJ, Strate RJ: Gentamicin dosage requirements: Wide interpatient variations in 242 surgery patients. Surgery 1980; 87:164–169.

## Counterpoint Discussion

# Aminoglycosides

Darwin E. Zaske, Pharm.D.

### Introduction

Aminoglycoside antibiotics are among the most useful group of antimicrobial agents for gram-negative infections. This group of antibiotics includes streptomycin, kanamycin, neomycin, paromomycin, gentamicin, tobramycin, and amikacin. In addition, netilmicin is presently in Phase III trials and will likely be marketed in the near future. Some agents have a higher risk of toxicity or higher incidence of bacterial resistance and are not currently used. Gentamicin, tobramycin, and amikacin are presently the most widely used aminoglycoside agents and this "counterpoint" will emphasize these agents.

The aminoglycosides are quite similar in physical, chemical, pharmacologic, and toxicologic properties. They are bactericidal and rapidly induce their lethal effects to the bacterial cells. Ototoxicity and nephrotoxicity are the most frequent and troublesome side effects of these agents. The following discussion describes the antibacterial activity, the pharmacokinetic parameters, factors related to elimination, methods for controlling serum concentrations, and the clinical results of controlling serum concentrations of these three commonly used agents.

**Clinical Indications.** The aerobic gram-negative bacilli are the primary pathogens for which aminoglycoside treatment is indicated. The spectrum of activity for the aminoglycosides include *Eschericha coli, Proteus* species, *Enterobacter* species, *Klebsiella* species, *Acinetobacter* species, *Pseudomonas* species, *Serratia* species, *Providencia* species, and *Staphylococcus aureus* (1). Other aerobic gram-negative bacilli are susceptible to aminoglycosides but are rarely indications for clinical use. These include *Neisseria gonorrhea, Neisseria meningitides,* and *Hemophilus influenzae.* Anaerobic bacteria are uniformly resistant to any of the aminoglycosides.

Several antibiotic groups have been demonstrated to have synergistic activity with aminoglycosides. This is especially true for the beta-lactam antibiotics such as the penicillins or cephalosporins. The proposed mechanism of synergy is an increase in the porosity of the bacterial cell caused by the beta-lactam antibiotic. This results in more of the aminoglycoside penetrating the bacterial cell and higher intracellular concentrations. This further increases the intracellular concentration of aminoglycosides and the antibacterial effect. Specific examples of synergistic activity include a combination of an amino-glycoside and penicillin with group-D *Streptococci* (2) and *Pseudomonas aeruginosa* (3). These combinations should be considered when these pathogens cause life-threatening infections such as endocarditis, pneumonia, or a bacteremia.

## Therapeutic Range

Improved treatment response has been associated with obtaining therapeutic serum concentrations of aminoglycosides early in a treatment course. Measuring serum concentrations and adjusting a patient's dosage regimen has been previously advocated (4,5,6). These drugs have a low therapeutic index, and concentrations necessary for optimal efficacy approximate those concentrations associated with a higher risk of toxicity. With large interpatient variation of pharmacokinetic parameters, serum concentrations resulting from recommended dosage regimens may have substantial variation. Measuring serum concentrations and adjusting an individual patient's dosage regimens are often necessary to achieve desired (therapeutic) serum concentrations.

Noone et al studied 68 episodes of gram-negative sepsis which were treated with gentamicin (4). They compared the treatment response in patients who had "subtherapeutic" serum concentrations to those who had "therapeutic" serum concentrations within the first 72 hours of treatment. The therapeutic concentrations were defined as peak concentrations greater than 5 µg/ml for patients with soft-tissue infections, gram-negative septicemias, or urinary tract infections. For patients with gram-negative pneumonia, peak concentrations greater than 8 µg/ml were considered therapeutic. The therapeutic responses for these two groups of patients were markedly different. Eighty-four percent of the patients who achieved therapeutic serum concentrations had an optimal treatment response while only twenty-three percent of the patients who had inadequate serum concentrations responded to treatment. Larger doses than those commonly recommended were frequently necessary to achieve desired concentrations. The authors concluded that the most direct and easiest way of ensuring adequate therapy within the first 72 hours of treatment is to measure serum concentrations and adjust the patient's dosage regimen. They further concluded that predictions of serum concentrations using estimates of renal function (i.e., serum creatinine or creatinine clearance) resulted in substantial error with individual patients.

Improved treatment response in burn patients with Pseudomonas ecthyma gangrenosum has been noted when patients received individualized doses of gentamicin (5,6). Ecthyma gangrenosum occurs infrequently in burn patients; however, it was universally fatal in these patients. This complication of Pseudomonas sepsis is characterized by the fulminant spread of Pseudomonas through the lymphatic and cardiovascular system and invasion of previously viable tissue. This metastatic spread of Pseudomonas occurs in visceral and cutaneous tissues. Recently, Loebl and coworkers described the successful treatment of three pediatric burn patients with this complication (5). They attributed the favorable response to administering inadvertently large doses of gentamicin. We have reported successful treatment in four of five patients with Pseudomonas ecthyma gangrenosum (6). These patients required excessively high doses to obtain "therapeutic" serum concentrations. One patient required 30 mg/kg/day to achieve the desired therapeutic concentration. The only patient who did not survive the course of ecthyma received a maximal daily dose of 12 mg/kg/day. However, the nonsurvivor achieved a peak serum concentration of only 4.5 µg/ml. The average daily dose required in these patients was 19 mg/kg/day. These burn patients thus required markedly increased dosages to achieve therapeutic serum concentrations, which in turn were associated with improved treatment response.

In patients with Pseudomonas bacteremias, subtherapeutic serum concentrations were identified as one of the major pharmacologic factors in explaining treatment failures with gentamicin (7). In addition, a large group of burn patients with predominantly pseudomonas bacteremia or burn wound sepsis were evaluated to determine the impact of individualized gentamicin dosage regimens (8). Sixty-six patients received individualized dosages and were compared to a retrospective control group of 39 patients who received conventional dosage regimens of 3 to 5 mg/kg/day. The patient groups were balanced in terms of independent variables which may affect patient survival, including percent burn, age, body weight, concurrent antibiotics, topical therapy, nutritional support, sex, complications, pre-existing disease, etc. Those patients who were given individualized gentamicin therapy required 7.4 mg/kg/day of gentamicin to ensure therapeutic concentrations (Figure 1), while patients given conventional dosages received an average daily dosage of 4.5 mg/kg/day. Patient survival for the first septic episode was 51% in patients receiving conventional dosage regimens and 86% for patients receiving individualized regimens ($x^2$ (1df) = 13.7; p< .001). Improved patient response for the first septic episode contributed to an overall improvement in patient survival for the entire hospital course. (Figure 2). Patients' survival for the entire hospital course was 33% for patients receiving conventional dosages compared to 64% in patients receiving individualized regimens. This difference was highly significant ($x^2$ (1df) 7.8; p< .005). A strong temporal relationship was found between the increased patient survival and the implementation of individualized regimens. In addition, further statistical analysis was also performed using multivariant techniques. From these analyses, measuring serum levels and adjusting dosages were found to be an important factor influencing patient survival.

The relationship between trough levels of antibiotics and treatment response was also evaluated. Anderson et al demonstrated a higher failure rate in patients who had excessively long periods of antibiotic serum concentrations below the inhibitory concentration for a particular pathogen (9). He referred to these treatment failures as "breakthrough bacteremias" attributed to long periods of the dosing interval where serum concentrations were below the inhibitory level. A large number of patients receiving aminoglycosides demonstrate an extremely short half-life (< 2 hours) of the drug resulting in serum concentrations below the minimum inhibitory concentration for selected pathogens early in the dosing interval. Thus, serum concentrations may be below the inhibitory level for many common gram-negative pathogens for 5 to 6 hours of the conventional 8-hour interval for gentamicin and tobramycin. For amikacin, this period of subinhibitory concentrations may be 9 to 10 hours of the conventional 12-hour dosing interval. Therefore, preventing excessively long periods of subinhibitory serum concentrations by adjusting the dosing interval according to the elimination rate may be an important factor in preventing treatment failures. This would appear to be more important in the patients who are a severely compromised host (neutropenic) with gram-negative sepsis.

**Inhibitory Concentrations.** The intrinsic activity of gentamicin and tobramycin is considerably higher than reported for amikacin. The minimum inhibitory concentration for most gram-negative pathogens is similar for gentamicin and tobramicin. Most gram-negative pathogens are susceptible to 2 to 3 µg/ml of gentamicin or tobramycin (Table 1). With amikacin, most pathogens are inhibited by concentra-

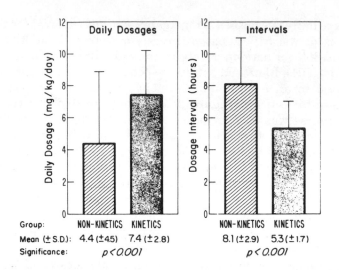

FIGURE 1. The daily dosage and dosage interval are illustrated for the patients receiving conventional dosages (non-kinetics) and patients who were individualized (kinetics). The patients who were individualized received approximately twice the daily dosage for the entire treatment period and received a dose more frequently.

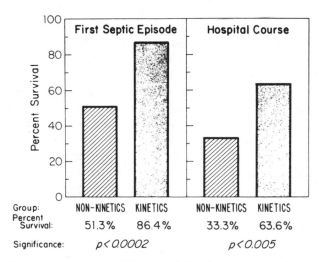

FIGURE 2. Patient survival is illustrated for the patients who received conventional dosages compared to those patients who received individualized regimens. Patient survival is indicated for the first septic episode and the entire hospital course. Thus, significant change in patient survival occurred for the first septic episode and entire hospital course after the implementation of individualized regimens.

214

TABLE 1. RELATIVE MINIMUM INHIBITORY CONCENTRATION TO INHIBIT 80% OF THE ISOLATES

| | Isolates tested | Gentamicin µg/ml | Tobramycin µg/ml | Amikacin µg/ml |
|---|---|---|---|---|
| E.coli | 300 | 1–1.5 | 1–1.5 | 4 |
| Klebsiella pneumoniae | 200 | 0.5–1 | 0.25–0.5 | 2–4 |
| Proteus mirabilis | 200 | 2–4 | 2–4 | 8–16 |
| Proteus rettgeri | 50 | R | R | 8 |
| Proteus morgani | 50 | 2–4 | 1–2 | 4–8 |
| Proteus vulgaris | 50 | 2–4 | 2–4 | 8–16 |
| Pseudomonas aeruginosa | 200 | 1–2 | 0.5–1 | 1–2 |
| Enterobacter aerogenes | 50 | 1–2 | 1–2 | 2–4 |
| Serratia marcescens | 25 | R | R | 8–16 |
| Providencia stuartii | 50 | R | R | 8–16 |

Summarized from Knothe et al: J Inf. Dis. 134:S272, 1976.
R = A large number of the isolates were resistant.

tions of 4 to 8 $\mu g/ml$. Many institutions are currently reporting susceptibility results from clinical isolates as a minimum inhibitory concentration. These values may be useful to the clinician in selecting desired peak and trough concentrations of an aminoglycoside for a specific patient.

**Desired Concentrations.** Treatment response is related to peak and trough concentrations. Several factors should be considered in selecting desired peak and trough concentrations for a specific patient. These factors include the patient's clinical condition, site of infection, and the relative sensitivity of the suspected or isolated pathogen. In patients with a higher risk of morbidity and mortality, higher peak and trough concentrations should be selected. For gentamicin and tobramycin, peak concentration should range between 5 and 8 $\mu g/ml$ for patients with soft-tissue infections or less severe gram-negative infections. In patients with more severe gram-negative sepsis or gram-negative pneumonias, the desired peak concentrations should range between 8 and 10 $\mu g/ml$. The trough concentrations for these two aminoglycosides should be less than 1 $\mu g/ml$ for less severe gram-negative infections and 0.5 to 1.5 for life-threatening infections. With amikacin, desired peak concentrations for moderately severe gram-negative sepsis range between 20 and 25 $\mu g/ml$, and 25 to 28 $\mu g/ml$ in patients with pneumonias or severe gram-negative sepsis. Desired trough concentrations for amikacin range between 1 and 4 $\mu g/ml$ for less severe infections; 4 to 8 $\mu g/ml$ for life-threatening infections. The peak level is the concentration post-infusion; the trough level is the concentration prior to an infusion at steady-state. These suggested values for peaks and troughs are guidelines which may need to be modified for specific patients.

## Toxicity

The two most frequent toxic effects occurring with aminoglycosides are ototoxicity and nephrotoxicity. When the aminoglycosides were originally introduced, the incidence of ototoxicity and nephrotoxicity was reported to range between 3 and 10%. More recently, however, markedly different incidences have been reported. Some of these differences may be attributed to different patient populations, different methods of evaluating toxicity, or different methods of administering aminoglycoside antibiotics. Some investigators have evaluated older patients in medical intensive care units. These patients are at a higher risk of toxicity due to their older age, concurrent medical complications (such as congestive heart failure), dehydration, hypotension, and concurrent drug therapy such as furosemide. Cochlear and vestibular function have been evaluated clinically for typical signs of ototoxicity such as vertigo, tinnitus, and hearing impairment. Audiometry and electronystagmography have been used to more objectively assess changes in eighth cranial nerve function and subclinical changes which may be associated with aminoglycoside treatment. However, several practical problems make these more objective measures difficult to perform in a clinical environment. Because of background noise or visual distractions, these tests should ideally not be performed in the patients' hospital room. Although these tests should be done in a sound-proof room, many patients receiving aminoglycosides cannot be transported because of isolation or supportive medical equipment. Moreover, many of these patients cannot cooperate with these tests because of altered states of consciousness secondary to sepsis or a physical injury such as facial burns or fractures. Thus, the results of audiometry and electronystagmography have day-to-day variations which may falsely be attributed to aminoglycoside toxicity. Various methods for the evaluation of nephrotoxicity were discussed in the previous chapter.

Aminoglycoside antibiotics have been administered by continuous infusion, bolus injections, and intermittent infusions. Each method of administration may have different risks of toxicity. Some investigators have monitored and controlled serum concentrations at one hour post-infusion. For gentamicin and tobramycin, the desired concentrations at the one-hour time point range between 5 and 10 µg/ml, and between 20 and 30 µg/ml for amikacin. A large number of patients have serum half-lives approximating one hour (Figure 8). In these patients with more rapid elimination, serum concentrations *immediately* post-infusion may have ranged between 10 and 20 µg/ml for gentamicin and tobramycin, and 40 to 60 µg/ml for amikacin. These concentrations may be associated with an increased risk of ototoxicity and nephrotoxicity.

Several risk factors have been identified which may be associated with a higher risk of oto- and/or nephrotoxicity. These include increasing age of the patient, compromised renal function, concurrent hemo- or peritoneal dialysis, increased peak or trough serum concentrations, total dose, duration of treatment, previous exposure to aminoglycosides, concurrent ototoxic or nephrotoxic drugs, concurrent use of rapid diuretics, and documented infection. Thus, a large number of variables seem to predispose patients to a higher risk of aminoglycoside toxicity. Some of these variables may be interrelated and the risk of ototoxicity and nephrotoxicity may be markedly reduced by controlling the peak and trough serum aminoglycoside concentrations.

Other side effects attributed to aminoglycosides include neuromuscular blockade, hypersensitivity reaction, and infrequent local gastrointestinal, hematologic, and central nervous system toxicity.

**Ototoxicity.** The incidence of overt clinical ototoxicity in the early experiences with gentamicin ranged between 3 and 10% of treated patients. Since the identification of risk factors associated with increased ototoxicity, the incidence has decreased substantially to 1 to 3% of patients treated. During clinical trials of tobramycin and amikacin, the incidence of overt ototoxicity was similar to the risk of ototoxicity with gentamicin (10,11). The auditory dysfunction induced by aminoglycosides appears to be reversible in approximately 50% of patients. The vestibular dysfunction is generally overcome by other compensatory mechanisms.

**Nephrotoxicity.** Aminoglycoside nephrotoxicity is more complex and often difficult to separate from complications due to underlying disease. In patients with severe gram-negative sepsis, hypotension and shock may be complications due to sepsis which may also result in acute tubular necrosis. These complications present with a clinical course which is difficult to differentiate from aminoglycoside induced renal failure. Clinically and histologically, the changes in the kidney resulting from aminoglycosides and hypotension cannot be differentiated. Thus, the specific cause of changes in renal function during a course of therapy for gram-negative sepsis is complex and difficult to determine. In some instances, the changes in renal function may be due to underlying disease, which then affect aminoglycoside elimination, resulting in increased serum concentrations and further damage to the nephron.

The incidence of nephrotoxicity has ranged between 3 and 10% in most clinical studies (10,11). The clinical parameter used to assess renal function and further define aminoglycoside nephrotoxicity is a change in serum creatinine of 0.5 mg/dl or greater. Urinary enzymes, proteins, and casts may provide additional and more specific information regarding aminoglycoside toxicity. In most patients, the changes in renal function induced by aminoglycosides are reversed during therapy or shortly after discontinuing the drug. Two recent reports suggest that the incidence of nephrotoxicity may range between 12 and 25% in patients receiving aminoglycosides (12,13). In both studies, peak serum levels were obtained one hour post-infusion, and these concentrations were controlled between 4 and 10 µg/ml for gentamicin and tobramycin, and 20 and 30 µg/ml for amikacin. The trough concentrations were obtained five minutes prior to the next dose, and the desired levels were 0.5 to 2 μg/ml for gentamicin and tobramycin, and 2 to 5 μg/ml for amikacin. A substantial amount of variation may occur in the post-infusion peak concentration when the one-hour level is controlled between 4 and 10 μg/ml for gentamicin and tobramycin and 20 and 30 μg/ml for amikacin. If a hypothetical patient had a half-life of one hour, the peak concentration could range between 10 and 20 μg/ml for gentamicin and tobramycin and 40 and 60 μg/ml for amikacin. These concentrations are associated with a higher risk of toxicity (14,15). In addition, the treatment aminoglycoside was not randomized, but determined by the physician (12). The groups receiving different aminoglycosides were not well matched for risk factors such as concurrent cephalosporins, diuretics, steroids, prior aminoglycosides, and increased age. The trough concentrations for gentamicin were markedly higher than trough concentrations of tobramycin. Prior aminoglycosides may protect against nephrotoxicity, while cephalosporins, potent diuretics, and increasing age are risk factors that were not balanced between groups. Thus, differences in toxicity may be group differences rather than intrinsic differences in aminoglycosides. The high toxicity is likely related to the high peak and trough concentrations, a population with higher risks, the frequent concurrent use of nephrotoxic drugs, or the intensive monitoring for toxicity. [*Editors Note:* Inspection of references 12 and 13, and communication with their authors reveals that peaks were measured at one hour after the *start* of the infusion, not one hour after the end. There were no patients with one hour half-lives in either study, and gentamicin and tobramycin groups show no statistical differences in age, sex, weight, trough concentrations, concurrent cephalosporins and diuretics, dose, or duration of treatment in either study.] In our institution, the peak and trough concentrations are controlled within the guidelines discussed under "Desired Concentrations." The incidence of nephrotoxicity (increase in serum creatinine of >0.5 mg/dl) was less than 1% of the first 1065 patients receiving individualized regimens of gentamicin.

**Relationship of Concentration and Toxicity.** For gentamicin and tobramycin, there is increased risk of oto- and nephrotoxicity if peak concentrations are consistently above 12 to 15 μg/ml (14). For amikacin, peaks above 32 to 34 μg/ml have been associated with a higher risk of oto- and nephrotoxicity (15). For gentamicin, a higher risk of toxicity has been associated with trough levels consistently above 2 μg/ml (16). For amikacin, trough concentrations consistently exceeding 10 μg/ml appear to be associated with a higher risk of toxicity. These guidelines should be followed to reduce the risk of toxicity.

**Neuromuscular Blockade.** Neuromuscular blockade occurs more frequently when an aminoglycoside is administered intravenously and concurrently with neuromuscular blocking or anesthetic agents such as ether, tubocurarine, succinylcholine, decamethonium, or gallamine. Additionally, patients with hypocalcemia or myasthenia gravis are more susceptible to neuromuscular blockade. The mechanism of aminoglycoside induced neuromuscular blockade involves interference with calcium and immediate release of acetylcholine at the level of presynaptic membrane. The respiratory depression and apnea is quickly reversed by promptly administering calcium or an anticholinesterase agent such as neostigmine or endrophonium.

## Pharmacokinetic Parameters

**Administration.** The aminoglycoside antibiotics may be administered by either intramuscular injection or intravenous infusion. These agents are generally well absorbed after intramuscular injections; however, in patients with severe gram-negative sepsis, blood perfusion of the intramuscular site may be reduced due to hypotension. Additionally, repeated injections at the same intramuscular site may impair absorption and result in more variation in serum concentrations. However, the intramuscular route of administration may be desirable in patients who are relatively stable and as follow up to intravenous therapy. Peak serum concentrations after intramuscular injections are generally achieved within 45 to 120 minutes after the injection (17). In patients with compromised renal function, these peak levels will be achieved later depending upon the degree of renal impairment. Intravenous infusions of 30 to 60 minutes are reported to be safer, since high serum concentrations achieved after bolus infusions may be associated with a higher incidence of toxicity. Some data suggest tissue levels of aminoglycosides may be increased in *in vivo* infection models if the concentration gradient is maintained for a period of time as compared to bolus injections. Thus, 30 to 60 minute infusions may have a higher degree of safety and may potentially increase tissue concentrations of these agents.

**Pharmacokinetic Model.** Aminoglycoside antibiotics are characterized by linear pharmacokinetic principles indicating a direct proportionality between increasing dose and both increasing serum concentration and increasing area under the concentration time curve. The relationship between serum concentration and time has received considerable discussion. Following a one-hour infusion, the serum concentration time data decline in a mono-exponential manner and can be characterized by a one-compartment model within the concentration range encountered clinically. Thus, a linear relationship is observed between the log of concentration and time. If the drug is given by rapid bolus, an early distribution phase may occur, resulting in a biexponential decline. This distribution phase is very rapid and generally does not occur with 60 minute infusions except in patients with compromised renal function. A third phase may also occur, especially in patients with compromised renal function. This phase most likely results from tissue redistribution. This phase is proposed to explain the drug accumulation in patients receiving aminoglycosides and to be related to patients developing nephrotoxicity. This drug accumulation may have substantial effects in patients with renal function less than 25% of normal and who are treated for longer than 10 to 14 days. The rising concentrations should be prevented by monitoring peak and trough levels at five to seven day intervals and adjusting the dosing interval accordingly. A one-compartment model thus characterizes the disposition of aminoglycosides with minimal error. These dosage adjustments should be done early in the patient's treatment course to ensure therapeutic concentrations and improve efficacy (4). If performed early, high peak and trough serum concentrations are prevented, reducing one of the risk factors of toxicity.

**Distribution.** Aminoglycoside antibiotics distribute well into body fluids including synovial, peritoneal, and pleural fluids (18). These agents distribute poorly in the bile, feces, prostate, and amniotic fluid. Aminoglycosides also distribute poorly in the central nervous system and the vitreous humor of the eye. Binding to serum proteins is less than 10% and is not considered to be clinically significant.

Aminoglycoside antibiotics distribute to a pharmacologic space very similar to the physiologic space of the extracellular fluid compartment. In normal volunteers, the extracellular fluid compartment approximates 20 to 25% of body weight. This physiological space is quite susceptible to several changes that may occur during gram-negative sepsis such as dehydration, congestive heart failure, etc. Frequently patients in initial phases of gram-negative sepsis are febrile, nauseated, and vomiting, resulting in dehydration. Consequently, the extracellular fluid compartment and drug volume are decreased. In these patients, the drug's distribution volume is markedly lower than 20% of body weight (Figure 3). Additionally, several subgroups of patients have been identified which are likely to have changes in drug distribution volume. These include patients with congestive heart failure, patients with peritonitis, patients immediately postpartum, or patients receiving intravenous hyperalimentation. In addition, newborn infants are known to have a larger extracellular fluid volume

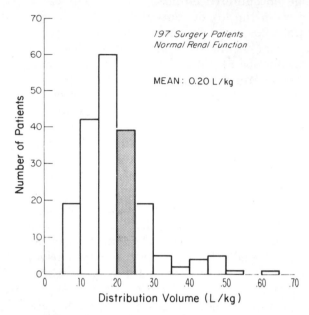

FIGURE 3. The distribution volume of gentamicin is illustrated for 855 patients who had a normal serum creatinine. The drug was originally thought to distribute into approximately 20 to 25% of body weight. However, substantially more variation occurred between patients as indicated.

per unit of body weight. Consequently, the drug's distribution volume in infants is frequently in the range of 50 to 70% of body weight (19). Initially, the distribution volume of aminoglycosides was thought to be consistent from patient to patient. However, the distribution volume demonstrates considerable variability between patients. This interpatient variation appears to be similar for all three aminoglycosides and have a substantial effect on serum concentrations and dosage requirements (Figure 4).

In addition to the interpatient variation, the drug's distribution volume may change during the course of antibiotic therapy. This is especially true for patients who are markedly dehydrated in the initial phases of sepsis or patients who have a large volume initially. During the course of therapy in a patient who is dehydrated, generally intravenous fluids are administered and consequently the fluid deficit is replaced. As the fluid deficit is replaced, the drug's distribution volume will increase. In contrast, patients with congestive heart failure or

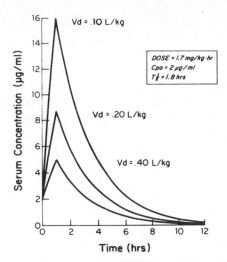

FIGURE 4. The wide interpatient variation in distribution volume has a marked effect on serum concentration-time data. If patients receive the same dosage, have the same starting concentrations, and the same half-life, the patient with the lower distribution volume achieves serum concentrations which are associated with a higher risk of toxicity. In contrast, patients with a larger distribution volume achieve serum concentrations with the same dose that only approach therapeutic levels. Thus, the variation in the distribution volume needs to be considered in individualizing a patient's dosage regimen.

peritonitis will eliminate their excess fluid during the course of therapy. In some patients, these changes can be substantial and require a marked change in the dosage regimen to control serum concentrations. This change in the distribution volume is independent of any change in renal function but will influence the drug's half-life if total body clearance remains constant within the patient (Figure 5). This change is a direct relationship and thus as the volume increases, the drug's half-life will also increase. With only *moderate* changes in the extracellular fluid volume and drug volume, the drug's clearance remains relatively constant. In a *severe* state of dehydration, the drug clearance may decrease secondary to a decrease in cardiac output and shunting of blood from the kidney. In patients with large volumes, the cardiac output, renal blood flow, glomerular filtration, and drug clearance may increase, providing the cardiovascular system can tolerate the extra fluid load without failing. Thus, cardiovascular hemodynamics and the drug's clearance may also change with the extracellular fluid compartment and drug volume. Clinically, monitoring of serum levels in patients with fluid changes is imperative to ensure therapeutic serum concentrations.

**Elimination.** Aminoglycoside antibiotics are primarily eliminated unchanged by the kidney via glomerular filtration. This route of elimination accounts for approximately 85 to 95% of the dose administered, and results in high urinary concentrations after recommended dosages. Small amounts of drug have been found in the bile and may represent an additional route of elimination (18). In the plot of aminoglycoside clearance versus creatinine clearance, a positive intercept occurs and is also suggested to support a non-filtration route of elimination. A small amount of the drug has been proposed to be actively secreted (20). The major route of elimination, however, is by glomerular filtration.

A wide interpatient variation in elimination of the three aminoglycosides has recently been recognized and is now a clinical problem of concern. This interpatient variation occurs in patients with normal serum creatinine or with a normal creatinine clearance. The magnitude of this variation seems greater in patients being treated for gram-negative sepsis than in normal volunteers. This variation may also be greater in the initial phases of treatment, rather than later in the treatment course when patients have stabilized.

In volunteers with normal renal function, the half-life of the gentamicin was initially reported to vary between 2.5 and 4 hours (21). The half-life of amikacin ranged from 0.8 to 2.1 hours (22), 2.1 to 2.4 hours (23), and 1.9 to 2.8 hours (24) in volunteers with normal renal function. The mean values ranged from 1.4 to 2.3 hours. In comparison, a large group of patients were studied in the early course of sepsis. For gentamicin, the half-life ranged from 0.4 to 32.7 hours in 855 patients with normal serum creatinine ($\leq$ 1.5 mg/dl) and 0.4 to 7.6 hours in 331 patients with normal serum creatinine clearance ($\geq$ 100 ml/min/1.73m$^2$). For tobramycin, the half-life ranged from 0.5 to 8.6 hours in 46 patients with a normal serum creatinine and from 0.5 to 5.1 hours in 16 patients with a normal serum creatinine clearance. For amikacin the half-life ranged from 0.68 to 14.4 hours in 67 patients with a normal serum creatinine (Figure 6) and from 0.68 to 7.2 hours in 37 patients with a normal creatinine clearance.

The total body clearance of the aminoglycosides also demonstrated considerable patient to patient variability. The total body clearance for gentamicin varied from 7.0 to 249 ml/hr/kg in 855 patients with a normal serum creatinine and from 8.4 to 242 ml/hr/kg in 331 patients with a normal creatinine clearance. For tobramycin, the total body

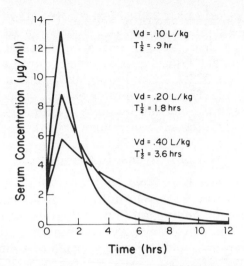

FIGURE 5.   When the distribution volume of aminoglycoside changes during the course of therapy, the half-life will also change *if* total body clearance remains constant. This change may substantially alter the dose and the dosing interval that a patient should receive to obtain therapeutic concentrations.

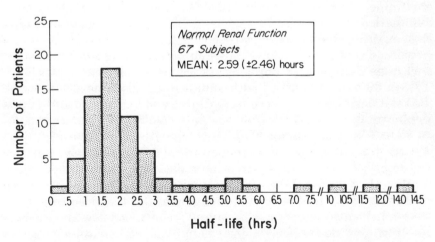

FIGURE 6.   The half-life of amikacin is illustrated for 67 patients who had a normal serum creatinine.

225

clearance varied from 14.8 to 222 ml/hr/kg in 46 patients with a normal serum creatinine and from 35.1 to 164 ml/hr/kg in 16 patients with a normal creatinine clearance. For amikacin, the total body clearance varied from 6.5 to 200 ml/hr/kg in 67 patients with a normal serum creatinine and from 37.8 to 200 ml/hr/kg in 37 patients with a normal creatinine clearance. Thus, considerable patient to patient variability occurred in the elimination and clearance of aminoglycosides, even in patients with normal serum creatinine or creatinine clearance.

## Factors Related to Aminoglycoside Disposition

Several factors have been reported to alter the disposition of aminoglycoside antibiotics and thereby influence serum concentrations and dosage requirements. Additionally, specific patient conditions seem to influence the elimination of aminoglycosides and dosage requirements. The following variables and their relationship to aminoglycoside disposition warrant discussion.

**Renal Function.** Most of the early pharmacokinetic studies of aminoglycosides were conducted in volunteers with varying degrees of renal function. Changes in renal function directly influenced the elimination rate of aminoglyclosides. In volunteers, approximately 80 to 90% of the variance ($r^2$) in elimination of aminoglycosides can be explained by changes of renal function. In patients with sepsis, less variance in aminoglycoside elimination can be explained by estimates of renal function. Barza et al reported that 52% of the variance in gentamicin elimination could be explained by changes in the serum creatinine (25). Kaye et al reported 50% of the variance in gentamicin elimination was explained by a change in creatinine clearance (26). For amikacin, similar statistical relationships were found with serum creatinine versus amikacin half-life, elimination rate constant versus creatinine clearance, and drug clearance versus creatinine clearance (27). In 98 patients treated with amikacin for gram-negative sepsis, the relationship between serum creatinine and amikacin half-life was significant ($p < 0.001$) (27). However, only 46% of the variance in amikacin half-life was explained with a change in serum creatinine. The statistical relationship with elimination rate vs. creatinine clearance and total body clearance vs. creatinine clearance for amikacin were similar. Thus substantial error may occur in predicting drug clearance or elimination rate from estimates of glomerular filtration rate.

**Age.** In healthy adults, cardiac output, renal blood flow and glomerular filtration decrease with increasing age. Pharmacologic agents which are primarily eliminated by glomerular filtration rate should be influenced by this physiologic change. The elimination of aminoglycosides decreases with increasing age. When the kinetic data are stratified according to age, the half-life in patients greater than 30 years is significantly longer. The average half-life in these older patients is approximately twice as long as the average half-life in patients less than 30 years of age. The clearance of aminoglycoside is markedly decreased with increasing age. The average clearance for amikacin in 24 younger patients ($<$30 yrs) was 113 ml/hr/kg compared to 60 ml/hr/kg in 50 older patients ($\geq$ 30 yrs) with normal renal function. The relationship of the elimination rate constant with age demonstrates that the rate of aminoglycoside elimination continually decreases with increasing age. The distribution volume (L/kg) for aminoglycosides was not related to age.

**Distribution Volume.** The relationship between the half-life and distribution volume was also significant with aminoglycosides (28). As the distribution volume of the drug increases, the half-life of the drug also increases. A nonlinear relationship occurred between the elimination rate constant and the distribution volume. However, a linear relationship appeared between the elimination rate constant and the reciprocal of the distribution volume. This relationship was stastically significant ($r = .52$; $p< 0.001$), indicating the elimination rate increased as the distribution volume decreased.

**Fever.** Fever also seems to be an important factor influencing serum concentrations and elimination of aminoglycosides (29). In dogs pretreated with endotoxin, a 25% decrease in serum gentamicin concentrations was observed at 60 minutes post-injection when compared to corresponding values in controls. In six human volunteers, serum concentrations of gentamicin were reduced by 40% at 1, 2, and 3 hours after intramuscular injection when compared to control values in the same subject. The half-life and renal clearance of gentamicin did not appear to be significantly affected by fever. However, fever was thought to be the principal factor associated with the lower levels of gentamicin. Physiologically, fever may change the elimination of aminoglycosides by increasing heart rate and cardiac output and thereby increasing renal blood flow and glomerular filtration. Thus, patients with high fevers may have a higher elimination rate of aminoglycosides due to underlying physiologic changes secondary to gram-negative sepsis.

**Hematocrit.** A curvilinear relationship was reported between the hematocrit and the half-life of gentamicin (25,30). The relationship of the reciprocal of the hematocrit and drug half-life was linear and explained 42% of the variance (25). In 976 patients, a significant relationship occurred between hematocrit and the gentamicin half-life ($r = - 0.12$; $p< 0.001$). However the degree of the association is low and explained only 1.4% of variance in half-life.

**Ideal Body Weight.** Aminoglycoside antibiotics were originally reported to distribute solely in ideal body mass, and prediction of serum levels was improved if methods used ideal body weight rather than total body weight. Recent data suggest these agents also distribute into excess weight or adipose tissue. Schwartz et al found the distribution volume of gentamicin and tobramycin to be significantly larger in healthy, obese volunteers when compared to controls (31). The relative distribution volume of gentamicin and tobramycin were similar in both groups if 40% of excess weight was added to ideal body mass to normalize weight. In 60 obstetric and gynecologic patients, gentamicin was found to distribute into 5 to 6% of excess weight (32). In ideal body mass, the distribution volume was 19% of body weight. Blouin et al has reported data indicating that tobramycin (33) and amikacin (34) also distribute into adipose weight. Thus, the drug's distribution volume increases with increasing excess weight, presumably due to distribution into adipose tissue. However, a substantial amount of variation in the distribution volume occurred at selected values of excess weight.

**Sex.** Barza et al reported an association between sex and the elimination rate of gentamicin (25). This relationship was only moderately significant. In 1,640 patients, females eliminated gentamicin more rapidly than males (3). The elimination rate constant, half-life, distribution volume, and clearances were significantly different for males and females. For the distribution volume, females had a lower volume per unit of weight than males. This observation is likely explained by the decreased muscle mass and decreased extracellular fluid per unit of weight in females.

**Obstetric Patients.** Several physiological factors occur antepartum and postpartum which may influence the elimination of aminoglycosides. The extracellular fluid compartment, total body water, cardiac output, renal blood flow, and glomerular filtration are all increased during the latter phases of pregnancy and require two to five days postpartum before the new equilibrium is re-established. Drugs such as the aminoglycosides, which distribute to the extracellular fluid and are dependent upon glomerular filtration, are markedly influenced during pregnancy. For gentamicin, the elimination was extremely rapid with 94% of the 55 patients having half-lives shorter than the reported range of 2.5 to 4 hours (35).

**Burn Patients.** Physiologically, burn patients appear to be "hypermetabolic." Their caloric expenditure can be as high as 10,000 to 12,000 calories daily. This figure can even be higher in patients who have concurrent gram-negative sepsis with fever. Hemodynamic changes secondary to the burn appear to explain why burn patients

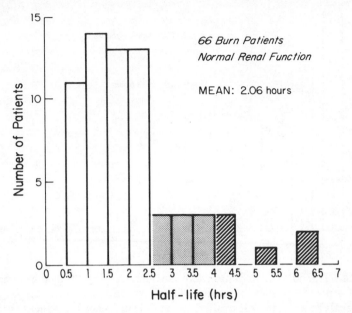

FIGURE 7. The half-life of gentamicin is illustrated in 66 burn patients who had a normal serum creatinine. A large majority of these patients had half-lives shorter than the previously reported range of 2.5 to 4 hours. However, an occasional patient had a half-life longer than 4 hours even though they had a normal serum creatinine.

have an extremely rapid rate of elimination. (Figure 7). In addition, the extracellular fluid compartment in burn patients can be extremely high immediately post-injury. Consequently, an occasional patient who develops gram-negative sepsis early in the course of burn resuscitation may have an extremely high distribution volume and a prolonged drug half-life even though renal function tests are normal (36).

**Pediatric Patients.** The elimination rate of aminoglycosides in pediatric patients is quite rapid (37,38). The half-life of gentamicin that we observed in 22 children was less than the reported range of 2.5 to 4 hours. This rapid rate of elimination is particularly apparent in pediatric patients with cystic fibrosis, burns, and leukemia.

**Internal Medicine Patients.** The half-life in 209 medicine patients with normal serum creatinines demonstrates substantial interpatient variation with gentamicin (Figure 8). A large number of patients had half-lives less than 2.5 hours. However, a substantial number of patients had prolonged elimination rates of the drug and required a

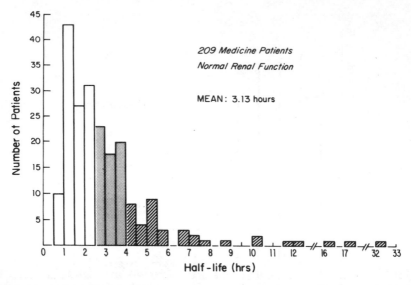

FIGURE 8.  The half-life of gentamicin is illustrated in 209 medicine patients who had a normal serum creatinine. These patients are markedly older and consequently their glomerular filtration rate is decreased. An increased number of patients had half-lives in excess of the usual range of 2.5 to 4 hours, indicating a need to measure serum concentrations and adjust dosages to prevent excessively high concentrations.

marked dosage reduction to prevent potentially toxic serum concentrations. This group of patients emphasizes the need for measuring serum concentrations and adjusting dosage regimens to prevent excessively high serum concentrations which may be associated with toxicity.

**Ascites.** The distribution volume of gentamicin was found to be markedly increased in patients with ascites (39). An expanded extracellular fluid volume attributed to the ascitic fluid explains the increase in distribution volume. Gentamicin appears to distribute rapidly into the ascitic fluid, however the large distribution volume necessitates a larger dose to achieve desired serum concentrations. The drug's half-life may be prolonged in these patients due to the large extravascular distribution volume. This prolonged half-life may occur even if patients have normal renal function.

**Effect of Interpatient Variation on Serum Concentrations.** The wide interpatient variation in aminoglycoside elimination has a marked effect on the serum concentration time profile. Patients with a short half-life eliminate more of the drug during a one-hour infusion.

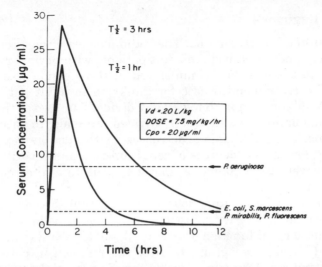

FIGURE 9.   The effect of the wide interpatient variation in amikacin half-life
on serum concentrations is illustrated. If two hypothetical patients received
the same dosage, had the same initial starting concentration, and had the
same distribution volume, the patient with a shorter half-life eliminates more
of the drug during the one hour infusion and has a lower peak level. In
addition, the serum concentration is below the inhibitory concentrations for
*Pseudomonas aeruginosa* for approximately 8 hours of the 12 hour interval.
Thus, the dosage interval of aminoglycosides should be adjusted according to
the patient's elimination rate of the drug.

Consequently, the peak level obtained after the same dose is lower
than obtained in patients with longer half-lives. In addition, the serum
concentrations are below the minimum inhibitory concentrations for
most gram-negative pathogens within the initial two hours of the
dosing interval. So with gentamicin and tobramycin, serum concentrations are below inhibitory concentration for 4 to 6 hours of the
usual 8 hour dosing interval. For amikacin, serum concentrations are
below the minimum inhibitory concentration for *Pseudomonas aeruginosa* for 9 to 10 hours of the recommended 12 hour interval (Figure
9). In patients with severe gram-negative sepsis and especially in
compromised hosts, the dosage interval should be decreased to prevent
these excessively long periods of subinhibitory concentrations. In addition, patients with a short half-life require a larger dose to achieve
therapeutic peak concentrations. In patients with a prolonged half-
life, the dosage interval should be prolonged to prevent excessively
high trough concentrations.

## Dosage Regimens

**Recommended Regimens.** The recommended dosage regimen for gentamicin and tobramycin in adult patients with normal renal function is 3 to 5 mg/kg/day administered in three equal doses every 8 hours. The recommended dose for amikacin in adult patients with normal renal function is 15 mg/kg/day divided into two or three equal doses and administered in equally divided intervals. In patients with compromised renal function, decreases in the dosage regimen are suggested for various degrees of renal function and severity of infection. However, these guidelines may have substantial error for individual patients.

**Nomograms.** Several methods have been published and suggested as an adequate means for adjusting dosage regimens in patients with compromised renal function. Cutler et al (40) and Hull et al (41) have developed dosing nomograms to alter the regimen in patients with compromised renal function. Cutler suggests multiplying the serum creatinine by a factor of 4 to estimate the drug's half-life and suggests a loading dose of 2 mg/kg of body weight to be repeated every third half-life of the drug. This approach may result in a long period of subinhibitory concentrations, especially in patients with severely compromised renal functions. Cutler also suggests a nomogram which uses serum creatinine to vary dose and/or dosage intervals. Other potentially important variables are not included in his nomogram. Hull's method utilizes estimates of renal function, lean body weight, age, and sex to predict required dosage regimens. The method allows the clinician to select a different dose and dosing interval for varying degrees of renal function and severity of infection.

**Precautions with Nomograms.** The use of nomograms to predict dosage requirements results in substantial variation in serum concentrations (25,26). Several assumptions are made in the dosage nomograms and probably explain the error in predicted dosages and serum concentrations. In patients with gram-negative sepsis, the correlation between predicted and measured creatinine clearance is markedly reduced. Results of a comparison of measured 24-hour creatinine clearance with a calculated creatinine clearance, estimated by four methods (42), suggest that predicted creatinine clearances are more variable in infected patients than previously reported in normal volunteers. Only 50 to 60% of the variance ($r^2$) in calculated creatinine clearance was explained by measured creatinine clearance for the four methods. Thus a substantial amount of error occurred when serum creatinine, age, body weight, and sex were used to estimate creatinine clearance in patients with severe gram-negative sepsis.

The distribution volume of aminoglycosides varies considerably between patients and may vary within the course of a patient's treatment. With nomograms, a constant volume of distribution is assumed for all patients. In addition, the relationship between drug clearance and creatinine clearance is only moderately correlated in patients with severe gram-negative sepsis (25). These factors explain the observed error in using these methods to predict dosage regimens. Several authors have suggested that measuring serum concentrations and titrating a patient's dosage regimen are necessary to ensure therapeutic concentrations (4,25,26). Although nomograms do provide the clinician with an initial dosage regimen, further dosage adjustments are essential to control serum concentrations. These adjustments depend on a measured peak and trough concentration.

## Individualizing Dosage Regimens with Serum Concentrations

**"Trial and Error" Method.** Therapeutic concentrations are frequently sought by measuring serum concentrations and making necessary dosage adjustments of aminoglycoside antibiotics. Unfortunately when serum samples are obtained clinically in an uncontrolled manner, important data such as the dose, time of sample and time of infusion are frequently not recorded. These errors of omission may lead to incorrect interpretation of serum levels and incorrect dosage adjustments (43). Many clinicians obtain a peak and/or trough level and make empirical dosage adjustments; besides the errors previously discussed, this results in a "trial and error period" with different dosage regimens until optimal serum concentrations are achieved. This empirical approach results in unnecessary patient cost and occasionally incorrect dosage adjustments (43). Thus, serum levels need to be obtained in a controlled manner and correctly interpreted to ensure optimal serum concentrations.

**Utilizing Pharmacokinetic Principles.** A method has been developed and applied in the patient care setting which utilizes serum concentration-time data from an individual patient to calculate an optimal dosage regimen (44,45). This method rapidly uses serum concentration-time data, preferably from the first dosing interval, to determine each patient's kinetic parameters. Dosages can be individualized within the first 12 to 24 hours of therapy. Patients achieve therapeutic serum concentrations early in the course of sepsis which may improve the likelihood of therapeutic success (4). In addition, the concentrations associated with a higher risk of toxicity are avoided, which may reduce the risk of toxicity. Patient safety and efficacy may thus be improved.

The drug's elimination rate constant and volume of distribution are determined from the serum concentration-time data. After the clinician has determined the desired peak and trough concentrations, the kinetic parameters are used to calculate the patient's dosage interval and dose. The use of this method allows the clinician to rapidly obtain these concentrations without the problems associated with the "trial and error" approach which uses a peak and/or trough level.

The kinetic parameters are estimated from serum concentration time data obtained from three serum samples. These samples are obtained over two to three estimated half-lives of the drug and preferably within the first dosage interval. For patients with normal renal function, the serum samples should be obtained over 3 to 5 hours postinfusion. For patients with impaired renal function, the half-life should be estimated using a factor of three times serum creatinine, and samples should be obtained over two to three estimated half-lives of the drug. A preinfusion serum sample is required if the patient has received prior doses. The times at which the infusion period was initiated and completed must be carefully recorded. The exact time that the serum samples were obtained must be carefully recorded. These samples should be rapidly analyzed; results should be available within the first 12 to 24 hours of therapy.

The serum concentration time data are fitted using least squares regression analysis assuming a one-compartment model. This fit can be either linear or nonlinear regression analysis. Linear regression analysis fits the log of serum concentration versus time. This simplified approach can be conducted with semilog graph paper or with a programmable hand-held calculator. The line of best fit is determined by the smallest vertical difference in the log of concentration. Nonlinear regression analysis fits the serum concentration versus time and requires more sophisiticated resources. With nonlinear regression analysis, the line of best fit is determined by the smallest vertical difference between the absolute concentration. With linear regression analysis, the vertical distance for 0.5 μg/ml will be greater at the lower end of the log cycle, and thus serum concentration time data may be weighted at lower values. In contrast, nonlinear fitting uses absolute values without weighting the data. Generally, the estimates of kinetic parameters obtained by either method are similar as long as the data fit well. It should be emphasized that the serum concentration time data should be plotted to visually inspect the data and the degree of fit. The visual inspection of the fit may alert the clinician to transcribing or analytical errors.

The drug's elimination rate constant (K) and the serum concentration on the regression line at zero time post-infusion $(C_{00})_{max}$ are estimated from the line of best fit. The drug's distribution volume (V) is calculated by the following equation which considers the amount of drug eliminated during the infusion period:

$$V = \frac{Ko}{K} \times \frac{1 - e^{-kt_i}}{[(C_{00})_{max} - (C_{00})_{min} \times e^{-kt_i}]}$$

(Eq. 1)

where Ko is the infusion rate, $T_i$ is the infusion period and $(C_{00})_{min}$ is the predose concentration.

The patient's dosing interval ($\tau$) is calculated knowing the desired peak level $(C_{00})_{max\text{-}D}$, desired trough level $(C_{00})_{min\text{-}D}$ and the infusion period $(t_i)$. These levels are based on the clinical status of the patient, site of infection, and pathogen isolated or suspected as previously discussed. The dosing interval is calculated by the following equation:

$$\tau = \frac{-1}{K} \left[ \ln \frac{(C_{00})_{min\text{-}D}}{(C_{00})_{max\text{-}D}} \right] + t_i$$

(Eq. 2)

The calculated dosage intervals are then rounded to clinically practical intervals of 4, 6, 8, 12, or 24 hours.

The infusion rate in mg/hr (Ko) required to produce a desired serum concentration is calculated by the following equation:

$$Ko = KV \, (C_{00})_{min\text{-}D} \times \frac{(1 - e^{-k\tau})}{(1 - e^{-kt_i})}$$

(Eq. 3)

This equation considers the fraction of the dose eliminated during the infusion period and the amount of drug remaining from the previous dose. These calculated dosages are rounded to practical increments for the nursing staff.

With the application of this method, desired peak and trough serum concentrations have been consistently obtained with gentamicin, tobramycin, and amikacin. The dosage requirements for these three aminoglycosides demonstrate substantial variability from patient to patient. The variability appears similar for each aminoglycoside. In our patients with normal renal function, the required dosage regimens ranged from 0.2 to 18.6 mg/kg/day for gentamicin (885 patients), from 0.9 to 15.3 mg/kg/day for tobramycin (46 patients), and from 3.7 to 53.3 mg/kg/day for amikacin (67 patients). Most patients required dosing intervals shorter than the recommended 8 to 12 hour intervals. However, a limited number of patients with normal renal function required dosing intervals beyond the recommended 8 to 12 hour interval to prevent excessively high trough concentrations. Thus, to achieve therapeutic serum concentrations, 35 to 45% of our patients treated with aminoglycosides require dosage regimens in excess of those commonly recommended. To prevent excessively high serum concentrations, 10 to 15% of our patients require dosages less than those commonly recommended, even though they have normal renal function. The use of conventionally recommended dosages results in a substantial number of patients who have subtherapeutic concentrations or achieve excessively high levels even though they have normal renal function.

**Intrapatient Variation.** A large number of factors may change during the course of aminoglycoside therapy and affect serum concentrations and dosage requirements. A change in glomerular filtration may occur during therapy and markedly change the elimination rate of aminoglycosides. Serum creatinine or blood urea nitrogen are common clinical tests used to monitor changes in renal function and assist the clinician in determining dosage changes of aminoglycosides. Occasionally, serum concentrations may rise before a change in serum creatinine is noted (see previous chapter). Tissue accumulation may also occur during therapy resulting in an apparent decrease in the drug's clearance (see previous chapter). The distribution volume of aminoglycosides may increase or decrease during therapy and can have a marked effect on serum aminoglycoside concentrations, half-life, and dosage regimens. Changes in physiologic parameters, which affect cardiac output, may be another means of changing the drug's clearance during therapy. Fever is an example where the heart rate and cardiac output may initially be increased and then return to normal as the infection is successfully treated. The intrinsic clearance of aminoglycosides appears to be flow dependent and changes in renal blood flow would likely cause a parallel change in aminoglycoside clearance. Thus, aminoglycoside clearance is likely to change during treatment due to changes in physiologic parameters such as cardiac output, renal blood flow, and glomerular filtration. These changes in drug clearance may not be apparent from concurrent changes in serum creatinine or blood urea nitrogen. Serum concentrations should be monitored periodically through the course of therapy and necessary dosage adjustments made to control serum concentrations.

## Cost Benefit

The additional expense of measuring serum concentrations can be substantial and should therefore be cost-effective. The costs of providing this service, including personnel, salaries, laboratory expenditures, operating costs, fixed costs, and physical equipment were assessed in a recent study (46). In this study, these costs were balanced by the benefit realized by the increase in patient survival (47). Moreover, the benefit from improved patient safety was not included in these analyses. Even so, the cost benefit ratio was positive, indicating that society realized a favorable outcome from these services. The cost benefit ratio was 1:4.5 to 1:24.0, indicating society realized 4.5 to 24 dollars for every dollar that the service cost. Several methods are available to estimate the benefit from the improved patient survival, and each method provides a different estimate of society's benefit. This ratio of cost to benefit was similar to the cost-benefit ratio reported for the measles vaccination program. Thus, this pharmacokinetic service has a very favorable impact on patient care and a favorable cost-benefit ratio.

## REFERENCES

1. Kagan BM: Applied pharmacology: *Antimicrobial Therapy*. Philadelphia, W.B. Saunders Company, 1974, Vol. 2, p. 44.
2. Moellering RC, Jr, Wennersben C, Weinburg AN: Studies on the antibiotic-synergism against enterococci. I Bacteriologic Studies. J Lab Clin Med 1971; 77:821–828.
3. Sonni M, Jawetz E: Combined action of carbenicillin and gentamicin on *Pseudomonas aeruginosa* in vitro. Appl Microbiol 1969; 17:893–896.
4. Noone P, Parson TNC, Pattison JR, et al: Experience in monitoring gentamicin therapy during treatment of serious gram-negative sepsis. Br Med J 1974; 1:477–481.
5. Loebl VC, Marvin JA, Curreri PW, et al: Survival with ecthyma gangrenosum: A previously fatal complication of burns. J Trauma 1974; 14:370–377.
6. Solem LE, Zaske DE, Strate RG: Ecthyma gangrenosum: Survival with individualized antibiotic therapy. Arch Surg 1979; 114:580–583.
7. Jackson GG, Riff LJ: Pseudomonas bacteremia: pharmacologic and other basis for failure of treatment with gentamicin. J Infect Dis 1971; 124:S185–191.
8. Zaske DE, Strate RG, Solem LE, et al: Improved patient survival with individualized gentamicin dosages, American Burn Association, 11th Annual Meeting, New Orleans, 1979.
9. Anderson ET, Young LS, Hewitt WL: Simultaneous antibiotic levels in "breakthrough" gram-negative rod bacteremia. Am J Med 1976; 61:493–497.
10. Smith CR, Baughman KL, Edwards CQ, et al: Controlled comparison of amikacin and gentamicin. N Eng J Med 1977; 296:349–351.
11. Feld R, Valdivieso N, Bodey GP, et al: Comparison of amikacin and tobramycin in the treatment of infection in patients with cancer. J Infect Dis 1977; 135:61–68.
12. Schentag JG, Plaut ME, Cerra FV, et al: Aminoglycoside nephrotoxicity in critically ill surgical patients. J Surg Res 1979; 26:270–279.
13. Smith CR, Lipsky J, Laskin O, et al: Tobramycin is less nephrotoxic than gentamicin: results of a double blind clinical trial. New Engl J Med 1980; 302:1106–1109.
14. Falco FG, Smith HM, Arcieri GM: Nephrotoxicity of aminoglycosides in gentamicin. J Infect Dis 1969; 119:406–409.

15. Gooding PV, Bermin E, Lane AZ, et al: A review of results of clinical trials with amikacin. J Infect Dis 1976; 134:S441–445.
16. Dahlgren JG, Anderson ET, Hewitt WL: Gentamicin blood levels: in regard to nephrotoxicty. Antimicrob Agents Chemother 1975; 8:58–62.
17. Clarke JT, Libke RD, Regamey C, et al: Comparative pharmcokinetics of amikacin and kanamycin. Clin Pharmacol Ther 1974; 15:610–616.
18. Appel GB, New HC: Gentamicin in 1978. Ann Intern Med 1978; 89:528–538.
19. Howard JB, McCracken GH: Pharmacological evaluation of amikacin in neonates. Antimicrob Agents Chemother 1975; 8:86–90.
20. Kirby WM, Clarke JT, Libke RD, et al: Clinical pharmacology of amikacin and kanamycin. J Infect Dis 1976; 134:S312–315.
21. Gyselynck AM, Forrey A, Cutler R: Pharmacokinetics of gentamicin: distribution of plasma and renal clearance. J Infect Dis 1971; 124:S70–76.
22. Plantier J, Forrey AW, O'Neil NA, et al.: Pharmacokinetics of amikacin in patients of normal or impaired renal function: radioenzymatic acetylation assay. J Infect Dis 1976; 134:S323–330.
23. Lode H, Grunert K, Koeppe P, et al: Pharmacokinetic and clinical studies of amikacin, a new aminoglycoside antibiotic. J Infect Dis 1976; 134:S316–322.
24. Clarke JT, Libke RD, Regamey C, et al: Comparative pharmacokinetics of amikacin and kanamycin. Clin Pharmacol Ther 1974; 15:610–616.
25. Barza M, Brown RB, Shen D, et al: Predictability of blood levels of gentamicin in man. J Infect Dis 1975; 132:165–174.
26. Kaye D, Levison ME, Labovitz ED: The unpredictability of serum concentrations of gentamicin: pharmacokinetics of gentamicin in patients with normal and abnormal renal function. J Infect Dis 1974; 130:150–154.
27. Zaske DE, Strate RG: Amikacin pharmacokinetics: wide interpatient variation in 98 patients. (In review).
28. Zaske DE, Cipolle RJ, Strate RG, et al: Increased gentamicin dosage requirements: rapid elimination in 249 gynecology patients. (In review).
29. Pennington JE, Dale DC, Reynolds HY, et al: Gentamicin and sulfate in pharmacokinetics: lower levels of gentamicin in blood during fever. J Infect Dis 1975; 132:270–275.
30. Zaske DE, Cipolle RJ, Strate RG: Gentamicin pharmacokinetics in 1640 patients: a method to control serum concentrations. (In review).
31. Schwartz SN, Pazin GJ, Lyon JA, et al: A controlled investigation of the pharmacokinetics of gentamicin and tobramycin in obese subjects. J Infect Dis 1978; 138:499–505.
32. Sketris I, Lesar T, Zaske DE, et al: Effect of obesity on gentamicin pharmacokinetics. (In review).
33. Blouin RA, Mann HJ, Griffen WO, et al: Tobramycin pharmacokinetics in markedly obese patients. Clin Pharmacol Ther 1979; 26:508–512.
34. Bauer LA, Blouin RA, Griffen WO, et al: Amikacin pharmacokinetics in morbidly obese patients. Am J Hosp Pharm 1980; 37:519–522.
35. Zaske DE, Cipolle RJ, Strate RG, et al: Rapid gentamicin elimination in obstetric patients. (In review).
36. Zaske DE, Cipolle RJ, Solem LD, et al: Rapid individualization of gentamicin dosage regimens in 66 burn patients. Burns, In press.
37. Siber G, Echeveria P, Smith A, et al: Pharmacokinetics of gentamicin in children and adults. J Infect Dis 1975; 132:637–649.
38. Evans WE, Feldman SF, Barker LF, et al: Use of gentamicin serum levels to individualize therapy in children. J Pediatr 1978; 93:133–137.

39. Gill MA, Kern JW: Altered gentamicin distribution in ascitic patients. Am J Hosp Pharm 1979; 36:1704–1706.
40. Cutler RE, Gyselyneck AM, Fleet WP, et al: Correlation of serum creatinine concentration in gentamicin half-life. JAMA 1972; 219:1037–1041.
41. Hull JH, Sarubbi FA: Gentamicin serum concentrations: pharmacokinetic predictions. Ann Intern Med 1976; 85:183–189.
42. Lott RF, Uden DL, Wargin WA, et al: Correlation of predicted versus measured creatinine clearance values in burn patients. Am J Hosp Pharm 1978; 35:713–720.
43. Anderson AC, Hodges GR, Barnes WG: Determination of serum gentamicin sulfate levels. Arch Intern Med 1976; 136:785–787.
44. Sawchuk RJ, Zaske DE: Pharmacokinetics of dosing regimens which utilize multiple intravenous infusions: gentamicin in burn patients. J Pharmacokin Biopharm 1976; 4:183–195.
45. Sawchuk RJ, Zaske DE, Cipolle RJ, et al: Kinetic models for gentamicin dosing with the use of individual patient parameters. Clin Pharmacol Ther 1977; 21:362–369.
46. Bootman JL, Zaske DE, Wertheimer AI, et al: Cost of individualizing aminoglycoside dosing regimens. Am J Hosp Pharm 1979; 36:368–370.
47. Bootman JL, Wertheimer AI, Zaske DE, et al: Individualizing gentamicin dosage regimens in burn patients with gram-negative septicemia: a cost-benefit analysis. J Pharm Sci 1979; 68:267–272.

# 8

# Cephalosporins

Charles H. Nightingale, Ph.D.
Margaret A. French, Pharm.D.
Richard Quintiliani, M.D.

## INTRODUCTION/BACKGROUND

Over the past few years a relatively large number of cephalosporins became available for general physician use: cephalothin (Keflin®) in 1964; cephaloridine (Loridine®) in 1966; cephaloglycin (Kafocin®) in 1970; cephalexin (Keflex®) in 1971; cefazolin (Ancef®, Kefzol®) in 1973; cephapirin (Cefadyl®) and cephradine (Velosef®, Anspor®) in 1974; cefamandole (Mandol®) and the cephamycin, cefoxitin (Mefoxin®) in 1978; and cefadroxil (Duricef®) and cefaclor (Ceclor®) in 1979. Many new agents are in various stages of development and are expected to be released for general use within the next three to five years. Clinicians have found it difficult to identify any particular merit of one of these drugs over another. This monograph presents a comparison of the pharmacokinetics of the agents commercially available and commonly used in the United States. In this section, the absorption, distribution and metabolism (when applicable) of first the oral agents, and then the parenteral agents will be presented. Then the excretion of all the cephalosporins will be discussed.

### Absorption, Distribution and Metabolism

**Oral Agents.** The pharmacokinetics of the oral cephalosporins are shown in Table 1, where it is obvious that more similarities exist between these drugs than differences. Since cephalexin and cephradine are the "older" agents, it is of interest to compare these to each other and then to the newer drugs cefadroxil and cefaclor.

*Cephalexin and Cephradine.* The oral cephalosporins, cephalexin (Keflex®) and cephradine (Velosef®, Anspor®) (Figure 1), differing in structure by only two hydrogen atoms in a six-membered ring, not

TABLE 1. PHARMACOKINETIC PARAMETERS OF THE ORAL CEPHALOSPORINS

| Parameter | Cephalexin[a] Mean ± SD | Cephradine[b] Mean ± SD | Cefadroxil[c] Mean ± SD | Cefaclor[d] Mean ± SD |
|---|---|---|---|---|
| $\alpha$, hr$^{-1}$ | 4.35 ± 0.32 | — | — | — |
| $\beta$, hr$^{-1}$ | 0.85 ± 0.17 | 0.86 ± 0.16 | 0.48 ± 0.06 | 0.98 ± 0.17 |
| $k_a$, hr$^{-1}$ | 2.38 ± 1.15 | 2.12 ± 1.03 | 2.30 ± 0.86 | 2.35 ± 0.07 |
| $k_{12}$, hr$^{-1}$ | 1.15 ± 0.02 | — | — | — |
| $k_{21}$, hr$^{-1}$ | 2.45 ± 0.30 | — | — | — |
| $k_e$, hr$^{-1}$ | 1.62 ± 0.02 | — | — | — |
| Lag time, hr | 0.34 ± 0.09 | 0.32 ± 0.09 | 0.36 ± 0.01 | 2.0 |
| t½$\alpha$, hr | 0.16 ± 0.01 | — | — | — |
| t½$\beta$, hr | 0.84 ± 0.15 | 0.83 ± 0.13 | 1.48 ± 0.18 | 0.73 ± 0.13 |
| $V_c$, liters | 10.95 ± 2.04 | — | — | — |
| Vd$_{ss}$, liters | 25.60 ± 8.63 | — | — | — |
| Vd$\beta$, liters | 20.51 ± 5.38 | — | — | — |
| Vdext, liters | 24.29 ± 5.47 | 20.27 ± 1.96 | 20.65 | — |

[a] compiled from references 1, 5, 6, 15, 16, 18, 24, 85, 100
[b] compiled from references 1, 6, 16, 24, 85
[c] compiled from references 15, 23, 24, 25
[d] compiled from references 16, 17, 18, 59, 101

unexpectedly have almost identical pharmacokinetic properties, microbiological activities, and clinical effectiveness.

We recently studied the pharmacokinetics of these agents in normal volunteers after the administration of one gram (two 500 mg capsules) of cephalexin, one gram (two 500 mg capsules) of cephradine and one gram (one 1.0 gm tablet) of cephalexin in a three-way crossover study (1). The results of this analysis (Figure 2) show that no significant pharmacokinetic differences exist between cephalexin or cephradine. The extent of absorption, effect of food, peak serum concentrations, time to reach the peak, rates of absorption and elimination, clearances, lack of metabolism, urinary recovery, urinary concentrations and protein binding [≤20% (2)] are either indistinguishable or the differences e.g., protein binding, are not important with these two cephalosporins.

The only apparent difference between these agents is the effect of food on the absorption process in children and infants. It is well established that when these drugs are administered with food to adults, the rate of absorption (as reflected in the peak serum concentration and the time to reach the peak), is altered, but the extent of absorption, as measured by the area under the serum concentration time curve (AUC), is not. This is also true for cephradine absorption in infants and children (3), but not for cephalexin (4). The AUC for cephalexin is also reduced. This is a surprising finding given the almost identical molecular structure and the tendency for cephradine to convert into cephalexin in solution. Further study is necessary to explain this finding.

A review of the literature (5,6) reveals that although both agents are widely distributed into a variety of tissues, their concentrations are not particularly high. For example, levels of 2 to 40 µg/ml are observed in the bile after a single 500 mg dose (5,6). This is a relatively low concentration compared to that obtained after equal doses of cefazolin or cefamandole. Spinal fluid levels are low (5,6), as with all cephalosporins, and this class of agents is generally not recommended in the treatment of CNS infections. Levels in amniotic fluid (5,7,8), breast milk, (5,6,8) aqueous humor (5,6) and saliva (5) were also not outstanding although recent reports demonstrated exudate levels of approximately 50% of serum concentrations for cephalexin (9) and that cephradine lung tissue concentrations were 42% of serum levels (10). Two other recent studies (11,12) indicate that cephalexin levels in synovial fluid, joint tissues and mandibular alveolar bone were high enough to be clinically useful. Rapid transport of cephradine into the fetus (10 min.) from maternal blood has been observed (13).

Although not well established, it appears that tissue levels are proportional to serum concentrations. Therefore, low tissue levels with cephalexin-cephradine are not unexpected, considering their lack of protein binding. Other, similar oral agents with a prolonged serum half-life should yield sustained tissue concentrations that are greater than those obtained with cephalexin-cephradine. A sustained release cephalexin dosage form was recently developed but is not commercially available (14). Based upon all measurable parameters, it is

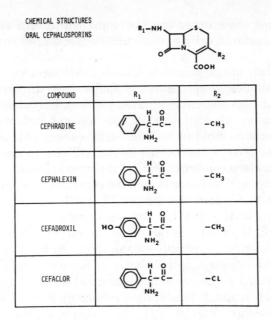

FIGURE 1.  Chemical structures of oral cephalosporins.

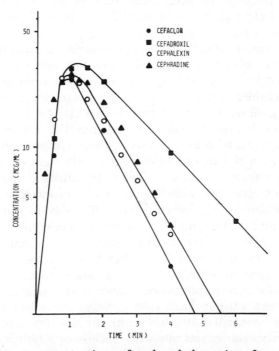

FIGURE 2.  Serum concentrations of oral cephalosporins after a 1.0 gm dose.

concluded that these drugs are not significantly different from each other pharmacokinetically and should be considered equivalent antibiotics.

*Cefaclor.* Only minor pharmacokinetic differences exist between cefaclor and cephalexin-cephradine. Cefaclor, like the other oral cephalosporins exhibits negligible binding (<20%). Examination of Table 1 and Figure 2 reveals that cefaclor has a somewhat shorter half-life than cephalexin-cephradine but this difference is only about six minutes. Dosage adjustments because of this difference are not required. Serum and urinary concentrations and percent of dose excreted in the urine are lower with cefaclor than with cephalexin-cephradine in both adults (15,16,17,18) and children (1,7) (Table 2). This is not due to metabolic loss of the drug in the body; rather, it is caused by an instability which appears to be pH-dependent (19). These differences between cefaclor and cephradine-cephalexin in blood and urine concentrations are not large and probably of little clinical significance in light of cefaclor's enhanced microbiological activity. Other pharmacokinetic studies (20,21), although non-comparative, support these findings. In essence, cefaclor is similar to cephalexin-cephradine with regard to rate and extent of absorption, effect of food on absorption, and protein binding characteristics. McCracken et al (22) reported that food had somewhat less of an effect on cefaclor absorption than it did on cephalexin absorption in children.

There is a paucity of data on the tissue penetration of cefaclor. Only two reports are available and neither one is a comparative study. In one report (22) cefaclor saliva and tear levels were determined in infants and children after a 15 mg/kg dose. Tear levels were reported to be >1.0 μg/ml while saliva levels were stated to be equal to serum concentrations. It cannot be determined from this report whether the authors demonstrated that the saliva concentrations were not due to residual drug in the mouth after oral administration of suspended solid particles (suspension) of cefaclor. In adults we have observed saliva concentrations of ampicillin after a 5 ml mock administration of the suspension (unpublished data). These levels were frequently above 100 μg/ml initially and >1 μg/ml for up to 6 hours after dosing. This was in spite of a mouth rinse with water to remove adhering suspension in the oral cavity. The other report concerns cefaclor penetration into sputum after 0.5 and 1 gm doses (18). At the peak, the ratio of cefaclor serum:sputum concentrations was 26:1 and 33:1 for the 0.5 gm and 1.0 gm doses respectively. The mean peak sputum concentrations were 0.4 and 0.6 μg/ml for the low and high doses. Non-peak saliva concentrations were as low as a fourth (0.14 μg/ml)

TABLE 2. BIOAVAILABILITY, URINARY CONCENTRATIONS AND PERCENT OF DOSE RECOVERED FOLLOWING 0.5 & 1.0 GRAM ORAL CEPHALOSPORIN DOSES

| | Urinary Concentration (μg/ml) (0.5g Dose) | | | | | % Recovered in Urine | | | | Bioavailability | | | |
| | | | | | | 0.5g[16] | | 1.0g[1] | | FD/V[16] (μg/ml) | | AUC (μg-h/ml) | |
| | 0-6h[16] | 6-12h[16] | 0-3h[24] | 3-6h[24] | 6-12h[24] | 0-6h | 6-12h | 0-6h | 0-24h | 0.5g | 0.5g | 0.5g[24] | 1.0g[1] |
|---|---|---|---|---|---|---|---|---|---|---|---|---|---|
| Cephalexin | 684.0 | 14.7 | 1783 | 607 | 78 | 85.2 | 1.7 | 94.5 | 90.6 | 23.9 | 32.0 | 29.0 | 52.7 |
| Cephradine | 830.0 | 14.8 | 2136 | 582 | 61 | 86.3 | 1.8 | 84.5 | 85.5 | 21.9 | 27.4 | 27.5 | 61.8 |
| Cefaclor | 388.0 | 4.7 | — | — | — | 53.8 | 0.4 | — | — | 18.4 | 16.1 | — | — |
| Cefadroxil | — | — | 1211 | 1113 | 167 | 78.7[26] | 6.8[26] | — | — | — | — | 47.4 | — |

[1] E. Finkelstein et al: J Pharm Sci 1978; 67:1447–50.
[16] P.G. Welling et al: Int J Clin Pharmacol & Biopharm 1979; 17:397–400.
[24] M. Pfeffer et al: Antimicrob Agents Chemother 1977; 11:331–38.
[26] D.M. Hennes et al: Clin Therap 1977; 1:263–73.

those of the peak concentrations. The pharmacokinetic profile of cefaclor in serum and urine suggests that tissue penetration will be equal to, or less than, that of older agents.

*Cefadroxil.* Cefadroxil, another oral agent, differs from cephalexin by the addition of a para-hydroxyl group on the aromatic ring (Figure 1). This manipulation does not alter the drug's microbiological spectrum although it does decrease its rate of elimination (15,23,24,25,26) (Table 1). Therefore, serum and urine concentrations (Figure 2, Table 2) of cefadroxil are higher and prolonged compared with cephalexin (15,23,24,25,26,27). An additional advantage of this drug is that its absorption is less affected by the presence of food (24,28) in the stomach when compared to cephalexin and cephradine. (However, the entire dose of these drugs is recovered in the urine regardless of meals.) Like cefaclor, cefadroxil penetration into tissue cannot be evaluated since sufficient data has not been published. Saliva levels in infants and children were reported in one study (28).

**Parenteral Agents.** The parenteral cephalosporins can be historically classified into the older "first generation" agents (cephalothin, cephapirin, and cefazolin) and the newer "second generation" agents (cefoxitin, cefamandole). They can also be classified as those which undergo metabolism and those which do not.

*Metabolized Cephalosporins: cephalothin and cephapirin.* The metabolized cephalosporins, (Figure 3) have similar pharmacokinetic properties (Tables 3 and 4). Intramuscular absorption of these drugs is complete with a peak concentration of 20 μg/ml after a one gram dose. This peak occurs approximately 30 to 40 minutes after dosing (Table 4). Both drugs are bound to serum proteins to a moderate extent: 60.4% (2,6,29) and 55.7% (6,29,30) for cephalothin and cephapirin respectively. Limited pharmacokinetics have been reported in children (6,31). In adults the biological half-life after intravenous administration is 32 and 41 minutes, while the apparent half-life after intramuscular administration increases to 47 and 51 minutes for cephalothin and cephapirin respectively. These relatively short half-lives (Figure 4) are due to metabolism to desacetyl compounds as well as elimination via the kidney. The metabolites possess 20% and 54% of the microbiological activity of the parent drugs for cephalothin and cephapirin respectively (6). The metabolism of these drugs by esterases occurs in virtually all tissues, with minor metabolism also occurring in serum.

There are few studies which compare the tissue penetration of cephalothin and cephapirin. In two recent studies comparing the tissue penetration characteristics of these drugs in adults (32) and children

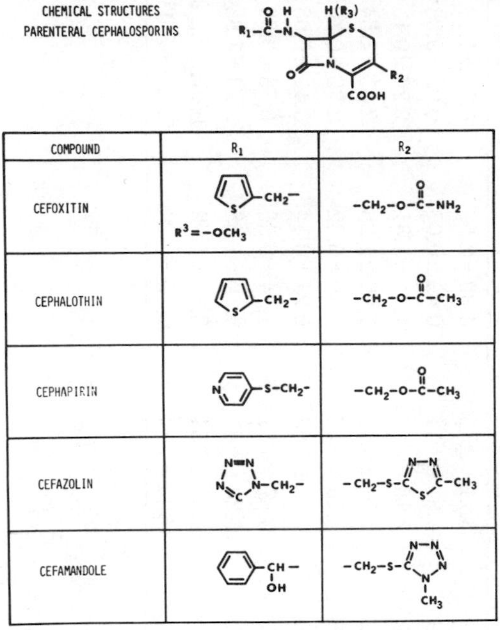

CHEMICAL STRUCTURES
PARENTERAL CEPHALOSPORINS

| COMPOUND | $R_1$ | $R_2$ |
|---|---|---|
| CEFOXITIN | (structure) $-CH_2-$  $R^3=-OCH_3$ | $-CH_2-O-\overset{O}{\underset{\|}{C}}-NH_2$ |
| CEPHALOTHIN | (structure) $-CH_2-$ | $-CH_2-O-\overset{O}{\underset{\|}{C}}-CH_3$ |
| CEPHAPIRIN | (structure) $-S-CH_2-$ | $-CH_2-O-\overset{O}{\underset{\|}{C}}-CH_3$ |
| CEFAZOLIN | (structure) $-CH_2-$ | $-CH_2-S-$ (structure) $-CH_3$ |
| CEFAMANDOLE | (structure) $-\overset{}{\underset{OH}{C}}H-$ | $-CH_2-S-$ (structure) $CH_3$ |

FIGURE 3.   Chemical structures of parenteral cephalosporins.

(33) undergoing open heart surgery, it was found in adults that cephapirin achieved slightly higher levels than those of cephalothin in pericardial fluid and right atrial appendage, whereas, in children these levels were identical.

Several new cephalosporin tissue penetration studies have been reported, such as prostate and seminal vesicles (34), ascitic fluid (6), bronchial secretions (6), pleural fluid (6), spinal fluid (6) and placental cord blood (6), in addition to previously reviewed work (5). Although tissue concentration comparisons between the metabolized and non-metabolized cephalosporins are difficult to assess because of experimental differences in study design and methodology, it appears that the metabolized drugs in general exhibit lower tissue concentrations than the non-metabolized agents, e.g., aqueous humor (18), ascitic fluid (6), heart (26,32,33,35,36) bone (37,38,39,40,41) synovial fluid (5,6,39) and amniotic fluid (18). This is partially due to the fact that at equal doses the serum concentrations are lower compared to the non-metabolized drugs. Cephalothin and cephapirin do not penetrate well through non-inflamed meninges (5,6). Penetration through in-

TABLE 3. PHARMACOKINETIC PARAMETERS OF THE PARENTERAL CEPHALOSPORINS

| Parameter | Cephalothin[a] Mean** ±SD | Cephapirin[b] Mean** ±SD | Cefoxitin[c] Mean ±SD | Cefamandole[d] Mean ±SD | Cefazolin[e] Mean** ±SD | Cephradine[f] Mean ±SD |
|---|---|---|---|---|---|---|
| $\alpha$, $h^{-1}$ | 6.95±1.93 | 5.31±0.44 | 5.82±0.48 | 3.21±0.45 | 4.30±2.56 | 6.39±1.39 |
| $\beta$, $h^{-1}$ | 1.50±0.48 | 1.05±0.12 | 0.94±0.09 | 0.81±0.11 | 0.42±0.08 | 0.99±0.38 |
| $k_{12}$, $h^{-1}$ | 1.82±0.83 | 1.15±0.18 | 2.01±0.20 | 0.76±0.06 | 1.72±1.31 | 2.26±0.13 |
| $k_{21}$, $h^{-1}$ | 2.52±0.88 | 1.53±0.26 | 1.92±0.32 | 1.31±0.15 | 2.00±1.28 | 2.81±1.54 |
| $k_e$, $h^{-1}$ | 4.12±0.87 | 3.67±0.36 | 2.83±0.05 | 2.15±0.37 | 1.00±0.32 | 2.32±0.10 |
| $t_{1/2}\alpha$, h | 0.11±0.03 | 0.13±0.01 | 0.12±0.00 | 0.22±0.03 | 0.23±0.14 | 0.11±0.03 |
| $t_{1/2}\beta$, h | 0.53±0.28 | 0.67±0.08 | 0.75±0.07 | 0.87±0.11 | 1.74±0.36 | 0.76±0.03 |
| $V_c$, L | 8.08±2.68 | 9.58±0.65 | 7.38±0.71 | 6.20±2.81 | 4.10±1.68 | 9.23±1.88 |
| $VD_{ss}$, L | 14.61±5.59 | 16.85±1.13 | 14.80±1.29 | 9.81±4.51 | 8.32±1.92 | 16.04±2.22 |
| $V_D$,ext L | 23.54±8.48 | 33.21±3.52 | 22.25±3.09 | 15.62±5.68 | 12.38±4.43 | 21.20±3.03 |

[a] compiled from references 5, 82*, 102
[b] compiled from references 5, 65, 82*, 102
[c] compiled from references 5, 67*, 83
[d] compiled from references 103, 104*, 105, 106
[e] compiled from references 5, 82*
[f] compiled from reference 5
* data re-analyzed using a two compartment model
** means obtained by individually averaging all data found in review articles

TABLE 4. INTRAMUSCULAR ABSORPTION

| | Cephalothin[a] Mean ± SD | Cephapirin[b] Mean ± SD | Cefoxitin[c] Mean ± SD | Cefamandole[d] Mean ± SD | Cefazolin[e] Mean ± SD | Cephradine[f] Mean ± SD |
|---|---|---|---|---|---|---|
| Serum peak μg/ml (500 mg dose) | 9.6±2.0 | 11.2±2.0 | 12.0±1.4 | 13.0±1.7 | 34.3±3.9 | 9.5 |
| Serum Peak μg/ml (1000 mg dose) | 18 | 20.0±4.4 | 24.8±4.8 | 23.8±7.5 | 68.2±0.2 | 12 |
| t max, hr | 0.62±0.33 | 0.55±0.25 | 0.31±0.15 | 1.0±0.4 | 0.98±0.22 | 0.88±0.18 |
| $k_a$, hr$^{-1}$ | — | — | 1.39 | 6.47 | 2.07±0.22 | 1.1 |
| t½ abs, min | — | — | 30 | 6 | 24 | 36 |
| t½ (IM), hr | 0.78±0.16 | 0.85±0.14 | 1.0±0.4 | 1.28±0.31 | 2.09±0.61 | 1.37±0.18 |
| 24 hr urine (% recovery) | 57.1±11.2 | 70.2±1.6 | 90–99 | — | 80.4±7.4 | 91.9 |
| Bioavailability | 98 | 98 | 95 | — | — | 100% |

[a] compiled from references 6, 29, 102, 107
[b] compiled from references 6, 29, 102, 107
[c] compiled from references 6, 83, 107, 108
[d] compiled from references 6, 29, 106, 108, 109
[e] compiled from references 6, 29, 107, 110
[f] compiled from references 6, 29

flammed meninges is somewhat better, but does not yield reliably high CSF levels to safely treat serious infection. These drugs are generally not recommended for the treatment of CNS infections.

Based upon all measurable parameters (e.g., microbiological activity, pharmacokinetic characteristics, therapeutic effectiveness, and toxicity), it can be concluded that cephalothin and cephapirin are not significantly different from one another and can be considered therapeutic alternatives.

*Non-Metabolized Cephalosporins: cefamandole and cefoxitin.* Cefamandole and cefoxitin are newer, "second generation" cephalosporins. Cefoxitin is often referred to as a cephamycin rather than a cephalosporin antibiotic, yet the differences in its basic nuclei are so small that it seems reasonable to consider this drug as another cephalosporin derivative.

Examination of Table 3 and Figure 4, reveals that although the pharmacokinetic parameters of cefoxitin and cefamandole are not identical, they are sufficiently similar to each other and different from cephalothin-cephapirin or cefazolin that it is also reasonable to discuss these drugs together. After intramuscular administration of 1.0 gm of either drug, a peak serum concentration of about 20 μg/ml is observed. This peak occurs approximately 20 minutes to one hour after dosing with cefoxitin and cefamandole respectively. Both drugs are equally bioavailable after IM injection. Their half-lives are shorter than that of cefazolin and closer to that of cephalothin-cephapirin. The half-lives for cefamandole and cefoxitin after intravenous administration are 55 and 45 minutes respectively; after intramuscular injection the apparent half-lives increase to 78 and 60 minutes respectively. Since the protein binding of cefamandole is relatively high, i.e. approximately 77% (6 and unpublished data), it is surprising that the half-life is not longer, as is the case with cefazolin (binding: 83%; $t^{1/2}$: 1.7h). The shorter half-life of cefamandole is apparently due to the fact that its renal elimination occurs primarily by secretion which is not dependent on the degree of protein binding (42). Cefoxitin is only 50 to 60% protein bound (6) and probably undergoes a smaller amount of active secretion. Therefore, the half-life is shorter and serum concentrations as a function of time are somewhat, but probably not significantly, reduced (Figure 4).

The protein binding differences between cefamandole and cefoxitin do not appear to result in significantly different tissue levels of these drugs. For example, it was observed that cefamandole and cefoxitin had approximately the same atrial appendage tissue concentrations and tissue composite half-life in patients undergoing open heart surgery (43). Other authors have also observed good heart tissue (35,36) but poor aqueous humor (44) concentration with cefamandole; cefoxitin exhibited penetration into breast milk (45). Like the other cephalosporins, cefamandole and cefoxitin do not penetrate well into non-inflammed meninges in adults (46,47) or children (48). Cefoxitin, presumably because it is less protein bound, achieves higher concentrations in non-inflammed meninges than cefamandole (47). Treatment of patients with CNS infections with cefoxitin resulted in measurable CSF concentrations, but the levels were not within a therapeutic range. In children, cefamandole was found to penetrate into CSF in low (1.2 μg/ml) concentrations (48). Neither cefamandole or cefoxitin is recommended for the treatment of CNS infections in children or adults.

Walker and Gahal (48) reported the typical age–t½ relationship for cefamandole. In infants less than three months of age the half-life was approximately 2 hours. This declined to approximately 1.5 hr in children older than one year. The half-life in adults is 0.87 hrs (Table 3).

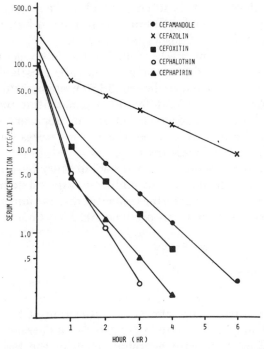

FIGURE 4. Serum concentrations of parenteral cephalosporins after a 1.0 gm bolus intravenous dose.

*Cefazolin.* In contrast with cephapirin and cephalothin, which are metabolized to a varying degree to the less microbiologically active desacetyl form, cefazolin remains unchanged in the body. Comparative pharmacologic studies in adults show that at equivalent dosage, cefazolin achieves serum concentrations that are significantly greater than those achieved by the other cephalosporins (5,6). The peak serum concentration after a 500 mg intramuscular dose of cefazolin is about 34 μg/ml, compared with 9.6, 11.3, 9.5, 12.0 and 12.0 μg/ml after a similar injection of cephalothin, cephapirin, cephradine, cefoxitin and cefamandole respectively (Table 4).

The serum half-life of cefazolin after an intravenous dose is 1.7 hr (Table 5). Cefazolin's lower rate of elimination through the kidneys, higher protein binding in serum, i.e. 83% (2,6,29,49), and smaller volume of distribution (Table 3) are mainly responsible for its higher and more prolonged blood concentrations (Figure 4). Although the high protein binding theoretically has a potential disadvantage in reducing the amount of free or microbiologically active drug, this problem is partially offset by its longer half-life and higher total serum levels. Because of these pharmacokinetic properties, cefazolin can frequently be administered half as often or in half the amount of the other parenteral cephalosporins.

Studies demonstrating high cefazolin tissue concentrations have recently been reported for aqueous humor (6), tonsils (5), peritoneal fluid (6), skeletal muscle (50), heart (36,51), pleural fluid (6,52) bone (37,38,39,53) and synovial fluid (39). Poor penetration into breast milk (54) and spinal fluid was observed (6,55). The apparent volume of distribution of cefazolin may also be affected by stress (56). Additional studies (5,7) were previously reviewed.

Cefazolin pharmacokinetics can be adequately described by a two compartment open model (5). In addition, a physiological perfusion model can also be used to describe cafazolin disposition, and this model has been successfully used to predict cefazolin bone concentrations (57).

## Renal Excretion

The mechanism of renal clearance for the cephalosporins is glomerular filtration of free drug, and active secretion of total drug. Since both processes may decrease in renal disease, a decrease in creatinine clearance will coincide with a prolongation of the half-life of all of these drugs. Probenecid (which blocks the tubular secretion of organic acids) will decrease excretion of all of these compounds.

The instability of cefaclor in biological fluids results in a lack of accumulation when this drug is used to treat patients with impaired renal function or chronic renal failure. In chronic renal failure the half-life ratio (t½ renal failure: t½ normal) of cephalexin increases to 16 (58). With cefaclor, the ratio increases to only 3.6 (58,59,60,61). Doses of 500 mg of cefaclor administered every six hours do not result in drug accumulation. The relationship between cefaclor elimination and creatinine clearance has been characterized by several investigators (58,61). Hemodialysis was found to decrease the elimination half-life by only 25 to 30% (59,60,62).

The higher and more prolonged excretion of cefadroxil compared to cephalexin does not mean that more cefadroxil is eliminated via the urine. The urinary recovery of both drugs is essentially the same (Table 2). After 12 hours, urinary recoveries of 89%, 85% and 100% have been reported for cefadroxil, cephalexin and cephradine, respectively. However, the excretion kinetics of these drugs are not similar. After administration of equivalent doses, cefadroxil urinary concentrations are initially ( 0 to 3 hrs) lower than those of cefalexin and cephradine (Table 2), and at all other time intervals cefadroxil concentrations are higher (24,26,27). The mechanisms for this change in elimination are not clear. Since the protein binding characteristics of these agents are not significantly different, this is not a possible mechanism. Cefadroxil, like cephalexin and cephradine, will accumulate in patients with impared renal function. The half-life ratio of normals compared to patients with renal dysfunction is 10 to 18% (23,63), which is similar to that of cephalexin (23,58) and the relationship between cefadroxil half-life and renal function has been well characterized (63). Hemodialysis (6 to 8 hrs) has decreased serum concentrations by 75% (23).

The 24 hour urinary recovery for unmetabolized parenteral caphalosporins ranges from 80 to 100% of a given dose (see Table 5). The desacetyl metabolites of cephalothin and cephapirin are also excreted renally, with 43% of a cephalothin dose and 45.3% of a cephapirin dose appearing as metabolite in the urine after 6 hours. This is 44% and 48% respectively of total drug recovered (64,65). However, in uremic patients only 4.7% of a cephalothin dose was recovered after 14 hours and 78.2 to 94.4% of total drug recovered was the metabolite. (64) It has been postulated that cephalosporins which are metabolized possess an advantage over non-metabolized cephalosporins in the treatment of uremic patients, since the parent compound does not accumulate. Unfortunately, the metabolite does accumulate (64) and until the toxicity of the metabolites is fully understood and the potential for resistant organisms explored, the same care in dosage adjustment is necessary for the metabolized and non-metabolized cephalosporins. The renal clearance of cefazolin (protein binding ~85%) is less than the other cephalosporins (Table 5). Cefamandole is also highly protein bound (~80%), but is renally excreted more rapidly, probably due to the high degree of active secretion (42).

As a consequence of their high renal clearance, urinary concentrations of the cephalosporins are relatively high. Even in renal failure, they remain many times above the MIC's for the common urinary tract pathogens. For example, in patients with creatinine clearances of 5 to 20 ml/min, 30% of a cefamandole dose was excreted in the urine in 24 hours and the concentrations in the urine ranged from 230 ± 33 μg/ml initially, to 66 ± 15 μg/ml at 24 hours (66). In patients with similar creatinine clearance values, the lowest concentration of cefamandole has been reported as 53 μg/ml (7). Rather than comparing concentrations which are dependent on urine volume, the percent of dose excreted may be compared. The percent of dose excreted in 24 hours, even with severe renal failure, is around 20% for all the unmetabolized cephalosporins (See Table 5).

The reported half-life of these antibiotics in various degrees of renal failure is quite variable. This is probably because at creatinine clearance values <20 ml/min, very small changes in drug clearance will markedly prolong half-life (66,67,68). In spite of this, most studies group patients into relatively broad categories and report mean half-life values for each group, e.g. 5–20 ml/min or <10 ml/min may be one category. Furthermore, creatinine clearance is not always measured, and the number of evaluated patients is often small.

Cephalothin, using a microbiological assay method, has been found to have a mean half-life of 3.7 hours in patients with creatinine clearances below 10 ml/min. (64) However, when investigated with an HPLC assay, the desacetyl metabolite was found to be accumulating in these patients given 1.0 gm every 12 hours. Furthermore, there was no apparent decline in the metabolite concentration 14 hours after a dose. In contrast, the half-life of unmetabolized cephalothin was 0.47 hours with normal renal function and no desacetyl metabolite was detected at 6 hours after dosing. Hemodialysis has little affect on the clearance of cephalothin, with a reported half-life during dialysis of 2.6 to 3.3 hours (5,69), which is not very different than that observed with severe renal insufficiency. Serum concentrations have been reported to be reduced by 50% with peritoneal dialysis (69).

At a mean creatinine clearance of 12.6 ml/min, the half-life of cephapirin was reported as 1.59 hours, while during hemodialysis the half-life was found to be 1.8 hours. (5) No information is available on the clearance of cephradine in renal failure.

A mean half-life of 14.9 ± 2.9 hours for cefazolin in 13 patients with creatinine clearance values of 10 to 35 ml/min (moderate renal failure

TABLE 5. RENAL EXCRETION

| | Cephalothin[a] | Cephapirin[b] | Cefoxitin[c] | Cefamandole[d] | Cefazolin[e] | Cephradine[f] |
|---|---|---|---|---|---|---|
| TBC-normal ml/min/1.73m² | 472 | 580 | 247–331 | 193–303 | 52–63 | 435 |
| RCL-normal ml/min/1.73m² | 274 | 342–360 | 225–329 | 160–250 | 42–64 | 367 |
| % normally excreted unchanged in 24 hr. | 50–70 | 41 | 84–100 | 65–96 | 80–100 | 79–96 |
| % excreted in 24 hr in renal failure | (<5 ml/min) 2.5 | 19 | (<10 ml/min) 26.6 | 8.6–30 | 22.1±14.0 | — |
| t½—MRF* | 1.4 | 1.6 | — | 3.0±0.3 | 14.9±2.9 | — |
| t½—SRF** | 3.7 | — | 15.0±5.3 | 10.4±2.4 | 35.3±9.6 | — |
| Hemodialysis t½ | 2.6–3.3 | 1.8 | 3.9±0.2 | 5.6±1.1 | 5.5±1.9 | — |
| Peritoneal Dialysis t½ | → serum concentration by 50% | 20% removed in 6 hr. | — | 8.7±2.4 | 32.5 | — |

a compiled from references 5, 6, 64, 69
b compiled from references 5, 6, 30, 69, 107
c compiled from references 5, 6, 67, 69, 75
d compiled from references 6, 65, 66, 69, 71, 72, 73, 74, 84, 107, 109
e compiled from references 5, 6, 69, 70
f compiled from reference 5

MRF—moderate renal failure ($Cl_{CR}$ 10–35 ml/min)
SRF—severe renal failure ($Cl_{CR}$ <5 ml/min)

- MRF) has been calculated by compilation of published data (69). This was also done for patients with creatinine clearance values <5 ml/min (severe renal failure - SRF) (69) and by adding subsequent data, a mean half-life of 35.3 ± 9.6 hours (31 patients) can be calculated. Hemodialysis, with a twin coil dialyzer, will decrease this half-life to 5.54 ± 1.86 hours (69,70) (37 patients). Peritoneal dialysis, on the other hand, affects the half-life of cefazolin very little (32.5 hrs), even though 19% of the dose is recovered in the dialysate (69).

With IM cefamandole, the mean half-life in nine patients in MRF was calculated as 3.0 ± 0.3 hours (69). In patients with SRF, the mean half-life can be calculated from various references (27 patients) to be 10.4 ± 2.4 hours (66,71,72,73,74). The effect of hemodialysis on cefamandole relative to cefazolin is interesting. The mean half-life during dialysis for cefamandole (twin coil and single pass dialyzer data grouped, since no appreciable difference was seen) is 5.64 ± 1.11 hours (66,71,72,73,74) (29 patients). This is very similar to cefazolin's hemodialysis half-life and both drugs are highly protein bound. However, *relative to half-life in SRF,* hemodialysis clearance appears less pronounced with cefamandole (i.e., decreasing the half-life by about 50% vs. 84% for cefazolin). Peritoneal dialysis seems to affect half-life very little with cefamandole, as the half-life during dialysis was reported to be 11.75 ± 2.05 hours in two patients (74).

In patients with creatinine clearances between 10 and 30 ml/min, the mean half-life of cefoxitin was found to be 6.3 hours. This increased to 13.2 hours in five other patients with creatinine clearances <10 ml/min but not requiring hemodialysis (67). In patients with SRF, the mean half-life between dialysis was calculated to be 15.0 ± 5.3 hours (67,69,75). During hemodialysis, the mean half-life was 3.89 ± 0.25 hours (67,75).

In summary, renal excretion is the most significant means of elimination for all these cephalosporins except cephalothin and cephapirin. Dosing must be adjusted when creatinine clearance is less than 20 to 30 ml/min. Peritoneal dialysis is ineffective in removing the drugs. Hemodialysis will decrease the half-life in patients with severe renal failure, but the half-life in this situation is still not comparable to that in patients with normal clearance.

## Biliary Excretion

In addition to biliary studies which were previously reviewed (5,17), several new studies describe the biliary excretion of cephalosporins in the presence of biliary disease (6,76,77,78,79,80). Due to differences in experimental design and patient population, these studies are extremely difficult to evaluate and compare. Fortunately, two comparative studies are helpful in elucidating the differences in biliary excretion between these agents. Brogard et al (76) compared cephalexin, cefazolin and cephalothin biliary concentrations. Peak concentrations after a 1.0 gram I.V. dose were approximately 28 and 11 µg/ml for cefazolin and cephalothin, respectively (representing 0.13 and 0.03% of the administered dose, respectively). Cephalexin 1.0 gm administered orally yields concentration of 26 µg/ml (0.28% of the dose). Ratzan et al (80) compared cefamandole, cefazolin and cephalothin. After a 1.0 gm intravenous dose of cefamandole, cefazolin and cephalothin, bile concentrations were approximately 352, 40 and 10 µg/ml, representing 0.4%, 0.12% and 0.025% of the administered dose, respectively. It is clear that cefamandole yields the highest bile concentrations, followed by cefazolin, cephalexin and cephalothin. In two patients with T-tubes, cefoxitin also produced high biliary concentrations (227.6 µg/ml two hours after a 2 gm intravenous dose) (45).

The higher bile concentrations of cefamandole compared with first generation cephalosporins are often mentioned as a therapeutic advantage; yet there is no evidence of any difference in the eradication of biliary tract infection with any cephalosporin. Perhaps the concentration of the cephalosporin in tissue, like gallbladder wall, is more important than the actual concentrations in bile. For instance, although cefamandole achieves much higher bile levels than those of cefazolin, the concentrations in the gallbladder wall are similar (81).

## Tissue Metabolism

Cephalothin and cephapirin undergo considerable tissue metabolism via esterases to produce desacetyl metabolites. A seldom appreciated aspect of this tissue metabolism is that it occurs both *in vivo* as well as *in vitro*. Recently, we determined that the usual procedures of homogenization, certrifugation and assay of placental tissue causes almost total conversion of cephalothin to its metabolite (unpublished data). This confirms earlier findings in bone tissue (38) where cephalothin recoveries were unacceptably low, necessitating a change in our method of extraction. In virtually every study reporting tissue concentrations of cephalothin and cephapirin, recovery values were not provided, nor was any mention made of special techniques to prevent drug metabolism during sample handling. We must assume that no special measures such as reduced temperature, short homogenization, or rapid protein precipitation were taken. In addition, almost all studies used a microbiological assay. In our estimation, cephalothin, in the absence of measures to prevent *in vitro* metabolism, will be converted by tissue esterases to the desacetyl form during the extraction procedure. Measurement of parent compound and metabolite concentration by microbiological techniques, using parent compound standard solutions, will grossly underestimate cephalothin concentrations if *in vitro* conversion to the metabolite is not prevented. In essence, it is highly likely that most cephalothin tissue penetration studies reported artifactual data that underestimated the true tissue penetration of cephalothin. Insufficient cephapirin data are available to determine whether tissue metabolism is also a problem with this drug. However, the similarities in pharmacokinetics (as measured via microbiological assay) suggest that cephapirin tissue concentrations were also underestimated.

It should also be noted that the pharmacokinetic parameters shown in Tables 3 and 4 are somewhat artifactual, since they were obtained from studies where drug concentrations were determined by microbiological analysis. These studies did not separate the biologically active metabolites from the parent compound. Since concentrations of parent drug-metabolite mixtures were determined using standard solutions of parent compound, the concentration time relationship (31) and pharmacokinetic parameters are in error. Thus, the serum concentration-time curve for cephalothin-cephapirin (Figure 4) should be considered as a "microbiologically active" concentration-time curve.

## CONCENTRATION VERSUS RESPONSE AND TOXICITY

### Usual Therapeutic Concentrations

The concentrations of cephalosporins required to eradicate an infection are generally exceeded in serum by a factor of 5 to 1000. However, effective concentrations in the interstitial fluid of infected tissue must also be considered. In a series of experiments investigating concentrations in atrial appendage tissue of patients undergoing open heart surgery (unpublished data), it was observed that tissue concentrations generally are proportional to serum concentrations (Table 6). Many factors, however, might affect the drug's ability to penetrate into interstitial fluid or tissue (e.g., serum protein binding).

In a study comparing heart tissue and pericardial fluid concentrations of the highly protein bound cefazolin to the negligibly bound cephradine in patients undergoing open heart surgery (51), it was found that the free (unbound) concentrations of cephradine in pericardial fluid were higher than those of cefazolin. The free cefazolin concentrations however, were within the therapeutic range. Since pericardial fluid contains albumin (approximately 50% of the serum concentration) to which cefazolin can bind, it is expected that the total (unbound plus bound) cefazolin concentrations would be greater than the free concentration. Furthermore, the observation that atrial appendage homogenate concentrations of cefazolin were higher than those of cephradine suggests that cefazolin also binds to tissue protein. Higher total cefazolin concentrations were also observed in synovial fluid and knee bone (unpublished data) as well as hip bone (38), and occurred even though the free serum concentrations of cefazolin were lower than those of cephradine.

The area under the serum concentration-time curve (AUC) for *free* drug can be used as an "availability index," since it takes into account all processes such as absorption, distribution, and elimination from the body. Such an analysis was done by Bergen (82), who found that the AUC for cefazolin was slightly higher (54.2) than that for cephalothin (47.6) and cephapirin (49.0). Thus, the high serum protein binding of cefazolin is not a disadvantage compared with the other cephalosporins, provided the concept of free AUC is proven to be a valid predictor of therapeutic equivalence.

The AUC can be increased by the co-administration of probenecid. One gram of probenecid was found to double the peak serum concentrations of cephalothin (5); increase the peak serum concentrations of cephradine by 40 to 70% (6); increase the peak serum concentration of cefoxitin 3½-fold, prolong the half-life to 83 minutes (83) and decrease renal clearance to 80 ml/min/1.73 $m^2$ (6); increase serum concentrations of cefamandole by about 80% and also decrease renal clearance of this drug (42,84). Two grams of cefazolin plus one gram of probenecid will give an AUC value equal to a three gram dose of cefazolin alone (5).

TABLE 6. RELATIONSHIP OF PROTEIN BINDING
TO SERUM AND TISSUE PEAKS OF CEPHALOSPORINS

|  | % Bound | C°p (μg/ml) | Tissue Peak (μg/gm) |
|---|---|---|---|
| Cephradine | 10–20 | 100 | 30–40 |
| Cephapirin | 50 | 150 | 30–40 |
| Cefoxitin | 60 | 150 | 30–40 |
| Cephalothin | 65 | 150 | 30–40 |
| Cefamandole | 74 | 160 | 50 |
| Cefazolin | 85 | 200 | 60 |
| Ceforanide* | 90 | 240 | 80 |

* Investigational cephalosporin

In some instances, oral administration of cephalosporins can yield higher serum concentrations than parenteral (intramuscular) injections. It has been shown that cephalexin and cephradine achieve excellent serum concentrations after oral administration (1). These peak serum concentrations of approximately 32 μg/ml far exceed those obtained with cephradine, cephalothin, and cephapirin after an equal intramuscular dose (5).

This observation prompted another study in which we compared the pharmacokinetics of cephalexin and cephradine after the administration of a 2.0 gm dose in a multiple dose regimen (85). Again it was found that the pharmacokinetics of these drugs are identical. Of possible clinical relevance was the attainment of peak serum concentrations of approximately 50 μg/ml, a concentration that is essentially similar to that observed after a 1.0 gm intravenous dose of cephradine, cephalothin or cephapirin (85). The peak serum concentrations obtained after a one gram dose of these oral cephalosporins (~32 μg/ml) are almost 10 times their usual minimum inhibitory concentrations for penicillin-resistant staphylococci (~3.4 μg/ml). Theoretically, in the treatment of staphylococcal infections therapeutic results should be similar to those obtained with parenteral cephalosporins. This was supported by a recent study (86) in which excellent clinical results were obtained in the therapy of staphylococcal osteomyelitis and suppurative arthritis in children with an initial one week course of a parenteral cephalosporin followed by three weeks of an oral cephalosporin.

Another factor influencing effective cephalosporin concentrations at the site of infection is beta-lactamase inactivation. There has been considerable controversy regarding the use of cefazolin in serious staphylococcal infections, such as bacterial endocarditis, owing to the in-vitro observations (87,88,89) that cefazolin is more easily inactivated than cephalothin by staphylococcal beta-lactamase. Incomplete and conflicting data currently prevent resolution of this controversy. All of these studies involve in-vitro testing for antibiotic hydrolysis in the presence and absence of beta-lactamase-producing Staph aureus. In every case it was shown that cefazolin was inactivated more rapidly than cephalothin, but even with cefazolin the viable bacterial cell count either decreased for 6 to 8 hours or remained relatively constant for 12 hours after incubation of the drug with the beta-lactamase-producing organisms. This occurred even though the concentration of cefazolin was rapidly declining due to inactivation. If the viable bacterial cell count decreased for 6 to 8 hours and the normal dosing interval is 6 to 8 hours, the clinical significance of the more rapid rate of cefazolin hydrolysis must be questioned.

Another factor that confuses the issue is the effect of the growth medium on the rate of inactivation (90). The MIC's for cefazolin are higher when the organisms are grown in trypticase soy broth than in Mueller-Hinton broth. Likewise, the rate of antibiotic degradation is lower when the drug is incubated with beta-lactamase-producing *Staph aureus* in Mueller-Hinton broth compared with trypticase soy broth. This is presumably related to the high dextrose content of trypticase soy broth, which may stimulate greater production of beta-lactamase. Another recent study (91) showed a large disparity between MIC's and minimum bactericidal concentrations (MBC's) of anti-staphylococcal antibiotics, including cephalothin and cefazolin. In this study, 87% of staphylococcal strains tested showed an eight-fold or greater difference in MBC when tested in Mueller-Hinton or in brain heart infusion broth. Moreover, because micro-organisms in the body are exposed to serum or interstitial fluid, and not to artificial media, the interpretation and extrapolation of these *in-vitro* data to the clinical situation may not be possible.

Another factor determining effective cephalosporin serum concentrations is the degree of protein binding among the cephalosporins. It is possible that the susceptibility of protein bound drug to beta-lactamase inactivation is different from that of the free drug. This subject was not addressed in the *in vitro* broth studies but was investigated (unpublished data) and it was found that cefazolin inactivation at 37° in serum without bacteria present was so rapid that the addition of beta-lactamase producing organisms to the incubating serum did not appreciably increase the rate of degradation.

Skeptics of the use of cefazolin in bacterial endocarditis point out that there are three case reports (92,93) of supposed failure of cefazolin in the treatment of staphylococcal endocarditis. However, because these cases occurred in heroin addicts, two of whom had splenic abscesses and one of whom had received two weeks of cephalothin before the introduction of cefazolin, they certainly cannot be considered true therapeutic failures. Moreover, even if all three cases are real failures, the number is not surprising, because it is well known that therapeutic failures in staphylococcal endocarditis are not unusual with any antibiotic. In a study of the treatment of experimental staphylococcal endocarditis in rabbits with methicillin, cefazolin, or cephalothin, no differences were observed in the cure rates (94).

Clearly the relevance of different rates of beta-lactamase inactivation with the cephalosporins is still uncertain. However, the bulk of scientific information favors the optimistic view that there is as yet no direct evidence for the hypothesis that these differences will result in any greater likelihood of a therapeutic failure if the clinician uses one cephalosporin over another in the therapy of serious staphylococcal infection.

## Toxic Interaction

It has been stated that patients receiving aminoglycoside and a cephalosporin have an increased risk of nephrotoxicity over that incurred when an aminoglycoside is given alone. But the evidence linking the association, however, is inferential. In fact, in one experimental animal study (95), cephalosporins partially protected kidneys from aminoglycoside nephrotoxicity. In this experiment the dose of cephalothin in rats (500 mg/kg) that was required to partially protect against the nephrotoxicity of gentamicin was equivalent to a dose in man of about 35 to 40 grams. Obviously, this amount of cephalothin is rarely, if ever, used in man, and hence, one would not expect to observe the protective effect of cephalothin in a clinical situation. Interestingly, the same investigators noted that the dose of carbenicillin in rats (100 mg/kg) that partially protected against the nephrotoxicity of gentimicin was equivalent to about 15 grams in man, a dose that is within the customary range used in serious infection. Therefore, it is not surprising that clinical studies (96,97,98) comparing the relative nephrotoxicity of the combination of gentamicin and cephalothin with the combination of gentamicin and carbenicillin have uniformly noted a higher incidence of adverse reaction with the former combination. It appears that with the gentamicin-cephalothin combination, one merely observes the inherent nephrotoxicity of the aminoglycoside; whereas, with gentamicin-carbenicillin, one obtains partial protection from the nephrotoxicity of the aminoglycoside.

## CLINICAL APPLICATION OF PHARMACOKINETIC DATA

The cephalosporins exhibit a biphasic decline in blood concentrations as a function of time, indicating that at least a two compartment pharmacokinetic model is required to describe the kinetics of these drugs. Since the cephalosporins have a relatively wide therapeutic index, use of multi-compartmental modeling for the purpose of dosage regimen calculations is unnecessary. Pharmacokinetic management of patients is generally restricted to patients with severe renal failure, which can be adequately handled by treating this class of agents as if they had one compartment model characteristics. In the treatment of patients with infections that present antibiotic penetration problems, pharmacokinetic dosage adjustments are not precise because of the paucity of information regarding the rate and extent of drug transport to the site of action. Under these conditions, use of the two compartment model offers no advantage in patient management.

## Dosing

Expected cephalosporin serum concentrations over time after a single dose are shown in Figures 2 (oral agents) and 4 (parenteral agents - I.V.). These values were achieved with a dosage of 15 mg/kg, using the average pharmacokinetic parameters in Tables 1 and 3, for a 70 kg adult with normal renal function. Cephalosporin serum concentrations are not routinely obtained clinically and the degree of correlation between average literature values (from normal volunteers) and actual patient data in various disease states is unknown. Steady-state concentrations would not differ significantly since the half-life of cephalosporins is relatively short compared to the usual dosing interval. In this situation, significant accumulation of drug does not occur.

The cephalosporin antibiotics have a wide "margin of safety" and dosage adjustments based on patient specific pharmacokinetic parameters are infrequently done. One case where a cephalosporin dose should be adjusted is in patients with renal failure. Even then, dosage changes do not become a critical requirement with cephalosporins until creatinine clearance is <20 to 30 ml/min. In such circumstances, one half the normal dose should be given approximately every half-life (or at the normal interval if this is longer than the half-life) (Table 5). This approach may avoid prolonged periods of relatively low serum concentrations. This also holds true for patients on intermittent hemodialysis. The dose of cephalosporin can be given after dialysis, and then approximately every half-life off dialysis. Peritoneal dialysis does not significantly remove cephalosporins, and dosing does not need to be changed from the regimen selected for severe renal failure.

## When To Obtain Blood Levels

Instances where it may be necessary to check the serum concentration of cephalosporins are: (i) whenever there is a question of lack of response or toxicity, (ii) in the patient with changing renal dysfunction and (iii) when using oral dosing for a serious infection such as osteomyelitis (86). In this latter case, a pharmacokinetic study should be done to document absorption and attainment of adequate serum concentrations. When using these drugs parenterally, checking a peak, a 4 hour and a trough serum concentration should be reasonable to answer questions regarding adequacy of dose, and to determine half-life. The 4 hour serum concentration is necessary because (except for cefazolin) drug may be undetectable or below the sensitivity of the assay at 6 hours (trough) (Figure 4).

With oral dosing, absorption becomes a concern and more frequent serum sampling may be necessary. If samples are obtained at 0.5 hour, 1 hour, 1.5 hours, 2 hours and 4 hours, the absorption rate constant $(k_a)$ and half-life can be calculated. Except for cefadroxil, drug may not be detectable at 6 hours (Figure 2). If an estimation of the absorption half-life is not required, it might be assumed that the peak concentration occurs after one hour in fasting patients and subsequent samples 1½, 3, and 4 hours post-dose will allow an estimation of the drug's half-life.

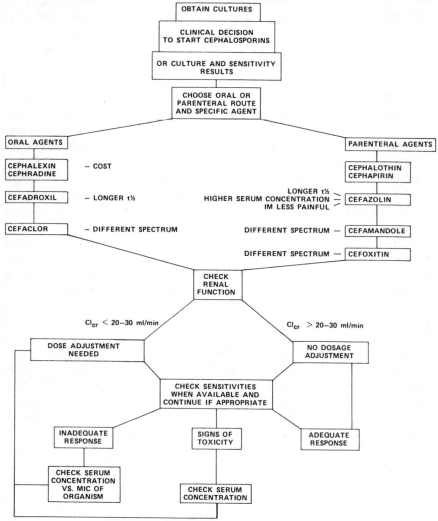

FIGURE 5. Algorithm for the application of pharmacokinetics to cephalosporin therapy.

## ASSAY METHODS

**Sample Collection.** Patient blood samples (approximately 3.0 ml) should be collected in non-heparinized tubes and maintained on ice. The blood should be allowed to clot and then centrifuged at 2500 rpm for 10 minutes at 4°C. The serum can then be transferred to polypropylene tubes and stored at − 70°C until assay.

Tissue samples should be blotted to remove excess blood and immediately frozen in liquid nitrogen and stored at − 70°C.

**Preparation of Serum Standards.** A standard curve may be prepared by diluting the test drug in normal serum, usually at a range of concentrations similar to those expected in clinical samples. This range must be linear when log concentration is plotted against zone diameter. If necessary, patient samples may be diluted with normal serum to fall into this range. Protein precipitation may be desired, and can be accomplished by using substances such as ethanol, acetone or acetonitrile. For the high pressure liquid chromatographic (HPLC) analysis of cephalosporins, acetonitrile is recommended as a protein precipitant.

**Assay of Serum Samples.** In our laboratory, samples are allowed to thaw and then maintained on ice along with the standards. Samples and standards are spotted on Scheicher and Scheule paper discs, 6.35 mm in diameter. Exactly 20 μl of solution is applied to the disc. Three discs (one should be a standard) are spotted on every plate. Plates are incubated for 6 hours at 37°C. Zones of inhibition are read to the nearest 0.1 mm on a Fisher-Lilly zone reader. A linear regression analysis is performed relating the log of each standard concentration to its zone size. Sample concentrations can be determined directly from this linear regression line.

**Tissue Homogenization.** Tissue samples are allowed to thaw, then kept on ice whenever possible during the procedure. The samples are gently blotted to remove excess blood, and fat is trimmed off. The exact weight is recorded and approximately 100 mg of tissue is used. Unused tissue is re-frozen in a labelled container.

With forceps and scalpel, the tissue is minced to expose a maximum amount of surface area, then transferred to a cold 7-ml Pyrex homogenizer. The tissue is homogenized as quickly as possible in a volume of buffer using a fixed volume to tissue-weight ratio. The homogenate is transferred to a small plastic tube and spun at 20,000 rpm for 15 minutes at 4°C. The supernatant is transferred to a small vial and frozen at − 70°C until assayed. If the tissue is very bloody, a correction should be made for the amount of drug due to blood in the sample (99).

## Microbiological Assay

The cephalosporins can be assayed using the agar diffusion technique on Antibiotic Medium 1 (Difco) using *Bacillus subtilis* as the assay organism. Other organisms that are susceptible to the cephalosporin can be used, such as *Sarcina lutea*. The choice of organism depends on the cephalosporin, and the required assay sensitivity. In most instances *B. subtilis* can be employed, providing the advantages of an easily handled spore forming organism.

**Preparation of Seeded Plates.** Antibiotic Medium 1 is rehydrated, autoclaved, cooled and maintained at 48°C in a water bath. Using proper aseptic technique, 0.15 ml of suspended *B. subtilis* spores are then added for each 100 mls of agar being prepared. The agar is mixed thoroughly to distribute the spores. A sterile cornwall syringe is used to deliver 6 mls of seeded agar into each sterile plastic petri dish, and the plates are swirled to evenly distribute the agar. Each plate is set on a level surface to solidify. Lids are kept slightly ajar to allow moisture to escape. Plates are stored in the refrigerator and are good for approximately two weeks.

*Comments.* The microbiological system described above utilizes paper discs for spotting the drug samples. Other techniques, such as the use of cylinders and wells punched in the agar can also be used. The cylinder plate method requires larger sample sizes and generally yields larger zone sizes, but does not necessarily increase assay sensitivity. Microbiologic assay systems are associated with an error rate of approximately 10%, however they allow a relatively large number of samples to be assayed at low cost. Technician time required to assay 20 serum samples is estimated to be approximately 3 hours, excluding incubation time. The incubation time can vary from 6 to 12 hours. The approximate minimum one time cost of equipment necessary for this assay technique is $4,000.

## High Pressure Liquid Chromatography

In general, cephalosporins exhibit a fairly high intrinsic absorbtivity at a wavelength of 254 nm. Chromotographic separations are performed using a column packed with a reverse phase material consisting of lipophilic C-18 chain units bonded to a microparticulate silica support. A solvent system of methanol/water/1% acetic acid is adequate as a mobile phase for chromatographing most of the cephalosporins. The amount of methanol is determined by the properties of the cephalosporin in question (e.g., lipophilicity, hydrogen bonding, ionic characteristics at pH of mobile phase). In general, the solvent system can be determined empirically by adjusting the amount of methanol until a convenient retention time is obtained (usually about 10 minutes).

The concentrations of MeOH: $H_2O$: AcOH listed in table 7 should afford retention times of about 6 to 10 minutes. There will be some column to column variation. In addition, there may be some day to day variation using the same column.

The detector response is a linear function of the concentration of drug in the sample. Therefore, a linear regression analysis of peak height (obtained from a strip chart recorder connected to the detector) vs. concentration for the standard samples produces a standard curve, from which the concentrations of patient samples may be determined.

*Comments.* The HPLC technique is a rapid and more accurate method of analysis compared to microbiological analysis. Delays in obtaining results do not occur because incubation of organisms is not necessary. This method, however, does not allow for rapid processing of large numbers of samples and is therefore more expensive than the microbiological techniques (Table 8). Technician time required to assay 20 serum samples is estimated to be approximately 8 hours. The minimum one time cost of equipment necessary for this assay technique is $11,000 to $12,000.

TABLE 7. SOLVENT RATIOS FOR VARIOUS CEPHALOSPORINS

| | % $H_2O$ | % MeOH | % AcOH |
|---|---|---|---|
| Cephalothin | 60 | 39 | 1 |
| Cefaperazone | 64 | 35 | 1 |
| Cefamandole | 66 | 33 | 1 |
| Cephalexin | 75 | 24 | 1 |
| Cefoxitin | 75 | 24 | 1 |
| Cephradine | 75 | 24 | 1 |
| Cefazolin | 75 | 24 | 1 |
| Cephapirin | 85 | 14 | 1 |
| Ceforanide | 85 | 14 | 1 |
| Cefaclor | 90 | 9 | 1 |
| Cefadroxil | 95 | 4 | 1 |

TABLE 8. COMPARISON OF THE RELATIVE ADVANTAGES AND DISADVANTAGES OF THE VARIOUS CEPHALOSPORIN ASSAY METHODS*

| Analytical Method | Limit of Sensitivity | Assayable Samples | | | | | | Estimated Reagent and Tech. Cost per Assay | Analysis** Costs | |
| | | Metabolite Analysis | Plasma/Serum | Urine | Saliva | Minimum Sample Volume Required | Analysis Time | | Initial Equipment Costs | Specialized Operator Training |
| --- | --- | --- | --- | --- | --- | --- | --- | --- | --- | --- |
| Microbiological | .5–1 | only if microactive | 3 | 3 | 3 | 60 µl | 9–15h (6–12 h is incubation time) | $0.98 | $4000 | none |
| HPLC | 0.1–0.5 | yes | 1 | 1 | 1 | 30 µl | 8h | $2.60 | $12,000 | none |

* Arbitrary Ranking Scale of 1 (Excellent) to 5 (Poor) with a score of 3 being average or nominal

** Estimated on basis of 20 samples

268

# REFERENCES

1. Finkelstein E, Quintiliani R, Lee R, Bracci A, Nightingale CH: Pharmacokinetics of oral cephalosporins: cephradine and cephalexin. J Pharm Sci 1978; 67:1447–50.
2. Singhvi SM, Heald AF, Schreiber EC: Pharmacokinetics of cephalosporin antibiotics: protein-binding considerations. Chemotherapy 1978; 24:121–33.
3. Ginsburg CM, McCracken GH Jr: Pharmacokinetics of cephradine suspension in infants and children. Antimicrob Agents Chemother 1979; 16:74–76.
4. McCracken GH Jr, Ginsburg CM, Clarkson JC, Thomas ML: Pharmacologic evaluation of orally administered antibiotics in infants and children: effect of feeding on bioavailability. Pediatrics 1978; 62:738–43.
5. Nightingale CH, Greene DS, Quintiliani R: Pharmacokinetics and clinical use of cephalosporin antibiotics. J Pharm Sci 1975; 64:1899–1927.
6. Brogard JM, Comte F, Pinget M: Pharmacokinetics of cephalosporin antibiotics. Antibiotics Chemother 1978; 25:123–62.
7. Quintiliani R, Nightingale CH: Cefazolin. Ann Intern Med 1978; 89:650–56.
8. Mischler TW, Corson SL, Larranaga A, Bolognese RJ, Neiss ES, Vakovich RA: Cephradine and epicillin in body fluids of lactating and pregnant woman. J Reproductive Med 1978; 21:130–36.
9. Gillett AP, Wise R: Penetration of four cephalosporins into tissue fluid in man. Lancet 1978; 962.
10. Kiss JJ, Farango E, Pinter J: Serum & lung tissue levels of cephradine in thoracic surgery. Br J Clin Pharmacol. 1976; 3:891–95.
11. Jalava S, Saarimoa H, Elfoing R: Cephalexin levels in serum synovial fluid and joint tissues after oral administration. Scand J Rheumatology 1977; 6:250–52.
12. Shuford GM: Concentration of cephalexin in mandibular alveolar bone, blood and oral fluids. J Amer Dental Assoc 1979; 99:47–50.
13. Craft I, Forster TC: Materno-fetal cephradine transfer in pregnancy. Antimicrob Agents Chemother 1978; 14:924–926.
14. Schneider H, Nightingale CH, Quintiliani R, Flanagan DR: Evaluation of an oral prolonged release antibiotic formulation. J Pharm Sci 1978; 67:1620–22.
15. Lode H, Stahlmann R, Koeppe P: Comparative pharmacokinetics of cephalexin, cefaclor, cefadroxil and CGP 9000. Antimicrob Agents Chemother 1979; 16:1–6.
16. Welling PG, Dean S, Selen A, Kendall MJ, Wise R: The pharmacokinetics of the oral cephalosporins cefaclor, cephradine and cephalexin. International J Clin Pharmacol and Biopharmacy 1979; 17:397–400.
17. Korzeniowski OM, Scheld WM, Sande MA: Comparative pharmacology of cefaclor and cephalexin. Antimicrob Agents Chemother 1977; 12:157–62.
18. Simon C, Gutzemeier U: Serum and sputum levels of cefaclor. Postgrad Med J 1979; 55:(Suppl 4)30–34.
19. Foglesong MA, Lamb JW, Dietz JV: Stability and blood level determinations of cefaclor, a new oral cephalosporin antibiotic. J Antimicrobial Therapy 1978; 13:49–52.
20. Glynne A, Goulbourn RA, Ryden R: A human pharmacology study of cefaclor. J Antimicrobial Chemother 1978; 4:343–48.
21. Meyers BR, Hirschman SZ, Wormser G, Gartenberg G, Surlevitch E: Pharmacologic studies with cefaclor, a new oral cephalosporin. J Clin Pharmacol 1978 :174–79.
22. McCracken GH Jr, Ginsburg CM, Clarkson JC, Thomas ML: Pharmacokinetics of cefaclor in infants and children. J Antimicrobial Chemother 1978; 4:515–21.

23. Humbert G, Leroy A, Fillastre JP, Godin M: Pharmacokinetics of cefadroxil in normal subjects and in patients with renal insufficiency. Chemotherapy 1979; 25:189–95.

24. Pfeffer M, Jackson A, Ximens J, Perde DeMenezes J: Comparative human oral clinical pharmacology of cefadroxil, cephalexin and cephradine. Antimicrob Agents Chemother 1977; 11:331–38.

25. Jolly ER, Hennes DM, Richards D Jr: Human safety, tolerance and pharmacokinetic studies of cefadroxil, a new cephalosporin antibiotic for oral administration. Current Therap Res 1977; 22:727–36.

26. Hennes DM, Richards D, Santella PF, Rubinfeld J: Oral bioavailability of cefadroxil, a new semisynthetic cephalosporin. Clinical Therapeutics 1977; 1:263–73.

27. Hartstein AI, Patrick KE, Jones SR, Miller MJ, Bryant RE: Comparison of pharmacological and antimicrobial properties of cefadroxil and cephalexin. Antimicrob Agents Chemother 1977; 12:93–97.

28. Ginsburg CM, McCracken GH Jr, Clarkson JC, Thomas M: Clinical pharmacology of cefadroxil in infants and children. Antimicrob Agents Chemother 1978; 13:845–48.

29. Paradelis AG, Stalhopoulos G, Trianthoplyllidis C, Logaras G: Pharmacokinetics of five cephalosporins in healthy male volunteers. Arzneim-Forsch 1977; 27:2167–70.

30. Arvidsson A, Borga O, Alvam G: Renal excretion of cephapirin and cephaloridine: evidence for saturable renal absorption. Clin Pharmacol Ther 1979; 25:870–76.

31. Rolewicz TF, Mirkin BL, Cooper MJ, Anders MW: Metabolic disposition of cephalothin and deacetyl-cephalothin in children and adults: comparison of high-performance liquid chromatographic and microbial assay procedures. Clin Pharmacol Ther 1977; 22:928–35.

32. Quintiliani R, Klimek J, Nightingale CH: Penetration of cephapirin and cephalothin into the right atrial appendage and pericardial fluid of patients undergoing open-heart surgery. J Infect Dis 1979; 139:348–52.

33. Green E, Subramanian S, Faden H, Quintiliani R, Nightingale CH: The penetration characteristics of cephapirin and cephalothin into the right atrial appendage, fat, skeletal muscle and pericardial fluid in children undergoing open heart surgery. Ann Thoracic Surg 1980; in press.

34. Rubi R, Galan HM: Cephapirin concentrations in prostatic and seminal vesicle tissue. Int J Clin Pharm Biopharm 1979; 17:87–89.

35. Archer GL, Polk RE, Duma RJ, Lower R: Comparison of cephalothin and cefamandole prophylaxis during insertion of prosthetic heart valves. Antimicrob Agents Chemother 1978; 13:924–29.

36. Eigel P, Tschirkov A, Satter P, Knothe H: Assays of cephalosporin antibiotics administered prophylactically in open heart surgery. Infection 1978; 6:23–28.

37. Wiggins CE, Nelson CL, Clarke R, Thompson CH: Concentrations of antibiotics in normal bone after intravenous injection. J Bone & Joint Surg 1978; 60-A:93–96.

38. Cunha BA, Gossling HR, Pasternak HS, Nightingale CH, Quintiliani R: The penetration characteristics of cefazolin, cephalothin and ᶦcephradine into bone in patients undergoing total hip replacement. J Bone & Joint Surg 1977; 59-A:856–59.

39. Schurman DJ, Hirshman HP, Kajiyama G, Moser K, Burton DS: Cefazolin concentrations in bone and synovial fluid. J Bone & Joint Surg 1978; 60-A:359–62.

40. Fitzgerald RH, Kelly PJ, Snyder RJ, Washington II JA: Penetration of methicillin, oxacillin and cephalothin into bone and synovial fluid. Antimicrob Agents Chemother 1978; 14:723–26.

41. Patel D, Moellering RC, Thrasher K, Fahmy NR, Harris WH: The effect of hypotensive anesthesia on cephalothin concentrations in bone and muscle of patients undergoing total hip replacement. J Bone & Joint Surg 1979; 61-A:531–38.
42. Greene DS, Quintiliani R, Thompson MA, Nightingale CH: Effect of probenecid on the renal excretion of cefamandole. Current Ther Res 1977; 22:737–40.
43. Olson N, Nightingale CH, Quintiliani R: Penetration characteristic of cefamandole into right atrial appendage and pericardial fluid in patients undergoing open heart surgery. Ann Thoracic Surg 1980; 29:104–106.
44. Axelrod JL, Kochman R: Cefamandole levels in primary aqueous humor in man. Am J Opth 1978; 85:342–48.
45. Geddes AM, Schnurr LP, Ball AP, McGhie D, Brookes GR, Wise R, Andrews J: Cefoxitin: a hospital study. Br Med J 1977; 1:1126–28.
46. Steinberg EA, Overturf GD, Baraff LJ, Wilkins J: Penetration of cefamandole into spinal fluid. Antimicrob Agents Chemother 1977; 11:933–35.
47. Liu C, Hinthorn DR, Hoges GR, Harms JL, Conchonnal G, Dworzack DL: Penetration of cefoxitin into human cerebrospinal fluid: comparison with cefamandole, ampicillin and penicillin. Rev Inf Dis 1979; 1:127–31.
48. Walker SH, Gahol VP: Pharmacokinetics of cefamandole in infants and children. Antimicrob Agents Chemother 1978; 14:315–17.
49. Greene DS, Quintiliani R, Nightingale CH: Rate of binding of antibiotics to serum protein. J Pharm Sci 1977; 66:1663.
50. Sinagowitz E, Pelz K, Burgert A, Kaczkowski W: Concentrations of cefazolin in human skeletal muscle. Infection 1976; 4:192–195.
51. Nightingale CH, Klimek J, Quintiliani R: The effect of protein binding on the penetration of non-metabolized cephalosporins into atrial appendage and pericardial fluid in patients undergoing open heart surgery. Antimicrob Agents Chemother 1980; 17:595–597.
52. Cole DR, Pung J: Penetration of cefazolin into pleural fluid. Antimicrob Agents Chemother 1977; 11:1033–35.
53. Cunha BA, Quintiliani R, Nightingale CH: The penetration characteristics of cefazolin and cephradine into bone in patients undergoing knee replacements. Manuscript in preparation.
54. Yoshioka H, Cho K, Masatoshi T, Maruyama S, Shimizer T: Transfer of cefazolin into human milk. J Pediatrics 1979; 94:151–52.
55. Bassaris HR, Quintiliani R, Maderazo E, Nightingale CH: Pharmacokinetics and penetration characteristics of cefazolin in human spinal fluid. Curr Ther Res 1976; 19:110.
56. Nightingale CH, Bassaris H, Tilton R, Quintiliani R: Changes in the pharmacokinetics of cefazolin due to stress. J Pharm Sci 1975; 64:712.
57. Greene DS, Quintiliani R, Nightingale CH: Physiological perfusion model for cephalosporin antibiotics I. Model selection based on blood-drug concentrations. J Pharm Sci 1978; 67:191–194.
58. Spyker DA, Thomas BL, Sande MA, Bolton WK: Pharmacokinetics of cefaclor and cephalexin: dosage normograms for impaired renal function. Antimicrob Agents Chemother 1978; 14:172–77.
59. Santoro J, Agarwal BN, Martinelli R, Wenger N, Levinson ME: Pharmacology of cefaclor in normal volunteers and patients with renal failure. Antimicrob Agents Chemother 1978; 13:951–54.
60. Levison ME, Santoro J, Agarwal BN: *In vitro* activity and pharmacokinetics of cefaclor in normal volunteers and patients with renal failure. Postgrad Med J 1979; 55 (Supp 4):12–16.

61. Bloch R, Szwed JJ, Sloan RS, Luft FC: Pharmacokinetics of cefaclor in normal subjects and patients with chronic renal failure. Antimicrob Agents Chemother 1977; 12:730–32.

62. Berman SJ, Boughton WH, Sugihara JG, Wong EGC, Sato MM, Siemsen AW: Pharmacokinetics of cefaclor in patients with end stage renal disease and during hemodialysis. Antimicrob Agents Chemother 1978; 14:281–83.

63. Cutler RE, Blair AD, Kelly MR: Cefadroxil kinetics in patients with renal insufficiency. Clin Pharmacol Ther 1979; 25:514–21.

64. Nilsson-Ehle I, Nilsson-Ehle P: Pharmacokinetics of cephalothin: accumulation of its deacetylated metabolite in uremic patients. J Infect Dis 1979; 139:712–16.

65. Cabana BE, VanHarken DR, Hottendorf GH: Comparative pharmacokinetics and metabolism of cephapirin in laboratory animals and humans. Antimicrob Agents Chemother 1976; 10:307–17.

66. Czerwinski AW, Pederson JA: Pharmacokinetics of cefamandole in patients with renal impairment. Antimicrob Agents Chemother 1979; 15:161–64.

67. Fillastre JP, Leroy A, Godin M. Oksenhendler G. Humbert G: Pharmacokinetics of cefoxitin sodium in normal subjects and in uraemic patients. J Antimicrob Chemother 1978; 4(suppl B):79–83.

68. Craig WA, Welling PG, Jackson TC, Kunin CM: Pharmacology of cefazolin and other cephalosporins in patients with renal insufficiency. J Infect Dis 1973; 128 (suppl):S347–53.

69. Andriole VT: Pharmacokinetics of cephalosporins in patients with normal or reduced renal function. J Infect Dis 1978; 137:S88–99.

70. Brogard JM, Pignet M, Brandt C, Lavillaureix J: Pharmacokinetics of cefazolin in patients with renal failure, special reference to hemodialysis. J Clin Pharmacol 1977; 225–230.

71. Ahern MJ, Finkelstein FO, Andriole VT: Pharmacokinetics of cefamandole in patients undergoing hemodialysis and peritoneal dialysis. Antimicrob Agents Chemother 1976; 10:457–61.

72. Appel GB, Neu HC, Parry MF, Goldberger MJ, Jacov GB: Pharmacokinetics of cefamandole in the presence of renal failure and in patients undergoing hemodialysis. Antimicrob Agents Chemother 1976; 10:623–625.

73. Campillo JA, Lanao JM, Dominguez-Gil, Tabernero JM, Rubina F: Pharmacokinetics of cefamandole in patients undergoing hemodialysis. Int J Clin Pharm Biopharm 1979; 17:416–20.

74. Meyers BR, Hirschman SZ: Pharmacokinetics of cefamandole in patients with renal failure. Antimicrob Agents Chemother 1977; 11:248–50.

75. Garcia MJ, Dominguez-Gil, Tabernero JM, Bondia RA: Pharmacokinetics of cefoxitin in patients undergoing hemodialysis. J Clin Pharm Biopharm 1979; 17:366–70.

76. Brogard JM, Dorner M, Pinget M, Adloff M, Lavillaureix J: The biliary excretion of cefazolin. J Infect Dis 1975; 131:625–33.

77. Ram MD, Watanatillan S: Cephalothin levels in human bile. Arch Surg 1974; 108:187–89.

78. Ram MD, Watanatillan S: Biliary excretion and concentration of cefazolin. Arch Surg 1974; 108:540–45.

79. Ratzan KR, Ruiz C, Irvin III GL: Biliary tract excretion of cefazolin, cephalothin and cephaloridine in the presence of biliary tract disease. Antimicrob Agents Chemother 1974; 6:426–31.

80. Ratzan KR, Baker HB, Lauredo I: Excretion of cefamandole, cefazolin and cephalothin into T-tube bile. Antimicrob Agents Chemother 1978; 13:985–87.

81. Quinn EL, Madhaven T, Wixon R, et al: Cefamandole: observations on its spectrum, concentration in bone and bile, excretion in renal failure and clinical efficiency. Current Chemotherapy 1978; 2:803–04.
82. Bergan T: Comparative pharmacokinetics of cefazolin, cephalothin, cephacetril and cephapirine after intravenous administration. Chemotherapy 1977; 23:389–404.
83. Schrogie JJ, Davies RO, Yeh KC, Rogers D, Holmes GI, Skeggs H, Martin CM: Bioavailability and pharmacokinetics of cefoxitin sodium. J Antimicrob Chemother 1978; 4(suppl B):69–78.
84. Griffith RS, Black HR, Brier GL, Wolny JD: Effect of probenecid on the blood levels and urinary excretion of cefamandole. Antimicrob Agents Chemother 1977; 11:809–12.
85. Chow M, Quintiliani R, Cunha BA, Thompson M, Finkelstein E, Nightingale CH: Pharmacokinetics of high dose cephalosporins. J Clin Pharmacol 1979; 19:185–94.
86. Tetzloff TR, McCracken GH, Nelson JD: Oral antibiotic therapy for skeletal infections in children. J Pediatrics 1978; 91:485.
87. Fong IW, Engelking ER, Kirby WMM: Relative inactivation by *staphylococcus aureus* of eight cephalosporin antibiotics. Antimicrob Agents Chemother 1976; 9:939–44.
88. Sabath LD, Gardner C, Wilcox C, Finland M: Effect of inoculum on the antistaphylococcal activity of thirteen penicillins and cephalosporins. Antimicrob Agents Chemother 1975; 8:344–49.
89. Regamey C, Libke RD, Engelking ER, Clarke JT, Kirby WMM: Inactivation of cefazolin, cephaloridine and cephalothin by methicillin-sensitive and methicillin-resistant strains of *staphyloccoccus aureus*. J Infect Dis 1975; 131:291–94.
90. Pursiano TA, Misied M, Leitner F, Price KE: Effect of assay medium on the antibacterial activity of certain penicillins and cephalosporins. Antimicrob Agents Chemother 1973; 3:33–39.
91. Peterson LR, Gerding DN, Hall WH, Schierl EA: Medium-dependent variation in bactericidal activity of antibiotics against susceptible *staphylococcus aureus*. Antimicrob Agents Chemother 1978; 13:665–68.
92. Bryant RE, Alford RH: Unsuccessful treatment of staphylococcal endocarditis with cefazolin. J Am Med Asso 1977; 237:569–70.
93. Quinn EL, Pohold D, Madhaven T, Burch K, Fisher E, Cox F: Clinical experience with cefazolin and other cephalosporins in bacterial endocarditis. J Infect Dis 1973; 128(suppl):S386–89.
94. Carrizosa J, Santoro J, Kaye D: Treatment of experimental *staphylococcus aureus* endocarditis: comparison of cephalothin, cefazolin and methicillin. Antimicrob Agents Chemother 1978; 13:74–77.
95. Bloch R, Luft FC, Rankin LJ, Sloan RS, Yum M, Maxwell DR: Protection from gentamicin nephrotoxicity by cephalothin and carbenicillin. Antimicrob Agents Chemother 1979; 15:46–49.
96. EORTC International Antimicrobial Therapy Project Group: Three antibiotic regimens in the treatment of infection in febrile granulocytopenic patients with cancer. J Infect Dis 1978; 137:14–29.
97. Klastersky J, Debusscher L, Ruhl-Weerts D, Prevost JM: Carbenicillin, cefazolin and amikacin as an empiric therapy for febrile granulocytopenic patients. Cancer Treat Reports 1977; 61:1433–39.
98. Lau WK, Young LS, Black RE, Winston DJ, Linne SR, Weinstein RJ, Hewitt WL: Comparative efficacy and toxicity of amikacin/carbenicillin versus gentamicin/carbenicillin in leukopenic patients. Am J Med 1977; 62:959–1006.

99. Lowry OH, Hastings AB: Histochemical changes associated with aging 1. method and calculations. J Biol Chem 1942; 143:257–69.
100. Greene DS, Flanagan DR, Quintiliani R, Nightingale CH: Pharmacokinetics of cephalexin and evaluation of one and two compartment model pharmacokinetics. J Clin Pharmacol 1976; 16:257–64.
101. Hodges GR, Chien L, Hinthorn DR, Harris JL, Dworzack DL: Pharmacological evaluation of cefaclor in volunteers. Antimicrob Agents Chemother 1978; 14:454–56.
102. Lane AZ, Chudzik GM, Siskin SB: Comparative pharmacokinetic studies of cephapirin and cephalothin following intravenous and intramuscular administration. Curr Ther Res 1977; 21:117–27.
103. Brogard JM, Kopferschmitt, Spach MO, Grudet O, Lavillaureix J: Cefamandole pharmacokinetics and dosage adjustments in relation to renal function. J Clin Pharm 1979; 19:366–77.
104. Aziz NS, Gambertoglio JG, Lin ET, Grausz H, Benet LZ: Pharmacokinetics of cefamandole using a HPLC assay. J Pharm Biopharm 1978; 6:153–64.
105. Polk RE, Archer GL, Lower R: Cefamandole kinetics during cardiopulmonary bypass. Clin Pharmacol Ther 1978; 23:473–80.
106. Griffith RS, Black HR, Brier GL, Wolny JD: Cefamandole: *in vitro* and clinical pharmacokinetics. Antimicrob Agents Chemother 1976; 10:814–23.
107. Anderson KE: On the pharmacokinetics of cephalosporins antibiotics. Scand J Inf Dis 1978; 13(Suppl):37–46.
108. Sonneville PF, Albert KS, Skeggs H, Genter H, Kwan KC, Martin CM: Effect of lidocaine on the absorption, disposition and tolerance of intramuscularly administered cefoxitin. Europ J Clin Pharm 1977; 12:273–79.
109. Neu HC: Comparison of the pharmacokinetics of cefamandole and other cephalosporins compounds. J Inf Dis 1978; 137(Suppl):S80–87.
110. Bergan T, Digranes A, Schreiner A: Absorption, distribution and elimination of cefazolin in patients with normal renal function. Chemotherapy 1978; 24:277–82.

# 9

# Phenytoin

Thomas N. Tozer, Ph.D.
Michael E. Winter, Pharm.D.

## INTRODUCTION/BACKGROUND

Phenytoin (Dilantin®, formerly diphenylhydantoin, chemical name—5,5-diphenyl-2,4-imidazolidinedione) is a drug whose plasma concentration is frequently monitored, yet the concentration of phenytoin is unquestionably the most difficult to interpret pharmacokinetically. Although these statements appear to be contradictory, they have a common basis in the lack of predictability of the amount in the body or concentration-time profile of phenytoin when a patient receives a known dosage regimen.

Table 1 shows how phenytoin concentration varies among patients treated chronically with the same dose, 300 mg per day. Because concentrations associated with optimal therapy are usually between 10 and 20 µg/ml, it is apparent that there is a high incidence of concentrations for which subtherapeutic responses are probable and, at the same time, there is about a 16% incidence of concentrations at which toxic responses are probable.

The poor correlation between plasma concentration and the rate of phenytoin administration in chronic therapy is further demonstrated by the data in Figure 1. Clearly, there is no dosage at which the incidence of both subtherapeutic concentrations and potentially toxic concentrations is not high. These interindividual differences are explained in large part by capacity-limited metabolism. This mechanism also explains why the dosage adjustment required to achieve a therapeutic concentration in an individual patient is often quite small, that is, small relative to the required change in concentration. Needless to say, this mechanism makes evaluation and interpretation of phenytoin concentrations difficult.

This chapter explores the clinical pharmacokinetics of phenytoin. Particular emphasis is given to the mechanism and consequences of

TABLE 1.  DISTRIBUTION OF PHENYTOIN CONCENTRATIONS
IN PLASMA AMONG 100 AMBULANT PATIENTS
CHRONICALLY TREATED WITH 300 MG OF PHENYTOIN DAILY[a]

| Plasma Phenytoin Concentration (µg/ml) | Percent of Patients |
|---|---|
| 0–5 | 27 |
| 5–10 | 30 |
| 10–20 | 29 |
| 20–30 | 10 |
| >30 | 6 |

[a]Data abstracted from Figure 2 of reference 1.

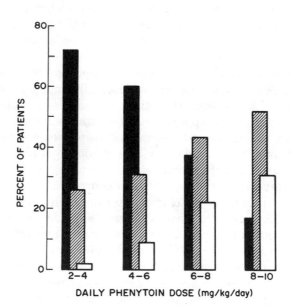

DAILY PHENYTOIN DOSE (mg/kg/day)

FIGURE 1.  The percent of patients with plasma phenytoin concentrations either below (dark bars) or above (light bars) the usual therapeutic concentration range of 10 to 20 µg/ml is large compared to the percent within the range (shaded bars), regardless of the daily phenytoin dose normalized to body weight. Data from Figure 1 of reference 2.

276

TABLE 2.   PHENYTOIN DOSAGE FORMS

| | Oral | | | Parenteral |
|---|---|---|---|---|
| | **Tablets** | **Capsules** | **Suspension** | **Solution** |
| Phenytoin Acid | 50 mg[a] | | 30 mg/5 ml[a] 125 mg/5 ml | |
| Phenytoin Sodium[b] (92% Phenytoin) | | 30 mg 100 mg | | 50 mg/ml |

[a] Pediatric dosage forms.
[b] The content is given in mg of phenytoin sodium.

capacity-limited metabolism and to the considerations needed for monitoring of plasma phenytoin concentrations.

Phenytoin is administered both orally and parenterally for management of epilepsy, and occasionally for treatment of cardiac arrhythmias, especially those associated with digitalis toxicity. Complications may be encountered in its administration because of problems with its absorption as well as its disposition.

## Absorption

The oral and parenteral routes of administration each has its own set of problems that primarily relate to the low solubility of phenytoin acid, 14 mg/liter at room temperature (2), and the relatively high pKa, 8.3.

**Oral Administration.** Three dosage forms are available for oral administration as listed in Table 2. Capsules of the sodium salt are by far the most commonly used. The tablet, containing phenytoin acid, is "chewable" and thus is a convenient pediatric dosage form. Phenytoin suspensions of the acid, available in two concentrations, have limited utility for two reasons. First, unless well-shaken before each dose the drug precipitates in the bottle giving rise to a lower than expected dose initially and the converse as the container is emptied. Second, the usual methods for measurement of liquids, especially with teaspoons, are inexact. Because small changes in the dosage can produce large changes in the concentration observed, the dosage must be carefully controlled. In addition, because two strengths of suspensions are available, there is a potential for error. The most dangerous is the mistaken administration to children of the 125 mg/5 ml preparation in place of the pediatric suspension containing 30 mg/5 ml.

The bioavailability of phenytoin has been reviewed (4). Several studies have shown bioavailability differences with products in general use. The salt is readily soluble in water, but in the acidic medium of the stomach it precipitates subsequent to its dissolution from a solid dosage form. The size of the acid crystals, aggregates, or particles entering the intestine is probably the most critical factor in determining the rate and extent of absorption. Thus, whether the acid or the sodium salt is administered, the absorption of the drug depends upon the product formulation.

The bioavailability of phenytoin is difficult to determine by conventional methods because of concentration dependence in the clearance of the drug. The area under the plasma concentration-time curve is less after oral than after intravenous administration (5). However, after correcting for the nonlinear elimination, Jusko et al (6) have shown that with quality products the bioavailability is essentially unity. Nonetheless, changes in dosage form or manufacturer should be avoided once a patient's dosage requirements are established, as a relatively small decrease or increase in bioavailability can greatly alter the plateau plasma concentration during chronic administration.

The rate of absorption varies considerably among dosage forms. The time at which the concentration peaks is 3 to 12 hours after a single oral dose of a capsule or tablet (3,5). However, for some preparations and in some individuals the time to peak may be even more than 12 hours. This slow absorption and the relatively slow elimination of the drug have led to the recommendation of once daily administration. The Food and Drug Administration, however, has cautioned against the use of any brand other than Dilantin® Kapseals® for once-a-day use (7), because many generic preparations are more rapidly absorbed and may produce an intolerable fluctuation in the plasma phenytoin concentration.

Although not thoroughly studied, the availability of phenytoin may be reduced in gastrointestinal diseases, particularly those associated with increased intestinal motility. The relatively slow absorption of drug suggests this possibility. Thus, in cases of severe diarrhea, malabsorption syndrome, or gastric resection, decreased availability should be considered even with products known to be well absorbed.

**Parenteral Administration.** Phenytoin sodium is given both intravenously and intramuscularly to patients who can not receive the drug orally or who require a rapid onset of drug effects. But both of these routes of administration have limitations.

The major disadvantage of the intravenous route is the requirement for slow administration of the 40% propylene glycol and 10% alcohol diluent which is adjusted to pH 12 with sodium hydroxide. This vehicle is required to maintain the phenytoin in solution at a concentration of 50 mg of the sodium salt per milliliter. Cardiovascular collapse and central nervous system depression are the major toxicities observed on intravenous administration. These reactions may be primarily due to the propylene glycol. To reduce or avoid these problems the rate of administration should never exceed 50 mg/min.

Because of the inconvenience of administering the drug slowly, there is often a desire to give phenytoin with other intravenous fluids. This is not recommended due to a lack of solubility with resultant precipitation of phenytoin acid (8). If phenytoin piggybacks are to be used, they should be carefully monitored for crystal growth and the infusion should be started immediately after making the admixture. Only normal saline or Lactated Ringers Solution should be used. The acid content of dextrose solutions has been a particular problem. Admixtures with all other drugs should be avoided to prevent pH-induced precipitation.

The intramuscular route of administration should be avoided because of precipitation of phenytoin at the site of injection. The tissue buffers the injection solution and the propylene glycol-alcohol solvent is absorbed from the injection site, resulting in the deposition of phenytoin crystals. Consequently, absorption from this site tends to be erratic and slow, often continuing for five days or more (9). Figure 2 shows the prolongation of the plasma phenytoin concentration on intramuscular administration compared to that observed following intravenous and oral administration.

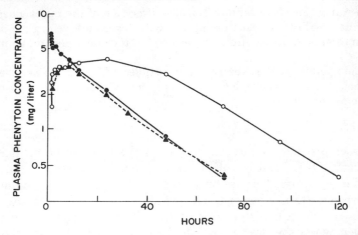

FIGURE 2.  The time course of the phenytoin concentration is quite different after intramuscular administration (500 mg, 0——0) compared to that after either intravenous (250 mg, ●——●) or oral (300 mg, ▲——▲) administration. The points shown are the averages of 12 subjects (IM and IV) and 6 (oral) subjects. Intramuscular and intravenous data from reference 9; oral data from reference 5.

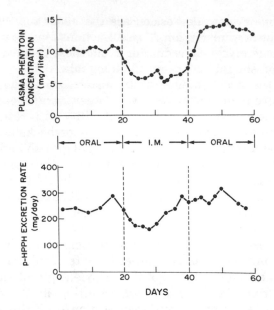

FIGURE 3.   *Top panel*: The plasma phenytoin concentration drops on changing from oral to intramuscular route of administration. On reverting to oral administration, the concentration rises and exceeds that previously observed with this route. Prolonged absorption from the intramuscular site produces this observation.
*Bottom panel*: The changes in the urinary excretion of the major phenytoin metabolite, p-HPPH, are small compared with those observed in the plasma concentration on changing from the oral to the intramuscular route and the converse.

The data points are the average of seven subjects. The dosage was the same throughout the time shown, but individually varied from 3.95 to 6.45 mg/kg. Data from reference 10.

A major problem is encountered when the route of administration is converted from oral to intramuscular, or the converse, as demonstrated in Figure 3. Because only 50 to 75% of an intramuscular dose is absorbed within 24 hours, the conversion from oral to intramuscular administration results in a drop in the plasma phenytoin concentration even when the dose is not changed. It has been suggested (10) that the intramuscular dose be increased over the oral dose by 50% for one week. On converting from intramuscular to oral administration, a reduction in the oral dose to one-third the intramuscular dose (one-half the original oral dose) for one week is also suggested. Because of interindividual and intersite variability in phenytoin absorption and varying periods of time on intramuscular administration, general rules for making dosage adjustment are difficult. Consequently, the intramuscular route should probably be totally avoided or, at the least, carefully monitored. In addition, this route of administration is painful and can cause muscle damage (11).

## Distribution

The rate and extent of phenytoin distribution are of therapeutic importance for entirely different reasons.

**Time for Tissue Equilibration.** Following an intravenous dose, phenytoin rapidly distributes to the tissues with distribution equilibrium being achieved in 30 to 60 minutes (9,12,14). The initially elevated concentration and the rapid distribution can be seen in Figure 2. The time required for attainment of distribution equilibrium partially explains why phenytoin should not be administered as a bolus dose, but rather infused at a rate not exceeding 50 mg/min. Thus, a loading dose of 500 to 1000 mg for a rapid antiarrhythmic or anticonvulsant response should not be administered over less than 10 to 20 minutes and is probably more safely administered over at least 30 to 60 minutes. Bigger et al (14) have suggested that in the treatment of cardiac arrhythmias 100 mg (50 mg/min) can be administered every 5 minutes until the arrhythmia is controlled. The total dose should probably not exceed 1000 mg (14 mg/kg).

The drug rapidly distributes to the brain (15,16) and the concentration in the brain is comparable to or slightly higher than that in plasma within 10 minutes after about a 10-minute infusion of a loading dose (16). The rapid distribution phase in plasma is not observed in either brain tissue or cerebrospinal fluid suggesting that the central nervous system effects initially observed, when a dose of phenytoin is given too rapidly by the intravenous route, may be associated with the propylene glycol vehicle and not the drug itself.

**Volume of Distribution.** Once distribution equilibrium is achieved, the drug appears to be diluted into a space comparable to the total body water, 0.6 to 0.7 liters/kg. This value is deceptive, however, in that the drug is highly bound to plasma proteins and to tissue components (The fraction unbound in plasma is usually about 0.1). The concentration in the brain is comparable to that in plasma and the concentration in the cerebrospinal fluid is the same as that in plasma water, suggesting that about 90% of the drug in brain is bound to tissue components.

Except for situations of rapid intravenous infusion, the distribution of phenytoin can be considered to be unicompartmental. This is particularly the case for oral and intramuscular administration.

Being bound primarily to albumin in plasma, a change in the albumin concentration alters the apparent volume of distribution. Based on the principles of protein binding and the assumption that tissue binding is unaltered, the volume of distribution, V, can be roughly estimated (authors) from serum albumin as follows:

$$V \text{ (liters/kg)} = 2.8/\text{Serum Albumin (gm/dl)} \qquad \text{(Eq. 1)}$$

This relationship applies to situations in which only the albumin concentration is altered.

Plasma protein binding is altered in renal failure. The fraction unbound is increased two- to threefold in uremia (17–22). Part of this change, on average, is accounted for by a decrease in serum albumin, but the majority of the decreased binding is caused by another, as yet unsubstantiated, effect. An altered albumin molecule or a decreased apparent affinity for albumin due to the accumulation of a substance which displaces the drug has been suggested (20–22).

Tissue binding does not appear to be affected by renal failure (18). The apparent volume of distribution is changed essentially in proportion to the change in plasma protein binding.

$$V \text{ (liters/kg)} = \frac{\alpha'}{\alpha} \cdot 0.65 \qquad \text{(Eq. 2)}$$

where $\alpha'$ is the fraction unbound in renal failure and $\alpha$ is the value of the fraction unbound in normal renal function (0.1). The value of V in renal failure is then, on average, about 1 to 2 liters/kg. The volume is, of course, also dependent on the serum albumin concentration.

A decrease in the plasma protein binding and hence an increase in the volume of distribution also occurs in chronic hepatic disease (23, 24). The change here is primarily a result of a reduction in serum albumin, although an increased concentration of bilirubin with associated displacement may also contribute. Estimates of the volume of distribution can therefore be approximated using Equation 1, except perhaps in jaundiced patients.

**Unbound Concentration.** The unbound concentration is undoubtedly a better correlate of phenytoin's efficacy and toxicity and should therefore be a better guide to therapy than the total plasma concentration. However, the current methods available for separating the unbound drug are too costly, time consuming, and irreproducible for routine clinical use.

One alternative method suggested is the measurement of the drug in saliva (25–27). The concentration here is about equal to that unbound in plasma. There is, however, considerable variability in the ratio of concentrations, saliva/unbound in plasma. Some of this variability is due to error in the measurement of plasma protein binding; the actual error is unknown. Experience is presently inadequate to advocate the routine use of saliva concentration measurements.

## Metabolism

Elimination of phenytoin occurs primarily by biotransformation to several inactive hydroxylated metabolites (28–29). Figure 4 shows the structures of phenytoin and several of its reported metabolites. Some of these metabolites, notably 5-(p-hydroxyphenyl)-5-phenylhydantoin (p-HPPH), are further metabolized by conjugation with glucuronic acid. The urinary recovery of p-HPPH and its glucuronide accounts for 60 to 90% of an oral dose of phenytoin (5,10,13)

The rate of any enzymatically-mediated reaction is expected to have an upper limit as the concentration of the substrate is increased; the enzyme has a limited capacity. For most drugs, the rate of metabolism at the concentrations associated with therapy is well below this limit and the rate of metabolism is, therefore, directly proportional to the plasma concentration. This is not the case for phenytoin; at therapeutic concentrations the rate of metabolism is close to the limit. For this reason, the metabolism of phenytoin is said to be capacity-limited or to show saturability.

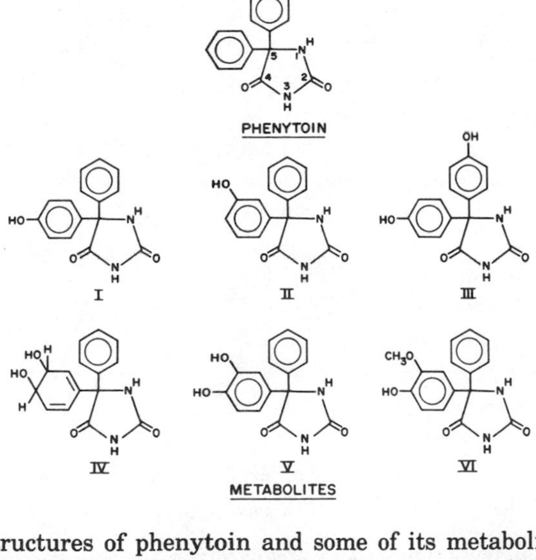

FIGURE 4. Structures of phenytoin and some of its metabolites: I, 5-(p-hydroxyphenyl)-5-phenylhydantoin: II, 5-(m-hydroxyphenyl)-5-phenylhydantoin; III, 5,5-bis-(p-hydroxyphenyl)-hydantoin; IV, 5-(3,4-dihydroxy-2,5-cyclohexadiene)-5-phenylhydantoin; V, 5-(3,4-dihydroxyphenyl)-5-phenylhydantoin; VI, 5-(3-methoxy-4-hydroxyphenyl)-5-phenylhydantoin.

Evidence for the capacity-limited metabolism of this drug is observed in many ways. For example, Figure 5 shows the semilogarithmic decline of plasma phenytoin concentration with time following the discontinuation of drug administration. The convex curvature indicates an increase in the fractional rate of elimination as the concentration decreases. This is consistent with capacity-limited metabolism, but other explanations are possible.

Perhaps the most compelling evidence of saturable metabolism is the disproportionate increase in the plasma phenytoin concentration at steady-state as the rate of administration is increased. Figure 6 shows this relationship for each of several patients. The consequence of this kind of elimination is apparent. For each individual the dosage required to achieve a steady-state concentration above 20 μg/ml is not much greater than that required for a concentration of 10 μg/ml.

Further evidence of capacity-limited metabolism is seen in Figure 3 in which only minor changes in the urinary excretion of p-HPPH (conjugated with glucuronic acid and unconjugated) occur in spite of large changes in the plasma phenytoin concentration. The rate of excretion of this major metabolite is limited by its rate of formation from phenytoin.

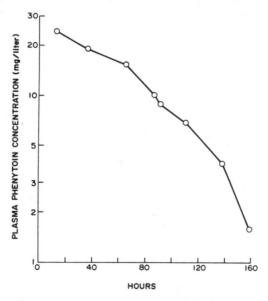

FIGURE 5. The plasma phenytoin concentration declines convexly on a semilogarithmic plot when a daily dose of 7.9 mg/kg is discontinued in an individual subject. This nonlinearity is evidence of dose-dependent kinetics. Data from reference 30.

To explain the kinetic behavior of phenytoin and to aid in predicting and evaluating dosage requirements and plasma concentrations, a model for phenytoin disposition is useful (Figure 7). In this model, metabolism is assumed to occur enzymatically to give an unstable intermediate, presumably an epoxide, which is further metabolized to other products. The only other route of phenytoin elimination is renal excretion. This pathway only contributes about 1 to 5% and is thus usually ignored.

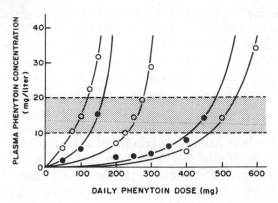

FIGURE 6. For each patient the plasma phenytoin concentration at steady state increases disproportionately with an increase in the rate of administration. In all patients the daily dose required to achieve a steady-state concentration of 20 mg/liter (μg/ml) is not much greater than that required to achieve a value of 10 mg/liter (μg/ml), the therapeutic concentration range. The five patients were selected in this study because their dosage needed to be changed several times to control their epileptic seizures. The lines are computer fits of the data using the model in Figure 7. Figure modified from that in reference 31.

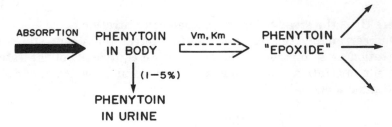

FIGURE 7. Pharmacokinetically, phenytoin elimination appears to be rate-limited by a single metabolic step, presumably to an epoxide intermediate, and characterized by the Michaelis-Menten enzyme kinetic parameters Km and Vm. Some elimination occurs by renal excretion, but its contribution is usually negligible.

**Characteristics of Capacity-limited Metabolism.** The rate-limiting enzymatic reaction is assumed to follow typical Michaelis-Menten kinetics in which the rate of the reaction ($v$) depends upon the substrate concentration, here the concentration in plasma, C, as follows:

$$v = \frac{Vm \cdot C}{Km + C}$$

(Eq. 3)

where Vm is the maximum rate of metabolism (metabolic capacity) with units of mg per day and Km, with units of μg/ml, is a constant equal to the plasma concentration at which the rate of metabolism is one-half the maximum. The values of these constants usually vary from 100 to 1000 mg/day for Vm and 1 to 15 μg/ml or more for Km (31–38). Our estimates of the average values in epileptic patients are about 500 mg/day or expressed relative to body weight, 7 mg/kg/day, and 4 μg/ml, respectively. The values are based upon the patients for whom an analysis of phenytoin kinetics was undertaken. Admittedly, this may have been a biased sample in that the kinetics were often pursued in patients with problems in controlling their therapy. Problem patients have a tendency toward lower values of Km and our bias may be in this direction.

The consequences of the capacity-limited metabolism of the drug are most readily observed under steady-state conditions, that is, when the drug is chronically administered at a fixed rate until the rate of elimination and the average rate of absorption are equal. Assuming conditions simulating an intravenous infusion, the rate in (R) must then be equal to the rate of elimination; thus,

$$R = \frac{Vm \cdot C_{ss}}{Km + C_{ss}}$$

(Eq. 4)

where $C_{ss}$ is the *steady-state* or *plateau* concentration.

On rearranging this relationship to express the steady-state concentration as a function of the rate in, the equivalent of the rate of oral administration when the availability is unity, the effect of capacity-limited metabolism is clear.

$$C_{ss} = \frac{Km \cdot R}{Vm - R}$$

(Eq. 5)

or

$$\frac{C_{ss}}{Km} = \frac{R}{Vm - R}$$

(Eq. 6)

As the rate of administration approaches the maximum rate of metabolism, the steady-state concentration increases disproportionately and approaches infinity. Values of R greater than Vm are not applicable because steady-state can not occur under these conditions. This relationship also shows that when the steady-state concentration is comparable to or greater than the value of Km, the value of R approaches Vm. For phenytoin, therapeutic concentrations almost always exceed the value of Km, thus capacity-limited metabolism is evident.

Equation 4 can be rearranged to give:

$$R = Vm - Km \cdot \frac{R}{C_{ss}}$$ 

(Eq. 7)

This is one of three ways to derive a linear relationship from the Michaelis-Menten equation. The value of $R/C_{ss}$ is conventionally called clearance as it is the parameter that relates the rate of elimination to the plasma concentration. A plot of R versus $R/C_{ss}$ (clearance) gives a straight line with a y-intercept of Vm and a slope of $-Km$. It is one of the more useful methods of treating steady-state concentrations obtained with two or more rates of administration as subsequently discussed and shown in Figure 14.

Expressing the last relationship as

$$VM = R + Km \ \frac{R}{C_{ss}}$$

(Eq. 8)

and treating Vm and Km as variables, it is apparent that a continuous set of Vm and Km values are consistent with a given steady-state concentration observed on administering the drug at rate R. On plotting Vm versus Km, the y-intercept is R and the x-intercept is $-C_{ss}$. This relationship is the basis of the subsequently described methods B, D, and E for estimating the values of the pharmacokinetic parameters, Vm and Km.

**Time to Plateau.** Because of phenytoin's nonlinear elimination, the time to reach a steady-state concentration varies with the rate of administration and depends upon the values of Vm and Km (39,40). To show this dependence, assume a constant rate of infusion of phenytoin, in which case the net rate of change of phenytoin in the body, $V \cdot dC/dt$, is the difference between the rates in and out, thus

$$V \cdot dC/dt = R - \frac{Vm \cdot C}{Km + C}$$

(Eq. 9)

which, on integrating and assuming C to be zero at time zero, is equal to

$$\frac{Km \cdot Vm}{(Vm - R)} \ \ln \left[ \frac{R \cdot Km}{R \cdot Km - (Vm - R)C} \right] - C = \frac{(Vm - R)}{V} \ t$$

(Eq. 10)

By appropriate substitution, the time required to achieve 90% of the steady-state value, $C = 0.9$ Km $\cdot$ R (Vm $-$ R), can be obtained and is equal to

$$t_{90\%} = \frac{Km \cdot V}{(Vm - R)^2} \cdot (2.303 \, Vm - 0.9 \, R) \qquad \text{(Eq. 11)}$$

The value of $t_{90\%}$ increases dramatically as the value of R approaches Vm. If they are equal, steady state is never achieved.

Using values of 4 µg/ml, 50 liters, and 500 mg/day for Km, V, and Vm, respectively, the approach to plateau is shown in Figure 8. The higher the rate of administration the longer it takes to approach steady state and, as expected, the steady-state concentration is increased disproportionately. Note that for steady-state concentrations of 10 and 20 µg/ml, the values of $t_{90\%}$ are about 8 and 21 days for the parameter values given.

The time to accumulate to a given plateau concentration varies with the values of Km and Vm. Table 3 lists the times to achieve 90% of a plateau of 16 µg/ml. The smaller the value of Km the longer it takes to reach plateau. Indeed, for patients with a small value of Km (2 µg/ml or less), several weeks of accumulation are required to achieve steady-state and the rate of administration required to maintain a concentration within the therapeutic range is close to the maximum rate of metabolism.

**Decline of Concentration on Discontinuing Drug.** The rate of decline of the phenytoin concentration is of importance when toxic effects (and levels) are observed. In this situation, discontinuance of drug administration is desirable to achieve the usual therapeutic concentrations most rapidly. The decline with time may be calculated from the relationship

$$Km \cdot \ln \left( \frac{C_1}{C_2} \right) + C_1 - C_2 = \frac{Vm}{V} \cdot t \qquad \text{(Eq. 12)}$$

Figure 9 shows the decline in the plasma phenytoin concentration when the drug is discontinued and the initial concentration is 50 µg/ml. At concentrations above 12 µg/ml the rate of metabolism is greater than 75% of the metabolic capacity, Vm (Equation 4), for this patient. The decline of the plasma concentration (solid line) is therefore approximately equal to Vm/V (dashed line). This measurement of the rate of decline is a reasonable method of estimating the value of Vm/V. The value can be more closely obtained from

$$\frac{Vm}{V} = \frac{C_1 - C_2 + Km \cdot \ln (C_1/C_2)}{t} \qquad \text{(Eq. 13)}$$

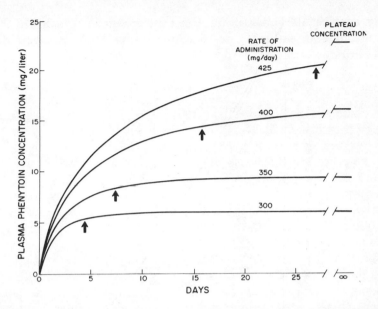

FIGURE 8. On administering the drug at a constant rate of 300, 350, 400, and 425 mg/day, the plasma concentration approaches steady-state values of 6, 9.3, 16, and 22.7 mg/liter (μg/ml), respectively. Not only are the steady-state concentrations disproportionately increased, but so is the time to approach the plateau. The arrows indicate the time required to reach 90% of the plateau value. An intravenous infusion is simulated in a patient with the following parameter values: Km, 4 mg/liter (μg/ml); Vm, 500 mg/day; V, 50 liters.

TABLE 3. TIME TO ACCUMULATE TO 90%
OF A PLATEAU CONCENTRATION OF 16 MG/ML
AS A FUNCTION OF THE VM AND KM VALUES[a]

| Situation | Km (μg/ml) | Vm (mg/day) | $t_{90\%}$ (days) |
|---|---|---|---|
| 1 | 1 | 425 | 50 |
| 2 | 2 | 450 | 27 |
| 3 | 4 | 500 | 16 |
| 4 | 8 | 600 | 10 |
| 5 | 12 | 700 | 8 |

[a]Calculated from Equations 8 and 11, using a daily dose of 400 mg and a value of 50 liters for V.

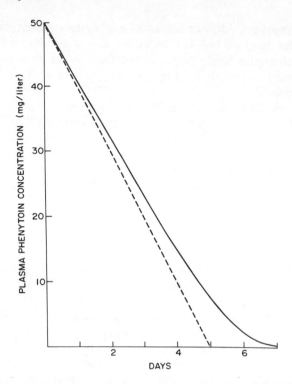

FIGURE 9. The decline of the plasma phenytoin concentration (solid line) following the discontinuance of the drug, when a concentration of 50 mg/liter (μg/ml) is present, appears to be almost linear and to approach the rate expected if the drug is continually eliminated at the maximum rate, Vm, of metabolism (stippled line). The parameter values in Figure 8 are used in the simulation.

by assuming a value of Km. Values for Km can only be calculated accurately (Equation 12) if several levels are measured, including one or more below the value of Km. This is an unlikely situation in the usual course of therapeutic monitoring.

When a high concentration is observed, knowledge of the time required to lower the level to 20 μg/ml is desirable to know how long to withhold the drug. The primary information needed is an estimate of Vm/V. Although it may seem appropriate to use the average value of 500 mg/day/50 liters, a more cautious approach is to reason why the level is high. If the level is high because the patient's metabolic capacity, Vm, is less than the rate of administration then a decreased estimate of Vm/V is in order. For an overdose of the drug, the average may be appropriate. Measurement of a plasma concentration one to two days later may be helpful; however, the possibility of absorption continuing after the first sample is obtained must be considered. We have observed reasonably stable concentrations for several days following overdoses.

**Effect of an Altered Bioavailability.** Because of capacity-limited metabolism of phenytoin, a small change in the bioavailability can produce a dramatic change in the steady-state concentration. To illustrate this point, consider a patient who has a steady-state concentration of 10 μg/ml on a daily dose of 400 mg and whose Km and Vm values are 4 μg/ml and 500 mg/day, respectively. On changing from a dosage form with a bioavailability of 0.9 to one with a value of 1.0, the steady-state concentration increases (Equation 5) from 10 to 16 μg/ml, a 60% increase in the concentration with only an 11% increase in the extent of absorption.

**Clearance and Half-life.** Clearance is the parameter that relates rate of elimination to the plasma concentration. From Equation 3, it can be seen that the clearance, Cl, of phenytoin is a function of the plasma concentration, that is,

$$Cl = \frac{Vm}{Km + C} \qquad \text{(Eq. 14)}$$

Because clearance depends on the concentration, it is of limited utility and probably should never be used. Furthermore, the measurement of bioavailability using the area under the curve is also inappropriate because clearance is not constant.

Half-life also is a parameter that has little utility for phenytoin. As the half-life depends upon how readily a drug is removed from plasma (Cl) and on how it is distributed (V), that is

$$t_{1/2} = 0.693 \ V/Cl \qquad \text{(Eq. 15)}$$

it follows from Equation 14 that,

$$t_{1/2} = 0.693 \ \frac{V}{Vm} \ (Km + C) \qquad \text{(Eq. 16)}$$

The half-life, $t_{1/2}$, is a function of the plasma concentration. It is not the time required to eliminate one-half of the drug in the body, but is rather an "instantaneous" value for the time required to eliminate half, if the fractional rate of elimination were to continue at the rate observed at a given concentration. Both clearance and half-life values should not be used for phenytoin. The most useful parameters are Vm, Km and V.

## Renal Excretion

Only 1 to 5% of a dose is recovered unchanged in the urine (41,42) when renal function is normal. The percent is higher at high concentrations than at low concentrations as a consequence of capacity-limited metabolism. The recovery is also greater at high urine flow rates because the renal clearance is urine flow dependent (42). In most clinical situations, however, the renal excretion of phenytoin is minor and can be neglected.

The major phenytoin metabolite, p-HPPH glucuronide, is actively secreted (42) into the renal tubule. Because its elimination is rate-limited by its formation from phenytoin, the rate of excretion of the metabolite is an index of the rate of metabolism of phenytoin. As this metabolite accounts for 60 to 90% of the total elimination of phenytoin, it can be used to assess compliance and bioavailability. For example, when a low phenytoin concentration is observed, measurement of the 24-hour p-HPPH excretion allows one to conclude whether the drug is being absorbed or not (43). If the excretion is low (less than 50% of dose) and bioavailability is not believed to be reduced, then compliance is a likely explanation. A high urinary output of the metabolite in spite of a low phenytoin concentration confirms rapid metabolism.

Because p-HPPH-glucuronide is renally eliminated, it accumulates in patients with compromised renal function. This accumulation appears to be unimportant since the metabolite is inactive. Except for patients with severe renal failure, the recovery of the metabolite can be used to test for drug input, regardless of renal function, as the compound is only eliminated by renal excretion.

## Hemodialysis

Only 2 to 4% of the phenytoin initially in the body is removed during an 8-hour period of hemodialysis by conventional methods (44). Administration of the drug therefore does not have to be altered because a patient undergoes intermittent (every two to three days) hemodialysis. Because of a low serum albumin concentration and renal failure, plasma protein binding is decreased. This requires an adjustment of the "therapeutic" concentration range, but has little effect on the dosage requirements of these patients.

## CONCENTRATION versus RESPONSE and TOXICITY

### Therapeutic Response

The usually accepted therapeutic range for plasma phenytoin concentrations is 10 to 20 µg/ml. These concentrations are usually effective in controlling both seizure disorders and cardiac arrhythmias (2,14,15,45,46). In the treatment of seizure disorders the response to phenytoin is graded, with 50% of the patients showing a decreased frequency at concentrations greater than 10 µg/ml and with 86% of the patients at concentrations greater than 15 µg/ml (47). Occasionally, there are patients who are seizure-free with concentrations below 10 µg/ml (48), indicating the need for clinical evaluation of the patient in addition to monitoring of the plasma concentration.

When phenytoin is used as an antiarrhythmic agent, 90% of the patients who are successfully treated have plasma concentrations below 18 µg/ml, with the majority having concentrations between 10 and 18 µg/ml (14). Serious consideration should be given to adding or changing to another antiarrhythmic or anticonvulsant agent, if a satisfactory therapeutic response is not achieved with a phenytoin concentration of 20 µg/ml.

### Toxicity

Phenytoin side effects such as hypertrichosis, gingival hypertrophy, carbohydrate intolerance, folic acid deficiency, peripheral neuropathy, Vitamin D deficiency, and systemic lupus erythematosus, do not appear to be readily related to the plasma phenytoin concentration. Central nervous system side effects, such as nystagmus, ataxia, and decreased mentation have been associated with elevated phenytoin concentrations, with the more severe symptoms occurring at higher concentrations. Far-lateral nystagmus occurs in the majority of patients with concentrations exceeding 20 µg/ml and nystagmus at a 45-degree lateral gaze as well as ataxia usually occur with concentrations exceeding 30 µg/ml. Significantly diminished mental capacity is usually apparent when phenytoin concentrations are above 40 µg/ml (49) as shown in Figure 10.

Elderly patients appear to have greater mental changes than do younger patients at the same concentration (49). Decreased plasma protein binding with age may explain some or all of this observation.

Nystagmus is usually accepted as the first sign of elevated phenytoin concentration, as it is probably the most frequent objective symptom that can be documented. Nystagmus, however, does not always

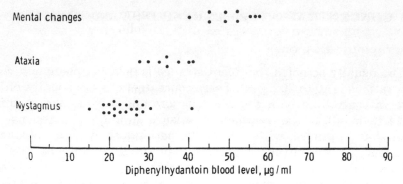

FIGURE 10. The onset of central nervous system side-effects in relation to phenytoin concentration is shown above. Far-lateral nystagmus is most frequently observed with a concentration of 20 μg/ml; however, this symptom is first observed occasionally at much lower or higher concentrations. Ataxia and gross mental changes are usually evident at concentrations of greater than 30 and 40 μg/ml, respectively. From reference 49.

occur first, and phenytoin toxicity should be considered in patients with unusual involuntary muscular movements, mental symptoms, or ataxia, even if nystagmus is not present (48–50).

Seizure activity and the induction of involuntary movements have also been described, when measured toxic phenytoin concentrations have been reported (51–53).

In addition to those side effects associated with phenytoin, additional precautions must be observed when the drug is given intravenously as the propylene glycol diluent is potentially a cardiac depressant (54). Symptoms associated with rapid intravenous injections of phenytoin include bradycardia, hypotension, and widening of the QRS and QT intervals on an electrocardiogram. These symptoms can be diminished or avoided by injecting the drug slowly as previously discussed.

## Target Phenytoin Concentrations

The usually accepted therapeutic or "target" concentration of 10 to 20 μg/ml assumes normal plasma protein binding. The unbound concentration, about 10% of the measured value, is probably more closely related to the drug effects than the total, because only the unbound drug can cross cell membranes to reach the sites of action and biotransformation.

The therapeutic unbound phenytoin concentration is approximately 1 to 2 µg/ml and can be calculated with the following formula:

$$C_u = \alpha \cdot C \qquad \text{(Eq. 17)}$$

where C is the total drug concentration, $C_u$ is the unbound concentration and $\alpha$ is the fraction of the total in plasma that is unbound.

In conditions of altered plasma protein binding, the therapeutic range or measured phenytoin concentration must be adjusted. Anticipation of altered binding, therefore, is critical in evaluating a phenytoin concentration.

## Adjustment of Target Concentration

In almost all conditions in which plasma protein binding is altered, a decrease is observed. Typical causes of decreased binding are: hypoalbuminemia, renal failure, and displacement by other drugs.

In patients with hypoalbuminemia the fraction unbound is increased. The observed concentration can be adjusted by using the following equation (55).

$$C_{normal} = \frac{C_{observed}}{0.9 \times \left( \dfrac{\text{Albumin Concentration}}{4.4} \right) + 0.1} \qquad \text{(Eq. 18)}$$

where $C_{observed}$ is the measured phenytoin concentration, the patient's albumin concentration is in gm/dl, and $C_{normal}$ is the phenytoin concentration that would have been observed if the patient's albumin concentration had been normal (4.4 gm/dl). This equation assumes that the unbound fraction is 0.1 when the albumin is normal.

In patients with renal failure, it appears that the unbound fraction is increased approximately two- to threefold (18,19). When the fraction unbound is doubled in a uremic patient, the expected therapeutic effect of a measured phenytoin concentration would be that of an approximately doubled concentration. For comparison, one could either double the measured phenytoin concentration or reduce the usual therapeutic range by one-half so that the target or desired phenytoin concentration would be from 5 to 10 µg/ml. This adjustment procedure applies only to patients with severe renal failure as it is in this type of patient that the change in binding has been measured. Unfortunately, there is little information upon which to predict changes, if any, in plasma binding for a patient with only moderately diminished renal function.

For patients with a low serum albumin and renal failure, the following equation (adapted from reference 55) can be used to adjust the measured or observed phenytoin concentration:

$$C_{normal} = \frac{C_{observed}}{0.1 \times \text{Albumin Concentration (gm/dl)} + 0.1} \quad \text{(Eq. 19)}$$

where $C_{normal}$ is the phenytoin concentration one would expect to measure if protein binding were normal. It is the value which should be used when comparing the phenytoin concentration to the usual therapeutic range of 10 to 20 µg/ml. In addition, $C_{normal}$ should be employed whenever a phenytoin nomogram is used.

Many of the drugs which have been shown to displace phenytoin from its albumin binding sites are weak acids, including phenylbutazone (56), salicylic acid (19), and valproic acid (57). Displacement of phenytoin from albumin by such drugs in the clinical setting is difficult to predict, as knowledge of not only the binding affinity but also the displacing drug's concentration is required. Because both of these factors are seldom known, evaluation of phenytoin concentrations in the presence of a displacing drug requires an empiric approach in which target concentration adjustments are made when usual concentration-patient responses are encountered.

In an effort to obtain unbound plasma phenytoin concentration estimates, saliva and erythrocyte phenytoin concentrations have been suggested (26,58). Neither of these methods has been used extensively for routine patient care, possibly because of inconvenience in performing the erythrocyte drug concentration and the necessary calculations or, as in the case of saliva concentrations, the variability from patient to patient in the ratio of free drug to salivary drug concentration (26).

## CLINICAL APPLICATION OF PHARMACOKINETIC DATA

### Achieving a Therapeutic Concentration

When phenytoin therapy is initiated, it is necessary to decide if rapid achievement of therapeutic concentrations is necessary. If slow accumulation towards a therapeutic concentration is unsatisfactory, a loading dose can be calculated with the following equation:

$$\text{Loading Dose} = \frac{V \cdot (C_{desired} - C_{observed})}{F} \quad \text{(Eq. 20)}$$

where $C_{desired}$ is the phenytoin concentration desired, $C_{observed}$ is the phenytoin concentration prior to administering the loading dose, V is the apparent volume of distribution, and F is the bioavailability, which is assumed to be 1.0. If no phenytoin has been previously administered, $C_{observed}$ is assumed to be zero.

For patients, the values of $C_{desired}$ and V are assumed to be 20 µg/ml, and 0.65 liter/kg (13,20,54), respectively. The loading dose of phenytoin to achieve approximately 20 µg/ml is 910 mg or about 1000 mg for the average 70 kg patient.

If the dose is to be given by the intravenous route, it should be administered slowly to avoid the cardiac toxicities associated with the propylene glycol diluent (14,54). If the loading dose is to be given orally it has been suggested that the dose be divided and administered at two-hour intervals to avoid the gastrointestinal distress associated with large doses of phenytoin (59). Following administration of an oral loading dose, the peak level does not occur for several hours and it is substantially lower than the expected peak concentration following intravenous administration (59,60).

If a patient has a known or estimated phenytoin concentration prior to the administration of the loading dose, that value ($C_{observed}$) should be subtracted from the desired concentration ($C_{desired}$) and the adjusted loading dose calculated from Equation 20.

Confusion often arises about the need for a change in the loading dose when binding to albumin is altered. Little or no change is required because the volume of distribution and the therapeutic concentration range change inversely with each other. For example, when the serum albumin concentration is reduced, the volume of distribution is increased (Equation 1) and the target concentration is decreased (Equation 17) by virtually the same factor, resulting in little or no change in the loading dose as calculated from Equation 20.

## Maintenance of a Therapeutic Concentration

Phenytoin is difficult to administer properly. The capacity-limited metabolism results in a relatively narrow dosage range for an individual patient. The most commonly prescribed dosage is 300 mg daily, even though the majority of patients appear to have phenytoin concentrations that are less than 10 µg/ml on this regimen (45,61). This average maintenance dose may be the result of a reasonably high percentage of patients developing side effects or toxicities on 400 mg daily and a large number of adult patients who are not therapeutically controlled on 200 mg/day (See Figure 1.).

There have been reports that the dose may be administered once daily because of slow absorption characteristics following oral administration (62). As stated previously, once daily dosing should be reserved for Dilantin® Kapseals® at the present time. Even here, it would seem reasonable to administer the drug more frequently than once daily to those patients who require a large daily dose of phenytoin.

## Initial Individualization of Phenytoin Dosage

When a patient varies significantly from the average weight of 70 kg, some adjustment in the customary daily maintenance dose of 300 mg is likely to be required. Frequently, 5 mg/kg is used to determine doses for small adults or pediatric patients. This approach tends to underdose these patients, as the measured phenytoin concentrations are usually lower than those seen in the adult population (63,64).

Body surface area is an alternative to weight for estimating dosage requirements. The maintenance dose is then estimated by the following:

$$\begin{array}{l}\text{Patient's} \\ \text{Maintenance} \\ \text{Dose (mg/day)}\end{array} = \begin{array}{l}\text{Usual Adult} \\ \text{Maintenance} \\ \text{Dose (mg/day)}\end{array} \times \frac{\text{Patient's Body Surface Area (M}^2)}{1.73 \text{ M}^2}$$

$$\begin{array}{l}\text{Patient's} \\ \text{Maintenance} \\ \text{Dose (mg/day)}\end{array} = \begin{array}{l}\text{Usual Adult} \\ \text{Maintenance} \\ \text{Dose (mg/day)}\end{array} \times \left[\frac{\text{Patient's Weight} \\ \text{(kg)}}{70 \text{ kg}}\right]^{0.7} \quad \text{(Eq. 21)}$$

as weight to the 0.7 power is approximately proportional to body surface area (3).

Following the selection and initiation of a maintenance dose, the patient is evaluated for efficacy and toxicity. In this evaluation it is important to remember that one to two weeks or longer may be required for steady state to be achieved (7,39,65). Moreover, the higher a measured plasma concentration, the less likely that steady state has been achieved.

A patient's response is evaluated by recording seizure frequency, watching for adverse reactions, and by obtaining phenytoin plasma concentrations. The maintenance dose can then be adjusted, but care should be taken to avoid manipulating the dose based on the plasma phenytoin concentration without considering the clinical response of the patient. Because of the capacity-limited metabolism, dose adjustments of less than 100 mg/day are frequently required, and adjustments of more than 100 mg/day should only be undertaken with caution.

## Monitoring of Plasma Concentration and Dosage Adjustment

**Data Collection.** A complete evaluation of a plasma phenytoin concentration requires an accurate history of the phenytoin dosing regimen and the other drugs the patient is receiving, as well as pertinent laboratory data. Important laboratory data include serum creatinine, or a measurement of the creatinine clearance, and the serum albumin; these factors are associated with altered plasma protein binding. If renal failure or hypoalbuminemia is present, the measured phenytoin concentration will require adjustment (See Concentration versus Response and Toxicity). Additional laboratory data, such as serum bilirubin, liver enzymes, and prothrombin time may give some indication of hepatic function. In severe chronic hepatic disease a decreased ability to metabolize phenytoin is anticipated, as is diminished plasma protein binding. The latter is primarily a consequence of the hypoalbuminemia associated with chronic liver disease.

The sensitive relationship between the daily dose of phenytoin and the steady-state concentration make even relatively slight modifications in either absorption or elimination clinically significant. Compliance and bioavailability are more critical than usual. Drugs such as chloramphenicol, isoniazid, diazoxide, and disulfiram have been shown to increase phenytoin concentration (45,66,67). Carbamazepine and, occasionally, phenobarbital have been associated with a reduction in phenytoin concentration, presumably because of enzyme induction, that is, an increase in the maximum metabolic rate (Vm) (45,66,68).

Serum phenytoin concentrations are decreased during pregnancy, presumably due to enzyme induction (69,70) but diminished serum albumin may also contribute. Dosage requirements during pregnancy are difficult to predict, but an increase may be necessary to avoid the increased frequency of seizures observed in pregnant epileptic women (70).

The monitoring of outpatients is particularly difficult as compliance here is always suspect. Even in a controlled environment care should be taken to ensure that all doses are administered.

**When to Obtain a Phenytoin Concentration.** A fairly strong case can be made for monitoring phenytoin concentrations in all patients, because of the difficulty in estimating appropriate dosage regimens and the problems associated with distinguishing some of the central nervous system side effects of phenytoin from those of other anticonvulsant drugs or the disease state itself. At a minimum, patients who have not achieved optimal seizure control or who have developed symptoms consistent with phenytoin toxicity should have phenytoin concentrations measured.

The average steady-state concentration is important for determining the pharmacokinetic parameters Vm and Km. It is also required when a nomogram is used to adjust the maintenance dose. When a patient has achieved steady state on an oral dosing regimen, the fluctuation in peak to trough phenytoin concentration is relatively small. Thus, it makes little difference when a plasma sample is obtained and it can be assumed that the trough approximates the average concentration. The relative error in assuming the trough to be the average concentration is greater and potentially important when the drug is given once daily and the trough concentration is less than 5 μg/ml or the dose more than 400 mg.

If the drug is given by an intermittent short-term intravenous infusion, the average concentration at steady state ($C_{ss}$) can be estimated with the following equation:

$$C_{ss} = \frac{F \times Dose}{2 V} + \text{Trough Concentration}$$

(Eq. 22)

This equation assumes steady state has been achieved and that the average concentration is approximately half-way between the peak and trough concentrations. When given orally the average concentration may be approximated by the following Equation.

$$C_{ss} = \frac{F \times Dose}{4 V} + \text{Trough Concentration}$$

(Eq. 23)

This approximation assumes that the fluctuation at steady state following oral dosing is about half that observed with intravenous administration. In general, most patients receiving 300 mg of phenytoin orally once a day have an average concentration that is 1 to 2 μg/ml higher than the trough.

## Estimation of Pharmacokinetic Parameters (Vm, Km)

Estimation of the maximum metabolic rate (Vm) and the Michaelis-Menten constant (Km) for phenytoin usually requires that steady state has been achieved and that the average concentration ($C_{ss}$) during a dosing interval is known or can be approximated. In addition, most approaches require that the plasma protein binding is normal ($\alpha = 0.1$). If abnormal binding is present, a correction should be made so that the adjusted concentration represents the total phenytoin concentration that would be observed if binding were normal (see Equations 18 and 19).

### Dosage Adjustment Based on a Single Steady-state Concentration.

Case History: R.J., a 37-year-old 70 kg male, has been receiving 300 mg of phenytoin once daily at bedtime for several months. He has noted a decreased seizure frequency but still has one or more per week. He has no symptoms that might be associated with an elevated phenytoin concentration. His serum albumin and renal functions are normal as are his liver function tests. He is receiving no other medications. A plasma sample was obtained and a phenytoin concentration of 8 µg/ml was reported. *What would be an appropriate maintenance dose of phenytoin to achieve a steady-state concentration of 15 µg/ml?*

Several methods can be used to answer this question.

*Method A.* Equation 8 can be used to calculate Vm, if the value of Km is assumed or known. In this equation the phenytoin dose and Vm are in units of mg/day and Km and $C_{ss}$ are in µg/ml. Using the average value of 4 µg/ml for Km, the estimated value of Vm for R.J. would be

$$Vm = 300 \text{ mg/day} + 4 \text{ µg/ml} \times \frac{300 \text{ mg/day}}{8 \text{ µg/ml}} = 450 \text{ mg/day} \qquad \text{(Eq. 24)}$$

With the estimates of Vm and Km, a new maintenance dose can be calculated using Equation 4.

$$R = \frac{Vm \times C_{ss}}{Km + C_{ss}} = 355 \text{ mg/day} \qquad \text{(Eq. 25)}$$

Adjustment of the maintenance dose to this specific calculated value would be inappropriate as the calculated values of Km and Vm are only estimates. The most reasonable dose to administer would be 350 mg/day. This administration rate may be approximated with 300 and 400 mg on alternate days. Taking a more conservative approach, a Km value below 4 µg/ml could have been selected. The calculated maintenance dose to achieve 15 µg/ml would then have been less than 355 mg/day.

*Method B.* An alternative method is an approach developed by Sheiner as shown in Figure 11. This method allows estimation of the most probable values of Vm and Km for the individual patient based upon information previously obtained in a patient population. If the procedure outlined in the figure is followed, the most probable estimates of Vm and Km are 7 mg/kg/day (490 mg/day/70 kg) and 5 µg/ml, respectively. A new maintenance dose can be determined using Equation 4 or Figure 11. In this case, 5.2 mg/kg/day or 364 mg/70 kg/day is obtained. Again, a daily dose of 350 mg would probably be prescribed (300 and 400 mg on alternate days) because of convenience and the uncertainty that exactly 364 mg/day is required.

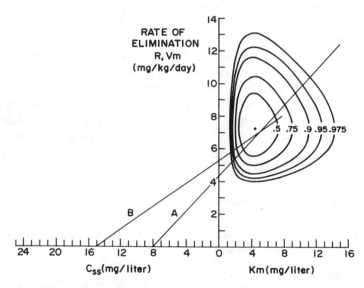

FIGURE 11. The most probable values of Vm and Km for a patient may be estimated using a single steady-state phenytoin concentration and a known dosing regimen. The eccentric circles or "orbits" represent the fraction of the sample patient population whose Km and Vm values are within that orbit. *Use of graph*: 1. Plot the daily dose of phenytoin (mg/kg/day) on the vertical line (rate of metabolism). 2. Plot the steady-state concentration, $C_{ss}$, on the horizontal line. 3. Draw a straight line connecting $C_{ss}$ and daily dose through the orbits (line A). The coordinates of the midpoint of the line crossing the innermost orbit through which the line passes are the most probable values for the patient's Vm and Km. 4. To calculate a new maintenance dose draw a line from the point determined in step 4 to the new desired $C_{ss}$, (line B). The point at which line B crosses the vertical line (rate of elimination) is the new maintenance dose (mg/kg/day). The line A represents a $C_{ss}$ of 8 mg/liter on 300 mg/day for a 70-kg patient. Line B was drawn assuming the new desired steady-state concentration was 15 mg/liter (μg/ml). Modified and reproduced with the permission of Dr. Lewis B. Sheiner, University of California, San Francisco.

*Method C.* Figure 12 shows a nomogram published by Rambeck et al (71). The use of this nomogram is similar to the first approach in that the author has selected a representative Km value. In general, the nomogram approach is reasonably satisfactory but it does not allow the user to adjust the Km value. If a more conservative dose adjustment is desired, a lower steady-state phenytoin concentration may be selected.

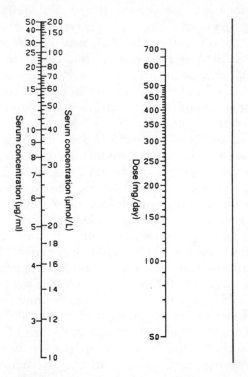

FIGURE 12. *Phenytoin nomogram.* Given a single reliable serum concentration on a given daily dose of phenytoin, the dose required to achieve a desired serum concentration can be predicted. A line is drawn connecting the observed serum concentration (left-hand scale) with the dose administered (center scale) and extended to intersect the right-hand vertical line. From this point of intersection, another line is drawn back to the desired serum level (left-hand scale). The dose required to produce this level can be read off the center scale.

Note: This nomogram will give misleading predictions if the serum concentration measurement is inaccurate, if the patient's compliance is in doubt, or if a change in concurrent treatment has been made since measurement of the serum concentration. From reference 71. Reproduced with permission.

Using the nomogram and the information provided, a new dosing regimen of 360 mg/day can be calculated. Again, since the suggested maintenance dose is inconvenient, the patient could be started on an average of 350 mg/day and then be re-evaluated at some future date to ensure that a reasonable therapeutic response and phenytoin concentration are achieved.

**Dosage Adjustment Based on Two or More Steady-state Concentrations at Different Dosing Rates.**

> Previous case history continued: The daily dose of 300 mg (previous $C_{ss}$ of 8 μg/ml) was increased to 350 mg/day. Two months later R.J. returned to the clinic with excellent seizure control but complained of an inability to concentrate. A phenytoin concentration was obtained and reported to be 20 μg/ml. *How should his dosage be adjusted to achieve a phenytoin concentration of 14 μg/ml?*

*Method D.* Figure 13 demonstrates the method suggested by Mullen (72) for multiple steady-state phenytoin concentrations. The values for Vm and Km, satisfying both observations, are 5.6 mg/kg/day (392 mg/70kg/day) and 2.5 μg/ml. Substituting these parameter values into Equation 4 yields a new maintenance dose of 333 mg to obtain a steady-state concentration of 14 μg/ml. Using the alternative approach of constructing line B gives 4.8 mg/kg/day, the same value.

Although a daily dose of 333 mg is not convenient, the two steady-state values indicate the need for a fine dosage adjustment to achieve the target concentration of 14 μg/ml. If 325 mg were prescribed, the expected $C_{ss}$ would be about 12 μg/ml as calculated from Equation 4.

If more than two dosing regimens and corresponding steady-state concentrations are obtained and plotted on Figure 13, multiple points of intersections are likely. These discrepancies may be the result of assay error, noncompliance, changes in the pharmacokinetic parameters, or using concentrations not truly at steady state.

*Method E.* Figure 14 shows another approach to obtain information from two or more steady-state levels. The method involves plotting the daily maintenance dose of phenytoin (R) versus the phenytoin clearance (daily maintenance dose divided by the steady-state concentration, $R/C_{ss}$) (35,36,73).

By calculation, clearance values for the daily doses of 300 mg and 350 mg are 37.5 liters/day and 17.5 liters/day, respectively. When the daily doses are plotted versus these values on Figure 14, a Vm of 390 mg/day is obtained. A value of 2.5 μg/ml for Km is obtained from the slope of the line. Using the Vm and Km values derived from Figure

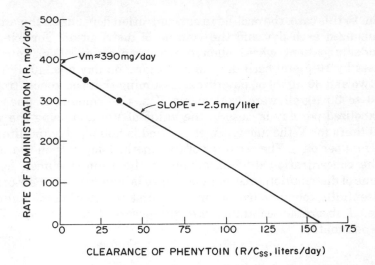

FIGURE 13. Determination of Vm and Km values for a patient, when steady-state phenytoin concentrations on two or more dosing regimens are known. *Use of graph*: 1. Draw lines A₁ and A₂, using steps 1 through 3 in Figure 11 for two separate dosing regimens and corresponding steady-state concentrations. The point of intersection for lines A₁ and A₂ are the coordinates for Vm and Km of the patient. 2. Draw a line from the point of intersection to the desired C$_{ss}$ (line B) to estimate the required dosage rate (mg/kg/day). This rate is where line B crosses the vertical line (rate of elimination). Line A₁ represents a C$_{ss}$ of 8 mg/liter on 300 mg/day and line A₂ a C$_{ss}$ of 20 mg/liter (µg/ml) on 350 mg/day for a 70-kg patient. Line B was drawn assuming the new desired C$_{ss}$ was 14 mg/liter (µg/ml).

14, a new dosing regimen of 331 mg/day can be calculated from Equation 4 to achieve a steady-state concentration of 14 µg/ml.

The approaches used in Methods D and E are essentially the same; any differences in the estimates of the pharmacokinetic parameters or dosing regimens are due to errors in plotting or interpreting the data. If more than two steady-state concentrations are obtained, the line of best fit should be used to approximate the parameter values.

**Evaluation of Nonsteady-state Phenytoin Concentrations.** Nonsteady-state concentrations of phenytoin are difficult to evaluate and, in most cases, it is not possible to accurately derive pharmacokinetic parameters (Vm, Km) when phenytoin concentrations are changing with time. One exception to this rule is when a high phenytoin concentration is allowed to decline with no additional doses being given. In this case, the decline in concentration depends on the amount metabolized each day and the volume of distribution. For example, consider a patient whose phenytoin concentration of 50 µg/ml decreases by 10 µg/ml each day, i.e., 50 µg/ml on day one, 40 µg/ml on day two and 30 µg/ml on day three. Assuming that the concentrations of 50 to 30 µg/ml were well above Km, the amount of phenytoin metabolized per day is close to the value of Vm and using the value of 50 liters for V the amount metabolized is 500 mg/day (50 liters × 10 µg/ml per day). The accuracy of this method depends on the errors in the concentration difference and in the value assumed for the volume of distribution. Also of importance is whether or not absorption is essentially complete by the time the first observation (50 µg/ml) is made. If absorption continues into the observed decay phase, Vm is underestimated.

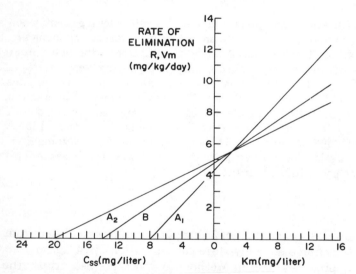

FIGURE 14. An alternative method for determination of Vm and Km values from steady-state concentrations on two or more dosing regimens.
*Use of graph*: 1. Plot the rate of administration (mg/day) vs. clearance of phenytoin (liter/day) for two or more steady-state concentrations. 2. Draw a straight line of best fit through the points plotted. The intercept on the rate of administration axis is Vm (mg/day) and the slope of the line

$$\left( \frac{(R_1 - R_2)}{\dfrac{R_1}{C_{ss_1}} - \dfrac{R_2}{C_{ss_2}}} \right)$$ is the negative value of Km.

In the clinical setting, Km can seldom be accurately estimated from a phenytoin decay curve as concentrations above and below Km are needed. Most patients have Km values that are below the therapeutic range, (34,35,73) and a maintenance dose is usually reinstituted before concentrations below Km are achieved.

A more complex situation is one in which phenytoin concentrations are rising or falling towards steady state, while the patient receives a fixed daily dose.

> Now consider a 70 kg patient who is receiving 300 mg/day, who has a steady-state phenytoin concentration of 8 μg/ml, and who is subsequently placed on 350 mg of phenytoin. Fourteen days later a phenytoin concentration of 20 μg/ml is measured. *Is the concentration likely to represent a steady-state value?*

Assuming an average Km of 4 μg/ml, the expected Vm for the patient is 450 mg/day (Equation 8). Using these parameter values the expected steady-state concentration for this patient on 350 mg/day is 14 μg/ml (Equation 5). Furthermore, 10 days are required to achieve 90% of this value. This time is calculated from the difference between the time to reach the plateau (Equation 11) and the time to reach 8 μg/ml from a concentration of zero (Equation 10). A volume of distribution of 0.65 liters/kg is assumed.

Thus, a concentration in excess of the expected steady-state value was achieved in about the same time interval. This information leads to the conclusion that the rate of metabolism is much less than expected, and continued accumulation is anticipated.

Some additional information might be gained from the dosing history and measured phenytoin concentrations. It is possible to estimate the average rate of metabolism over the 14-day period by subtracting the amount accumulated from the total dose administered. Over this interval the plasma concentration rose by 12 μg/ml. Assuming an average volume of distribution of 45.5 liters (0.65 liter/kg) for the patient, the amount of phenytoin accumulated per day is 39 mg. The rate of metabolism is then the difference between the administration rate and the accumulation rate, or 311 mg/day (350 mg/day − 39 mg/day). This estimate confirms that the maximum rate of metabolism in this patient is limited to something slightly greater than 300 mg/day, and that a daily dose of 310 mg should result in a steady-state concentration between 8 and 20 μg/ml. Obviously, it is very difficult to estimate the exact dose for a patient who is this sensitive to phenytoin dose adjustment.

## ALGORITHM

Figure 15 is an algorithm summarizing the principal steps in monitoring phenytoin therapy. Both the pharmacologic effects (therapeutic and toxic) and the plasma phenytoin concentration are considered. When an adjustment in dosage is required, a pharmacokinetic analysis, as previously discussed with a few examples in the last section, is helpful to estimate the values of Vm and Km in the individual patient.

## ASSAY METHODS

Phenytoin has been analyzed using spectrophotometric, colorimetric (with derivatization), gas chromatographic, high-pressure liquid chromatographic and immunologic methods. Gas chromatography is probably the most common procedure for routine monitoring, although the use of high-pressure liquid chromatography and immunologic methods is increasing.

Both chromatographic and immunologic techniques can be accurately performed with coefficients of variation of less than 10% at concentrations within the therapeutic range. They are, in general, specific and sensitive to a concentration of 1 μg/ml or less. Unfortunately, these assays have been shown (74,75) to be improperly handled in many laboratories. In large part, inadequate attention to quality control is probably responsible for the wide interlaboratory variability reported (74). To be of clinical value, laboratory results must be reliable. A much greater effort is needed to assure this goal in all laboratories.

The user of plasma phenytoin concentrations must be cognizant of assay error when interpreting measured values. An allowance of ± 20% is often in order. For example, a measured value of 20 μg/ml can be considered to be 16 to 24 μg/ml. Calculations of the pharmacokinetic parameters Vm and Km for these limits permit dosages to be adjusted based on the more conservative estimate.

---

FIGURE 15. Algorithm for monitoring and adjusting phenytoin therapy using steady-state plasma concentrations. The algorithm assumes patient compliance, achievement of steady state, constant bioavailability, and no change in the patient's clinical condition (e.g. renal function) or other drug therapy. It can be used to monitor additional steady-state concentrations obtained subsequent to a dose adjustment or monitoring period. ⟶

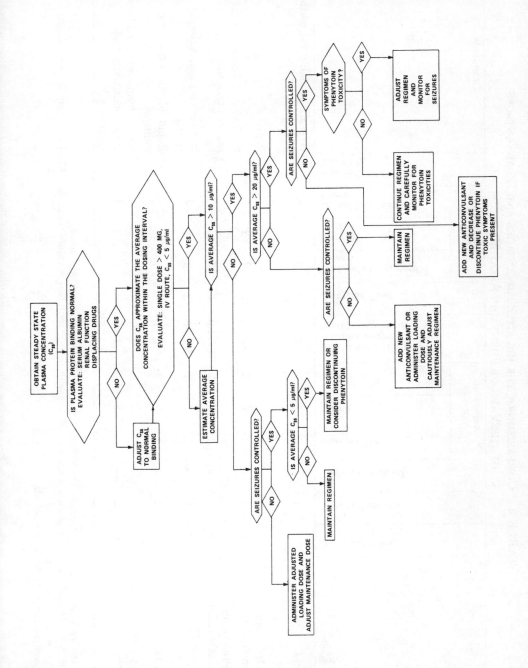

OBTAIN STEADY STATE PLASMA CONCENTRATION ($C_{ss}$)

IS PLASMA PROTEIN BINDING NORMAL? EVALUATE: SERUM ALBUMIN RENAL FUNCTION DISPLACING DRUGS

NO — ADJUST $C_{ss}$ TO NORMAL BINDING

YES — DOES $C_{ss}$ APPROXIMATE THE AVERAGE CONCENTRATION WITHIN THE DOSING INTERVAL?

EVALUATE: SINGLE DOSE > 400 MG, IV ROUTE, $C_{ss}$ < 5 $\mu$g/ml

NO — ESTIMATE AVERAGE CONCENTRATION

YES — IS AVERAGE $C_{ss}$ > 10 $\mu$g/ml?

NO — ARE SEIZURES CONTROLLED?

ARE SEIZURES CONTROLLED?
NO — ADMINISTER ADJUSTED LOADING DOSE AND ADJUST MAINTENANCE DOSE
YES — IS AVERAGE $C_{ss}$ < 5 $\mu$g/ml?
NO — MAINTAIN REGIMEN
YES — MAINTAIN REGIMEN OR CONSIDER DISCONTINUING PHENYTOIN

YES — IS AVERAGE $C_{ss}$ > 20 $\mu$g/ml?

NO — ARE SEIZURES CONTROLLED?
NO — ADD NEW ANTICONVULSANT OR ADMINISTER LOADING DOSE AND CAUTIOUSLY ADJUST MAINTENANCE REGIMEN
YES — MAINTAIN REGIMEN

YES — ARE SEIZURES CONTROLLED?
NO — CONTINUE REGIMEN AND CAREFULLY MONITOR FOR PHENYTOIN TOXICITIES
YES — SYMPTOMS OF PHENYTOIN TOXICITY?
NO — ADJUST REGIMEN AND MONITOR FOR SEIZURES
YES — ADJUST REGIMEN AND MONITOR FOR SEIZURES

ADD NEW ANTICONVULSANT AND DECREASE OR DISCONTINUE PHENYTOIN IF TOXIC SYMPTOMS PRESENT

309

TABLE 4. COMPARISON OF THE RELATIVE ADVANTAGES AND DISADVANTAGES OF THE VARIOUS PHENYTOIN ASSAY METHODS[a]

| Analytical Method[b] | Specificity for Phenytoin | Limit of Sensitivity | Metabolite Analysis | Assayable Samples | | | Minimum Sample Volume Required for Plasma/Serum | Analysis Time | Analysis Costs | | | Specialized Operator Training | Comments |
|---|---|---|---|---|---|---|---|---|---|---|---|---|---|
| | | | | Plasma/Serum | Urine | Saliva | | | Estimated Reagent Costs | Tech. Cost Per Assay | Initial Equipment Costs | | |
| HPLC | 1 | 1 | c | 1 | 2 | 2 | 0.2 ml | 2 | 3 | 3 | 3 | 3 | Overall, probably the method of choice. |
| GC | | | | | | | | | | | | | |
| On column methylation | 1 | 1 | c | 1 | 2 | 2 | 0.5 ml | 2 | 2 | 2 | 2 | 4 | } Method used in most of the recent literature. |
| Precolumn methylation | 1 | 1 | c | 1 | 2 | 2 | 0.5 ml | 3 | 2 | 2 | 2 | 4 | |
| RIA | 2 | 1 | — | 1 | ? | ? | 0.2 ml | 2 | 4 | 2 | 4 | 2 | Requires a scintillation counter. |
| EMIT | 2 | 1 | — | 1 | ? | ? | 0.2 ml | 1 | 4 | 1 | 2 | 1 | Rapid. Minimal training required. |
| SP | 4 | 3 | — | 2 | 3 | — | 1 ml | 3 | 1 | 2 | 1 | 2 | Now infrequently used because of less sensitivity and specificity. |

[a] Arbitrary Ranking Scale of 1 (Excellent) to 5 (Poor) with a score of 3 being average or nominal.
[b] HPLC = high performance liquid chromatography, GC = gas chromatography, RIA = radioimmunoassay, EMIT = enzyme immunoassay, SP = spectrophotometry.
[c] Hydrolysis and separate assay required.

# REFERENCES

1. Koch-Weser J: The serum level approach to individualization of drug dosage. Europ J Clin Pharmacol 1975; 9:1–8.
2. Lund L: Effects of phenytoin in patients with epilepsy in relation to its concentration in plasma. In: Davis DS, Pritchard BNC, eds. *Biological Effects of Drugs in Relation to Their Concentration in Plasma*. Baltimore: University Park Press 1972: 227–39.
3. Dill WA, Kazenko A, Wolf LM, Glazko A: Studies on 5,5-diphenylhydantoin (Dilantin[R]) in animals and man. J Pharmacol Expt Ther 1956; 118:270–9.
4. Neuvonen PJ: Bioavailability of phenytoin: clinical pharmacokinetic and therapeutic implications. Clin Pharmacokin 1979; 4:91–103.
5. Gugler R, Manion CV, Azarnoff DL: Phenytoin: pharmacokinetics and bioavailability. Clin Pharmacol Ther 1976; 19:135–42.
6. Jusko WJ, Koup JR, Alvan G: Nonlinear assessment of phenytoin bioavailability. J Pharmacokin Biopharm 1976; 4:327–36.
7. Food and Drug Administration: New prescribing directions for phenytoin. FDA Drug Bull 1978; 8:27–8.
8. Bauman JL, Siepler JK, Fitzloff J: Phenytoin crystallization in intravenous fluids. Drug Int Clin Pharm 1977; 11:646–9.
9. Kostenbauder HB, Rapp RP, McGovern JP, Foster TS, Perrier DG, Blacker HM, Hulon WC, Kinkel AW: Bioavailability and single-dose pharmacokinetics of intramuscular phenytoin. Clin Pharmacol Ther 1975; 18:449–56.
10. Wilder BJ, Serrano EE, Ramsey E, Buchanan RA: A method for shifting from oral to intramuscular diphenylhydantoin administration. Clin Pharmacol Ther 1974; 16:507–13.
11. Serrano EE, Wilder BJ: Intramuscular administration of diphenylhydantoin. Histologic follow-up. Arch Neurol 1974; 31:276–8.
12. Suzuki T, Saitoh Y, Nishihara K: Kinetics of diphenylhydantoin disposition in man. Chem Pharm Bull 1970; 18:405–11.
13. Glazko AJ, Chang T, Baukema J, Dill BS, Goulet JR, Buchanan RA: Metabolic disposition of diphenylhantoin in normal human subjects following intravenous administration. Clin Pharmacol Ther 1969; 10:498–504.
14. Bigger T, Schmidt DH, Kutt H: Relationship between the plasma level of diphenylhydantoin sodium and its cardiac antiarrhythmic effects. Circulation 1968; 38:363–74.
15. Vajda F, Williams FM, Davidson S, Falconer MA, Breckenridge A: Human brain, cerebrospinal fluid, and plasma concentrations of diphenylhydantoin and phenobarbital. Clin Pharmacol Ther 1974; 15:597–603.
16. Wilder BJ, Ransay RE, Willmore LJ, Feussner GF, Perchalski RJ, Shumate JB: Efficacy of intravenous phenytoin in the treatment of status epilepticus; kinetics of central nervous system penetration. Ann Neurol 1977; 1:511–18.
17. Shoeman DW, Azarnoff DL: The alteration of plasma proteins in uraemia as reflected in their ability to bind digitoxin and diphenylhydantoin. Pharmacology 1971; 7:169–77.
18. Odar-Cederlof I, Borga O: Kinetics of diphenylhydantoin in uraemic patients: consequences of decreased plasma protein binding. Europ J Clin Pharmacol 1974; 7: 31–7.
19. Odar-Cederlof I, Borga O: Impaired protein binding of phenytoin in uremia and displacement effects of salicylic acid. Clin Pharmacol Ther 1976; 20:36–47.
20. Odar-Cederlof I: Plasma binding of phenytoin and warfarin in patients undergoing renal transplantation. Clin Pharmacokin 1977; 2:147–53.

21. Sjoholm I, Kober A, Odar-Cederlof I, Borga O: Protein binding of drugs in uremia and normal serum: the role of endogenous binding inhibitors. Biochem Pharmacol 1976; 25:1205–13.
22. Boobis SW: Alteration of plasma albumin in relation to decreased drug binding in uremia. Clin Pharmacol Ther 1977; 22:147–53.
23. Hooper WD, Bochner F, Eadie MJ, Tyrer JH: Plasma protein binding of diphenylhydantoin. Effects of sex hormones, renal, and hepatic disease. Clin Pharmacol Ther 1974; 15:276–82.
24. Wallace S, Brodie MJ: Decreased drug binding in serum from patients with chronic hepatic disease. Europ J Clin Pharmacol 1976; 9:429–32.
25. Bochner F, Hooper WD, Sutherland JM, Eadie MJ, Tyrer JH: Diphenylhydantoin concentrations in saliva. Arch Neurol (Chicago) 1974; 31:57–9.
26. Reynolds F, Ziroyanis P, Jones N, Smith SE: Salivary phenytoin concentrations in epilepsy and in chronic renal failure. Lancet 1976; 2:384–6.
27. Paxton JW, Whiting B, Stephen KW: Phenytoin concentrations in mixed parotid and submandibular saliva and serum measured by radioimmunoassay. Brit J Clin Pharmacol 1977; 4:185–92.
28. Glazko AJ: Antiepileptic drugs: biotransformation, metabolism, and serum half-life. Epilepsia 1975; 16:367–91.
29. Witkin KM, Bius DL, Teague BL, Wiese LS, Boyles LW, Dudley KH: Determination of 5(p-hydroxyphenyl)-5-phenylhydantoin and studies relating to the disposition of phenytoin in man. Therap Drug Monitoring 1979; 1:11–34.
30. Arnold K, Gerber N: The rate of decline of dephenylhydantoin in human plasma. Clin Pharmacol Ther 1970; 11:121–34.
31. Richens A, Dunlop A: Serum phenytoin levels in the management of epilepsy. Lancet 1975; 2:247–8.
32. Eadie MJ, Tyrer JH, Bochner F, Hooper WD: The elimination of phenytoin in man. Clin Exp Pharmacol Physiol 1976; 3:217–24.
33. Houghton GW, Richens A, Leighton M: Effect of age, height, weight, and sex on serum phenytoin concentration in epileptic patients. Br J Clin Pharmacol 1975; 2:251–6.
34. Mawer GE, Mullen PW, Rodgers M, Robins AJ, Lucas SB: Phenytoin dose adjustment in epileptic patients. Br J Pharmacol 1974; 1:163–8.
35. Ludden TM, Allen JP, Valutsky WA, Vicuna AV, Nappi JM, Hoffman SF, Wallace JE, Lalka D, McNay JL: Individualization of phenytoin dosage regimens. Clin Pharmacol Ther 1977; 21:287–93.
36. Martin E, Tozer TN, Sheiner LB, Riegelman S: The clinical pharmacokinetics of phenytoin. J Pharmacokin Biopharm 1977; 5:579–96.
37. Allen JP, Ludden TM, Burrow SR, Clementi WA, Stavchansky SA: Phenytoin cumulation kinetics. Clin Pharmacol Ther 1979; 26:445–8.
38. Gerber N, Wagner JG: Explanation of dose-dependent decline of diphenylhydantoin plasma levels by fitting to the integrated form of the Michaelis-Menten equation. Res Commun Chem Pathol Pharmacol 1972; 3:455–66.
39. Ludden TM, Allen JP, Schneider LW, Stavchansky SA: Rate of phenytoin accumulation in man: a simulation study. J. Pharmacokin Biopharm 1978; 6:399–415.
40. Wagner JG: Time to reach steady state and prediction of steady-state concentrations for drugs obeying Michaelis-Menten elimination kinetics. J Pharmacokin Biopharm 1978; 6:209–25.
41. Karlen B, Garle M, Rane A, Gutova M, Lindeborg B: Assay of diphenylhydantoin (phenytoin) metabolites in urine by gas chromatography. Metabolite pattern in humans. Europ J Clin Pharmacol 1975; 8:359–63.

42. Bochner F, Hooper WD, Sutherland JM, Eadie MJ, Tyrer JH: The renal handling of diphenylhydantoin and 5-(p-hydroxyphenyl)-5-phenylhydantoin. Clin Pharmacol Ther 1973; 14:791–6.

43. Kutt H, Haynes J, McDowell F: Some causes of ineffectiveness of diphenylhydantoin. Arch Neurol 1966; 14:489–92.

44. Martin E, Gambertoglio JG, Adler DS, Tozer TN, Roman LA, Grausz H: Removal of phenytoin by hemodialysis in uremic patients. JAMA 1977; 238:1750–3.

45. Lund L: Anticonvulsant effects of diphenylhydantoin relative to plasma levels: a prospective three year study in ambulant patients with generalized epileptic seizures. Arch Neurol 1974; 31:289–94.

46. Vajda FJE, Prineas RJ, Lovell RRH, Sloman JG: The possible effects of long-term high plasma levels of phenytoin on mortality after acute myocardial infarction. Europ J Clin Pharmacol 1973; 5:138–44.

47. Buchthal F, Svensmark O, Schiller PJ: Clinical and electroencephalographic correlations with serum levels of diphenylhydantoin. Arch Neurol 1960; 2:624–30.

48. Lascelles PT, Kocen RS, Reynolds EH: The distribution of plasma phenytoin levels in epileptic patients. J Neurol Neurosurg Psych 1970; 33:501–5.

49. Kutt H, Winters W, Kolenge R, McDowell F: Diphenylhydantoin metabolism, blood levels and toxicity. Arch Neurol 1964; 11:642–8.

50. Ahmand S, Laidlaw J, Houghton GW, Richens A: Involuntary movements caused by phenytoin intoxication in epileptic patients. J Neurol Neurosurg Psych 1975; 38:225–31.

51. Levy L, Fenichel GM: Diphenylhydantoin activated seizures. Neurol 1969; 15: 716–22.

52. Shuttleworth E, Wise G, Paulson G: Choreoathetosis and diphenylhydantoin intoxication. JAMA 1974; 230:1179–1.

53. Chalhub EG, Devivo DC, Volpe JJ: Phenytoin-induced dystonia and choreoathetosis in two retarded epileptic children. Neurol 1976; 26:494–8.

54. Louis S, Kutt H, McDowell F: The cardiovascular changes caused by intravenous Dilantin and its solvent. Am Heart J 1967; 74:523–9.

55. Sheiner LB, Tozer TN: Clinical pharmacokinetics: the use of plasma concentrations of drugs. In: Melmon KL, Morrelli HF, eds. *Clinical Pharmacology: Basic Principles in Therapeutics.* New York: Macmillan 1978: 71–109.

56. Lunde PKM, Rane A, Yaffe SJ, Lund L, Sjoquist F: Plasma protein binding of diphenylhydantoin in man: interactions with other drugs and the effect of temperature and plasma dilution. Clin Pharmacol Ther 1970; 11:844–55.

57. Mattson RH, Cramer JA, Williamson PD, Novelly RA: Valproic acid in epilepsy: clinical and pharmacological effects. Ann Neurol 1978; 3:20–5.

58. Kurata D, Wilkinson GR: Erythrocyte uptake and plasma binding of diphenylhydantoin. Clin Pharmacol Ther 1974; 16:355–62.

59. Wilder BJ, Serrano EE, Ramsay E: Plasma phenytoin levels after loading and maintenance doses. Clin Pharmacol Ther 1973; 14:797–801.

60. Hvidberg E, Dam M: Clinical pharmacokinetics of anticonvulsants. Clin Pharmocokin 1976; 1:161–88.

61. Wilson JT, Wilkinson CR: Delivery of anticonvulsant drug therapy in epileptic patients assessed by plasma level analysis. Neurology 1979; 24:614–23.

62. Strandjord RE, Johannessen SI: One daily dose of diphenylhydantoin for patients with epilepsy. Epilepsia 1974; 15:317–27.

63. Borofsky LG, Louis S, Kutt H, Roginsky M: Diphenylhydantoin: efficacy, toxicity and dose-serum level relationship in children. Ped Pharmacol Ther 1972; 81:995–1002.

64. Svensmark O, Buchthal F: Diphenylhydantoin and phenobarbital. Am J Dis Child 1964; 108:82–7.
65. Richens A: Clinical pharmacokinetics of phenytoin. Clin Pharmacokin 1979; 4: 153–69.
66. Kutt H: Interactions of antiepileptic drugs. Epilepsia 1975; 16:393–402.
67. Roe TF, Podosin RL, Blaskovics M: Drug interactions: diazoxide and diphenylhydantoin. J Pediatr 1975; 87:480–4.
68. Molholm-Hansen J: Carbamazepine-induced acceleration of diphenylhydantoin and warfarin metabolism in man. Clin Pharmacol Ther 1971; 12:539–43.
69. Dam M, Christiansen J, Munck O, Mygind KI: Antiepileptic drugs: metabolism in pregnancy. Clin Pharmacokin 1979; 4:53–62.
70. Knight AH, Rhind EG: Epilepsy and pregnancy: a study of 153 pregnancies in 59 patients. Epilepsia 1975; 16:99–110.
71. Rambeck B, Boenigk HE, Dunlop A, Mullen PW, Wadsworth K, Richens A: Predicting phenytoin dose: a revised nomogram. Ther Drug Monitoring 1980; 1: 325–354.
72. Mullen RW: Optimal phenytoin therapy: a new technique for individualizing dosage. Clin Pharmacol Ther 1978; 23:228–32.
73. Lambi DG, Nanda RN, Johnson RH, Shakir RA: Therapeutic and pharmacokinetic effects of increasing phenytoin in chronic epileptics on multiple drug therapy. Lancet 1976; 2:386–9.
74. Pippenger CE, Penry JK, White BG, Daly DD, Buddington R: Interlaboratory variability in determination of plasma antiepileptic drug concentrations. Arch Neurol 1976; 33:351–5.
75. Richens A: Drug level monitoring—quantity and quality. Br J Clin Pharmacol 1978; 5:285–8.

*Counterpoint Discussion*

# Phenytoin

### Thomas M. Ludden, Ph.D.

Drs. Tozer and Winter have expertly and thoroughly described the relevant factors concerning the clinical pharmacokinetics of phenytoin. These are only additional comments that may lend assistance to the clinician responsible for the design of individual phenytoin dosage regimens. These comments are organized under the same headings used in the primary chapter so as to provide easy cross reference.

## INTRODUCTION/BACKGROUND

### Absorption

**Oral Administration.** The problems related to the administration of phenytoin (Dilantin®) suspension, 125 mg/5 ml have been examined (1). This product was reformulated a few years ago such that if the drug is initially well suspended by the dispensing pharmacist, minimal agitation is required before the measurement of each dose. Of course, the difficulty of accurate dose measurement is still present. The use of a large bore measuring syringe may help reduce dosing errors.

## CONCENTRATION VERSUS RESPONSE AND TOXICITY

### Adjustment of Target Concentration

Recent reports concerning the *in vivo* displacement of phenytoin by valproate (2) and salicylate (3,4) point out that while the free fraction of phenytoin in plasma is increased, the concentration of free drug is likely to remain unchanged and the total concentration is decreased. This requires a compensatory adjustment of the therapeutic range for total drug concentration. There is as yet insufficient data to permit an accurate prediction of the quantitative aspects of such an interaction and measurement of the free phenytoin concentration would be most helpful.

The finding that the concentration of unchanged phenytoin in urine may closely approximate the free plasma phenytoin concentration (5) deserves attention. If additional studies confirm this finding, determination of the phenytoin concentration in urine may provide a convenient indicator of circulating free drug in patients with adequate urine output. On a theoretical basis, significant deviations between urine and free concentrations are most likely to occur if the urinary pH becomes quite alkaline, i.e. approaching 8.

## CLINICAL APPLICATION OF PHARMACOKINETIC DATA

### Monitoring of Plasma Concentration and Dosage Adjustment

As Drs. Tozer and Winter described, the optimization of phenytoin therapy can be long and tedious. The following method of dose titration and plasma concentration monitoring may facilitate the achievement of phenytoin levels within the usual therapeutic range. An appropriate oral loading dose designed as previously described to achieve a serum concentration of 10 to 15 µg/ml is administered and followed in 6 to 12 hours by determination of the plasma phenytoin concentration and initiation of maintenance dosing, usually 300 mg daily. The phenytoin concentration serves as a reference for future determinations. After two to three days of maintenance therapy, a second plasma concentration may indicate the need for an adjustment in daily dosage. The size of the adjustment depends upon the magnitude of the change in concentration. For example, if the level has dropped from over 10 µg/ml to less than 7 µg/ml, a 1 to 1.5 mg/kg or greater increase in dose would be indicated. A partial load may be required if the decrease in concentration is too great. Again, the postload serum concentration should be measured. If only a moderate drop has occurred, then a 0.5-1 mg/kg increase in daily dose would be more appropriate. On the other hand, if the levels are stable or only slowly increasing and are within the usual therapeutic range, monitoring should be continued at weekly intervals for at least two weeks to detect possible excessive accumulation. Finally, if the concentration has shown a rapid rise, then a decrease in dose is indicated. A decrease in drug dose of about 0.5 mg/kg is usually an appropriate adjustment under these circumstances.

In any case, if a change in dosage is made, the phenytoin concentration should be monitored after another two to four days to assess the initial result of the dosage change. An additional adjustment may be required at this time. For example, the post-load plasma phenytoin concentration is 10.2 µg/ml. A maintenance dose of 300 mg/day is initiated. After three days the phenytoin concentration has dropped to 7.0 µg/ml. At this time the daily dose is increased to 400 mg/day and after four days the serum concentration has risen to 9.4 µg/ml. Since it is quite unlikely that this value represents the eventual steady-state concentration, additional monitoring is clearly indicated. After an additional two weeks the concentration is 12.0 µg/ml. If a further small increase in concentration is desired the dosage must be changed cautiously. Given the solid oral dosage forms available, the next convenient titration step is 430 mg/day. This dosage is instituted and monitoring continued as described above.

If appropriate monitoring is performed and titration increments or decrements made with a clear understanding of Michaelis-Menten pharmacokinetic behavior, an appropriate maintenance dosage should be established fairly rapidly in most subjects while the serum concentration is maintained within or close to the usual therapeutic range. The use of equations describing the time course of phenytoin concentrations during continued dosing (6) may also prove useful in combination with the above procedure for evaluating the appropriateness of a given regimen.

Once the serum concentration appears to be stabilizing, the monitoring of serum concentrations every week or every other week for a month should permit the detection of most patients who may slowly accumulate phenytoin. Very slow accumulation of drug may only be detectable if the monitoring of serum concentrations is continued at one to two month intervals for two or three months (6).

### Estimation of Pharmacokinetic Parameters (Vm,Km)

**Dosage Adjustment Based on Two or More Steady-State Concentrations at Different Dosing Rates.** As noted recently (7,8) and as pointed out by Drs. Tozer and Winter, the different mathematical or graphical techniques used for estimating a new dosage regimen based upon two or more previous steady-state concentrations at different dosing rates are essentially equivalent when only two or three data pairs are available, as in the clinical situation. Compliance, assay accuracy, concurrent drug therapy, disease states, product formulation and the assessment of steady-state are much more important factors to be considered. In addition, there is very little information concerning the stability of kinetic parameters as a simple function of time. For example, a patient with a low Km value whose steady-state plasma phenytoin concentration is initially within the therapeutic range may show large fluctuations in phenytoin concentration in response to only small changes in the Vmax value or the extent of drug absorption. Regardless of what pharmacokinetic techniques are used for dosage individualization, the appropriate and accurate monitoring and interpretation of plasma phenytoin concentrations is essential for the rational therapeutic use of phenytoin.

## REFERENCES

1. Taylor JW and Ludden TM. (Unpublished results).
2. Mattson RH, Cramer JA, Williamson PD, Novelly RA: Valproic acid in epilepsy: clinical and pharmacological effects. Ann Neurol 1978; 3:205.
3. Fraser DG, Ludden TM, Evens RP, Sutherland III EW: Displacement of phenytoin from plasma binding sites by salicylate. Clin Pharmacol Ther 1980; 27:165–9.
4. Paxton JW: Effects of aspirin on salivary and serum phenytoin kinetics in healthy subjects. Clin Pharmacol Ther 1980; 27:170–8.
5. Borga O, Hoppel C, Odar-Cederlof I, Garle M: Plasma levels and renal excretion of phenytoin and its metabolites in patients with renal failure. Clin Pharmacol Ther 1979; 26:306–314.
6. Ludden TM, Allen JP, Schneider LW, Stavchansky SA: Rate of phenytoin accumulation in man: A simulation study. J Pharmacokin Biopharm 1978; 6:399–415.
7. Ludden TM: Individualization of phenytoin therapy. J Pharm Pharmacol 1980; 32:152.
8. Schumacher GE: Using pharmacokinetics in drug therapy VI: Comparing methods for dealing with nonlinear drugs like phenytoin. Am J Hosp Pharm 1980; 37:128–32.

# 10

# Digoxin

Philip W. Keys, Pharm.D.

## INTRODUCTION/BACKGROUND

### Absorption

Digoxin is absorbed from the gastrointestinal tract by a passive, nonsaturable transport process (1–2). Absorption, which is independent of gastric acidity and the presence of bile, occurs twice as fast in the proximal as it does in the distal small intestine. Forty to sixty percent of the total dose is absorbed in the stomach, duodenum, and upper jejunum (1–2) and only approximately 10% is absorbed in the stomach. The first order rate constant for absorption is several times greater than the elimination rate constant (3) and, therefore, variation in the rate of absorption has little clinical relevance. Once absorbed, digoxin is transported to a greater extent by the portal vein than by the lymphatic system (1). The low hepatic clearance of digoxin as compared to hepatic blood flow suggests negligible metabolism during "first pass" through the liver (4).

Earlier studies demonstrated extreme variability in the percentage of total dose absorbed from the tablets of various manufacturers. Further investigation demonstrated that much of the variance was associated with differences in dissolution rate (5–7). Shaw et al (5) reported a correlation coefficient of 0.89 ($p < 0.05$) between percentage dissolution at 30 minutes and steady-state plasma concentration. Federal regulations now require that all tablets meet dissolution rate standards of greater than 55% in one hour.

Compilation of several studies shows that the average bioavailability of tablets which meet dissolution rate standards is 68% to 70% and the average bioavailability of the elixir is approximately 77% (8–9). [Lanoxin® tablets (Burroughs-Wellcome) were employed throughout this text unless otherwise stated.] Marcus et al (9) suggest that the average percentage of absorption from tablets is closer to 80%; however, their findings may be an artifact of their analytic procedures (10). As might be expected with a drug which is incompletely absorbed, marked variation in bioavailability occurs between subjects. Huffman et al (11) showed completeness of absorption to range from 50% to 93% in six healthy subjects who were receiving daily maintenance doses of digoxin tablets. Between-subject variability in percentage absorption is also seen with the elixir (range of 70% to 100%) and with tablets which have high (98% in one hour) dissolution rates (12–14). In addition, some patients appear more sensitive to differences in the rate of tablet dissolution. When two patients were switched from a tablet (Macarthy's) with a dissolution rate of 57% to a tablet with a dissolution rate of 100%, the serum concentration of one patient remained unchanged, whereas the serum concentration of the other rose from 1.5 ng/ml to 1.8 ng/ml (5).

Individual differences in absorptive capacity most likely account for much of the variance observed in digoxin bioavailability. Other factors, however, may influence digoxin bioavailability. Rapid gastrointestinal transit time favors incomplete dissolution and has been shown to reduce absorption of tablets (Orion Company; dissolution rate not stated) (15). However, when patients received tablets known to meet present dissolution rate standards, no effect from increased gastrointestinal motility was seen (16). Of interest is one case study which reports a patient who experienced a marked reduction in digoxin absorption (from 84% to 16%) during an acute transient diarrheal episode (17).

Absorptive defects may decrease the absorption of digoxin tablets. Nine patients with a malabsorption syndrome associated with either sprue, small bowel resections or hypermotility showed reduced absorption of digoxin tablets (18). In contrast, seven patients with malabsorption of fat and d-xylose secondary to jejunoileal bypass surgery had no evidence of digoxin malabsorption (19). Patients with pancreatic insufficiency also do not appear to malabsorb digoxin (18). Radiation therapy to the abdomen, whether resulting in signs of a malabsorption syndrome or not, has been shown to decrease absorption of digoxin tablets (20–21). Absorptive defects apparently have a less pronounced effect on the bioavailability of digoxin elixir. Absorption was not diminished when digoxin was administered as a solution to patients with either a malabsorption syndrome or partial gastrectomy (22–23). Furthermore, administration of digoxin elixir to a patient with radiation-induced malabsorption resulted in approximately 40% absorption, whereas practically no absorption occurred from tablets (21).

Bioavailability was not altered when digoxin was administered either with or after a usual breakfast (4,24); however, it may be reduced by as much as 17% when digoxin is given with a breakfast of high fiber content (25). Co-administration of digoxin and cholestyramine 4 grams and 8 grams resulted in decreased digoxin absorption of 17% and 31%, respectively (25). No effect was seen when digoxin was given eight hours before cholestyramine. Concomitant antacid administration reduced digoxin bioavailability by approximately 30% (26); and kaolin-pectin, when given concurrently, resulted in a decrease in digoxin absorption of 42% in one study (26) and 62% in another study (27). Kaolin-pectin, and most likely antacids, should be administered two hours after digoxin (27). Two other drugs, sulfasalazine and neomycin, have been shown to markedly decrease the extent of digoxin absorption (28–29). Alteration of administration times did not eliminate the interactive effect, and when possible, these latter two drugs should be avoided in patients receiving oral digoxin.

Physiologic factors which affect absorptive capacity have not been well-studied with regard to digoxin. Elderly patients with mild heart failure absorbed digoxin as well as young patients with mild heart failure (30). The presence of severe right-sided congestive heart failure does not appear to decrease digoxin absorption (31).

### Distribution

Digoxin's disposition is adequately described by a two-compartment, open model (32–34), where the central compartment represents the blood and well-perfused body fluids and tissue and the peripheral compartment represents the remaining, slowly-perfused body space. The steady-state volume of distribution ($V_{ss}$) of digoxin is large and extremely variable. Differences in renal function account for some of the intersubject variation. The $V_{ss}$ averages 510 liters in subjects with normal renal function, whereas in patients with renal impairment, the average is only 330 liters (32). Although $V_{ss}$ appears to covary with renal function, marked variation still exists in individuals with similar creatinine clearances. Koup et al (33–34) observed a range of 386 liters to 1026 liters in subjects with creatinine clearances of 101 $\pm$ 13 ml/min/1.73 $m^2$ and a range of 189 liters to 481 liters in patients with creatinine clearances less than 8 ml/min/1.73 $m^2$.

The apparent volume of the central compartment remains approximately one-fourth that of the steady-state volume of distribution regardless of renal function (32). Digoxin is approximately 25% bound to serum protein in subjects with moderate (50 to 75 ml/min) to normal creatinine clearances (32,34). The extent of binding is diminished to approximately 18% in patients with severe renal impairment (34) and to approximately 13% in patients receiving heparin concomitantly (35). Reduction in binding is most likely due to displacement secondary to the build-up of endogenous binding inhibitors in the former and rise in serum free fatty acids in the latter. Any change in the free fraction of digoxin in the serum would be transient and have minimal effect on tissue concentration.

Serum digoxin is bound almost entirely to albumin with an association constant of approximately $9 \times 10^2$ liter/mole at 37° C (36). The degree of metabolite binding progressively decreases with stepwise removal of digoxin's sugar moieties (see Metabolism) resulting in only 14% of digoxigenin being bound to serum albumin (36).

The larger fraction of digoxin in the peripheral compartment is due to a high degree of tissue binding. Concentration of digoxin differs throughout the body and is greatest in the heart (37). As might be expected, some studies have shown a relatively constant ratio between serum and myocardium concentrations of digoxin. The ratio of serum to right atrium concentration was 1:24 with a range of 1:18 to 1:29 (38). Serum to papillary muscle concentration correlated highly ($r = 0.957$; $p < 0.001$) and had a ratio of 1:67 (39). Other investigators, however, have noted appreciable intersubject variation in serum to myocardium ratios (40). Approximately 50% of this variability can be accounted for by variation in renal function. Jusko and Weintraub (40) report a correlation coefficient of 0.715 ($p < 0.01$) between creatinine clearance and the ratio of serum to left ventricle digoxin concentration. This finding further supports the observation of reduced $V_{ss}$ in patients with severe renal impairment. Whether reduced binding is due to the accumulation of endogenous binding inhibitors or other factors such as reduced tissue perfusion or changing ratios of digoxin metabolites is unknown.

Morphological changes in the myocardium due to an underlying cardiac disease may also alter the extent of digoxin tissue binding and thus cause variability in serum to myocardium concentration ratios. Coltart et al (41) found that when histological change was minimal in the four chambers of the heart, digoxin was homogenously distributed in the myocardium, and concentrations tended to be higher in patients with higher serum concentrations. Conversely, digoxin concentration in a fibrotic left ventricle of one patient was only 25% of the concentration in the right ventricle which had a normal histological appearance. Of particular interest is the finding that digoxin concentration in the microsomal fraction of the heart of two patients was almost identical to the serum concentration regardless of the morphological structure of surrounding tissue. This may imply a more constant ratio between serum digoxin and the active receptor site and help explain the relationship between serum concentration and pharmacologic effect (see Concentration versus Response and Toxicity).

The ratio of serum to skeletal muscle varies from 1:16 in subjects with normal renal function to 1:5 in patients with compromised renal function (37,39). The majority of digoxin's body store is bound to skeletal muscle since its mass may reach 40% of total body weight (37). Digoxin distributes poorly into adipose tissue and thus, lean body weight provides a better estimate of volume of distribution than does total body weight (42).

## Metabolism

Digoxin's chemical structure (Figure 1) consists of digoxigenin coupled with three sugar (digitoxose) moieties. Digoxigenin has a steroid nucleus with a five-membered, α, β unsaturated lactone ring at C17, and a β-oriented hydroxyl group at the C3, C12 and C14 positions. The sugar moieties are attached to each other and to digoxigenin through the hydroxyl group at the C3 position of digoxigenin.

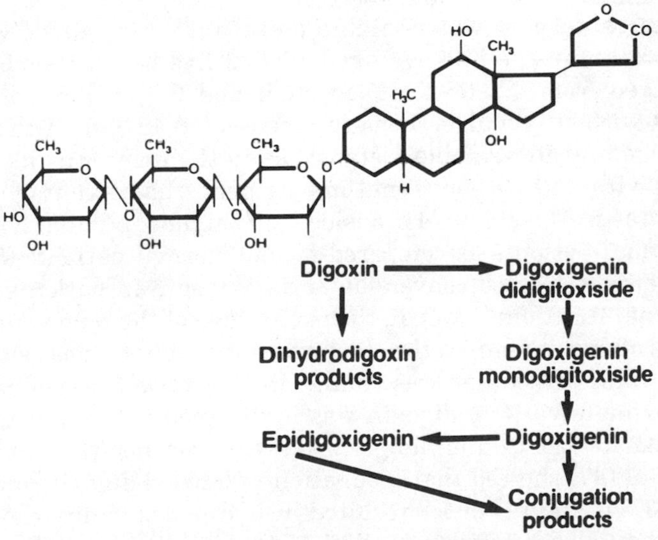

FIGURE 1.   Digoxin's Chemical Structure and Metabolic Pathways

The metabolism of digoxin follows two pathways (Figure 1). One pathway is the stepwise cleavage of the three sugars to form digoxigenin didigitoxiside, digoxigenin monodigitoxiside and digoxigenin (43). Following removal of the sugar portions, digoxigenin is converted to 3-keto digoxigenin in the liver by NAD-dependent 3 β-hydroxysteroid dehydrogenases (44). The 3-keto intermediate is further reduced to the 3-epimer of digoxigenin by 3 α-hydroxysteroid dehydrogenases. Both digoxigenin and epidigoxigenin are conjugated into sulfate and glucuronide products.

Various percentages of these metabolites are found in bile and stool as well as urine. Beerman et al (2) reported that only 37% to 48% of the radioactivity of labeled digoxin in duodenal bile was in the form of the parent compound. The mono- and didigitoxisides of digoxigenin comprised 9.4% of the total recovery of digoxin and metabolites in the bile of one patient who was described as representative of all six study patients (45). Chromatographic analysis of stool from two patients without cardiac, renal or hepatic disease showed an average of 19.4% digoxigenin monodigitoxiside and 19.7% digoxigenin didigitoxiside (46). The partition of metabolites in the urine of the same two patients showed 3.5% digoxigenin monodigitoxiside and 10.9% digoxigenin didigitoxiside. Others (47) have found no greater than between 9 and 14% digoxigenin and its mono- and didigoxisides in the urine of over 20 subjects; whereas, one patient in another study (48) excreted 32% of these metabolites in the urine.

The percentage of water-soluble metabolites (presumedly conversion products) in the bile averaged 32% in five healthy subjects (50), and ranged from 4.2 to 20.1% in stool and 0.9 to 10% in urine of patients without renal or hepatic disease (46,48–49). Although the percentage of water-soluble metabolites in the urine was identical in patients with and without renal impairment, the percentage of these metabolites in the stool was considerably higher (p value not stated) in two renal patients as compared to four normal patients (51). This may mean accelerated conversion of digoxigenin in patients with reduced renal function; however, the percentage of the mono- and didigitoxisides of digoxigenin in the stool was noticeably reduced suggesting that the total percentage was similar in these two types of patients.

Approximately 7% of digoxin was hydrolyzed in the gut to digoxigenin and its mono- and didigitoxisides in two healthy subjects (2). Gault et al (47) showed that incubation of labeled digoxin and gastric juice at 37° C and pH of 1.2 resulted in hydrolysis to digoxigenin and its two digitoxisides with only 34% of the activity remaining as digoxin in 30 minutes. Analysis of the gastric contents of one patient revealed that intragastric hydrolysis can occur at the same rate with a pH of 0.9. Hydrolysis of digoxin on exposure to gastric acid may be of clinical significance since pH may fall below 1 in certain conditions (e.g., Zollinger-Ellison Syndrome). Furthermore, digoxigenin appears to be absorbed to the same extent as digoxin (2,47).

The other digoxin metabolic pathway involves reduction of the lactone ring to form dihydrodigoxin with subsequent cleavage of the sugars to produce the monodigitoxiside and didigitoxiside of dihydrodigoxigenin and dihydrodigoxigenin itself (43,52). Formation of these reduction metabolites varies considerably between individuals. Of 50 patients who were receiving digoxin maintenance therapy, 15 had greater than 15% dihydrodigoxin in the urine (48). The average was 13% with a range of 1 to 47%. Peters et al (52) found an average of 12.4 ± 11% (SD) in the urine of 100 patients on chronic digoxin therapy. There was no relationship between the percentage of reduction products in the urine and sex, age, renal function or serum digoxin concentration. Seven of the 100 patients had greater than 35% dihydrometabolites in the urine and the urine of one patient contained 27% digoxin, 21% digoxigenin and its two digitoxisides, and 52% dihydrodigoxin metabolites. Obviously, digoxin is not always excreted primarily as the unchanged glycoside.

The stepwise cleavage of the sugar moieties progressively decreases the cardioactivity of the digoxin-related compounds (53). Epimerization and conjugation renders the metabolites almost completely cardioinactive. All dihydrometabolites are substantially less cardioactive than the parent compound, digoxin. The potency ratios of the various metabolites in comparison to digoxin have been determined from intravenous administration of lethal doses to animals and are presented in Table 1. The order of potency is the same for inotropy as it is for toxicity (54). Comparison of ratios is difficult because of the different animal species used in the experiments.

TABLE 1.   POTENCY RATIOS OF DIGOXIN METABOLITES

| Digoxin Metabolite | Potency Ratio (compared to digoxin) | Ref. |
|---|---|---|
| Digoxigenin didigitoxiside | 1/1.3 | 53 |
| Digoxigenin monodigitoxiside | 1/1.5 | 53 |
| Digoxigenin | 1/4.8; 1/23 | 53, 54 |
| 3-epidigoxigenin | 1/10 | 53 |
| Dihydrodigoxin | 1/16; 1/41 | 54, 55 |
| Dihydrodigoxigenin | < 1/46 | 54 |

In summary, for any given body load of digoxin, the average percentage of the various metabolites excreted in the urine by patients with normal hepatic and renal function is 12 to 13% dihydrometabolites (cardioinactive), 1 to 10% conversion products (cardioinactive) and 9 to 14% digoxigenin and its sugars (cardioactive). Similar patients excreted in the stool an average of 40% digoxigenin and its mono- and digitoxisides, 4 to 20% conversion products and an undetermined percentage of the dihydrometabolites.

## Excretion

Digoxin is cleared from the blood primarily by renal excretion and metabolism, where the overall rate of elimination is proportional to the serum concentration. Total body clearance ($Cl_B$) varies greatly from individual to individual depending on both the degree of renal function and extent of metabolism. In eight subjects with normal renal and hepatic function (33), total clearance averaged 188 ± 44 ml/min/1.73 m$^2$ with renal clearance comprising 75% of the total; whereas, in four patients with severe renal impairment and apparently normal hepatic function (34), total clearance averaged only 49 ml/min/1.73 m$^2$ with nonrenal clearance (primarily metabolism) comprising 75% of the total. It follows that determination of $Cl_B$ in patients with mild to moderate reduction in renal function (e.g., the aged and/or suffering from heart failure) requires consideration of both the renal and metabolic routes of elimination.

The mechanisms of digoxin renal clearance include glomerular filtration as well as both tubular reabsorption and secretion. Creatinine clearance, which provides an estimate of glomerular filtration rate, has been shown by several investigators (56–58) to approximate renal clearance of digoxin. Although the clearance of digoxin and creatinine appear similar, digoxin clearance may differ by as much as 30 to 40 ml/min in any two individuals with similar creatinine clearance. In addition, Baylis et al (59), in a study of 31 randomly selected patients (aged 58 to 91) with creatinine clearances ranging from 8 to 123 ml/min, reported an extremely poor correlation (r = 0.240) between creatinine and digoxin renal clearance. In two studies (57,59) of patients with varying degrees of renal function, digoxin clearance was consistently lower than creatinine clearance. This might be expected if glomerular filtration was the sole mechanism since serum digoxin is 25% protein bound and digoxin clearances are usually calculated from total serum concentration. However, other studies (33,34) of patients with varying degrees of renal function report digoxin clearances which were greater than creatinine clearances.

Differences between the renal clearance of digoxin and creatinine reflect the operation of renal tubular mechanisms. The renal clearance of unbound serum digoxin in 13 patients with good renal function was almost twice (1.94) that of inulin (mean 64 ml/min, range 25–110 ml/min) suggesting active tubular secretion of about 50% of the digoxin excreted in the urine (58). Apparently, this secretory mechanism is saturable at high serum concentrations (60). It should be noted that inulin and creatinine clearances are comparable except in patients with renal impairment where creatinine clearances overestimate inulin clearance because of tubular secretion of creatinine (61). Studies (33,58) showing good correlation between digoxin and creatinine renal clearances with no evidence of tubular reabsorption of digoxin are based on subjects without clinical signs of congestive heart failure. In patients with cardiovascular disease and signs of prerenal azotemia, however, renal clearance of digoxin appears to be further reduced because of passive tubular reabsorption. Halkin et al (62) reported a relationship between digoxin renal clearance and urine flow rate, which was independent of creatinine clearance, in patients with low urine flow rates (<1 ml/min in 50% of the patients) and urea clearances well below (average 36%) creatinine clearances. Thus, creatinine clearance may overestimate digoxin renal clearance in patients with reduced renal function and signs of prerenal azotemia.

The nonrenal clearance of digoxin consists primarily of metabolism and is the major route of elimination in patients with severe renal impairment. The mean value was 42.8 ml/min/1.73 m$^2$ (0.56 ml/min/kg) in five patients with creatinine clearances less than 5 ml/min/1.73 m$^2$ and no signs of cardiac failure (34). In eight healthy subjects with normal renal function, the average nonrenal clearance was 47.7 ml/min/1.73 m$^2$. The similarity between these two values suggests that renal failure alone does not alter digoxin metabolism (34). Waldorff et al (60) report an average value of 0.63 ml/min/kg ($\sim$ 44 ml/min/1.73 m$^2$) in four patients with arteriosclerotic heart disease, aged 64 to 75 years, versus 1.03 ml/min/kg ($\sim$ 70 ml/min/1.73 m$^2$) in four healthy individuals, aged 28 to 52 years.

Biliary excretion accounts for some nonrenal clearance. Approximately 30% of labeled digoxin was eliminated in the bile of five healthy subjects during the first 24 hours following intravenous administration (50). Since only 10% of an orally administered dose of digoxin is absorbed in the stomach, as much as 60 to 70% of digoxin and metabolites excreted in the bile may be reabsorbed. At least one-half of digoxin products in the stool are metabolites and thus, fecal excretion of digoxin, itself, is approximately 6% of total clearance and 20% of nonrenal clearance in healthy subjects.

Marked intersubject variation in nonrenal clearance is evidenced by a reported range of 0.19 to 1.13 ml/min/kg in one study (60). Variability is further documented by the wide range in percentages of the various metabolites present in the urine and stool of patients (see Metabolism). Metabolic clearance may be altered by hepatocellular damage resulting from hepatic congestion (31). Koup et al (34) note a nonrenal clearance of only 23.3 ml/min/1.73 m², in a patient with congestive heart failure. In addition, these investigators showed a slightly improved prediction of serum digoxin concentrations when estimated nonrenal clearance in patients with a history of congestive heart failure was reduced by 50%.

Spironolactone 100 mg twice daily is reported to decrease (p < 0.02) digoxin renal clearance by inhibiting tubular secretion (58,60). Both renal and total body clearance were reduced by an average of 26% indicating a similar decrease in nonrenal clearance. Percentage reduction in $Cl_B$ ranged from 0 to 74%. In addition, $V_{ss}$ was significantly (p < 0.01) reduced (range 3 to 59%) suggesting decreased tissue binding of digoxin.

A transient and most likely clinically-insignificant rise in both glomerular filtration rate and digoxin renal clearance, due to increased renal cortical blood flow, may occur following rapid, intravenous administration of furosemide (63). Daily maintenance doses of furosemide 40 mg had no effect on digoxin renal clearance (64–65). However, should chronic administration of this diuretic result in decreased glomerular filtration and prerenal azotemia secondary to volume depletion, an appreciable decrease in renal clearance of digoxin would be expected. Furosemide-induced hypokalemia has been reported to reduce tubular secretion of digoxin. When low serum potassium (range 2.6 to 3.0 mEq/L) was elevated to above 3.6 mEq/L in four congestive heart failure patients, the total body clearance of digoxin increased (p < 0.01) from an average of 85 ml/min to 144 ml/min while glomerular filtration rate remained unchanged (66).

Concurrent administration of quinidine 200 mg every six hours resulted in average reduction of 35% (range 7 to 52%) in total body clearance of digoxin (67). Renal and hepatic clearance as well as volume of distribution were reduced, on an average, to the same extent. The reduction in renal clearance was apparently due to decreased tubular secretion since no change in creatinine clearance was seen.

The biologic half-life (t½) of digoxin in healthy individuals with normal renal and hepatic function is about 1.6 days. Reduction in renal clearance results in prolongation of t½; however, the relationship between t½ and renal function is confounded by concurrent reduction in volume of distribution and variability in nonrenal clearance. Patients with severe renal impairment have been noted to have a digoxin half-life which ranged from 2.2 to 4.9 days (34). The t½ was normal (1.9 days) in one patient despite a creatinine clearance of only 20 ml/min (56). In a study (30) of seven elderly patients with mild congestive heart failure and normal (< 1.3 mg%) serum creatinine, t½ varied from 1.0 to 5.4 days.

The mean t½ of digoxigenin didigitoxiside, digoxigenin monodigitoxiside, digoxigenin and dihydrodigoxin in six healthy subjects with creatinine clearances greater than 95 ml/min was 11.5 hours, 8.5 hours, 2.0 hours and 1.2 hours, respectively (68). Except for digoxigenin monodigitoxiside, t½ of metabolites was approximately 4 to 5 times longer in six patients with creatinine clearances less than 8 ml/min.

## CONCENTRATION VERSUS RESPONSE AND TOXICITY

### Therapeutic and Toxic Concentrations

Digoxin has an inotropic and electrophysiologic action on the heart. Electrophysiologic effects, and most likely inotropy, result from suppression of transmembrane transport of sodium and potassium ions by means of inhibition of $(Na^+, K^+)$-ATPase (69). A high-affinity binding of digoxin to $(Na^+, K^+)$-ATPase has been identified in the microsomal fraction (light membrane fragments) of heart tissue minces (69–70). This microsomal fraction is regarded by some as the source of digoxin's receptor sites (70). Whether binding of digoxin to the enzyme-mediated receptor sites takes place on the cell plasma membrane or in the sarcoplasmic reticulum is not clear.

The extent of $(Na^+, K^+)$-ATPase inhibition by digoxin is related to serum concentration and increases with dosage increments (69). It might be expected that serum concentration would be related to myocardial concentration which, in turn, would be related to the drug's myocardial effects. However, digoxin binds to lipid membrane sites as well as $(Na^+, K^+)$-ATPase (69), and it is therefore doubtful that total myocardial digoxin is bound to the active receptor sites. In addition, myocardial content of digoxin decreases with both diminishing renal function and the presence of fibrotic tissue, making serum to myocardium ratios highly variable (40–41). These observations have led some investigators to suggest that serum digoxin may equilibrate differently with the receptor sites than with total myocardial stores (40).

There is some limited evidence in humans to support this supposition. Coltart et al (41) have determined the steady-state plasma concentration of digoxin along with left ventricular microsomal and myocardial concentration in the hearts of three patients following cardiac transplantation (Table 2). At least for these patients, the ratios of plasma to microsomal concentration appear more consistent than the ratios of plasma to myocardial concentration. A more constant ratio of serum to microsomal concentration would explain the relationship between serum concentration and inhibition of $(Na^+, K^+)$-ATPase.

In any event, clinical studies have shown that serum digoxin concentrations bear a close relationship to the drug's myocardial effects. Changes in left ventricular ejection time correlated moderately ($r = -0.55$; $p < 0.01$) with steady-state serum digoxin concentrations when daily doses were varied from 0 to 0.75 mg in nine patients with congestive heart failure (71). Redfors (72) observed a progressive decrease in ventricular rate at both rest and high work loads as serum digoxin concentrations were gradually increased in 11 patients with atrial fibrillation. Several studies have reported a statistically significant difference in serum digoxin concentrations of toxic versus non-toxic patients (73). Furthermore, when 116 patients on digoxin maintenance doses were classified as (1) non-toxic, in congestive heart failure; (2) non-toxic, not in congestive heart failure; (3) possibly toxic; and, (4) definitely toxic, the mean serum digoxin concentrations of each group were noted to progressively increase from one group to the next (74). The mean values differed significantly ($p \leq 0.05$) from each other and were 0.95 ng/ml, 1.49 ng/ml, 2.53 ng/ml and 3.32 ng/ml, respectively. Analysis of several variables which might predict therapeutic versus toxic response revealed that serum digoxin concentration alone was the best indicator of the patient's clinical response.

Therapeutic serum concentrations of digoxin range from 0.9 ng/ml to 2.0 ng/ml (74). Concentrations in excess of 2.0 ng/ml usually, but not always, are associated with toxicity. Smith and Haber (75) found in a study of 179 patients that 87% of the patients with cardiac signs of toxicity had serum digoxin concentrations above 2.0 ng/ml, while 90% of the patients without evidence of toxicity had serum concentrations below 2.0 ng/ml. Overlap between the two groups ranged from 1.6 to 3.0 ng/ml. Inotropy begins at concentrations less than 0.9 ng/ml and increases with increasing serum concentrations until toxicity is encountered. A usual serum concentration range for inotropic action is between 0.9 ng/ml and 1.5 ng/ml. Chronotropic serum concentrations are normally slightly higher than those recommended for inotropy. Chamberlain et al (76) found that patients with an acceptable ven-

## TABLE 2. PLASMA AND LEFT VENTRICULAR CONCENTRATION OF DIGOXIN

| Patient | Plasma Conc. ng/ml | Microsomal Conc. ng/mg | Ratio of Plasma to Microsomal | Myocardial Conc. ng/Gm | Ratio of Plasma to Myocardial |
|---------|--------------------|------------------------|-------------------------------|------------------------|-------------------------------|
| 1 | 1.0 | 1.2 | 1/1.2 | 120.0 | 1/120 |
| 2 | 1.8 | 1.9 | 1/1.1 | 19.2 | 1/10 |
| 3 | 2.6 | 2.5 | 1/1.0 | 75.2 | 1/29 |

tricular response (60 to 85 beats/min) to atrial fibrillation had a mean ($\pm$ SD) serum digoxin concentration of 1.6 $\pm$ 0.7 ng/ml. Others (77) have reported similar mean serum concentrations which controlled ventricular rate between 60 and 100 beats/min in patients with uncomplicated atrial fibrillation.

## Exceptions

Although studies have defined a clinically-useful therapeutic range, the serum digoxin concentration which optimizes response without producing toxicity can be divergent for some patients. Beller et al (78) report that 29% of the patients (N = 34) in their study who were diagnosed as definitely digoxin toxic had serum concentrations below 1.7 ng/ml. Several factors may predispose a patient to toxicity even though the serum concentration is in the therapeutic range. Of 16 toxic patients with serum concentration below 2.0 ng/ml, 15 had coronary artery disease, and of these, half had a history of myocardial infarction (75,78). Studies in animals also suggest that the presence of myocardial infarction reduces the toxic dose of digoxin. The severity of cardiac disease is apparently related to toxicity (73). Approximately three-quarters of the toxic patients in the study by Beller et al (78) were in functional class III or IV (New York Heart Association's Classification). This might be expected since increased automaticity is seen more frequently in the presence of ventricular dilatation and failure (69,73). Toxicity has also been associated (p $<$ 0.05) with an increased prevalance of pulmonary disease and may be related to the occurrence of hypoxia (73).

The serum concentrations of certain electrolytes have long been known to influence myocardial sensitivity to digoxin. Hypokalemia has been shown to result in cardiac toxicity when serum digoxin concentrations were in the therapeutic range. Six of 12 congestive heart failure patients (average serum digoxin 1.3 ng/ml) developed cardiac arrhythmias when their serum potassium concentrations fell from a mean of 4.37 mEq/L to 3.41 mEq/L (11% loss of total body potassium) (79). Brater and Morrelli (80) report that 28 normokalemic patients with metabolic alkalosis had a significantly (p $<$ 0.05) higher incidence of digoxin-related arrhythmias than 14 nonalkalotic patients. Ninety-three percent of the alkalotic patients were receiving potassium-losing diuretics as compared to only 29% of the nonalkalotic patients. The mean ($\pm$ SD) serum digoxin concentration in the toxic patients was 1.3 $\pm$ 0.4 ng/ml; one toxic patient had a serum concentration under 1.0 ng/ml. These investigators note that potassium-losing diuretics may cause a deficit in total body potassium which presents as a secondary alkalosis with normokalemia and further suggest that clinicians should be alert to conditions, such as hypochloremic alkalosis with paradoxical aciduria, which might signal potassium depletion.

Hypomagnesemia has been associated with increased sensitivity to digoxin in animals and should be considered in toxic patients with normal serum digoxin concentrations. Enhanced myocardial sensitivity to digoxin also has been observed in hypercalcemic animals; however, extremely high concentrations of serum calcium were required to elicit toxicity (73).

In contradiction to sensitive patients, some patients with atrial fibrillation or other supraventricular tachycardia require serum concentrations well above 2.0 ng/ml for an appropriate degree of atrioventricular blockade (76,81). Goldman et al (82) report several patients with atrial fibrillation who required serum concentrations between 2.0 to 4.0 ng/ml to control (60 to 100 beats/min) ventricular response. In five instances, ventricular response was not controlled with these high concentrations. Furthermore, there was no evidence of toxicity in any of these patients. Resistance to digoxin's electrophysiologic effects may be related to the patient's clinical status since most patients with stable, chronic atrial fibrillation were well controlled with serum concentrations less than 2.0 ng/ml; whereas, most patients who were not controlled with therapeutic serum concentrations had acute or chronic atrial fibrillation with unstable conditions such as postoperative state, sepsis or pulmonary embolism (82). It is suggested that the decreased sensitivity seen in these seriously ill patients was related to an increased release of circulating beta-adrenergic stimulators. Of further note is a case report of a patient with hypocalcemia (6.7 mg%) and atrial fibrillation who was refractory to serum digoxin concentrations between 1.5 and 3.0 ng/ml (83). When the hypocalcemia was corrected, the ventricular rate dropped from 160/min to 80/min, despite no change in serum digoxin concentration.

Hyperthyroid patients are notoriously resistant to digoxin while hypothyroid patients appear extremely sensitive. Although several investigators have studied this phenomenon, the mechanism of interaction still remains controversial. Croxson and Ibbertson (84) observed significantly (p < 0.001) higher steady-state serum concentrations of digoxin in 16 hypothyroid patients as compared to 17 hyperthyroid patients. Creatinine clearance differed significantly (p < 0.01) between groups and correlated highly (r = 0.94) with digoxin renal clearance suggesting slightly altered renal elimination in thyroid disease. Malabsorption may also be partially responsible for differing serum concentrations (85). One hyperthyroid patient, who presented with hyperactive bowel sounds, was noted to absorb only 40% of orally administered digoxin (86). This could suggest decreased absorption in hyperthyroidism; healthy patients, however, have also been reported to absorb as little as 40% (12). It is interesting to note that if the fraction of dose absorbed is reduced to 0.4 for the hyperthyroid patients in the study by Croxson and Ibbertson (84), the difference between the estimated mean total clearance and renal clearance is the same (approximately 95 ml/min) for both hyper- and hypothyroid patients. Lawrence et al (87) found no consistent difference in either absorption or clearance between nine hyperthyroid and four hypothyroid patients with varying degrees of altered thyroid function. Renal function did improve dramatically when two patients with primary hypothyroidism became euthyroid; however, no change in renal function was seen when the hyperthyroid patients became euthyroid. Nonrenal clearance varied from 109 ml/min in a 34-year-old, moderately thyrotoxic patient to only 7 ml/min in a 65-year-old hyperthyroid patient with atrial fibrillation. One finding common to most studies is an increased volume of distribution in hyperthyroidism (reduced in hypothyroidism) which might be related to increased tissue $(Na^+, K^+)$-ATPase activity (73,87). At best, one can say that patients with thyroid disease usually have an altered response to digoxin, the etiology of which may vary from patient to patient depending on the severity of the disease and the presence of other underlying diseases.

## CLINICAL APPLICATION OF PHARMACOKINETIC DATA

### Maintenance Dose

The relationship between steady-state serum concentration $(\bar{C})$, maintenance dose $(X_o/day)$ and total body clearance $(Cl_B)$ is shown in Equation 1 where F is the fraction of the dose absorbed and $\tau$ is the dosing interval:

$$\bar{C}(ng/ml) = \frac{X_o\ (mg/day) \cdot 10^6 \cdot F}{Cl_B(ml/min) \cdot \tau(min)}$$ (Eq. 1)

For patients with no evidence of altered bioavailability (see Absorption), F can be assumed to be 0.68 for tablets and 0.77 for elixir. Equation 1 can then be rearranged and written as follows:

$$X_o\ (mg/day) = \frac{\bar{C}(ng/ml) \cdot Cl_B(ml/min)}{P_c}$$ (Eq. 2)

where $P_c$ is a proportionality constant and equals 472 for tablets, 535 for elixir, and 694 for intravenous administration.

Total body clearance ($Cl_B$) is a composite of renal clearance ($Cl_R$) and nonrenal clearance ($Cl_M$). Koup et al (34) have described the relationship between these clearances as:

$$Cl_B(ml/min/1.73m^2) = 1.101 \cdot Cl_R(ml/min/1.73m^2) + Cl_M(ml/min/1.73m^2)$$
$$(Eq.\ 3)$$

where $Cl_M$ equals 36 in patients with resolved or no history of congestive heart failure and equals 20 in patients with severe congestive heart failure. A reduction in $Cl_M$ would also apply to patients receiving either quinidine or high doses of spironolactone.

Digoxin renal clearance can be determined from a urine sample collected during the last 12 hours of a 24 hour dosing interval and a serum sample drawn midpoint in the urine collection period. Renal clearance is calculated using Equation 4:

$$Cl_R(ml/min) = \frac{\text{Urine concentration (ng/ml)} \cdot \text{urine vol. (ml)}}{720\ min \cdot C\ midpoint\ (ng/ml)} \quad (Eq.\ 4)$$

Urine concentration of digoxin can be determined by diluting a portion of urine to a concentration of approximately 3.0 to 5.0 ng/nl and then assaying a mixture of one milliliter each of diluted urine and digoxin-free plasma. To properly dilute the urine portion, an initial estimate of urine digoxin concentration can be made from the patient's estimated creatinine clearance (88) and rearrangement of Equation 4. Use of Equations 1 through 4 has been shown to account for 85% of the variance in serum digoxin concentrations of 16 patients with varying degrees of renal function (34).

Digoxin renal clearance is reported to be similar to creatinine clearance. Figure 2 shows the relationship between creatinine and digoxin renal clearances for 44 hospitalized patients (unpublished observations) with congestive heart failure. Both clearances were determined from one 24 hour urine collection for each patient. Digoxin concentrations in the serum and urine were assayed by radioimmunoassay (RIA) using a common commercial kit. Lean body weight (89) was used to determine body surface area in patients whose actual weight was greater than ideal body weight.

Patient characteristics are noted in Table 3. Visual inspection of the scatterplot shows that many of the patients with a digoxin renal clearance less than creatinine clearance were either receiving quinidine or were hypokalemic (values of 2.8 mEq/L and 3.1 mEq/L). Other sources of variance include renal tubular mechanisms and possibly the percentage (reported as 0 to 32%) of hydrolytic products in the urine. Since these metabolites are measured by RIA (see Assay Methods) and their half-life is shorter than the half-life for digoxin, it is possible that actual digoxin renal clearance is overestimated in some patients.

The nomogram of Siersback-Nielsen et al (88) can be used to estimate creatinine clearance ($Cl_{cr}$) from serum creatinine when a urine collection is not available. The relationship between estimated $Cl_{cr}$ and digoxin renal clearance ($Cl_R$) is shown in Figure 3 for those patients (Table 3) who were neither hypokalemic nor receiving quinidine. Lean body weight (89) was used in the nomogram and again for body surface area. As shown in Figure 3, $Cl_R$ was usually overpredicted by estimated creatinine clearance in patients with severe congestive heart failure. Spurious values may have resulted from the inappropriate use of the nomogram. An assumption for its use is that the patient's renal function is stable; however, renal function in congestive heart failure patients may improve during the course of hospital treatment. When renal function is changing, $Cl_{cr}$ should be estimated by the method proposed by Jelliffe and Jelliffe (90).

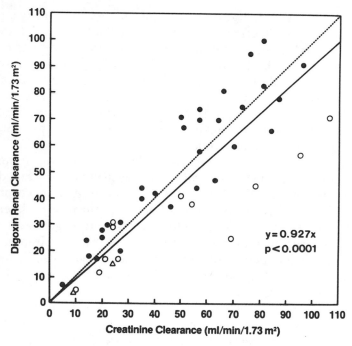

FIGURE 2. Relationship between Creatinine and Digoxin Renal Clearance in 44 Patients. Open circles depict patients receiving quinidine; triangles denote hypokalemic patients. The intercept in the regression equation (solid line) is set at zero. Dashed line is at 45° for reference only and is not a regression line.

Dobbs et al (91) have reported a relationship between total body clearance of digoxin and creatinine clearance (Equation 5) which is remarkably similar to that shown in Equation 3.

$$Cl_B = 1.104 \cdot Cl_{cr} + 28.9 \qquad \text{(Eq. 5)}$$

The study consisted of 51 patients with varying degrees of renal function and cardiac failure. In determining the regression line, estimations of $Cl_{cr}$ from the nomogram of Siersback-Nielsen (88) were used for 31 patients with mild cardiac failure and estimated clearances (mean 55.4 ml/min ± 6.8 SEM) similar to the measured values (mean 55.2 ml/min ± 6.5 SEM). Measured $Cl_{cr}$ was used for 20 patients with severe congestive heart failure. Evaluation of Equation 5 showed that digoxin doses were usually overpredicted in patients with severe cardiac failure. This supports the observations in Figure 3, and the findings of Halkin et al (62). The similarity between the slopes in Equation 3 and 5 suggests that creatinine and digoxin renal clearances share the same relationship to $Cl_B$. Furthermore, the intercept value of 28.9 is almost exactly midway between the range for $Cl_M$ in Equation 3.

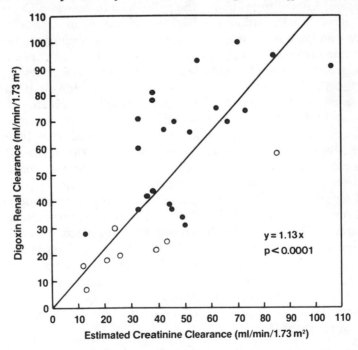

FIGURE 3. Relationship between Estimated Creatinine and Digoxin Renal Clearance in 30 Patients. Circles depict patients in functional Class IV. The intercept in the regression equation is set at zero.

TABLE 3. CHARACTERISTICS OF PATIENTS IN FIGURE 2

| Age (Years) | Sex | Serum Creatinine | NYHA[+] | Serum Albumin |
|---|---|---|---|---|
| Mean 67 | M 23 | Mean 1.71 mg% | (I-II) 14 | Mean 3.8 gm/dl |
| SD ± 11.9 | F 21 | SD ± 1.15 mg% | (III-IV) 30 | SD ± 0.53 gm/dl |

+ New York Heart Association's Classification

This intermediate value would be expected since patients with severe heart failure comprised 40% of the study sample. It should be noted that Equation 5 is estimated to account for 67% of variance in dosage requirements, whereas use of measured digoxin renal clearances and Equation 3 accounted for 85% of variance.

Although prediction of $Cl_B$ is improved when digoxin renal clearance is used, the requisite procedure of urine collection is not always practical. In these cases, creatinine clearance can be estimated from serum creatinine and then adjusted based on the presence of factors (see Excretion) known to influence the relationship between $Cl_{cr}$ and $Cl_R$. Most patients with either resolved or no history of congestive heart failure should have a digoxin renal clearance slightly higher than creatinine clearance. In patients with more advanced cardiac failure and signs of prerenal azotemia, digoxin renal clearance would be expected to be less than creatinine clearance. Many patients with mild to moderate congestive heart failure will conceivably have evidence of both tubular secretion and mild tubular reabsorption. It might be assumed that these latter patients would show little difference between creatinine and digoxin renal clearance. Based on the above considerations, the adjusted value of $Cl_{cr}$ can be used as $Cl_R$ in Equation 3 to determine $Cl_B$. Reduction in $Cl_M$ should probably be based on clinical evidence of right-sided failure. This is supported by the observation that cardiac failure patients categorized as severe in the study by Dobbs et al (91) had moderate to gross edema and marked hepatomegaly and distention of the jugular vein. The derived value for $Cl_B$ should be reduced in patients receiving quinidine and spironolactone (200 mg daily) by 35% and 25%, respectively.

In patients under stable conditions where F, $Cl_B$ and $\tau$ in Equation 1 remain fixed, the ratio of dose to steady-state serum concentration equals a constant ($P_x$):

$$\frac{X_o}{\bar{C}} = P_x \qquad \text{(Eq. 6)}$$

To change the steady-state serum concentration, the new dose is equal to the product of the desired $\bar{C}$ and $P_x$. Although convenient, the proper use of this ratio requires that the assumption of stable conditions be met. The first and probably most difficult task in verifying this assumption is determining if the patient has complied to the prescribed schedule (fixed $\tau$). Noncompliance is a common occurrence with digoxin (92) and obviously distorts the ratio of dose to serum concentration. In addition, some patients who are normally compliant may omit their dose on the day of admission to a hospital, and thus, a serum determination on the following day would not reflect $\bar{C}$. Of the various sources of variance in F (see Absorption), the concurrent administration of antacids probably occurs most commonly. Influences on $Cl_B$ are discussed above.

### Loading Dose

An approximation of loading dose $(X_o^*)$ can be calculated from lean body weight (LBW) with an appropriate reduction in the dose based on renal function. In patients with normal renal function, an average amount of digoxin in the body at steady-state $(\bar{X})$ of 0.008 to 0.01 mg/kg (LBW) and 0.011 to 0.013 mg/kg (LBW) should result in an average serum concentration of 1.0 to 1.4 ng/ml and 1.6 to 2.0 ng/ml, respectively (93). For patients with diminished renal function, $X_o^*$ should be reduced in accordance with reduction in volume of distribution. For digoxin, $V_{ss}$ can be assumed to be the same as $V_D$ (34). Jusko et al (56) have defined $V_D$ as a function of creatinine clearance using a Michaelis-Menten-type equation. The relationship is:

$$V_D(L/1.73m^2) = V_A + \frac{V_N \cdot Cl_{cr}(ml/min/1.73m^2)}{K_D + Cl_{cr}(ml/min/1.73m^2)} \qquad (Eq.\ 7)$$

where $V_A$ equals 225 liters/1.73m$^2$, $V_N$ equals 298 liters/1.73m$^2$ and $K_D$ equals 29.1 ml/min/1.73m$^2$. Loading dose can then be determined from Equation 8:

$$X_o^* (mg) = \frac{desired\ \bar{X}(mg) \cdot V_D(liters)}{450\ liters} \qquad (Eq.\ 8)$$

Thus, the loading dose in a patient with a creatinine clearance of 10 ml/min or less would be about 65% that of a patient with normal renal function and similar lean body weight. This is in agreement with the data of Reuning et al (32). No reduction in loading dose is necessary in patients with a creatinine clearance greater than 80 to 90 ml/min/1.73 m$^2$.

Since:

$$\beta(min^{-1}) = \frac{Cl_B(ml/min)}{V_D(ml)} \qquad (Eq.\ 9)$$

and,

$$X_o^* = \frac{X_o}{1 - e^{-\beta t}} \qquad \text{(Eq. 10)}$$

loading dose can also be determined from an estimate of $Cl_B$ (Equation 3), $X_o$ (Equation 2) and $V_D$ (Equation 7). The loading dose calculated from Equation 8 is for intravenous administration and should be divided by 0.68 for oral administration. Conversely, when $X_o^*$ in Equation 10 is for oral administration its value should be multiplied by 0.68 when given intravenously. It is recommended that loading dose be given in three divided doses about 5 to 6 hours apart. Further reduction in loading dose is necessary in patients who are hypothyroid or receiving either quinidine or spironolactone.

## When to Obtain Blood Samples

The relationship (32,34) between serum concentration (C) and time (t) after intravenous administration is shown in Figure 4 and is expressed as:

$$C = R_1 e^{-\alpha t} + R_2 e^{-\beta t} \qquad \text{(Eq. 11)}$$

where $R_1 e^{-\alpha t}$ primarily represents initial distribution of digoxin from central to peripheral compartment and $R_2 e^{-\beta t}$ represents elimination from the central compartment. Upon completion of the initial distribution phase ($R_1 e^{-\alpha t} = 0$), the slope of the curve becomes $\beta$ which equals the product of the elimination rate constant and the fraction of digoxin in the central compartment.

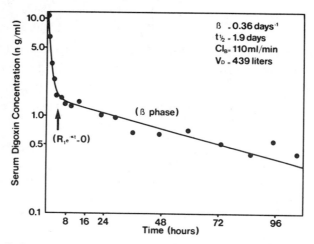

FIGURE 4. Relationship between serum digoxin concentration and time following a 1.0 mg intravenous dose. Adapted from Kleijn E. et al, Clinical Pharmacokinetics of Digoxin, in *Plasma Digitalis Concentration and Digitalis Therapy*, edited by Godfraind T, Editions Arscia, Brussels, 1977.

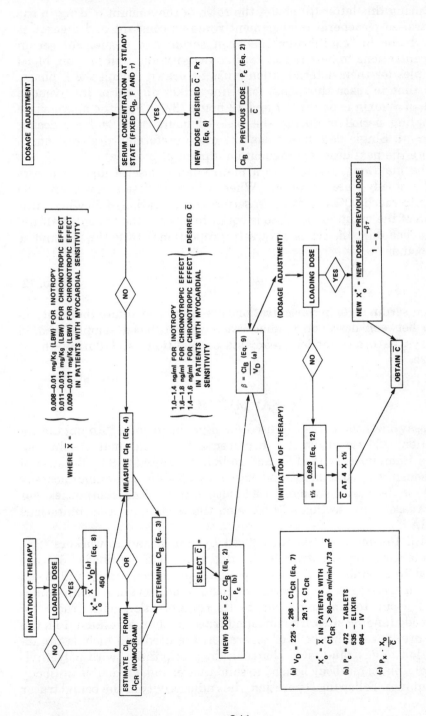

FIGURE 5. Algorithm for the application of pharmacokinetics to digoxin therapy.

341

During this latter (β) phase, the ratio of the amount of drug in the central to peripheral compartment remains constant and digoxin is said to be in "equilibrium" between serum and tissue. For serum concentrations to best reflect cardiac activity and elimination, blood samples for their determination must be drawn during the β phase. The time to reach this phase following either an oral or intravenous dose of digoxin is between 7 and 12 hours (32). Thus, the appropriate sampling period is during the last 12 hours of a 24 hour dosing interval. Single determinations are more preferably drawn 6 hours before the next dose (approximate midpoint of β phase).

The maximum response to a maintenance dose of digoxin occurs under steady-state conditions. When a loading dose is not given, the time to reach 90% steady-state serum concentrations following initiation of the maintenance dose is equal to 4 times the biologic half-life ($t\frac{1}{2}$). For digoxin, $t\frac{1}{2}$ is inversely proportional to β (Eq. 9) and is defined as:

$$t\frac{1}{2} = \frac{0.693}{\beta} \qquad \text{(Eq. 12)}$$

When serum digoxin concentrations are used to evaluate the relationship between dose and cardiac response, the blood samples should always be drawn under steady-state conditions and during the β phase.

## ASSAY METHODS

Assay methods currently used for digoxin include [86]Rb-uptake inhibition, ATPase enzymatic displacement, gas chromatography, enzyme immunoassay (EMIT) and radioimmunoassay (94). Because of its sensitivity, specificity and speed (81,95–96), radioimmunoassay (RIA) is the most commonly used method in clinical laboratories. For this reason, this section will focus on the techniques and limitations of RIA.

With the method first introduced by Smith and co-workers (95), radiolabeled digoxin (tracer) and digoxin-specific antibody (81) are added to a buffered solution of patient serum containing unlabeled digoxin. During a short period of incubation, serum digoxin (unlabeled) competes in proportion to its concentration with tracer for antibody binding sites. The unbound tracer is then separated from the mixture. Several methods of separation are used and include (a) adsorption to dextran-coated charcoal; (b) precipitation with polyethylene glycol; (c) antibody bonded to solid phase; and, (d) double antibody techniques. Following separation, the radioactivity of the bound tracer is counted and compared to a standard curve to determine the serum concentration of unlabeled digoxin. The more tracer that is bound, the higher the count, and thus, the lower the serum digoxin concentration of the patient.

Several RIA kits are now commercially available. Depending on the kit, results are usually ready in less than three hours. The necessary sample size is extremely small (0.1 ml of serum) and the assay can accurately measure concentrations as low as 0.5 ng/ml (97).

Commercial kits use either tritium (beta-emitting) or radioactive iodine (gamma-emitting) as the tracer. Comparison of 11 different kits showed a range in the percentage of digoxin recovery (accuracy) of 91% to 104% for five kits with tritium-labeled tracer and 85% to 101% for six kits with $^{125}$I label (97). Precision within each assay as determined by the coefficient of variation for low therapeutic to high therapeutic concentrations ranged from an average of 11.1% to 7.4% for the tritium-labeled kits and from 11.4% to 8.8% for the iodine-labeled kits. It should be noted that the iodinated kits showed greater variation from kit to kit than did the tritium kits.

Various conditions are known to alter assay results (98). Beta counting of the tritium label, which requires a liquid scintillation system, is subject to interference by both chemiluminescence from serum of uremic patients (underestimation) and color quenching (overestimation) from hyperbilirubinemia and products of hemolysis (98). These errors are not seen with a gamma counting technique. Diagnostic tests (e.g., liver and lung studies) which use a gamma-emitting radioisotope will interfere with the assay whether gamma or liquid scintillation counting techniques are used (98). Hypoalbuminemia is associated with an increase in binding of both tracers to the antibody (98–99). Falsely low or high results may occur depending on whether the patient's sample or pooled serum for preparation of standard curves is hypoalbuminemic (99–100). This effect apparently varies not only between commercial kits, but between patients as well. Antibody binding of a common $^{125}$I-labeled tracer, 3-0-succinyl-digoxigenin-$^{125}$I-labeled tyrosine, has been shown to be significantly (p < 0.01) higher in patients with low serum concentration of thyroxine (101). No effect on binding was seen when $^{125}$I-labeled tyrosine-methyl-ester-digoxin was used as the tracer.

Although antibodies show a high specificity for digoxin, compounds with a similar molecular structure such as digoxin metabolites and other cardenolides may cross-react with the antibody. Digoxigenin and its two digitoxisides have a binding affinity for antibody similar to that of digoxin (102). This should not influence the clinical interpretation of serum digoxin concentrations since these metabolites are cardioactive and are not present to any appreciable extent in serum. Dihydrodigoxin has been shown to cross-react with digoxin antibody; however, the degree of cross-reactivity varied (0 to ⅓) between commercial kits (103). Serum concentrations of dihydrodigoxin (cardoinactive) may be as high as 1.6 ng/ml (52) in some patients, making serum digoxin concentrations difficult to interpret when kits with a high degree of cross-reactivity are used. Deslanoside is capable of binding to the antibody to the same extent as digoxin, whereas, the average percentage of cross reactivity with digitoxin is only 11% (95,104). Spironolactone and physiologic steroids apparently do not cross react even when present in extremely high amounts (95,104).

Because of interference problems associated with the tritium label, RIA kits using radioactive iodine may be preferable. In addition, gamma counting techniques are quicker and less costly. Problems with separation may be reduced with kits using a solid phase or double-antibody technique. More recently, a homogeneous enzyme immunoassay method of digoxin assay has been introduced which eliminates the need for separation (105). This method also offers the speed, specificity and sensitivity of radioimmunoassay (105–106). Although interference from gamma-emitting radioisotopes is not seen with enzyme immunoassay, digoxin metabolites and other cardiac glycosides will cross react. Although the digoxin EMIT assay differs from other EMIT procedures by being a batch method, it can still be completed in about one hour. General statements about specificity may or may not apply to a specific kit for either radioimmunoassay or enzyme immunoassay. For example, a common radioimmunoassay kit used by our laboratory reports a 1.03% cross reactivity for digitoxin. Information on antibody specificity and affinity constants should be obtained from the manufacturer of each kit; however, even then, unsuspected interferences may occur since specificity may vary between lots from the same manufacturer (96).

## ACKNOWLEDGMENTS

The author is indebted to Dr. William Jusko and Dr. Bruce Martin for their support in developing a pharmacokinetic service at Mercy Hospital of Pittsburgh; to Dr. Jeanne Cooper and Dr. Arthur Katoh for providing laboratory facilities; to Dr. Thomas Strauss for assistance in preparing the section on assay; and to Ms. Linda Mascara Livengood for typing the manuscript.

# REFERENCES

1. Greenberger NJ and Caldwell JH: Studies on the intestinal absorption of [3]H-digitalis glycosides in experimental animals and man, in *Basic and Clinical Pharmacology of Digitalis,* edited by Marks BH, Weissler AM, Springfield, Illinois, Charles C. Thomas, 1972.
2. Beerman B, Hellstrom K and Rosen A: The absorption of orally administered [12α - [3]H] digoxin in man. Clin Sci 1972; 43:507–518.
3. Jelliffe RW: A mathematical analysis of digitalis kinetics in patients with normal and reduced renal function. Math Biosci 1967; 1:305–325.
4. Greenblatt DJ, Smith TW and Koch-Weser J: Bioavailability of drugs: the digoxin dilemma. Clin Pharmacokinet 1976; 1:36–51.
5. Shaw TRD, Raymond K, Howard MR and Hamer J: Therapeutic non-equivalence of digoxin tablets in the United Kingdom: correlation with tablet dissolution rate. Br Med J 1973; 4:763–766.
6. Lindenbaum J, Butler VP, Murphy JE and Cresswell RM: Correlation of digoxin-tablet dissolution-rate with biological availability. Lancet 1973; 1:1215–1217.
7. Binnion PF: The absorption of digoxin tablets. Clin Pharmacol Ther 1974; 16:807–812.
8. Colaizzi JL: Bioavailability monograph—digoxin. J Am Pharm Assoc 1977; 17:635–638.
9. Marcus FI, Dickerson J, Pippin S, Stafford M and Bressler R: Digoxin bioavailability: formulations and rates of infusions. Clin Pharmacol Ther 1976; 20:253–259.
10. Stoll RG and Wagner JG: Intravenous digoxin as a bioavailability standard. Clin Pharmacol Ther 1975; 17:117–118.
11. Huffman DH, Manion CV and Azarnoff DL: Absorption of digoxin from different oral preparations in normal subjects during steady state. Clin Pharmacol Ther 1974; 16:310–317.
12. Johnson BF and Bye C: Maximal intestinal absorption of digoxin and its relation to steady state plasma concentration. Br Heart J 1975; 37:203–208.
13. Manninen V, Reissel P and Ojala K: Maximal bioavailability of digoxin from tablets and oral solution in steady state. Acta Med Scand 1976; 199:487–489.
14. Mallis GI, Schmidt DH, and Lindenbaum J: Superior bioavailability of digoxin solution in capsules. Clin Pharmacol Ther 1975; 18:761–768.
15. Manninen V, Melin J, Apajalahti A, and Karesoja M: Altered absorption of digoxin in patients given propantheline and metoclopramide. Lancet 1973; 1:398–400.
16. Manninen V, Apajalahti A, Simonen H and Reissel P: Effect of propantheline and metoclopramide on absorption of digoxin. Lancet 1973; 1:1118–1119.
17. Kolibash AJ, Kramer WG, Reuning RH and Caldwell JH: Marked decline in serum digoxin concentrations during an episode of severe diarrhea. Am Heart J 1977; 94:806–807.
18. Heizer WD, Smith TW, Goldfinger SE: Absorption of digoxin in patients with malabsorption syndrome. N Engl J Med 1971; 285:257–259.
19. Marcus FI, Quinn EJ, Horton H, Jacobs S, Pippin S, Stafford M and Zukoski C: The effect of jejunoileal bypass on the pharmacokinetics of digoxin in man. Circulation 1977; 55:537–541.
20. Sokol GH, Greenblatt DJ, Lloyd BL, Georgotas A, Allen MD, Harmatz JS, Smith TW and Shader RI: Effect of abdominal radiation therapy on drug absorption in humans. J Clin Pharmacol 1978; 18:388–396.
21. Jusko WJ, Conti DR, Molson A, Puritsky P, Giller J and Schultz RW: Digoxin absorption from tablets and elixir: the effect of radiation-induced malabsorption. JAMA 1974; 230:1554–1555.

22. Hall WH, Doherty JE, Gammill J, Sherwood J: Tritiated digoxin XXII: absorption and excretion in malabsorption syndromes. Am J Med 1974; 56:437–442.

23. Beermann B, Hellstrom K, Rosen A: The gastrointestinal absorption of digoxin in seven patients with gastric or small intestinal reconstructions. Acta Med Scand 1973; 193:293–297.

24. Johnson BF, O'Grady J, Sabey GA, Bye C: Effect of standard breakfast on digoxin absorption in normal subjects. Clin Pharmacol Therp 1978; 23:315.

25. Brown DD, Juhl RP, Warner SL: Decreased bioavailability of digoxin due to hypocholesterolemic intervention. Circulation 1978; 58:164–172.

26. Brown DD, Juhl RP: Decreased bioavailability of digoxin due to antacids and kaolin-pectin. N Engl J Med 1976; 295:1034–1037.

27. Albert KS, Ayres JW, DiSanto AR, Weidler DJ, Sakmar E, Hallmark MR, Stoll RG, DeSante KA and Wagner JG: Influences of kaolin-pectin suspension on digoxin bioavailability. J Pharm Sci 1978; 67:1582–1586.

28. Juhl RP, Summers RW, Guillary JK, Blang SM, Cheng FH and Brown DD: Effect of sulfasalazine on digoxin bioavailability. Clin Pharmacol Ther 1976; 20:387–394.

29. Lindenbaum J, Maulitz RM and Butler VP: Inhibition of digoxin absorption by neomycin. Gastroenterology 1976; 71:399–404.

30. Cusack B, Kelly J, O'Malley K, Noel J, Lavan J and Hargan J: Digoxin in the elderly: pharmacokinetic consequences of old age. Clin Pharmacol Ther 1979; 25:772–776.

31. Benowitz NL, Meister W: Pharmacokinetics in patients with cardiac failure. Clin Pharmacokinet 1976; 1:389–405.

32. Reuning RH, Sams RA, Notari RE: Role of pharmacokinetics in drug dosage adjustment. I. Pharmacologic effect kinetics and apparent volume of distribution of digoxin. J Clin Pharmacol 1973; 13:127–141.

33. Koup Jr, Greenblatt DJ, Jusko WJ, Smith TW and Koch-Weser J: Pharmacokinetics of digoxin in normal subjects after intravenous bolus and infusion doses. J Pharmacokinet Biopharm 1975; 3:181–192.

34. Koup JR, Jusko WJ, Elwood CM, Kohli RK: Digoxin pharmacokinetics: role of renal failure in dosage regimen design. Clin Pharmacol Ther 1975; 18:9–21.

35. Storstein L and Janssen H: Studies on digitalis. VI. The effect of heparin on serum protein binding of digitoxin and digoxin. Clin Pharmacol Ther 1976; 20:15–23.

36. Lukas DS and DeMartino AG: Binding of digitoxin and some related cardenolides to human plasma proteins. J Clin Invest 1969; 48:1041–1053.

37. Doherty JE, Perkins WH, Flanigan WJ: The distribution and concentration of tritiated digoxin in human tissues. Ann Intern Med 1967; 66:116–124.

38. Gullner HG, Stinson EB, Harrison DC and Kalman SM: Correlation of serum concentrations with heart concentrations of digoxin in human subjects. Circulation 1974; 50:653–655.

39. Hartel G, Kyllonen K, Merikallio E, Ojala K, Manninen V and Reissel R: Human serum and myocardium digoxin. Clin Pharmacol Ther 1976; 19:153–157.

40. Jusko WJ and Weintraub M: Myocardial distribution of digoxin and renal function. Clin Pharmacol Ther 1974; 16:449–454.

41. Coltart DJ, Gullner HG, Billingham M, Goldman RH, Stinson EB, Kalman SM and Harrison DC: Physiological distribution of digoxin in human heart. Br Med J 1974; 4:733–736.

42. Ewy GA, Groves BM, Ball MF, Nimmo L, Jackson B and Marcus F: Digoxin metabolism in obesity. Circulation 1971; 44:810–814.

43. Doherty JE: Metabolism of digitalis in man, in *Basic and Clinical Pharmacology of Digitalis,* edited by Marks BH, Weissler A. Springfield, Illinois, Charles C. Thomas, Pub., 1972.

44. Lukas DS: Some aspects of the distribution and disposition of digitoxin in man. Ann NY Acad Sci 1971; 179:339–361.
45. Doherty JE, Flanigan WJ, Murphy ML et al: Tritiated digoxin XIV. Enterohepatic circulation, absorption and excretion studies in human volunteers. Circulation 1970; 42:867–873.
46. Marcus FI, Burkhalter L, Cuccia, C et al: Administration of tritiated digoxin with and without a loading dose. Circulation 1966; 34:865–874.
47. Gault MH, Charles JD, Sugden DL, Kepkay DC: Hydrolysis of digoxin by acid. J Pharm Pharmac 1977; 29:27–32.
48. Clark DR, Kalman SM: Dihydrodigoxin: A common metabolite of digoxin in man. Drug Metabolism Disposition 1974; 2:148–150.
49. Marcus FI, Kapadia GJ, Kapadia GG: The metabolism of digoxin in normal subjects. J Pharmacol Exp Ther 1964; 145:203–209.
50. Caldwell JH, Cline CT: Biliary excretion of digoxin in man. Clin Pharmacol Ther 1976; 19:410–415.
51. Marcus FI, Peterson A, Salel A et al: The metabolism of tritiated digoxin in renal insufficiency in dogs and man. J Pharmacol Exp Ther 1966; 152:372–382.
52. Peters U, Falk LC, Kalman SM: Digoxin metabolism in patients. Arch Intern Med 1978; 138:1074–1076.
53. Lage GL, Spratt JL: Structure-activity correlation of the lethality and central effects of selected cardiac glycosides. J Pharmacol Exp Ther 1966; 152:501–508.
54. Brown BT, Stafford A, Wright SE: Chemical structure and pharmacological activity of some derivatives of digitoxigenin and digoxigenin. Br J Pharmacol 1962; 18:311–324.
55. Bach EJ, Reiter M: The difference in velocity between the lethal and inotropic action of dihydrodigoxin. Arch Exp Path Pharmak 1964; 248:437–449.
56. Jusko WJ, Szelfer SJ and Goldfarb AL: Pharmacokinetic design of digoxin dosage regimens in relation to renal function. J Clin Pharmacol 1974; 14:525–535.
57. Ewy GA, Kapadia GG, Yao L, Lullin M, Marcus FI: Digoxin metabolism in the elderly. Circulation 1969; 39:449–453.
58. Steiness E: Renal tubular secretion of digoxin. Circulation 1974; 50:103–107.
59. Baylis EM, Hall MS, Lewis G, Marks V: Effects of renal function on plasma digoxin levels in elderly ambulant patients in domiciliary practice. Br Med J 1972; 1:338–341.
60. Waldorf S, Anderson JD, Heeboll-Nielsen N, Nielsen OG, Moltke E, Sorensen U, Steiness E: Spironolactone-induced changes in digoxin kinetics. Clin Pharmacol Ther 1978; 24:162–167.
61. Bennett WM, Porter GA: Endogenous creatinine clearance as a clinical measure of glomerular filtration rate. Br Med J 1971; 4:84–86.
62. Halkin H, Sheiner LB, Peck CC, Melmon KL: Determinants of the renal clearances of digoxin. Clin Pharmacol Ther 1975; 17:385–394.
63. McAllister RG, Howell SM, Gomer MS, Selby JB: Effect of intravenous furosemide on the renal excretion of digoxin. J Clin Pharmacol 1976; 16:110–117.
64. Brown DD, Dormois JC, Abraham GN: Effect of furosemide on the renal excretion of digoxin. Clin Pharmacol Ther 1976; 20:395–400.
65. Duarte JE: Digoxin kinetics during furosemide administration. Clin Pharmacol Ther 1977; 21:567–574.
66. Steiness E: Suppression of renal excretion of digoxin in hypokalemic patients. Clin Pharmacol Ther 1978; 23:511–514.
67. Hager WD, Fenster P, Mayersohn M, Perrier D, Graves P, Marcus F, Goldman S: Digoxin-quinidine interaction: pharmacokinetic evaluation. N Engl J Med 1979; 300:1238–1241.

68. Gault MH, Sugden D, Maloney C, Ahmed M and Tweeddale M: Biotransformation and elimination of digoxin with normal and minimal renal function. Clin Pharmacol Ther 1979; 25:499–513.
69. Smith TW, Haber E: Digitalis (first of four parts). N Engl J Med 1973; 289:945–1010.
70. Marks BH: Factors that affect the accumulation of digitalis glycosides by the heart, in *Basic and Clinical Pharmacology of Digitalis,* edited by Marks BH, Weissler AM, Springfield, Illinois, Charles C. Thomas, 1972.
71. Hoeschen RJ, Cuddy TE: Dose-response relation between therapeutic levels of serum digoxin and systolic time intervals. Am J Cardiol 1975; 35:469–472.
72. Redfors A: Plasma digoxin concentration—its relation to digoxin dosage and clinical effects in patients with atrial fibrillation. Br Heart J 1972; 34:383–391.
73. Smith TW: Digitalis toxicity: epidemiology and clinical use of serum concentration measurements. Am J Med 1975; 58:470–476.
74. Huffman DH, Crow JW, Pentikainen P, Azarnoff DL: Association between clinical cardiac status, laboratory parameters and digoxin usage. Am Heart J 1976; 91:28–34.
75. Smith TW, Haber E: Digoxin intoxication: the relationship of clinical presentation to serum digoxin concentration. J Clin Invest 1970; 49:2377–2386.
76. Chamberlain DA, White RJ, Howard MR, Smith TW: Plasma digoxin concentration in patients with atrial fibrillation. Br Med J 1970; 3:429–432.
77. Dobbs SM, Rodgers EM, Kenyon WI, Livskin D, Slater E, Godsmark B: Digoxin prescribing in perspective. Br J Clin Pharmacol 1977; 4:327–335.
78. Beller GA, Smith TW, Abelmann WH, Haber E, Hood WB: Digitalis intoxication, a prospective clinical study with serum level correlation. N Engl J Med 1971; 284:989–997.
79. Steiness E, Olesen KH: Cardiac arrhythmias induced by hypokalemia and potassium loss during maintenance digoxin therapy. Br Heart J 1976; 38:167–172.
80. Brater DC, Morrelli HF: Digixon toxicity in patients with normokalemic potassium depletion. Clin Pharmacol Ther 1977; 22:21–33.
81. Butler VP, Lindenbaum J: Serum digitalis measurements in the assessment of digitalis resistance and sensitivity. Am J Med 1975; 58:460–469.
82. Goldman S, Probst P, Selzer A, Cohn K: Inefficacy of therapeutic serum levels of digoxin in controlling the ventricular rate in atrial fibrillation. Am J Cardiol 1975; 35:651–655.
83. Chapra D, Janson PJ, Sawin CT: Insensitivity to digoxin associated with hypocalcemia. N Engl J Med 1977; 296:917–918.
84. Croxson MS, Ibbertson HK: Serum digoxin in patients with thyroid disease. Br Med J 1975; 3:566–568.
85. Watters K, Tomkin GH: Serum digoxin in patients with thyroid disease. Br Med J 1975; 4:102.
86. Huffman DH, Klaassen CD, Hartman CR: Digoxin in hyperthyroidism. Clin Pharmacol Ther 1977; 22:533–538.
87. Lawrence JR, Summer DJ, Kalk WJ, Ratcliffe WA, Whiting B, Gray K, Lindsay M: Digoxin kinetics in patients with thyroid dysfunction. Clin Pharmacol Ther 1977; 22:7–13.
88. Siersbaek-Nielsen K, Hansen JM, Kampmann J, Kristensen M: Rapid evaluation of creatinine clearance. Lancet 1971; I:1133–1134.
89. Diem K, Lentner C: *Documenta Geigy Scientific Tables,* 7th ed., Basel, Switzerland, JR Geigy, 1974, p 712.

90. Jelliffe RW, Jelliffe SM: A computer program for estimation of creatinine clearance from unstable serum creatinine levels, age, sex, and weight. Math Biosci 1972; 14:17–24.

91. Dobbs SM, Mawer GE, Rodgers EM, Woodcock BG: Can digoxin dose requirements be predicted? Br J Clin Pharmac 1976; 3:231–237.

92. Weintraub M, Au WY, Lasagna L: Compliance as a determinant of serum digoxin concentration. JAMA 1972; 224:481–485.

93. Jelliffe RW, Buell J, Kalaba R: Reduction of digitalis toxicity by computer-assisted glycoside dosage regimens. Ann Int Med 1972; 77:891–906.

94. Smith TW: Contribution of quantitative assay techniques to the understanding of the clinical pharmacology of digitalis. Circulation 1972; 46:188–199.

95. Smith TW, Butler VP, Haver E: Determination of therapeutic and toxic serum digoxin concentrations by radioimmunoassay. N Engl J Med 1969; 281:1212–1216.

96. Kostenbauder HB, McGovren JP, Perrier DG: Digoxin radioimmunoassay in patient monitoring, in *Clinical Pharmacokinetics*, edited by Levy G, American Pharmaceutical Association, 1974.

97. Kubasik NP, Brody BB, Barold SS: Problems in measurement of serum digoxin by commercially available radioimmunoassay kits. Am J Cardiol 1975; 36:975–977.

98. Cerceo E, Elloso C: Factors affecting the radioimmunoassay of digoxin. Clin Chem 1972; 18:539–543.

99. Voshall DL, Hunter L, Grady HJ: Effect of albumin on serum digoxin radioimmunoassays. Clin Chem 1975; 21:402–406.

100. Kuczala ZJ, Ahluwalia GS: Evaluation of two digoxin radioimmunoassay procedures in which $^{125}$I-labeled digoxin is used. Clin Chem 1976; 22:193–197.

101. Kroening BH, Weintraub M: Reduced variation of tracer binding in digoxin radioimmunoassay by use of $^{125}$I-labeled tyrosine-methyl-ester derivative: Relation of thyroxine concentration to binding. Clin Chem 1976; 22:1732–1734.

102. Greenwood H, Snedden W, Hayward RP, Landon J: The measurement of urinary digoxin and dihydrodigoxin by radioimmunassay and by mass spectroscopy. Clinica Chimica Acta 1975; 62:213–224.

103. Kramer WG, Linnear NL, Morgan HK: Variability among commercially available digoxin radioimmunoassay kits in cross reactivity to dihydrodigoxin. Clin Chem 1978; 24:155–157.

104. Muller H, Brauer H, Resch B: Cross reactivity of digitoxin and sprinolactone in two radioimmunoassays for serum digoxin. Clin Chem 1978; 24:706–709.

105. Rosenthal AF, Vargas MG, Klass CS: Evaluation of enzyme-multiplied immunoassay technique (EMIT) for determination of serum digoxin. Clin Chem 1976; 22:1899–1902.

106. Sun L, Spiehler V: Radioimmunoassay and enzyme immunoassay compared for determination of digoxin. Clin Chem 1976; 22:2029–2031.

# 11

# Lidocaine

John H. Rodman, Pharm.D.

## INTRODUCTION/BACKGROUND

Lidocaine is the most frequently used drug for the initial parenteral therapy of acute ventricular arrhythmias (1). Recent investigations (2,3,4) evaluating the effectiveness of lidocaine in the prevention of primary ventricular fibrillation in acute myocardial infarction have led to recommendations (5) that may markedly increase the use of lidocaine. Lidocaine is also widely used as a local anesthetic and significant systemic absorption often occurs (6). An understanding of lidocaine pharmacokinetics will help to optimize therapy and minimize the risk of toxicity for both of these indications. However, this chapter will focus on lidocaine as an antiarrhythmic agent.

A fundamental prerequisite for the clinical utility of pharmacokinetics is a quantitative, although not necessarily constant, relationship between amount of drug present and effect. Recent reviews (1,7) support such a relationship between both the antiarrhythmic effect and toxicity of lidocaine and its measured blood concentrations. (The term blood concentration, when used here, will refer to whole blood, plasma, or serum measurements interchangeably, and specific note will be made if this distinction is clinically important.)

The need for a more quantitative, pharmacokinetic approach, incorporating the knowledge of a concentration-effect relationship, is determined by the efficacy and toxicity (therapeutic index) of standard dosage regimens. Standard dosage regimens for lidocaine anti-arrhythmic therapy are usually an initial bolus (0.5 to 1.5 mg/kg) followed by a continuous infusion (10 to 50 µg/kg/min). Incremental boluses and increases in infusion rates are given if response to initial therapy is not adequate (1,7). Empirical dosage adjustments are suggested for presence of cardiac or liver disease (8). Using such standard regimens, the incidence of toxicity is about 15% (3,9), even when high risk patients with congestive heart failure, shock, and ventricular

350

tachycardia or fibrillation are excluded (3). The therapeutic failure rate with standard dosage regimens in a large series was 18% (10), even with the administration of two to four supplemental boluses. When blood concentrations were measured in a smaller group of patients (9), 38% were reported as being above or below the generally accepted therapeutic range. Thus, there is strong evidence that more precisely controlled blood concentrations would improve the clinical outcome of lidocaine therapy.

## Absorption

Despite rapid and relatively complete absorption, oral administration of lidocaine is not clinically useful. Sixty to seventy percent of an oral dose is metabolized by the liver before reaching the general circulation (11). Thus, lidocaine blood concentrations in normal volunteers (11) and patients (12) are usually too low to be effective. However, significant toxicity thought to be associated with high metabolite blood concentrations produced from first-pass metabolism is commonly observed (11).

The role of first-pass hepatic metabolism in limiting the bioavailability of lidocaine has been investigated in both dogs (13) and man (14). Bioavailability in nine normal volunteers was estimated to be 39%. Lidocaine concentrations were subtherapeutic, yet central nervous system toxicity was observed. However, in 12 cirrhotic patients and five patients with end-to-side portacaval shunts, bioavailability was greater than 90% (14).

Intramuscular administration of lidocaine avoids the first-pass effect of portal circulation. The ability to achieve potentially therapeutic blood concentrations within 10 to 30 minutes using intramuscular (IM) doses of 200 to 400 mg has been demonstrated in patients and volunteers (16–19). Deltoid muscle administration provides faster absorption than gluteal injections (17–19) or lateral thigh injections (17,18,20). Peak blood concentrations occur at about 10 to 15 minutes with deltoid injections, and usually between 30 and 45 minutes with lateral thigh or gluteal injections. Evidence from an early study (17) suggesting that concentration of the solution injected affects absorption has not been borne out by subsequent work (18,22).

Several uncontrolled studies (20,21,23–25) have shown a reduction in the frequency of ventricular ectopics with the administration of IM lidocaine. In each study, measured blood concentrations correlated reasonably well with the reduction of ectopics. A comparison of 300 mg lidocaine (10% injected in lateral thigh) with an infusion regimen of 75 mg followed by 2 mg/minute suggested the IM and IV regimens were equally effective in controlling the number of ventricular ectopics for the initial 2 hours of therapy (25). It is particularly interesting to note that the IM dose produced significantly higher mean blood concentrations than the IV regimen during the first hour of therapy. A controlled double-blind study (26) in patients with acute myocardial infarction has provided additional evidence for the effectiveness of IM lidocaine in reducing the frequency of ventricular ectopics with minimal toxicity.

Despite the demonstrated effectiveness of IM lidocaine in controlling ventricular ectopics, the exact role of this route of administration remains to be defined. The primary goal in the use of IM lidocaine will most often be the prevention of primary ventricular fibrillation and sudden death in the pre-hospital phase of acute myocardial infarction. A large double-blind, placebo-controlled study using 300 mg of IM lidocaine demonstrated a significant reduction in the frequency of deaths in the first 2 hours after injection (27). However, several major methodological faults have limited extrapolating this study to clinical practice.

In a subsequent study (28), 300 patients with a documented acute myocardial infarction were given 300 mg IM lidocaine or placebo within 6 hours of onset of symptoms and heart rhythm was continuously monitored. Blood concentrations of lidocaine were measured for the first hour. IM lidocaine (deltoid) was no more effective than placebo in preventing ventricular fibrillation. Mean lidocaine concentrations were 1.7 to 1.9 $\mu$g/ml during the first hour. Although these results are discouraging, alternative dosage regimens providing higher blood concentrations may still prove to be useful in the pre-hospital phase of myocardial infarction. Careful consideration of absorption kinetics will be helpful in developing dosage regimens providing potentially therapeutic yet safe lidocaine blood concentrations.

Substantial absorption occurs when lidocaine is used as a local anesthetic (15). A recent review (1) includes a useful referenced tabular listing of lidocaine blood concentrations achieved for varying doses and administration sites. The site of injection, use of epinephrine, and dose rate significantly alter blood concentration profiles (29). A linear dose to maximum blood concentration relationship has been shown for local administration. No correlation was found with weight or age. Epidural administration of lidocaine, commonly used for abdominal procedures, seems to have absorption rates similar to IM administration (15,29) and usual doses commonly produce blood concentrations which exceed 6 $\mu$g/ml. The total doses and duration of therapy require very careful monitoring during epidural administration.

Pulmonary administration of lidocaine is common for bronchoscopy or during intubation. Blood concentrations after doses of 280 to 400 mg are commonly in the therapeutic (30,31) and sometimes the toxic (32) range. Intermittent positive pressure techniques may produce somewhat higher blood concentrations than ultrasonic nebulization.

## Distribution

Lidocaine is extensively distributed in tissues (33–35) and the distribution process is clinically important in describing blood concentration profiles in man (8,11,34–39). Tissue and blood concentrations have been measured in several animal studies (33–35,40,41), providing some insight into probable tissue distribution in man. Lidocaine is about 50 to 70% protein bound and binding is linear up to about 6 μg/ml. Above 10 μg/ml, binding appears to become saturable (57). Plasma to whole blood ratios have been estimated to be from 1.1 (33,36) to 1.5 (57) and variable with concentration (57). This could cause some confounding of response versus concentration data unless recognized.

Benowitz et al (33–34) determined organ concentrations in rhesus monkeys and, using a perfusion-limited model and scaleup, performed computer simulations of lidocaine behavior in humans. Following an IV bolus dose, high blood:tissue ratios were predicted in spleen, lungs, kidney, and adipose tissue. Brain and myocardial concentrations are approximately those found in blood, while musculoskeletal tissue had partition coefficients of less than one. Rapid uptake was predicted for the brain, heart, kidney, and splanchnic organs. Skeletal tissue, skin and muscle accumulated drug slowly. However, the large mass of muscle has the potential to sequester significant amounts of lidocaine. The quantitative application of physiological models is not yet feasible for clinical problems. However, blood concentration profiles of lidocaine in man are consistent with these simulations. The major clinical importance of the extensive distribution of lidocaine in planning therapy is selecting a sufficiently precise model for prediction of changes in blood concentrations associated with measurable clinical effects.

The initial rigorous pharmacokinetic analyses of lidocaine in normal volunteers (11,36) postulated a two-compartment open model (Figure 1). A three-compartment model was used for fitting lidocaine data from anesthetized patients (37), but no quantitative comparison of two- and three-compartment model fits was provided. Refitting these data (unpublished) to both two- and three-compartment models using a recently developed nonlinear least squares program for pharmacokinetic parameter estimation (42), no significant difference was

## Two Compartment Model for Lidocaine

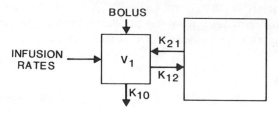

$K_{10}$ = Elimination Rate Constant from Compartment 1
$K_{12}$ = Transfer Rate Constant from Compartment 1 to Compartment 2
$K_{21}$ = Transfer Rate Constant from Compartment 2 to Compartment 1
$V_1$ = Volume of Compartment 1

FIGURE 1. Lidocaine pharmacokinetics are most often described using a linear two-compartment pharmacokinetic model.

found when comparing residual sum of squares. A two-compartment open model can adequately describe lidocaine's blood concentration profile (8,11,26,102) and can be useful in planning dosage regimens (42). More complex models (34) may be useful in the future as more is learned about the kinetics of lidocaine and its metabolites.

### Metabolism

A summary of lidocaine's proposed metabolic fate (43,45,50,55) is shown in Figure 2. The hepatic extraction ratio for lidocaine is estimated as 70% (38), indicating very avid metabolism. Sequential oxidative N-dealkylation by the cytochrome P450 system in the hepatic microsomes produces monoethylglycinexylidide (MEGX) and glycineylidide (GX) (43). Measurable blood concentrations of these metabolites are commonly found in man (44–49) and have demonstrable pharmacological effect (11,45,47,50–52). In animal models, MEGX appears to be slightly less potent than lidocaine as an antiarrhythmic (50,52) and a more potent emetic. GX has been estimated as having only one-tenth the potency of lidocaine as an antiarrhythmic (53) or convulsant agent (52). The convulsant effects of MEGX and lidocaine may be additive (51) and GX could contribute to the convulsive effects of lidocaine and MEGX even though it is not as potent.

MEGX and GX are intermediate metabolites and are found in small

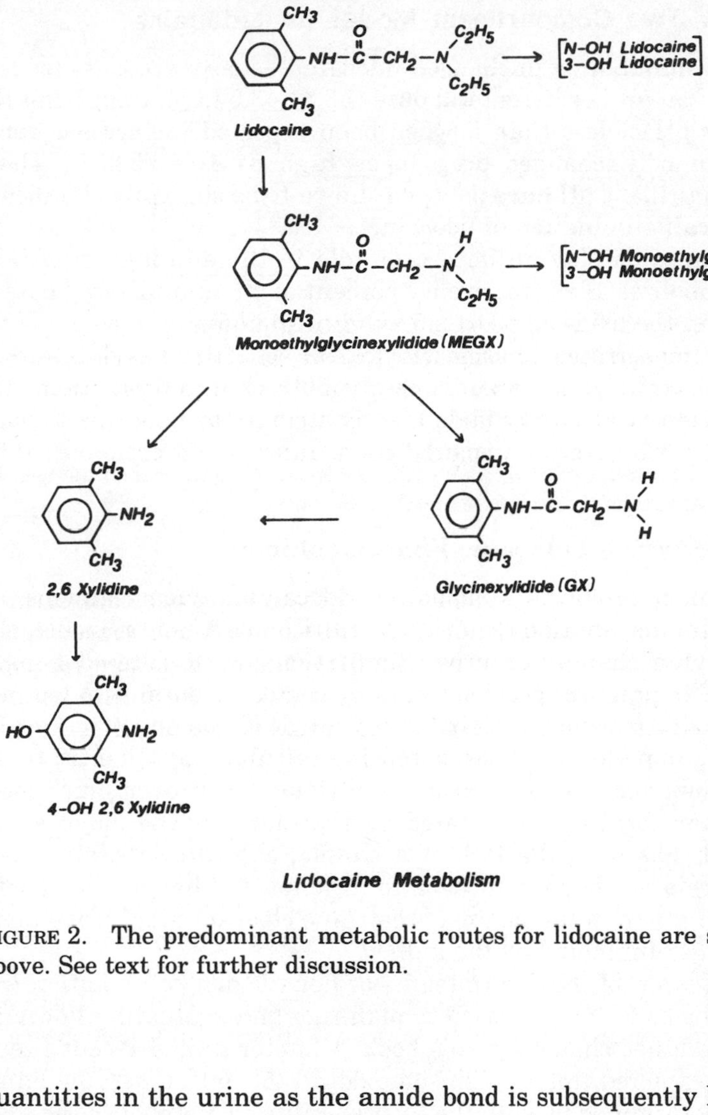

**Lidocaine Metabolism**

FIGURE 2. The predominant metabolic routes for lidocaine are summarized above. See text for further discussion.

quantities in the urine as the amide bond is subsequently hydrolyzed to yield 2,6 xylidine. 2,6 Xylidine is then hydroxylated to the primary urinary metabolite of lidocaine, 4-OH 2,6 xylidine (53–55). Other lidocaine metabolites which are found in man, but are of unknown clinical significance, include 3-OH lidocaine and 3-OH MEGX (33,55), N hydroxy derivatives of lidocaine and MEGX (54), and a cyclic intermediate in the N-dealkylation of lidocaine (56).

## Excretion

Renal elimination of unchanged lidocaine usually accounts for less than 5% of an oral or parenteral dose (36,41,43,54,55). Acidifying the urine to a pH of less than 5.5 has been reported to increase renal elimination of unchanged drug to as high as 10% (53,54). These changes in urinary pH have not been shown to be clinically significant in the overall elimination of lidocaine.

The kidneys do play an important role in the elimination of lidocaine metabolites. Sixty to seventy percent of an administered dose is recovered in the urine as 4-OH 2,6 xylidine (43,55), a compound without any demonstrated pharmacological effect. Glycinexylidide does rely on the kidneys for approximately 50% of its elimination (45). Accumulation of glycinexylidide may contribute to lidocaine toxicity in patients with severely impaired renal function on prolonged infusions (46).

## Factors Affecting Lidocaine Pharmacokinetics

The primary problems in adjusting lidocaine dosage regimens are 1) significant distribution requiring a multicompartmental model, and 2) quantifying changes in drug elimination due to altered hepatic function. The practical problems of multicompartmental behavior are largely model parameter estimation and development of clinically useful tools to perform tedious, extensive calculations. Quantitatively predicting change in hepatic drug elimination has proven much more difficult than for drugs eliminated by the kidneys. The major stumbling block has been the lack of a simple, accurate laboratory test which correlates changes in hepatic function to changes in hepatic drug elimination, in the manner creatinine clearance has proven useful for drugs eliminated by the kidney.

A brief review of the determinants of hepatic drug elimination will provide a basis for an approach to planning and evaluating lidocaine therapy. Another chapter in this book (Chapter 4) and recent literature have explored this area in some detail (58–60). Lidocaine elimination is determined by both the liver's ability to metabolize the drug (61,62) and the rate of delivery of drug to the liver. For drugs with high extraction ratios, such as lidocaine, changes in hepatic blood flow produce profound effects on disposition (59) and blood flow effects may dominate changes in metabolizing capacity (58). This behavior has been referred to as perfusion-limited (34,58,59).

The hepatic elimination of a drug can be conceptualized as being determined by the functionally perfused hepatic tissue. Approximately 25% of the cardiac output goes to the liver via the hepatic artery and portal vein. Alteration in cardiac output associated with congestive heart failure (8,9,38), age (102), or myocardial infarction (39,79) can impair hepatic blood flow and, thus, lidocaine elimination. The fall in hepatic blood flow in heart failure has been shown to be proportional to the fall in cardiac output (38). In addition to impaired cardiac output directly decreasing hepatic perfusion, the presence of intrahepatic and extrahepatic shunts may bypass the metabolic site within the liver, even though total hepatic blood flow is normal (64). Thus, "effective hepatic blood flow" is reduced. A summary of factors affecting lidocaine elimination is shown in Table 1.

Hepatic blood flow can be affected by several drugs, including anesthetics (65,66), propranolol (67), and norepinephrine (35). A recent report (68) demonstrated increased hepatic blood flow with lidocaine infusion rates of 2 and 4 mg/minute for 150 minutes in normal volunteers, when compared to controls receiving normal saline. It is unclear whether similar changes would occur in patients. Moreover, the clinical significance of such changes in hepatic blood flow remain undefined. If confirmed, these changes could be a consideration in pharmacokinetic studies, especially if longterm. In contrast to this report, most studies have reported little or no change in cardiovascular hemodynamics with usual doses of lidocaine in patients (69–71). Systolic time intervals measured after a 100 mg IV dose of lidocaine given over one minute suggested a small, negative inotropic effect but no change in blood pressure (72). Although there is definite potential for drugs with cardiovascular effects to alter lidocaine pharmacokinetics, corroborating clinical reports do not currently exist.

Although the effect of perfusion is important, changes in hepatocellular metabolism can also affect lidocaine disposition (8,61,62). Animal studies have shown lidocaine metabolism to be slowed by an enzyme inhibitor (73) and accelerated by induction with phenobarbital (74). It has been suggested (75), based on a very limited study, that anticonvulsants can slightly increase lidocaine elimination.

TABLE 1. FACTORS AFFECTING LIDOCAINE ELIMINATION

1). Decreased hepatic blood flow associated with decreased cardiac output (e.g., congestive heart failure, myocardial infarction, age, shock).
2). Portal-systemic and intrahepatic shunts in liver disease.
3). Hepatocellular liver disease.
4). Drugs which decrease hepatic blood flow (propranolol, anesthetics, norepinephrine).

Irrespective of whether the mechanism altered is effective hepatic perfusion or impaired hepatic metabolism, patients with proven liver disease can have markedly compromised lidocaine elimination (8,61,62,76) and are likely to develop toxicity with normal dosage regimens. However, not all patients with hepatomegaly, a clinical diagnosis of liver disease, or a long history of alcoholism will demonstrate abnormal lidocaine elimination. Liver histology has been suggested to be useful in predicting drug metabolism in liver disease (77). Obviously, liver histology is not routinely available and other simpler laboratory tests are needed. Indocyanine green has a high hepatic extraction ratio, similar to lidocaine, and indocyanine green clearances are relatively easy to measure. Indocyanine green clearances have been reported to be highly predictive of lidocaine clearance in heart failure (9) but of little quantitative use in viral hepatitis (61). While positive correlations between indocyanine green clearance and serum albumin, bilirubin, and prothrombin time have been shown, the overlap between normals and patients with liver disease was too great for any useful predictive capability (101). The presence of both an abnormal prothrombin time and serum albumin in chronic liver disease (62) was associated with a lidocaine half-life of 10.3 hours (range 4.5 to 19 hours).

Careful clinical assessment of each patient will help identify factors, such as those summarized in Table 1, which suggest qualitatively the likelihood of altered lidocaine pharmacokinetics. Quantitative adjustments in dosage regimens are available for the presence of heart failure (9,80,100). Additional studies with careful characterization of liver disease are needed to critically assess the effect of hepatic disease on lidocaine kinetics. There appear to be major differences between the effects of viral hepatitis, cirrhosis, acute alcoholic hepatitis, and alcohol-induced fatty livers with regards to changes in lidocaine kinetics.

## CONCENTRATION VERSUS RESPONSE AND TOXICITY

With the common concept of a "therapeutic range," the assumption is often made that a value above this range is "toxic" and values below are "subtherapeutic." This ignores the intersubject and intrasubject variability which is inherent in the concentration versus effect relationship and is often observed even in the most carefully controlled laboratory experiment. Rather than a therapeutic range, the most useful process in establishing a clinically appropriate therapeutic goal, or in evaluating an established dosage regimen based on an estimated or measured blood concentration, is to define the likelihood of therapeutic success, therapeutic failure, and toxicity for selected concentration increments. Then the probability of success or failure can be balanced against the clinical need(s) of the individual patient. Unfortunately, this sort of quantitative information is sadly lacking, even for drugs such as digoxin for which thousands of blood concentrations are measured each day. The following is a brief synopsis of published data on lidocaine blood concentrations, toxicity, and therapeutic effect. However, each clinical center should develop their own collected, documented experience with their patient population and particular analytical procedure.

## Reported Incidence of Toxicity

The Boston Collaborative Drug Surveillance Program (81) reported an incidence of lidocaine toxicity of 6.3% in 750 patients. Twenty-five percent of the reactions were considered life threatening, but in no case was lidocaine judged to be primarily responsible for a death. Toxicity was more common among older, smaller patients with prolonged hospitalizations. Sixty-eight percent of reactions were CNS, while 17% were cardiovascular. While no lethal adverse reactions were reported here, there are a significant number of lidocaine related deaths in the literature, including one paper with 13 fatal reactions (82) associated with its use as a local anesthetic.

The incidence of toxicity in studies where dosages were controlled and side effects were closely monitored appears to be substantially higher than reported in the Boston Collaborative Study. Prophylactic lidocaine administered for 48 hours at a rate of 2.5 mg/minute produced an incidence of toxicity of 16.7% and four episodes (3.3%) of coma or seizures (83). A similar study (3) used 3 mg/minute, excluded all patients with heart failure, shock, or major arrhythmias, and found a 15% incidence of toxicity. A dose of 75 mg of lidocaine given over 2 minutes to 70 patients produced mild, transient symptoms (dizziness, tinnitus, nausea, sleepiness, paraesthesias) in 27% (2).

## Antiarrhythmic Concentrations

One of the earliest reports on the use of lidocaine as an antiarrhythmic drug in patients with coronary artery disease suggested a therapeutic range of 2 to 5 µg/ml, based on whole blood determinations (84). Equivalent plasma concentrations would be as much as 20% higher than whole blood, although the whole blood to plasma ratio appears to be distinctly nonlinear as concentration increases. Eight of ten patients with frequent (> 6 per minute) premature ventricular contractions (PVC's) given 200 mg IM lidocaine showed a significant reduction in frequency when measured serum concentrations were between 2.4 and 2.8 μg/ml (23). Fifteen patients with suspected acute myocardial infarction and frequent PVC's were given 250 mg of IM lidocaine (21). A mean peak plasma concentration of 3.8 μg/ml was associated with a 50% or greater reduction in ectopic beats. Frequency of PVC's began to increase as plasma concentrations fell below 2 μg/ml. Plasma concentrations were measured in nine acute myocardial infarction patients after a 100 mg bolus followed by a 300 mg IM dose of lidocaine (85). Ectopic frequency began to return to control levels as plasma concentrations fell below 2.5 μg/ml. However, significant reduction in ectopics persisted with a mean plasma concentration of 1.7 μg/ml. When concentrations fell below 1.5 μg/ml, there was no apparent difference in the frequency of PVC's compared to that observed prior to therapy. A large controlled double-blind study (28) examined the efficacy of 300 mg of IM lidocaine in preventing primary ventricular fibrillation in acute myocardial infarction. Mean lidocaine plasma concentrations of 1.4 μg/ml (± 0.7) were not any more effective than placebo in preventing ventricular fibrillation.

A small group of patients receiving high doses of lidocaine and considered to have lidocaine-resistant arrhythmias were intensively evaluated with respect to their response to lidocaine (86). The results of the study demonstrated that some patients required plasma concentrations greater than 5.0 μg/ml to control their arrhythmias and several patients responded to concentrations above 6 μg/ml with no apparent toxicity. While this very small uncontrolled study does not provide quantitative concentration-response data, it does indicate that higher than normal lidocaine concentrations could be considered if alternatives are not available for the control of a major arrhythmia.

## Toxic Concentrations

Lidocaine blood concentrations appear to correlate reasonably well with central nervous system (CNS) signs of toxicity, even during initial therapy while distribution is still taking place. Mild CNS symptoms are common shortly after a bolus and often quickly resolve.

Lidocaine was given as an IV infusion at a rate of 0.5 mg/kg/minute (35 mg/minute for 70 kg) for an average of 12.8 minutes to 12 volunteers (87). This rate of administration is approximately 10 times maximum recommended dosage rates. Lidocaine mean plasma concentrations, measured by a colorimetric method, were 5.29 (± 0.55) μg/ml at the end of the infusions. All subjects manifested significant toxicity, most commonly muscular fasciculations, euphoria, and twitching; and one subject developed seizures. Other symptoms included dysarthria, disorientation, sweating, confusion, somnolence, and numb extremities. Cardiovascular effects observed were primarily increased heart rate and blood pressure.

While the data from this study are very useful and often used as the basis for defining the "toxic" level of lidocaine, it should be interpreted carefully. The assay procedure was colorimetric and is not as specific as the more recently developed chromatographic assays. Also, computer simulations of the doses administered in this study, using normal parameters from the literature (36), suggest that end of infusion levels would be approximately 50% higher than those measured. Measured levels consistent with the computer simulations were found for a dose of 5 mg/kg in anesthetized patients. Mean peak lidocaine plasma levels in this study were 12 µg/ml (88). The low levels measured in the former study might be explained in part if there was even a 5 minute delay in drawing the post infusion sample.

In contrast to the above study (87) suggesting frequent toxicity with concentrations of 5 to 6 µg/ml, are a number of subsequent reports with somewhat different rates of toxicity. A study of 31 patients receiving various rates of lidocaine infusions, with random lidocaine plasma samples measured, found concentrations greater than 6 µg/ml in 9 of 31 patients and only one of nine had symptoms of toxicity. Another investigation of the adverse effects of lidocaine (95) used a 6 mg/kg infusion over 22 minutes, producing mean plasma concentrations of 6.2 µg/ml (range 3.3 to 11.0 µg/ml). Side effects were considered severe (marked drowsiness) in only one of ten patients, and mild (dizziness, tinnitus, vomiting) in three of ten patients. There were no appreciable effects on blood pressure, heart rate or intraventricular conduction, despite pre-existing heart disease and intraventricular conduction delay in all ten patients studied. An early study (84) of 29 patients given variable doses of lidocaine reported three patients with major toxicity (stupor, focal seizures). Measured whole blood concentrations at the time of toxicity were 6.8, 10.9, and 22.8 µg/ml. An evaluation of the effects of high dose lidocaine in 12 patients with heart disease and ventricular arrhythmias (86) reported side effects (lethargy, grogginess) in three patients with measured concentrations over 9 µg/ml. Of the remaining nine patients, five had measured concentrations between 5.0 and 7.8 µg/ml with no apparent adverse effects.

It is unclear whether blood concentrations achieved by rapid administration produce toxicity similar to that observed at concentrations achieved by gradual accumulation with slower administration. Observations on long-term epidural blockade with intermittent superimposed IV boluses suggest that in either case concentrations above

6 µg/ml are required to produce major signs of CNS toxicity (89). In anesthetized patients administered lidocaine by various routes, major cardiovascular adverse effects (changes in blood pressure or heart rate) were not observed unless concentrations were greater than 9 µg/ml (66). These data are of limited use, since most patients were under general anesthesia and evaluation of toxicity was difficult.

As is true with most pharmacologic agents, individual patient response is dependent on concurrent pathology. There have been several reports of adverse electrophysiological effects after small (90–92) or moderate (93) doses of lidocaine in patients with impaired conduction or major coronary artery disease. The effects of lidocaine in the presence of conduction system disease (94–95) and on hemodynamics (68,70–71) are variable. Special caution is needed and blood concentrations should be monitored in the presence of conduction disturbances and severe heart failure.

Lidocaine metabolites may contribute appreciably to clinical toxicity, although quantitative data on blood concentrations are limited. GX concentrations above 2 µg/ml (44–45) and MEGX concentrations above 4 µg/ml (47,95) have been reported in patients with apparent toxicity and lidocaine concentrations less than 5 µg/ml. Patients with impaired renal function or severe liver disease receiving long-term infusions are at greatest risk.

General guidelines for interpreting lidocaine plasma concentrations are provided in Table 2. Concentrations less than 1.5 µg/ml are not likely to be effective and generally 2.0 µg/ml is required before appreciable antiarrhythmic effects are observed. Major toxicity is common above 8.0 µg/ml. When random lidocaine concentrations are measured, they must be interpreted very carefully. The rapid change of lidocaine blood concentrations over the course of distribution and prolonged accumulation in patients with cardiac and liver disease require interpretation of measured values in the context of the dosage administered and the patient's clinical status.

The majority of lidocaine's adverse effects involve the central nervous system and often precede major cardiovascular toxicity. Milder toxicity such as drowsiness, dizziness, transient paresthesias, and nausea are common after bolus doses and may resolve quickly. If these occur during a maintenance infusion, they should be regarded as evidence of drug accumulation and harbingers of more severe toxicity. However, accumulation and severe toxicity may occur without premonitory milder symptoms. Confusion, obtundation, severe tinnitus, euphoria, dysarthria, tremor, and muscle fasiculations generally represent high concentrations of lidocaine, and possibly metabolites, and

TABLE 2. LIDOCAINE PLASMA* CONCENTRATIONS AND EFFECTS

| Concentration | Antiarrhythmic Effect | Toxicity** |
|---|---|---|
| < 1.5 µg/ml | Rarely effective | Idiosyncratic |
| 1.5 – 4.0 µg/ml | Usually effective | Mild CNS and cardiovascular effects in few patients |
| 4 – 6.0 µg/ml | May be needed for major arrhythmias | Mild CNS effects common; cardiovascular in those with concomitant heart disease. |
| 6–8 µg/ml | Acceptable only if alternative therapy not possible. | Significant risk of CNS and cardiovascular depression. |
| > 8 µg/ml | | Seizures, obtundation, decreased cardiac output common |

* Plasma and serum measurements are similar. Whole blood concentrations may be 10 to 30% lower.
** Patients with significant conduction system abnormalities or marginal hemodynamic status may develop apparent toxicity even at very low lidocaine concentrations. Metabolites also can contribute to toxicity even with modest lidocaine plasma concentrations.

warrant temporarily stopping the drug and restarting at a lower infusion rate. It is not sufficient to simply adjust the rate downward, especially early in the course of therapy. At concentrations above 6 µg/ml, the risk of severe CNS and cardiovascular depression is substantial. Above 8 µg/ml, coma, seizures, respiratory depression, and hypotension are likely.

## CLINICAL APPLICATION OF PHARMACOKINETIC DATA

### Planning and Evaluating Lidocaine Therapy

In developing patient-specific lidocaine dosage regimens one must consider the drug's multicompartmental pharmacokinetics and must quantify changes in hepatic elimination associated with altered cardiac output. A two-compartment open model (Figure 1) has been used for fitting data after both single doses (36) and infusions (11) in man.

TABLE 3. LIDOCAINE PHARMACOKINETIC PARAMETERS

| | $K_{10}$ (Min$^{-1}$) | $K_{12}$ (Min$^{-1}$) | $K_{21}$ (Min$^{-1}$) | $V_c$ (L) | $V_{ss}$ (L) | $V_\beta$ (L) | $t_{½\alpha}$ (Min) | $t_{½\beta}$ (Min) | TBC (ml/min/kg) |
|---|---|---|---|---|---|---|---|---|---|
| Reference 11 | .025 | .093 | .050 | 31 | 157 | 177 | 4.7 | 88 | 18.2 |
| Reference 36 | .024 | .070* | .035 | 33 | 84 | 107 | 6.8 | 108 | 9.2 |
| Reference 42 (Mean) | .032 | .087 | .032 | 40 | 190 | 244 | 9.9 | 356 | 7.8 |
| Reference 42 (Median) | .013 | .047 | .019 | 40 | 173 | 207 | 8.3 | 274 | 6.7 |
| Reference 102 (#) | .023 | | | 24 | 46 | | | 81 | 7.6 |
| Reference 102 (##) | .028 | | | 24 | 77 | | | 140 | 8.1 |

* The rate constants $K_{12}$ and $K_{21}$ appeared to have been reversed for two patients (PE&FG) in Reference #36. Thus, the means reported there for $K_{12}$ (0.66) and $K_{21}$ (.038) are slightly different than the means shown in the above table.

\# Four normal subjects 22 to 26 years of age.

\#\# Six subjects 61 to 67 years of age.

This model has also been useful in the prediction and control of lidocaine concentrations in patients (100).The literature data on parameter estimates for a lidocaine two-compartment model are summarized in Table 3. References 11 and 36 represent data from normal subjects, while the parameters from reference 42 were determined in acutely ill patients. A comparative study of lidocaine kinetics in young normal volunteers and elderly patients without heart disease after a bolus dose is also shown (102). Significantly different parameters were found in the elderly patients (over 60) when compared to the young volunteers. The mean microscopic rate constants ($K_{10}$, $K_{12}$, $K_{21}$) are similar for these studies. However, the standard deviations are usually large, suggesting substantial inter-subject variability, even among normal volunteers. Our findings in acutely ill patients have shown a distinctly non-normal distribution for all parameters. Thus, the median parameters are significantly different than the mean values. The non-normal distribution may be due, in part, to a small number of patients with acute illness of varying severity.

Preliminary work in dogs (40) and man (90) suggests the possibility of either nonlinear or metabolite inhibition in the pharmacokinetic behavior for lidocaine, but the evidence is as yet too limited to be applied clinically. The linear two-compartment open model appears most appropriate for our current understanding of lidocaine pharmacokinetics. Additional studies are needed to more precisely define parameters for acutely ill patients.

The objectives in planning lidocaine dosage regimens are summarized in Table 4. The initial loading dose and the maintenance infusion can be calculated on the basis of a desired blood concentration and the severity of the patient's arrhythmia. The effectiveness of the initial dosage regimen can be determined by the response if the ectopics are frequent. However, when lidocaine is given prophylactically to prevent primary ventricular fibrillation or when the variable character of the arrhythmia makes evaluation of a clinical endpoint difficult or impossible, the blood concentration goals may be the primary immediate objective.

TABLE 4.   CLINICAL OBJECTIVES IN PLANNING LIDOCAINE THERAPY

1). Loading dose adequate for arrhythmia control or prophylaxis
2). Maintenance dosage regimen adjusted for altered elimination to prevent undesirable accumulation
3). Calculation of incremental doses during the course of distribution

## Calculation of Loading Infusions

The loading dose of lidocaine is commonly thought of as a bolus when, in fact, it is a short-term infusion. The loading dose, if given as a bolus, is calculated very simply as:

$$LD = C_{max} \times V_c \qquad \text{(Eq. 1)}$$

where LD is the loading dose, $C_{max}$ is the desired concentration, and $V_c$ is the volume of the central compartment of the two-compartment model.

. It must be emphasized that despite the terminology used, lidocaine loading doses should never be administered as an actual bolus but rather as a short infusion over 2 or 3 minutes. This will minimize transiently high lidocaine concentrations and the side effects often reported with "bolus" doses of lidocaine. There is no benefit to the very rapid administration of lidocaine, even in the presence of life threatening ventricular arrhythmias, and there is a high likelihood of producing appreciable toxicity.

The use of Equation 1 will underestimate the initial loading dose (LD) when it is administered as an infusion, because drug is "lost" from $V_c$ during infusion by both elimination and distribution. The correct equation for calculating a loading infusion for a two-compartment open model is:

$$K_0^{LD} = \cfrac{C_{max} \times K_{10} \times V_c}{1 + \cfrac{\beta - K_{10}}{\alpha - \beta} e^{-\alpha t} + \cfrac{K_{10} - \alpha}{\alpha - \beta} e^{-\beta t}} \qquad \text{(Eq. 2)}$$

where $K_0^{LD}$ is infusion rate for the loading dose, $C_{max}$ is the desired concentration at the end of the loading infusion, and t is the duration of the infusion. The remaining symbols are standard parameters for an open two-compartment first-order kinetic model (Figure 1). The error in using Equation 1 for calculation of the LD is shown in an example in Table 5. The parameters used are representative of those found in normal subjects and show the error would be approximately 10% or less for infusions of less than 3 minutes. The error becomes substantial when LD's are administered by infusions longer than 5 minutes in duration. Equation 2 is then more appropriate than Equation 1.

While it is intuitively appealing to calculate a volume of distribution on the basis of patient weight, the existing pharmacokinetic studies do not support such an approach for the volume of the central compartment ($V_c$) for lidocaine. A plot of $V_c$ versus weight is shown in Figure 3 for two published studies (11,36) of lidocaine pharmacoki-

TABLE 5. ERROR IN CALCULATING LOADING DOSE (LD) OF
LIDOCAINE BY $C_{max} \times V_c$ WHEN ADMINISTERED BY INFUSIONS OF
VARIOUS DURATION ASSUMING A TWO-COMPARTMENT MODEL

| Loading Dose Infusion Time | $K_o$ in mg/min (nearest mg) | Loading Infusion from Eq. 2 | Percent Error* using $C_{max} \times V_c$ |
|---|---|---|---|
| 0.5 minutes | 244 | 122 | 1.8% |
| 1.0 minutes | 125 | 125 | 3.6% |
| 2.0 minutes | 65 | 130 | 7.0% |
| 3.0 minutes | 45 | 134 | 10.3% |
| 5.0 minutes | 29 | 143 | 16.2% |

Calculations based on desired $C_{max}$ of 3 μg/ml, $\alpha = .1$ min$^{-1}$, $\beta = .008$ min$^{-1}$, $K_{10} = 0.25$ min$^{-1}$, and $V_c = 40$ liters. $C_{max} \times V_c = 120$.

* Percent error = $\dfrac{\text{Loading Infusion from Eq. 2} - 120}{\text{Loading Infusion from Eq. 2}}$

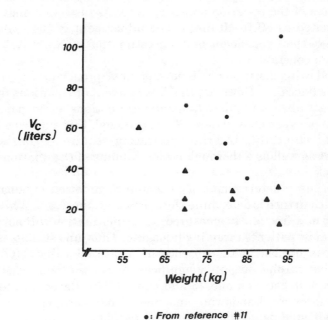

●: From reference #11
▲: From reference #36

FIGURE 3. The volume of the central compartment ($V_c$) for lidocaine is not positively correlated to weight. These data are taken from reference 11 (circles) and reference 36 (triangles).

netics in normal volunteers. Simple linear regression of this plot actually suggests a negative correlation between $V_c$ and weight.

It has been suggested that $V_c$ is smaller in the presence of heart failure (8); however, the data are limited. Initial loading infusions can probably be calculated on the basis of a mean value of 30 to 40 liters for adults. The smaller value should be used in the presence of severe heart failure and loading doses should be administered over a minimum of 3 minutes.

## Calculation of Maintenance Infusions

The maintenance infusion rate ($K_0^M$) for lidocaine will be determined by the clearance from the central compartment of the two-compartment open model, and the desired steady-state concentration ($C_{ss}$):

$$K_0^M = C_{ss} \times K_{10} \times V_c \qquad \text{(Eq. 3)}$$

where $K_{10} \times V_c$ determines clearance. This equation is consistent with Equation 2 as t approaches infinity, when the last two terms on the bottom of the equation approach zero. As discussed above, $V_c$ can be estimated as 30 to 40 liters. The adjustment of the maintenance infusion is then dependent only on estimation of $K_{10}$ if $K_{12}$, $K_{21}$, and $V_c$ remain constant.

The following discussion will develop an approach for the estimation of $K_{10}$ for lidocaine. However, the development of equations for dosage adjustment always requires limiting assumptions and depends on the precision of experimental data. Thus, although this approach has been evaluated clinically (42), the application requires rigorous clinical judgment as well as a thorough understanding of the pharmacokinetic principles.

The primary determinant of lidocaine elimination is hepatic blood flow, which in turn is determined by cardiac output (8,38). While cardiac output is now frequently measured, such information will not be available for most patients receiving lidocaine. Thus, an estimate of cardiac function is needed in the absence of measured values. It has been shown that cardiac output is significantly related to age and declines by about 50% between age 20 and age 80 (63). Based on the work of Brandfonþrenner, Landowne, and Shock (63), cardiac index (CI) can be age-adjusted using the following equation:

$$CI_{est} = 3.72 - 0.0232876\,(Age - 20) \qquad \text{(Eq. 4)}$$

or, simplified:

$$CI_{est} = 4.185752 - 0.0232876\,(Age) \qquad \text{(Eq. 5)}$$

where age must be at least 20 years. Estimation of the degree of impaired cardiac function in the absence of invasive measurements is difficult, but it has been suggested that reasonable approximations can be made (97). The algorithm shown in Table 6 has been used with an acceptable degree of precision to estimate CI and predict lidocaine plasma concentrations in 20 acutely ill patients (100). From this algorithm the cardiac index is estimated as a percent of normal. Thus, expressing the percent normal as a decimal fraction (e.g., 70% = 0.7), the decimal fraction (F) times Equation 5 will provide an age-adjusted clinical estimate of cardiac function:

$$\text{estimated cardiac index} = F(4.185752 - 0.0232876)(\text{age}) \quad \text{(Eq. 6)}$$

Based on previous work (8,9,38), the elimination rate constant from the central compartment ($K_{10}$) is assumed to change linearly with changes in cardiac output and hepatic perfusion. The data in Table 3 suggest a reasonable estimate of $K_{10}$ for a 45-year-old patient would be 0.024 min$^{-1}$ when cardiac index is 100% of normal (3.148 L/minute). If $K_{12}$ and $K_{21}$ are 0.066 min$^{-1}$ and 0.038 min$^{-1}$, respectively, the half-life would then be 91.5 minutes. Using this estimate of $K_{10}$ and Equations 5 and 6, the following relationship will adjust $K_{10}$ for age and degree of cardiac failure:

$$K_{10}^{adj} = \frac{F(CI_{est})(0.024)}{3.138} \quad \text{(Eq. 7)}$$

$$K_{10}^{adj} = F\left(\frac{4.18575 - .0232876\,(\text{Age})}{3.138}\right)(0.024) \quad \text{(Eq. 8)}$$

or, simplified:

$$K_{10}^{adj} = F(0.032 - 0.000178 \times \text{Age}) \quad \text{(Eq. 9)}$$

The estimate of $K_{10}$, adjusted for age and heart failure ($K_{10}^{adj}$), is expressed in min$^{-1}$.

Using Equation 3 and Equation 9 would allow calculation of an adjusted maintenance infusion rate:

$$K_0^M = C_{ss} \times V_c \times F(0.032 - 0.000178 \times \text{Age}) \quad \text{(Eq. 10)}$$

To increase lidocaine concentrations after a regimen has reached steady-state requires an additional incremental loading infusion and an increase in the maintenance infusion rate. The loading infusion can be calculated using Equation 1 (or Equation 2, if appropriate) only substituting the increment of change in concentration (Desired C-$C_{ss}$) desired for $C_{max}$:

$$\text{Incremental loading infusion} = (\text{Desired } C - C_{ss})V_c \quad \text{(Eq. 11)}$$

The new infusion rate is again calculated using Equation 10 but substituting the new desired $C_{ss}$.

TABLE 6. ESTIMATION OF CARDIAC FUNCTION INDEX
BASED ON CLINICAL CRITERIA

**Clinical Criteria**

| 1. Degree of Heart Failure | Points |
|---|---|
| S$_3$ present | 1 |
| Pulmonary Congestion: | |
| 1+–2+ Rales | 1 |
| 3+ Rales | 2 |
| Pulmonary Edema | 3 |
| Jugular Venous Distention: | |
| 1–3 cm | 2 |
| > 3 cm | 3 |
| Peripheral Edema: | |
| 1+ | 1 |
| 2+–4+ | 2 |
| Pre-renal Azotemia | 2 |

Total Points

| | Percent subtracted from 100% Normal |
|---|---|
| If total ÷ 5 is less than .2 then subtract | 0% |
| If total ÷ 5 is .2 to .49 then subtract | 5% |
| If total ÷ 5 is 0.5 to .9 then subtract | 10% |
| If total ÷ 5 is 1.0 to 1.49 then subtract | 15% |
| If total ÷ 5 is 1.5 to 1.99 then subtract | 20% |
| If total ÷ 5 is more than 2.0 then subtract | 25% |
| 2. Blood Pressure: Normal | 0% |
| Low | 10% |
| Palpable only | 15% |
| 3. Rhythm: Normal Sinus; Rate < 110 | 0% |
| Normal Sinus; Rate > 110 | 5% |
| Supraventricular Tachycardia; Rate < 110 | 10% |
| Supraventricular Tachycardia; Rate > 110 | 15% |
| 4. Urine Output: Normal (> 25 ml/hr) | 0% |
| Oliguria (< 25 ml/hr) | 10% |
| 5. Peripheral Vasoconstriction Present | 5% |
| 6. Acute Myocardial Infarction when #1 to #5 normal | 10% |

To determine the cardiac function index add the percent indicated in the right hand column for each of the clinical criteria present on the left hand side of the table. Subtract total from 100%. Maximal reduction in cardiac function index should not exceed 50%.

## Dosage Regimen and Two-Compartmental Behavior

The clinical consequence of the two-compartment behavior of lido-caine is a significant fall in concentration after the loading dose to values of one-half to one-third of the peak concentration, even when a continuous fixed rate maintenance infusion is begun immediately. A simulated example of lidocaine concentrations for a dosage regimen with two different rates of elimination $(K_{10})$ is shown in Figure 4. As equilibration occurs with the peripheral compartment, concentrations gradually rise to steady-state over 6 to 24 hours. Thus, with a loading dose and a maintenance infusion there will be a significant time during which the lidocaine concentration may not be adequate to control the arrhythmia or provide adequate protection against pri-mary ventricular fibrillation.

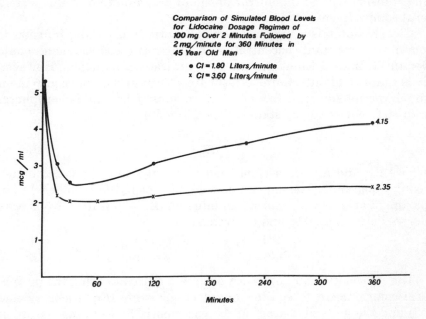

FIGURE 4. The primary determinant of lidocaine elimination is hepatic blood flow, which in turn is a function of cardiac output. The simulation shown here illustrates the potential effect of a fall in cardiac index (CI) from normal, approximately 3.6 liters per minute, to 1.8 liters per minute, a value consis-tent with marked heart failure. The heart failure patient would have a pre-dicted concentration of almost twice the concentration predicted for a patient with normal cardiac output.

The general approach required to maintain a constant concentration in the central compartment of a two-compartment open model has been developed by Kruger-Theimer (98). Maintaining a constant concentration in the central compartment during distribution can be thought of as requiring two continuous infusions. The first infusion replaces drug lost by elimination from the central compartment and is equal to

$$K_0^M = C_{ss} \times K_{10} \times V_c \qquad \text{(Eq. 3)}$$

A second infusion simultaneously replaces drug lost from the central compartment because of distribution to the peripheral compartment. The second infusion will decline exponentially as accumulation occurs in the peripheral compartment and equilibrium between the central and peripheral compartment is established. This exponentially declining infusion will be the mirror image of accumulation in the peripheral compartment.

Clearly, administering such an exponentially declining infusion to maintain a constant concentration in the central compartment would require tedious calculations and be technically impractical. However, it is quite straightforward to estimate the total dosage requirement for the peripheral compartment. The amount of drug in the peripheral compartment at steady state ($X_p^{ss}$) is defined by:

$$X_p^{ss} = \frac{K_{12}K_0^M}{K_{21}K_{10}} \qquad \text{(Eq. 12)}$$

where $K_{12}$ and $K_{21}$ are assumed not to change, and $K_{10}$ is calculated using Equation 9. The amount of drug present in the peripheral compartment at time t ($X_p$) during an infusion ($K_0$) of duration T has been derived elsewhere (99) and is given by:

$$X_p^t = \frac{K_{12}K_0(1-e^{\alpha t})}{-\alpha(\beta-\alpha)} e^{-\alpha t} + \frac{K_{12}K_0(1-e^{\alpha t})}{-\beta(\alpha-\beta)} e^{-\beta t} \qquad \text{(Eq. 13)}$$

The information on how much drug is required to bring the peripheral compartment to equilibrium at steady-state (Equations 12 and 13) and the general concept of the exponentially declining nature of the "second infusion" is very important. If the initial regimen does not provide an adequate clinical response, it is common clinical practice to give additional boluses and incrementally increase the maintenance infusion rate. However, during a period of time approximating three half-lives after starting therapy, upward adjustments of the maintenance infusion may not be needed or appropriate. Rather, additional lidocaine should be administered as short infusions up to the amount calculated with Equation 12. Immediately after a rapid infusion loading dose, this equation would give an estimate of the amount of drug needed to "fill up" the peripheral compartment. It must be remembered that as a maintenance infusion is begun, the peripheral compartment will gradually approach equilibrium. During the first half-life, as much as 75% of $X_p^{ss}$ could be administered without exceeding the $C_{max}^{ss}$ originally desired for any sustained time. If the total amount of lidocaine required to control the arrhythmia does exceed $X_p^{ss}$ in the first three half-lives, then an increased maintenance infusion rate will be required.

The half-life can be calculated from $K_{10}^{adj}$ as shown. An estimate can then be made as to when the patient will reach steady-state.

$$\beta = (K_{10}^{adj}) \left( \frac{K_{21}}{\alpha} \right)$$
(Eq. 14)

$$t_{\frac{1}{2}\beta} = \frac{.693}{\beta}$$
(Eq. 15)

The $\beta$ half-life is actually a function of not only $K_{10}$ but also the model parameters determining distribution. $t_{\frac{1}{2}\beta}$ as calculated in Equations 14 and 15 assumes that no changes in distribution occur and $K_{10}$ is the only parameter that changes with changes in cardiac output. While distribution of lidocaine may change, in the presence of heart failure such changes cannot yet be quantified or predicted. A change in $K_{10}$ also results in slight changes in $\alpha$. The magnitude of the change in $\alpha$ does not have a significant effect on calculation of $\beta$ in Equation 14.

### Other Factors Affecting Lidocaine Dosage Regimens

Patients with definite liver disease will require additional downward adjustment in maintenance infusion rates. There is no quantitative method for such dosage adjustment that has been clinically evaluated. Prothrombin times increased more than 1.5 times control after vitamin K replenishment and albumin concentrations less than 2.5 gm/dl are indicative of severe impairment of liver function and suggest a lidocaine half-life over 6 hours. The role of lidocaine metabolites in producing toxicity is a potential concern, especially in patients treated for more than 48 hours and with concurrent renal failure. Measurement of lidocaine and metabolites, if possible, should be obtained every 6 to 12 hours in such patients. Major alterations in distribution may occur in the presence of both heart failure and liver disease. The effect of age, apart from disease, may also alter distribution in patients over 60 (95). These and other factors remain to be quantified in a manner suitable for purposes of making dosage regimen adjustments.

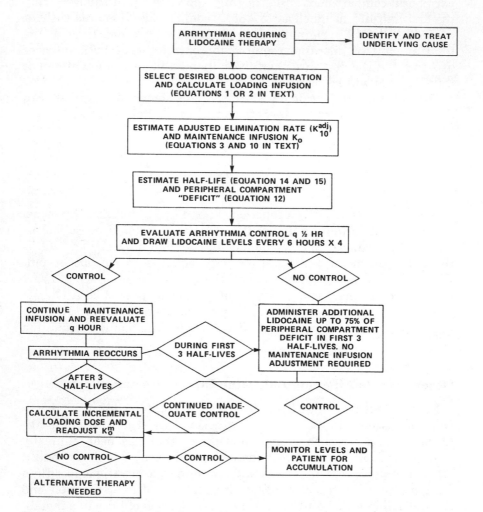

FIGURE 5.  Algorithm for the application of pharmacokinetics to lidocaine therapy.

## Computer-Assisted Lidocaine Therapy

The complexities of dosage regimen planning for a two-compartmental drug and the need for a more rigorous evaluation lend themselves to utilization of a computer. The basic approach outlined here has been incorporated into an interactive computer program currently used in a number of community hospitals. As can be observed in the sample patient calculation (Appendix 1), even a quite rigorous approach still produces a fluctuating concentration profile. With the assistance of a computer, it is possible to rapidly calculate a stepwise tapering regimen that closely approximates the theory of the declining exponential and maintain much tighter control of plasma concentrations during the distribution phase. In instances of complex past therapy and inadequate response or possible toxicity, the ability to retrospectively estimate concentrations can be extremely helpful in making clinical decisions.

A sample computer program can be found in Appendix 2. In this example, a patient had received four previous doses of lidocaine. An initial dose of 100 mg over 2 minutes followed by 2 mg per minute for 45 minutes failed to control the arrhythmia. A second rapid infusion of 100 mg over 2 minutes followed by 4 mg per minute abolished the arrhythmia. However, after 2 hours of infusion at the rate of 4 mg/minute, the patient was not easily arousable and muscle fasciculations were noted. The lidocaine infusion was then stopped. The past doses were entered in the computer and a printout of estimated plasma concentrations was provided. With this information an estimate of both the effective and possibly toxic concentrations were available. A dosage regimen was then calculated to maintain the concentration that appeared to control the arrhythmia without any side effects. Thus, the patient's clinical response and the estimated pharmacokinetic behavior of lidocaine could be integrated to aid in therapeutic management.

A computer is appropriate not only for complex but also mundane chores. As can be seen in the example, not only is a summary dosage regimen printed, but administration guidelines suitable for use by the nursing staff are provided. The tool that helped the patient is applied pharmacokinetics. The tool that helped the clinician is the computer. Computers are not mandatory for all pharmacokinetic problems, but in many instances they can expand capabilities as well as improve efficiency.

## ASSAY METHODS

The first method developed for measuring lidocaine in biological fluids was a modified methyl orange colorimetric method (41). This procedure lacks sufficient sensitivity and specificity for clinical monitoring and has been supplanted by chromatographic procedures. Gas liquid chromatography (43,48,103,104) has been the most commonly used assay for recent clinical studies and is generally regarded to be more specific and sensitive than the colorimetric procedure. Experience in our laboratory (104) and elsewhere (48) suggests that some problems with specificity persist with GLC because of the potential for extracting lidocaine metabolites with subsequent interference. The metabolite interference may be clinically significant unless care is taken in solvent selection and extraction.

The recent awareness of the importance of lidocaine metabolites has stimulated development of assays which measure the lidocaine metabolites monoethylglycinexylidide (MEGX) and glycinexylidide (GX). The most sensitive procedure for quantitatively identifying lidocaine metabolites is gas chromatography—mass fragmentography (106,107). The expense and technical problems in maintaining a mass spectrometer make this procedure of little practical value in routine clinical monitoring. However, pharmacokinetic studies may require the increased sensitivity for the measurement of metabolites at concentrations as low as 10 to 20 ng/ml.

There has been some success in the use of gas chromatography without mass spectroscopy for detecting lidocaine and metabolites, usually using a nitrogen sensitive flame ionization detector. An alkaline flame detector provides increased sensitivity and improves specificity by reducing interference from other hydrocarbons. Di Fazio and Brown (108) reported one of the initial procedures which allowed simultaneous measurement of GX and MEGX along with lidocaine. However, the chloroform extraction appeared to provide low recovery, peaks for GX and MEGX were not well resolved and no information on precision was provided. Keenaghan and Boyes (43) explored the use of hepatoflourobutyryl derivatives but assayed only urine without an internal standard and provided no quantitative information on precision.

The use of temperature programming combined with acetyl derivitization of lidocaine and the metabolites allowed detection of plasma and urine concentrations of down to 0.1 µg/ml with an intra-assay coefficient of variation of less than 10% (109). Although the peaks were symmetrical and fairly well separated, the retention time for GX is probably too long to make this assay practical for routine clinical

TABLE 7. COMPARISON OF THE RELATIVE ADVANTAGES AND DISADVANTAGES OF THE VARIOUS LIDOCAINE ASSAY METHODS*

| Analytical Method | Specificity for *LIDOCAINE* | Limit of sensitivity | Metabolite Analysis | Assayable Samples | | | | Minimum Sample Volume Required | Analysis Time | Analysis Costs | | | Comments |
|---|---|---|---|---|---|---|---|---|---|---|---|---|---|
| | | | | Plasma/Serum | Urine | Saliva | Other | | | Estimated Reagent and Tech. Cost Per Assay | Initial Equipment Costs | Specialized Operator Training | |
| Colorimetric | 4 | 4 | 5 | 4 | 4 | ? | 4 | 2 ml | 4 | 3 | 2 | 3 | obsolete; poor specificity |
| GC Mass Spec | 1 | 1 | 1 | 1 | 2 | ? | 2 | .5 ml | 5 | 4 | 5 | 5 | impractical for clinical work |
| GLC with alkali flame | 2 | 3 | 3 | 3 | 3 | ? | 4 | 1 ml | 3 | 3 | 3 | 3 | |
| HPLC | 2 | 2 | 3 | 2 | 3 | ? | ? | .5 ml | 2 | 2 | 3 | 3 | |
| EMIT | 3 | 3 | 5 | 2 | 5 | ? | ? | .5 ml | 1 | 1 | 3 | 1 | |

* Arbitrary Ranking Scale of 1 (Excellent) to 5 (Poor) with a score of 3 being average or nominal.

monitoring. Also described is a procedure for measuring 4-hydroxyxylidine, the major urinary product of lidocaine metabolism. An alternative method that avoids derivitization has been reported with detection down to 0.25 μg/ml of lidocaine and 0.1 μg/ml of MEGX and a coefficient of variation of less than 10% within run. However, GX was not measured and the extraction procedure is tedious and time consuming.

Our laboratory currently uses gas liquid chromatography with an alkali flame detector. Detection limits for lidocaine and MEGX are 0.05 μg/ml and 0.1 μg/ml for GX (105). Standard curves are linear from 0.1 to 10 μg/ml and the coefficient of variation is 7.5%. Derivitization with trifluoroacetic anhydride provides symmetrical peaks and adequate separation with only a preliminary extraction procedure. The liquid phase which provides the best separation from interfering endogenous substances is 3% OV-225 on Supelcort, 100/120 mesh. Retention time for the last compound eluted is 13.5 minutes. Temperature programming does not seem to be necessary or add much precision to the procedure. Mepivicaine has been found to be the most suitable internal standard. The use of a capillary column has recently been reported (111) with detection for lidocaine and metabolites down to 20 ng/ml and somewhat shorter retention times.

Several high pressure liquid chromatographic procedures have been reported for lidocaine simultaneously with other drugs (112,113) and with quantification of the de-ethylated metabolites (48,114). The advantages of the HPLC procedure include smaller sample size, simple extraction procedures, and no derivitization procedure is required. The procedure does require a variable wave length UV detector and area integration may be needed due to nonlinearity of standard curves when peak-height ratios are used (114). Lower limits of detection are reported as 0.1 μg/ml with coefficients of variation of 5% to 10% when sample size is 0.5 ml.

A major problem in using lidocaine blood concentrations for therapeutic management is the need for a rapid turnaround time. Normal clinical situations require a turnaround time of 4 to 6 hours and in some cases the results are needed even more rapidly. The recent development of a homogenous enzyme immunoassay (115,116) provides easy, rapid measurement of lidocaine with acceptable precision. Comparative studies have shown the enzyme immunoassay to correlate well with standard chromatographic procedures (115,116). The enzyme immunoassay is based on competitive binding principles similar to the radioimmunoassay. However, the lack of technical and logistical problems of dealing with a radioactive label and the simplicity of measurements done with a spectrophotometer make the procedure ideal for a test requiring rapid turnaround time and good reliability. The major disadvantage of the immunoassay is the inability to quantitate metabolites, although they do not appear to have significant cross-reactivity (115).

The most efficient assay for routine clinical monitoring is now the enzyme immunoassay. Although initial equipment and reagent costs may be higher, this disadvantage is offset by reduced technician time, less expertise required, and the ability to provide rapid turnaround time. The disadvantage of the immunoassay is the current inability to measure metabolites and variable spurious interference from plasma proteins. MEGX and possibly GX can be important in evaluating toxicity and in performing detailed pharmacokinetic studies. The measurement of metabolites can be accomplished with about equal precision using capillary column gas-liquid chromatography or high pressure liquid chromatography. The choice of chromatographic procedures is largely dependent on the expertise and equipment available. However, a good clinical laboratory should provide the analytical capabilities for measurement of metabolites as well as lidocaine.

A problem that is potentially troublesome for all assays is the artifacts in measured lidocaine concentrations when whole blood is collected in commercial blood collection tubes, such as Vacutainer® (Becton-Dickinson) or Monoject® (Sherwood Medical Industries). A plasticizer found in rubber stoppers has been suggested to be the cause for factitously low measured concentrations in both patient samples and *in vitro* spiked samples (113). This is not a problem when samples are collected in all glass containers.

## ACKNOWLEDGMENTS

Portions of the work reported here were supported by US Government Grant GM23826, and a Boehringer Fellowship in Clinical Pharmacology. The direction for further examining lidocaine pharmacokinetics was provided by the thoughtful and patient guidance of R. W. Jelliffe, M.D. Mrs. Georgene Denison provided expert secretarial assistance.

# APPENDIX 1

## Sample Lidocaine Dosage Calculation

A 65-year-old male was admitted to the coronary care unit with a 3-hour history of severe, crushing substernal chest pain radiating down both arms and an electrocardiogram consistent with an anterior myocardial infarction. Frequent multifocal ventricular ectopics and a short run of ventricular tachycardia were documented shortly after admission. The clinical estimate of cardiac index (Table 6) was 60% of normal. Lidocaine was ordered and a dosage regimen was calculated to achieve a plasma concentration of 3.0 µg/ml.

I.  *Loading Infusion to be Given over 5 Minutes:*

$$K_0^{LD} = C_{ss} \times V_c$$
$$= (3.0 \text{ mg/L}) (40 \text{ L})$$
$$= 120 \text{ mg @ 24 mg/minute}$$

II.  *Maintenance Infusion:*

a)  $K_{10}^{adj} = F(0.032 - 0.000178 \times \text{Age})$
$$= 0.6(0.032 - 0.000178 \times 65)$$
$$= 0.01226 \text{ min}^{-1}$$

b)  $K_0^M = (C_{ss})(K_{10}^{adj})(V_c)$
$$= (3)(0.01226)(40)$$
$$= 1.5 \text{ mg/minute}$$

III.  *Additional Lidocaine to be Administered Within First Three Half-lives if Arrhythmia Not Controlled:*

a)  $\beta = (K_{10}^{adj})\left(\dfrac{K_{21}}{\alpha}\right)$
$$\beta = (0.01226)(0.035/0.12)$$
$$\beta = 0.00358$$
$$T_{\frac{1}{2}\beta} = 0.693/0.00358 = 194 \text{ minutes}$$

b)  $X_p^{ss} = \dfrac{(K_{12})(K_0^M)}{(K_{21})(K_{10})}$
$$= \dfrac{(.07)(1.5)}{(.035)(.01226)} = 245 \text{ mg}$$

The 245 mg calculated here represents an estimate of the patient's lidocaine deficit immediately after the loading dose. Up to 75% of this amount can be administered in the first three half-lives without adjustment in the maintenance infusion.

IV.  *Interim Adjustment of Lidocaine Regimen:*

Ten minutes after the end of the loading dose of lidocaine another short run of ventricular tachycardia occurred and it was decided additional lidocaine was needed.

a) An additional dose of 50 mg was given by increasing the infusion rate from the maintenance rate of 1.5 mg/minute to 11.5 mg/minute for 5 minutes.

b) A second 50 mg was given by changing the infusion rate to 2.5 mg/minute for 50 minutes.

c) After 50 minutes at 2.5 mg/minute the maintenance rate was returned to 1.5 mg/minute.

# APPENDIX 2

## Sample Computer Program for Planning and Evaluating Lidocaine Therapy (approximate run time: 9 minutes)

```
        LASTname: PRACTICE          CHARTid: *              DATE: MAR 12, 1980
       FIRSTname: PATIENT              ROOM: *              TIME: 11:58 AM
             AGE: 55                 HEIGHT: 6            WEIGHT: 75K
             SEX: M        add'l INCHES: 1               GIRTH:
         program: LIDOCAINE                           BSA(msq): 1.98
        operator: RODMAN          , J

Is all of the above correct?


                                    Y

Are you an expert in running this program?
                                                  Y



VERSION OF 8/10/78....


DO YOU KNOW THE PATIENT'S CARDIAC OUTPUT
   ?N
THEN ESTIMATE PATIENT'S CARDIAC INDEX AS A PERCENT OF NORMAL:
   ?65
 65    % OF NORMAL
   ?Y
PATIENT'S ESTIMATED CARDIAC INDEX IS      1.88821    L/MIN/SQ METER;
DOES THIS SEEM REASONABLE TO YOU
   ?Y
```

```
HAS PATIENT HAD ANY RECENT PAST THERAPY WITH    LIDOCAINE
   ?Y
HOW MANY SERIAL DOSES WERE GIVEN
   ?4
DOSE   1     ROUTE    ?B
              ENTER     DOSE(MG),  IT ,  DI ,
            ?100,2,2
DOSE   2     ROUTE    ?I
              ENTER     RATE(MG/MIN),  IT ,  DI ,
            ?2,45,45
DOSE   3     ROUTE    ?B
              ENTER     DOSE(MG),  IT ,  DI ,
            ?50,2,2
DOSE   4     ROUTE    ?I
              ENTER     RATE(MG/MIN),  IT ,  DI ,
            ?4,120,120

WANT TO CHECK YOUR ENTRIES
   ?Y
I THINK YOU ENTERED:

DOSE ROUTE  DOSE   RATE     IT      DI
 NO. CODE   (MG)  (MG/MIN) (MIN)   (MIN)
   1  B    100.00  50.00    2.00    2.00
   2  I     90.00   2.00   45.00   45.00
   3  B     50.00  25.00    2.00    2.00
   4  I    480.00   4.00  120.00  120.00

ARE YOU SATISFIED WITH ALL OF THIS DATA
   ?Y

TIME(MIN) FROM START OF LAST DOSE TO START OF NEW(NEXT) REGIMEN
   ?180
WANT A PLOT OF PAST LEVELS REACHED
   ?Y
STANDARD PLOT(0-6 MCG/ML, 5 MIN INCREMENTS)
   ?Y
```

```
              B = LIDOCAINE BLOOD LEVEL, MCG/ML
                  (THERAPEUTIC LIMITS SHOWN AS DOTTED LINES)
              P = PERIPHERAL COMPARTMENT LEVEL, MCG/ML
   TIME       * = ADMINISTRATION RATE, MG/MIN                    DOSE

          0.00      1.00      2.00      3.00      4.00      5.00      6.00
  0---MIN-BP--------+-.-------+---------+---------+---------+----.----+    # 1
          I      P      .        * B                            .         # 2
          I           P.      B  *                              .
          I           . P B      *                              .
          I           .  BP      *                              .
          I           .  B P *                                  .
 30  MIN-+         +  .   B    P*         +         +         +  .   +
          I           .   B   *P                                .
          I           .   B  *  P                               .
          I           .    B  *   P                             .
          *           .        PB                               .         # 3
          I           .      B  P       *                       .         # 4
 60  MIN-+         +  .      B + P       *         +         +  .   +
          I           .        B      P    *                   .
          I           .        B       P  *                    .
          I           .        B       *P                      .
          I           .         B      *  P                    .
          I           .          B     *    P                  .
 90  MIN-+         +  .      +   B     *      P  +             .   +
          I           .          B     *        P             .
          I           .           B    *          P           .
          I           .            B   *            P .        .
          I           .            B   *              P        .
          I           .             B  *              . P      .
120 MIN-+         +  .      +        + B*       +        .  P + .
          I           .              B*                        . P
          I           .              *B                        .
          I           .              *B                        .
          I           .              * B                       .
          I           .              *  B                      .
150 MIN-+         +  .      +         + *   B   +         +     .   +
          I           .                *   B                   .
          I           .                *    B                  .
          I           .                *      B                .
          *           .                       B                .
          *           .                     B                  .
180 MIN-*         +  .      +         +     B   +         +     .   +
          *           .                  B                     .
          *           .                 B                      .
          *           .                B                       .
          *           .                B                       .
          *           .               B                        .
210 MIN-*         +  .      +        + B   +         +     .   +
          *           .                B                       .
          *           .               B                        .
          *           .              B                         .
230-MIN-*---------+-.-------+---------B---------+---------+----.---P+
          0.00      1.00      2.00      3.00      4.00      5.00      6.00
```

```
WANT ANOTHER PLOT(E.G., DIFFERENT SCALE, ETC.)
   ?N
WANT TO PLAN A DOSAGE REGIMEN OF     LIDOCAINE      NOW
   ?Y
WHAT IS THE PEAK SERUM LEVEL(MCG/ML) YOU WISH TO ACHIEVE
   ?3.5
DID YOU SPECIFY **********   3.50000  MCG/ML **********
   ?Y
WILL YOU BE USING THE DSII LABORATORIES    PROGRAMMABLE INFUSION PUMP
   ?N
THEN DESCRIBE HOW YOU WISH THE THERAPY TO BE GIVEN:

DOSE   1    ROUTE    ?I
              ENTER     IT ,  DI ,
            ?10,10
DOSE   2    ROUTE    ?R
              ENTER     IT ,  DI ,
            ?30,30
FOR DOSE   3    ?60,60
FOR DOSE   4    ?R,R

WANT TO CHECK YOUR ENTRIES
   ?N


CONSIDER:

       INFUSION #  1 ***    3.4 MG/MIN FOR    10.0 MIN IV, THEN
       INFUSION #  2 ***    2.0 MG/MIN FOR    30.0 MIN IV, THEN
       INFUSION #  3 ***    1.9 MG/MIN FOR    60.0 MIN IV, THEN
       INFUSION #  4 ***    1.9 MG/MIN FOR    60.0 MIN IV, THEN
       INFUSION #  5 ***    1.9 MG/MIN FOR    60.0 MIN IV, THEN

CONSIDER REPEATING INFUSION #  5 EVERY    60.0 MINUTES THEREAFTER.


WANT A PLOT OF PROBABLE LEVELS TO BE ACHIEVED WITH THIS REGIMEN
   ?N
WANT ADVICE ON HOW TO ADMINISTER THIS REGIMEN
   ?Y
DO YOU PLAN TO USE:

  1 - A SYRINGE IN A MOTORIZED SYRINGE DRIVE APPARATUS, OR
  2 - A BOTTLE WITH A DRIP SET
   ?1
IS THE SYRINGE YOU WILL BE USING:

     1 - A B-D PLASTIPAK 50 CC SYRINGE,
     2 - A MONOJECT 60 CC SYRINGE,
     3 - A STYLEX 50 CC SYRINGE, OR
     4 - SOME OTHER MAKE OR SIZE
   ?1
HOW MUCH    LIDOCAINE    WILL YOU PUT IN THE SYRINGE? E.G.,

   0.5 ,   1 , OR   2  GRAMS
   ?1
```

```
        YOUR SYRINGE WILL CONTAIN 1.0 GM(20.00 MG/ML) OF LIDOCAINE
IN A    50   CC VOLUME, WHICH IS A    2 % SOLUTION, CORRECT(Y/N)
    ?Y
THEN CONSIDER THE FOLLOWING SCHEDULE:

        INFUSION #  1 -  10.1 ML/HR(0.70 IN/HR) FOR  10.0 MIN, THEN
        INFUSION #  2 -   6.0 ML/HR(0.42 IN/HR) FOR  30.0 MIN, THEN
        INFUSION #  3 -   5.7 ML/HR(0.40 IN/HR) FOR  60.0 MIN, THEN
        INFUSION #  4 -   5.6 ML/HR(0.39 IN/HR) FOR  60.0 MIN, THEN
        INFUSION #  5 -   5.6 ML/HR(0.39 IN/HR) FOR  60.0 MIN, THEN

CONSIDER REPEATING INFUSION #  5 EVERY  60.0 MINUTES THEREAFTER.

WANT TO REVISE YOUR ADMINISTRATION PROCEDURE
    ?N
THEN CONSIDER USING THE FOLLOWING DIAGRAM(S) TO CHECK THE
INFUSION SPEED OF YOUR SYRINGE DRIVE.
        FROM 0 TO 50 ML SHOULD BE   3.50000  INCHES, CALIBRATED FOR A
PLASTIPAK OR MONOJECT 2 OUNCE SYRINGE, AND TYPED ON A STANDARD
MODEL 33 TELETYPE TERMINAL:


        HRS:MIN AFTER STARTING TO INFUSE SYRINGE #    1
          0:00.  1:36   3:23   5:11   6:58   8:46
        FOLD +......+......+......+......+......+ HERE
          50      40     30     20     10      0
                    ML LEFT IN SYRINGE


        HRS:MIN AFTER STARTING TO INFUSE SYRINGE #    2
          0:00   1:47   3:35   5:22   7:10   8:57
        FOLD +......+......+......+......+......+ HERE
          50      40     30     20     10      0
                    ML LEFT IN SYRINGE

THEN CONSIDER USING THE LAST DIAGRAM SHOWN ABOVE(#   2 ) TO CHECK
FOR PROPER INFUSION SPEED OF SUBSEQUENT SYRINGES USED TO
CONTINUE ADMINISTERING THE ABOVE DOSAGE RATE SCHEDULE.


WANT MORE ADVICE
    ?N
WANT TO REVISE YOUR DOSING STRATEGY
    ?N


        ALL INPUT AND OUTPUT HAS BEEN EVALUATED, CHECKED FOR ERRORS,
CHECKED FOR BEING CONSISTENT WITH THE PATIENT'S STATED CLINICAL
PICTURE, AND HAS BEEN VALIDATED BY THE RESPONSIBLE PERSON WHOSE
SIGNATURE APPEARS BELOW AS O.K. TO CONSIDER GIVING:



            .............................M.D. OR PHARM.D.
(OUTPUT NOT VALID UNLESS DECLARED SO BY BEING SIGNED ABOVE)
```

# REFERENCES

1. Benowitz NO and Meister W: Clinical pharmacokinetics of lidocaine. Clin Pharmacokin 1978; 3:177–201.
2. Mogenson L: Ventricular tachyarrhythmias and lignocaine prophylaxis in acute myocardial infarction. Acta Med Scand 1970; 513 (supp):1–80.
3. Lie KI, Wellens HJ, van Capelle FJ and Durrer D: Lidocaine in the prevention of primary ventricular fibrillation. N Engl J Med 1974; 291:1324–1326.
4. Wyman MG and Hammersmith L: Comprehensive treatment plan for the prevention of primary ventricular fibrillation in acute myocardial infarction. Am J Cardiol 1974; 33:661–667.
5. Harrison DC: Should lidocaine be administered routinely to all patients after myocardial infarction? Circ 1978; 58:581–584.
6. Covino BG: Local anesthesia. N Engl J Med 1972; 286:975–986 and 286:1035–1042.
7. Collinsworth KA, Kalman SM and Harrison DC: Clinical pharmacology of lidocaine as an antiarrhythmic drug. Circ 1974; 50:1217–1230.
8. Thomson PD, Melmon KL, Richardson JA et al: Lidocaine pharmacokinetics in advanced heart failure, liver disease, and renal failure in humans. Ann Int Med 1973; 78:499–508.
9. Zito RA and Reid PR: Lidocaine kinetics predicted by indocyanine green clearance. N Engl J Med 1978; 298:1160–1163.
10. Wyman MG, Lalka D, Hammersmith L, Cannon DS and Goldreyer BN: Multiple bolus technique for lidocaine administration during the first hours of an acute myocardial infarction. Am J Cardiol 1978; 41:313–317.
11. Boyes RN, Scott DB, Jepson PJ, Goodman MJ, and Julian DJ: Pharmacokinetics of lidocaine in man. Clin Pharmacol Therap 1971; 12:105–116.
12. Parkinson PI, Margolin L and Dickson DSP: Oral lignocaine: Its absorption and effectiveness in ventricular arrhythmia control. Brit Med J 1970; 2:29–30.
13. Gugler R, Lain P and Azarnoff DL: Effect of portacaval shunt on the disposition of drugs with and without first-pass effect. J Pharmacol Exp Therap 1975; 195:416–423.
14. Huet M, LeLorier J, Pomier G and Marlean D: Bioavailability of lidocaine in normal volunteers and cirrhotics. Clin Pharm & Therap 1979; 25:33.
15. Bromage PR and Robson JG: Concentrations of lidocaine in the blood after intravenous, intramuscular, epidural, and endotracheal administration. Anesth 1961; 16:461–478.
16. Scott DB, Jebson PJ, Vellani CW and Julian DG: Plasma levels of lignocaine after intramuscular administration. Lancet 1968; 2:1209–1210.
17. Cohen LS, Rosenthal JE, Horner DW, Atkins JM, Matthews OA and Sarnoff SJ: Plasma levels of lidocaine after intramuscular administration. Am J Cardiol 1972; 29:520–523.
18. Ryden L, Wasir H, Tor-Bjorn C and Olsson B: Blood levels of lignocaine after intramuscular administration to patients with proven or suspected myocardial infarction. Brit Heart J 1972; 34:1012–1017.
19. Zener JC, Kerber RG, Spivock AP and Harrison DC: Blood lidocaine levels and kinetics following high-dose intramuscular administration. Circ 1973; 48:984–987.
20. Schwartz ML, Meyer MB, Covino BG, Narang RM, Sethi V, Schwarter AJ and Kamp P: Antiarrhythmic effectiveness of intramuscular lidocaine: influence of different injection sites. J Clin Pharmacol 1974; 15:77–83.

21. Fehmers MCO and Dunning AJ: Intramuscularly and orally administered lidocaine in the treatment of ventricular arrhythmias in acute myocardial infarction. Am J Cardiol 1972; 29:514–519.
22. Jebson P: Intramuscular lignocaine 2% and 10%. Brit Med J 1971; 3:566.
23. Bellet S, Roman L, Kostis JB and Fleischman DB: Intramuscular lidocaine in the therapy of ventricular arrhythmias. Am J Cardiol 1971; 27:291–294.
24. Bernstein V, Bernstein M, Griffiths J and Peretz DI: Lidocaine intramuscularly in acute myocardial infarction. JAMA 1972; 219:1027–1031.
25. Ryden L, Waldenstrom A, Ehn L, Holmberg S and Husaini M: Comparison between the effectiveness of intramuscular and intravenous lignocaine on ventricular arrhythmias complicating acute myocardial infarction. Brit Heart J 1973; 35:1214–1131.
26. Singh JB and Kocot SZ: A controlled trial of intramuscular lidocaine in the prevention of premature ventricular contractions associated with acute myocardial infarction. Am Heart J 1976; 91:430–436.
27. Valentine PA, Frew JL, Mushford ML and Sloman JG: Lidocaine in the prevention of sudden death in the pre-hospital phase of acute infarction. N Engl J Med 1974; 291:1237–1331.
28. Lie KI, Lien KL, Lourditz WJ, Jamse MJ, Willebrands AF and Durrer D: Efficacy of lidocaine in preventing primary ventricular fibrillation within 1 hour after a 300 mg intramuscular injection. Am J Cardiol 1978; 42:486–488.
29. Scott DB, Jepson PJR, Braid DP, Ortengren B and Frisch P: Factors affecting plasma levels of lignocaine and prilocaine. Brit J Anaesth 1972; 44:1040–1048.
30. Chin WM, Zavala DC and Ambre J: Plasma levels of lidocaine following metabolized aerosol administration. Chest 1977; 71:346–348.
31. Karvonen S, Jokinen K, Karvumen P and Hollman A: Arterial and venous blood lidocaine concentration after local anesthesia of the respiratory tract using an ultrasonic nebulizer. Acta Anaesth Scand 1976; 20:156–159.
32. Credle WF, Smiddy JF and Elliott RC: Complications of fiberoptic bronchoscopy. Am Rev Respir Dis 1974; 109:67–72.
33. Ahmad K and Medzihradsky F: Distribution of lidocaine in blood and tissues after single doses and steady infusion. Res Comm Chem Path Pharmacol 1971; 2:813–828.
34. Benowitz N, Forsyth RP, Melmon KL and Rowland M: Lidocaine disposition kinetics in monkey and man. I. Prediction by a perfusion model. Clin Pharmacol Ther 1974; 16:87–98.
35. Benowitz N, Forsyth RP, Melmon KL and Rowland M: Lidocaine disposition kinetics in monkey and man. II. Effects of hemorrhage and sympathomimetric drug administration. Clin Pharmacol Ther 1974; 16:99–109.
36. Rowland M, Thomson PD, Guichard A and Melmon KL: Disposition kinetics of lidocaine in normal subjects. Ann NY Acad Sci 1971; 179:383–398.
37. Tucker GT and Boas RA: Pharmacokinetic aspects of regional anesthesia. Anesthesiology 1971; 34:538–549.
38. Stenson RE, Constantion RT and Harrison DC: Interrelationships of hepatic blood flow, cardiac output and blood levels of lidocaine in man. Circ 1971; 48:205–211.
39. LeLorier J, Gremon D, Latour Y, Caille G, Dumont G, Brosseau A and Solinger A: Pharmacokinetics of lidocaine after prolonged intravenous infusions in uncomplicated myocardial infarction. Ann Int Med 1977; 87:700–702.
40. LeLorier J, Moison R, Gagne J and Caile G: Effect of the duration of infusion on the disposition of lidocaine in dogs. J Pharmacol Exp Therap 1977; 203:507–511.

41. Sung CY and Truant AP: The physiological disposition of lidocaine and its comparison in some respects with procaine. J Pharmacol Exp Ther 1954; 112:432–443.
42. D'Argenio DZ and Schumitzky A: A program package for simulation and parameter estimation in pharmacokinetic systems. Comp Prog Biomed 1979; 9:115–134.
43. Keenaghan JB and Boyes RN: The tissue distribution, metabolism, and excretion of lidocaine in rats, guinea pigs, dogs and man. J Pharmacol Exp Ther 1972; 180:454–463.
44. Strong JM, Parker M and Atkinson AJ: Identification of glycinexylidide in patients treated with intravenous lidocaine. Clin Pharmacol Ther 1973; 14:67–72.
45. Strong JM, Mayfield DE, Atkinson AJ, Burris BC, Raymon F and Webster LT: Pharmacological activity, metabolism, and pharmacokinetics of glycinexylidide. Clin Pharmacol Ther 1975; 17:184–194.
46. Collinsworth KA, Strong JM, Atkinson AJ, Winkle RA, Perlroth F and Harrison DC: Pharmacokinetics and metabolism of lidocaine in patients with renal failure. Clin Pharmacol Therap 1975; 18:59–64.
47. Halkin H, Meffin P, Melmon KL and Rowland M: Influence of congestive heart failure on blood levels of lidocaine and its active monodeethylated metabolite. Clin Pharmacol Ther 1975; 17:669–676.
48. Narang PK, Crouthamel WG, Carliner NH and Fisher ML: Lidocaine and its active metabolites. Clin Pharmacol Ther 1978; 24:654–662.
49. Adjepon-Yamoah KK and Prescott LF: Lignocaine metabolism in man. Brit J Clin Pharmacol 1973; 47:672P–673P.
50. Smith ER and Duce BR: The acute antiarrhythmic and toxic effects in mice and dogs of 2-ethylamino-2', 6'-acetoxylidocaine (L-86), a metabolite of lidocaine. J Pharmacol Exp Ther 1971; 179:580–585.
51. Blumer J, Strong JM and Atkinson AJ: The convulsant potency of lidocaine and its N-dealkylated metabolites. J Pharmacol Exp Ther 1973; 186:31–36.
52. Burney RG, DiFazio GA, Peach MJ, Petrie KA and Sylvester MJ: Antiarrhythmic effects of lidocaine metabolites. Am Heart J 1974; 88:765–769.
53. Beckett AH, Boyes RN and Appleton PJ: The metabolism of and excretion of lidocaine in man. J Pharm Pharmacol 1966; 18:765–815.
54. Mather LE and Thomas J: Metabolism of lidocaine in man. Life Sciences 1972; 11:915–919.
55. Nelson SD, Garland WA, Breck GD and Trager WF: Quantification of lidocaine and several metabolites utilizing chemical-ionization mass spectrometry and stable isotope labeling. J Pharm Sci 1977; 66:1180–1189.
56. Breck GD and Trager WF: Oxidative N-dealkylation: a mannich intermediate in the formation of a new metabolite of lidocaine in man. Science 1971; 173:544–545.
57. Tucker GT, Boyes RN, Bridenbaugh PO and Moore DC: Binding of amilide type local anesthetics in human plasma. Anesthesiology 1970; 33:387.
58. Nies AS, Shand DG and Wilkinson GR: Altered hepatic blood flow and drug disposition. Clin Pharmacokin 1976; 1:135–155.
59. Pang KS and Rowland M: Hepatic clearance of drugs. I. Theoretical considerations of a "well stirred" model and a "parallel tube" model. Influence of hepatic blood flow, plasma and blood cell binding and the hepatocellular enzymatic activity on hepatic drug clearance. J Pharmacokin Biopharm 1977; 5:625–653.
60. Pang KS and Rowland M: Hepatic clearance of drugs. II. Experimental evidence for acceptance of the "well stirred" model over the "parallel tube" model using lidocaine in the perfused rat liver in situ preparation. J Pharmacokin Biopharm 1977; 5:655–699.

61. Williams RL, Blasche TF, Meffin PJ, Melmon KL and Rowland M: Influence of viral hepatitis on the disposition of two compounds with high hepatic clearance: lidocaine and indocyanine green. Clin Pharmacol Therap 1976; 20:290–299.

62. Forrest JAH, Finlayson NDC, Adjepon-Yamooh KK and Prescott LF: Antipyrine, paracetomol, and lignocaine elimination in man. Brit Med J 1977; 1:1384–1387.

63. Brandfonbrenner M, Landowne M and Shock NW: Changes in cardiac output with age. Circulation 1955; 12:557–566.

64. Grossman R, Kotelanski B, Cohn JN and Khatri IM: Quantification of portasystemic shunting from the splanchnic and mesenteric beds in alcoholic liver disease. Am J Med 1972; 53:715–722.

65. Cooperman LH: Effects of anesthetics on the splanchnic circulation. Brit J Anesthes 1972; 44:967–970.

66. Burney RG and DiFazio CA: Hepatic clearance of lidocaine during $N_2O$ anesthesia in dogs. Anesth Analg 1976; 55:322–325.

67. Branch RA, Shand DG, Wilkinson GR and Nies AS: The reduction of lidocaine clearance by dl-propranolol: an example of hemodynamic drug interaction. J Pharmacol Exp Ther 1973; 184:515–519.

68. Wiklund L: Human hepatic blood flow and its relation to systemic circulation during intravenous infusion of lidocaine. Acta Anesth Scand 1977; 21:148–160.

69. Rahimtoola SH, Sinno MZ, Loeb HS, Chuquimia R, Rosen KM and Gunnar RM: Lidocaine infusion in acute myocardial infarction. Effects on left ventricular function. Arch Intern Med 1971; 128:416–418.

70. Binnion PF, Murtagl G, Pollock AM and Fletchers E: Relation between plasma lignocaine levels and induced hemodynamic changes. Brit Med J 1969; 3:390–392.

71. Schumaker RR, Lieberson AD, Childress RH and William JF: Hemodynamic effects of lidocaine in patients with heart disease. Circulation 1968; 38:965–972.

72. Boudoulas H, Schall SF, Lewis RP, Welch TG, De Green P and Kates RE: Negative inotropic effect of lidocaine in patients with coronary arterial disease and normal subjects. Chest 1977; 71:70–175.

73. Lautt WW and Skelton FS: The effect of SKF-525A and of altered hepatic blood flow on lidocaine clearance in the cat. Can J Physiol Pharmacol 1977; 55:7–12.

74. Di Fazio CA and Brown RE: Lidocaine metabolism in normal and phenobarbital pretreated dogs. Anesthesiology 1972; 36:238–243.

75. Heinonon J, Takki S and Jahro L: Plasma lidocaine levels in patients treated with potential inducers of microsomal enzymes. Acta Anaesth Scandinav 1970; 14:89–95.

76. Adjepon-Yamoah KK, Nimmo J and Prescott LF: Gross impairment of hepatic drug metabolism in a patient with chronic liver disease. Brit Med J 1974; 4:387–388.

77. Sotaniemi EA, Ahlqvist J, Pelkonen RO, Pirttiaho HI and Luoma PV: Histological changes in the liver and indices of drug metabolism in alcoholics. Europ J Clin Pharmacol 1977; 11:295–303.

78. Pirttiaho HI, Sotaniemi EA, Ahlqvist J, Pitkonen U and Pelkomen RO: Liver size and indices of drug metabolism in alcoholics. Europ J Clin Pharmacol 1978; 13:61–67.

79. Prescott LF, Adjepom-Yamoah and Talbot RG: Impaired lignocaine metabolism in patients with myocardial infarction and heart failure. Brit Med J 1976; 1:939–941.

80. Jelliffe RW, Goicoechea FJ, Tuey DB, Wyman MG, Rodman J and Goldreyer B: An improved computer program for lidocaine infusion regimens. Clin Res 1975; 23:125A.

81. Pfeifer HJ, Greenblatt DJ and Koch-Weser J: Clinical use and toxicity of intravenous lidocaine. Am Heart J 1976; 92:168–173.
82. Deacock ARC and Simpson WT: Fatal reactions to lidocaine. Anesthesiology 1964; 19:217–221.
83. Pitt A, Lipp H and Anderson ST: Lignocaine given prophylactically to patients with acute myocardial infarction. Lancet 1971; 1:612–616.
84. Gianelly R, von der Gruben JO, Spivack AP and Harrison DC: Effect of lidocaine on ventricular arrhythmias in patients with coronary heart disease. N Engl J Med 1967; 277:1215–1219.
85. Sheridan DJ, Crawford L, Rawlins MD and Julian DG: Antiarrhythmic action of lignocaine in early myocardial infarction. Lancet 1977; 1:824–825.
86. Alderman EL, Kerber RE and Harrison DC: Evaluation of lidocaine resistance in man using intermittent large dose infusion techniques. Am J Cardiol 1974; 34:342–349.
87. Foldes FF, Molloy R, McNall PG and Koukal LR: Comparison of toxicity of intravenously given local anesthetic agents in man. JAMA 1960; 172:1493–1498.
88. Wikinski JA, Usubiaga JE, Morales RL, Torrieri A and Usubiaga LE: Mechanism of convulsions elicited by local anesthetic agents. Anesth Analg 1970; 49:504–510.
89. Sjogren S and Wright B: Blood concentrations of lidocaine during continuous epidural blockade. Acta Anaesth Scandinav 1972; 16:51–56.
90. Marriott HL and Bieza CF: Alarming ventricular acceleration after lidocaine administration. Chest 1972; 61:682–683.
91. Lichstein E, Chadda KD and Gupta PK: Atrioventricular block with lidocaine therapy. Am J Cardiol 1973; 31:277–281.
92. Chang TO and Wauhwa K: Sinus standstill following intravenous lidocaine administration. JAMA 1973; 223:790–792.
93. Jeresaty RM, Kahn AH and Landry AB: Sinoatrial arrest due to lidocaine in a patient receiving quinidine. Chest 1972; 61:683–685.
94. Gupta PK, Lichstein E, Chadda KD: Lidocaine induced heart block in patients with bundle branch block. Am J Cardiol 1974; 33:487–492.
95. Kunkel F, Rowland M and Scheinmann MM: The electrophysiologic effects of lidocaine in patients with intraventricular conduction defects. Circulation 1974; 49:894–899.
96. Lalka D, Manion CV, Berlin A, Baer DT, Dodd B and Meyer MB: Dose dependent pharmacokinetics of lidocaine in volunteers. Clin Pharmacol Therap 1976; 19:110.
97. Forrester JS, Diamond G, Chatterjee K and Swan HJC: Hemodynamic therapy of myocardial infarction. N Engl J Med 1976; 295:1404–1413.
98. Kruger-Thiemer G: Continuous intravenous infusion and multicompartment accumulation. Europ J Pharmacol 1968; 4:317–324.
99. Benet LZ: General treatment of linear mammillary models with elimination from any compartment as used in pharmacokinetics. J Pharm Sci 1972; 61:536–546.
100. Rodman J, Tuey DB, deGuzman M, Haywood LJ and Jelliffe RW: Clinical evaluation of a pharmacokinetic model and computer program for improving lidocaine dosage regimens. Clin Pharmacol Therap 1979; 25:245.
101. Branch RA, James JA and Read AE: The clearance of antipyrine and indocyanine green in normal subjects and patients with chronic liver disease. Clin Pharmacol Therap 1976; 20:81–89.
102. Nations RL, Triggs EJ and Selig M: Lignocaine kinetics in cardiac patients and aged subjects. Brit J Clin Pharmacol 1977; 4:439–448.
103. Keenaghan JB: The determination of lidocaine and prilocaine in whole blood by gas chromatography. Anesthesiology 1968; 29:110–112.

104. Benowitz N and Rowland M: Determination of lidocaine in blood and tissues. Anesthesiology 1973; 39:639–641.

105. Hisayasu GH, Dawson MF and Cohen JL: GLC determination of lidocaine and its deethylated metabolites in biological fluids using alkalai flame detection. 27th Annual Academy Pharmaceutical Sciences Proceedings, Kansas City, Mo., November 11–15, 1979.

106. Strong JM and Atkinson AJ: Simultaneous measurement of lidocaine and its desethylated metabolite by mass fragmentography. Anal Chem 1972; 44:2287–2290.

107. Hignite CE, Tschanz C, Steiner J, Huffman DH and Azarnoff DL: Quantification of lidocaine and its deethylated metabolites in plasma and urine by gas chromatography—mass fragmentography. J Chromatog 1978; 161:243–249.

108. DiFazio CA and Brown RE: The analysis of lidocaine and its postulated metabolites. Anesthesiology 1971; 34:86–90.

109. Adjepon-Yamoah KK and Prescott LF: Gas liquid chromatographic estimation of lignocaine, ethylglycylxylidide, glycylxylidide, and 4-hydroxyxlylidine in plasma and urine. J Pharm Pharmacol 1974; 26:889–893.

110. Nation RL, Triggs EJ and Selig M: Gas chromatographic method for the quantitative determination of lidocaine and its metabolite monoethylglycylxylidide in plasma. J Chromatog 1976; 116:188–193.

111. Rosseel MT and Bogaert MG: Determination of lidocaine and its desethylated metabolites in plasma by capillary column gas-liquid chromatography. J Chromatog 1978; 154:99–102.

112. Adams RF, Vandemark FL and Schmidt G: The simultaneous determination of lidocaine and procainamide in serum by high pressure liquid chromatography. Clin Chim Acta 1976; 69:515–524.

113. Massoud AM, Scratchly GA, Stohs SS and Wingard DW: Simultaneous determination of lidocaine and thiopental in plasma using high pressure liquid chromatography. J Liquid Chromatog 1978; 1:607–616.

114. Nation RL, Peng GW and Chiou WL: High pressure liquid chromatographic method for simultaneous determination of lidocaine and its N-dealkylated metabolites in plasma. J Chromatog 1979; 162:466–473.

115. Cobb ME, Buckley N, Hu MW, Miller JG, Singh P and Schneider RS: Homogenous enzyme immunoassay for lidocaine in serum. Clin Chem 1977; 23:1161.

116. Wahlberg CB: Lidocaine by enzyme immunoassay. J Analyt Toxicol 1978; 2:121–123.

117. Stargell WW, Roe CR, Routledge PA and Shand DG: Importance of blood collection tubes in plasma lidocaine determinations. Clin Chem 1979; 25:617–619.

*Counterpoint Discussion*

# Lidocaine

Laurence Green, Pharm.D.
Milford G. Wyman, M.D.
David Lalka, Ph.D.

**Clinical Pharmacokinetics of Lidocaine**

**Introduction.** Dr. Rodman has thoroughly summarized the classical view of lidocaine pharmacokinetics in his chapter (see sections dealing with the calculation of loading infusions, maintenance infusion selection and considerations relating to two-compartment behavior). However, there are several reports which are not adequately explained by classical kinetic theory. In this section a number of observations inconsistent with the classical view of lidocaine kinetics will be discussed. Furthermore, a summary of recent advances in the study of lidocaine plasma protein binding as well as a brief commentary on selected aspects of lidocaine metabolism are presented.

**Aclassical Features of Lidocaine Kinetics.** The classical view of lidocaine disposition suggests that the drug exhibits linear kinetics consistent with a two- *or* three-compartment open model. Following bolus administration to healthy young volunteers, the terminal phase half-life has been reported to be approximately 1.5 hours and the overall volume of distribution has been estimated to be about 1.5 liters/kg (1–3). Furthermore, evidence has been presented suggesting that chronic congestive heart failure and alcoholic liver disease cause a moderate prolongation of half-life as well as decreased clearance (2). However, little experimental data were available concerning lidocaine kinetics in the immediate post acute myocardial infarction (AMI) period. Because of this paucity of data, Prescott et al (4) performed the first detailed study of lidocaine kinetics in this group of patients. They reported that the half-life of lidocaine was 4.3 ± 0.8 hours in AMI patients without heart failure, while the presence of heart failure was associated with a prolongation of the half-life to 10.2 ± 2.0 hours (all data mean ± SEM). Furthermore, they reported that plasma

392

concentrations did not reliably reach steady-state following 46 hours of constant rate infusion in the presence *or* absence of heart failure. These data are quite contradictory to the classical view of lidocaine kinetics. Furthermore, several laboratories have provided data which clearly demonstrate that lidocaine does exhibit this strikingly increased half-life following *prolonged infusion* to AMI patients (5–8). The mechanism(s) responsible for the prolonged half-life of lidocaine is (are) presently unknown. However such factors as a "deep" compartment of large apparent volume which slowly releases drug back into the central compartment, the possibility of product and/or substrate inhibition of lidocaine metabolism and/or the expansion of lidocaine's apparent volume of distribution caused by its displacement from plasma protein binding sites (perhaps by metabolites) are all currently under investigation.

In the context of aclassical behavior following the administration of loading doses, we have reported (9) that a series of boluses yields lidocaine plasma concentrations which are much lower than would be expected on the basis of simulations using pharmacokinetic constants from normal or non-AMI patient volunteers (2,3). The mechanism which is responsible for this behavior is unclear. However, it could be related in part to the saturation of plasma protein binding sites or increased transport out of the blood secondary to altered organ perfusion. The plasma protein binding of lidocaine has been examined by several groups (10–13) and is discussed in detail below. Furthermore, the perfusion changes which have been reported secondary to brief infusion (60 to 240 min) of lidocaine have been rather impressive (14, 15). Specifically, Tucker et al (14) have shown that hepatic blood flow rate increased by about 35% in response to a 150 min infusion of 4 mg/min. Similarly, Vyden et al (15) have presented convincing evidence for major alteration in the perfusion of skeletal muscle. Thus, the "vasoactive" behavior of lidocaine should not be totally ignored.

Other pure kinetic studies in normal healthy volunteers have provided evidence suggesting dose dependence (16,17). However, these two studies were troubled by the fact that very small populations were examined (17) and/or that blood samples were drawn into Vacutainers® and hence "Vacutainer effects" yielding spuriously low plasma levels could have occurred (see ref. 22 and the section on Plasma Protein Binding for details).

Within the context of aclassical behavior of lidocaine kinetics in animal studies, LeLorier and coworkers have convincingly established that the hepatic extraction of lidocaine decreases from 0.79 to 0.26 between the second and twenty-fourth hours of constant rate infusion in dogs (18). Finally, we have provided evidence showing that pretreatment of dogs with a high dose (125 μg/kg/min × 240 min) of lidocaine reduces the clearance of the drug when it is subsequently infused at a lower rate (19). Elaboration of the mechanisms responsible for this observed aclassical behavior appears to be a fertile area for pharmacokinetic research.

Based upon these complexities and those cited below (see sections on Plasma Protein Binding and Dosing Guidelines), it seems possible that reliance upon a classical two-compartment open model for dosing predictions is unwise. Furthermore, based on pragmatic grounds (i.e., clinical success), it is reasonable to use the dosing guidelines described below (see Guidelines for Drug Administration) pending the identification of a model which accurately describes lidocaine kinetics in the setting of acute myocardial infarction.

**Plasma Protein Binding.** The binding of lidocaine to human serum proteins was first reported in 1963 by Sawinsky and Rapp (20). They observed significant binding of this drug to human serum albumin while little or no association with human gamma globulin was found. In the late 1960's another important publication appeared; Shnider and Way (10) reported extensive binding of lidocaine to plasma proteins from mothers and neonates at the time of delivery. Furthermore, these authors reported a significant increase in free fraction as lidocaine concentration was increased through the range usually observed in the treatment of ventricular arrhythmias. Tucker et al (11) reported the same effect approximately one year later but they observed a significantly attenuated relationship between free fraction and total lidocaine plasma concentration. More recently, others have reported a still more limited change in lidocaine free fraction with increasing plasma concentration (21). The authors of this last report made the interesting observation that lidocaine free fraction was sensitive to pH; a pH change from 7.4 to 7.0 caused the free fraction to increase from 0.52 to 0.65 when the lidocaine concentration was 5 μg/ml. We have confirmed this observation. Furthermore, we see a more substantial effect. Specifically, free fraction increased from 0.30 to 0.43 (a more than 40% increase) as pH decreased from 7.4 to 7.1 (12). Since much of our early protein binding data were rendered unusable because of Vacutainer®-related drug displacement, which has now been confirmed by others (22), we speculate that the rather high free fraction reported by these investigators (21) as well as the more modest pH effect may have resulted from a "Vacutainer effect"; i.e., a chemical leached out of some rubber stoppers displaces lidocaine from its plasma protein binding sites. Binding changes caused by these collection tubes can be enormous (i.e., doubling of free fraction).

Fortunately, the most serious error which collection tubes have been reported to cause in plasma concentration estimation is about a 25% decrease (see reference 22 for details). Thus, it is likely that much of the early lidocaine plasma concentration data are contaminated by a systematic error. However, this error is unlikely to exceed 25%.

There have been several recent advances in our understanding of lidocaine plasma protein binding. Piafsky and Knoppert provided convincing evidence that lidocaine binds to $\alpha_1$ acid glycoprotein (23). This protein has been implicated in the binding of a number of other drugs such as propranolol (24,25), chlorpromazine (24), quinidine (26), and imipramine (27). Thus, a realistic possibility of drug protein binding interactions appeared to exist. McNamara et al (12) have shown *in vitro* that several of these drugs (as well as their metabolites) can cause a 25 to 35% increase in lidocaine free fraction if concentrations of the displacing agent approximate the upper end of their therapeutic range. An increase in free fraction of this magnitude is probably of some clinical importance; however, its exact significance remains to be established. It should be noted that similar studies with four lidocaine metabolites (monoethylglycinexylidide, glycinexylidide, 3 hydroxylidocaine, and 4 hydroxylidocaine) at concentrations which might be observed in AMI patients demonstrated that they were *not* capable of significantly displacing lidocaine (12). Thus, it appears that although lidocaine is sensitive to displacement, the clinical importance of this phenomenon remains to be established *in vivo*.

A study of intersubject variability of lidocaine free fraction in normal subjects has recently been completed in this laboratory (13). In 16 fasting healthy volunteers, ages 23 to 72, it was observed that free fraction ranged from 0.208 to 0.342 (mean: 0.280) at a lidocaine concentration of 1.4 µg/ml. Part of this variability appeared to be related to the smoking status of the subjects. Smokers exhibited a trend toward lower free fractions; $0.258 \pm 0.039$ vs. $0.307 \pm 0.030$; $p < 0.02$. The mechanisms responsible for this behavior *may* be related to the fact that tobacco smoking is a sufficiently potent inflammatory stimulus to elevate plasma levels of $\alpha_1$ acid glycoprotein (28). Increased concentration of this binding protein would be expected to decrease the free fraction. It should be noted that our smoking and nonsmoking volunteers were well matched with respect to age, sex, serum albumin, and total serum protein concentration. Thus, it appears that normal volunteers exhibit a *relatively* narrow range of free fraction values. *However,* since Piafsky and coworkers (24) have shown that in a typical patient population (including renal disease, hepatic disease, inflammatory disease, etc.) a two to four fold range of $\alpha_1$ acid glycoprotein concentration exists and because detailed scatchard analysis by McNamara et al (12) suggests that a doubling of $\alpha_1$ acid glycoprotein levels would substantially reduce free fraction, it should be anticipated that abnormal and highly variable lidocaine free fractions will be observed in patient populations.

**Pharmacologic Effects of Lidocaine Metabolites.** As Dr. Rodman correctly indicated, a number of laboratories have reported data establishing that monoethylglycinexylidide (MEGX) and glycinexylidide (GX) exhibit pharmacologic activity in a variety of animal models (29–31). Furthermore, significant indirect evidence of the toxicologic and pharmacologic significance of these compounds has been reported (i.e., toxicological observations have been made in patients who had extraordinarily elevated plasma concentrations of MEGX and/or GX with what could be regarded as lidocaine concentrations at the lower end of the therapeutic range). However, the only unambiguous human toxicology data for either metabolite would appear to be those from Atkinson's Laboratory (32). They infused themselves with GX and achieved peak plasma concentrations in the range of 5 to 10 µg/ml with little or no objective toxicity. These concentrations are substantially above any seen in AMI patients during long-term lidocaine infusion. Beyond this observation, there are little data available for the direct assessment of the toxicologic or pharmacologic significance of any lidocaine metabolites in man.

One apparent toxicological observation attributed to lidocaine metabolite(s) is the anecdotal report by Boyes et al (2) in which "toxicity" was observed after the oral administration of 500 mg of lidocaine HCl. Since the lidocaine concentrations observed in these subjects were low and because 50 to 75% of the dose could be expected to be biotransformed as a result of first-pass effect, these toxicological events were attributed to "metabolite(s)". This explanation is difficult to accept if there is any correlation between plasma concentration (arterial or venous) of the metabolites and toxic effect, since the elegant studies of Nelson et al (33) have established that no known metabolite is observed in significant plasma concentrations following an oral dose in the range of 250 to 500 mg. Nelson et al assayed plasma for lidocaine as well as for essentially all known (and several postulated) metabolites. They demonstrated that only rather low concentrations of MEGX and GX were observed. Intuitively, one might expect that (if toxicity correlated with metabolite level) individuals loaded intravenously with 100 to 150 mg and infused at 2 to 4 mg/min for 24 to 72 hr would probably develop levels of metabolites which were substantially greater than could realistically be seen following oral administration of 500 mg of lidocaine HCl. Thus the toxic effects observed following an oral dose of lidocaine are not readily attributable to lidocaine metabolites.

## Guidelines for Drug Administration

**Dosing Guidelines.** Guidelines for the use of lidocaine in the prevention and treatment of ventricular ectopy and ventricular fibrillation have been based largely on the experience gained in coronary care units. The most aggressive of these guidelines have been used quite successfully (34,35). However, approximately 20% of treated patients fail to have their arrhythmias satisfactorily controlled (9). Some of these failures are very probably secondary to an inadequate drug concentration at the site of action. Thus, in the absence of signs of toxicity it is likely that substantial intersubject variability in lidocaine kinetics (3,6,7) is a significant cause of treatment failures. Since the clinical pharmacokinetics of lidocaine are very complex (see Aclassical Kinetics section) and because of the life-threatening nature of the condition being treated, comprehensive dosage guidelines are necessary to insure the most satisfactory treatment response. This need for guidelines may be satisfactorily fulfilled by a computer-assisted treatment program as suggested by Dr. Rodman. However, at present most coronary care units do not have access to the computers needed to establish dosage regimens as suggested in Dr. Rodman's chapter. Furthermore, since contemporary computer-assisted dosing recommendations rely on the validity of a model known to inadequately describe the observed data (see Aclassical Kinetics section), simple dosing recommendations which have been shown to be clinically effective (34) may well suffice until studies of the clinical kinetics of lidocaine in AMI patients allow the preparation of more comprehensive guidelines based on sufficient clinical and pharmacokinetic data. In the remainder of this section we will discuss data and philosophy relevant to the clinical utilization of lidocaine in the typical AMI patient. Reliable guidelines for the treatment of AMI patients with concurrent disease such as hepatic cirrhosis remain to be established.

**Loading Dose.** The goal of a standard loading dosage regimen should be to reach therapeutic plasma concentrations (i.e. achieve complete arrhythmia suppression and prevent ventricular fibrillation) in a very large fraction of all patients without producing toxicity. Furthermore, this loading dose must maintain plasma concentrations in the therapeutic range until the concentration (i.e., pharmacologic effect) can be maintained by a constant rate infusion.

A loading dose is usually based on a percent of body weight. However, it has been difficult up to this time to correlate body weight and the initial volume of distribution. For this reason it has proven practical to establish a fixed loading dose (rather than one based on percent body weight) that will provide lidocaine plasma concentrations that are both therapeutic and safe.

Loading may be accomplished by an infusion technique (36) or by using single or multiple bolus injections (9). The multiple bolus technique has proven to be simple and effective. This method has the advantage that a patient is not arbitrarily loaded with a standard infusion (which may represent much more drug than is needed) to sustain the desired effect. It has been our practice to give an initial 75 mg loading dose to these patients when they are first seen in the emergency room and to follow this bolus with a series of 50 mg boluses (given as 1 min infusions with 5 mins allowed between the initiation of each infusion) to a total of 225 mg if needed to control ectopy. Preliminary evidence suggests that some patients may benefit from doses of 275 or 325 mg. Thus, these techniques can be used to quickly establish whether a patient's arrhythmia will respond to lidocaine since they reliably produce lidocaine plasma concentrations in the therapeutic range (yet below toxic concentrations) even in patients with congestive heart failure (9). If transient central nervous system side effects occur, the bolus dosage can be reduced and/or infused more slowly.

**Maintenance Dose.** To maintain therapeutic plasma levels a constant rate infusion is initiated immediately following the commencement of the bolus regimen. The maintenance infusion should be delivered with an infusion pump. Selection of an infusion rate based on an estimated cardiac output (i.e., using nomograms) appears to be of some value. However, there is a substantial overlap between observed total body clearances in congestive heart failure (CHF) and noncongestive heart failure patients (6,7). In the absence of CHF and liver disease an initial infusion rate of 2 mg/min is highly effective (34) and rarely causes toxic effects (34,37). In patients with *severe* heart failure and reduced cardiac output the infusion rate should be decreased. Preliminary evidence (7) suggests that a 33% reduction of infusion rate given to patients having class III-IV heart failure would result in plasma concentrations similar to those observed in patients with class O-I failure (see reference 9 for detailed definitions of the severity of heart failure).

**Treatment of Breakthrough Arrhythmias.** The treatment of breakthrough ventricular arrhythmias is predicated on the fact that in the setting of acute ischemia or necrosis premature ventricular beats can cause ventricular fibrillation. If arrhythmias reappear during the course of an infusion after being initially suppressed, it is our policy to administer an additional 25 to 50 mg bolus injection. Furthermore, the infusion rate is increased 1 mg/min (up to a maximum of 4 mg/min) after each additional bolus that is needed to suppress the arrhythmia. The infusion rate increase is necessary to provide adequate plasma concentrations to maintain suppression of arrhythmias after the effect of the bolus injection has become insignificant. It is particularly important to observe the patient carefully for signs of central nervous system toxicity when multiple boluses of lidocaine are being given and the continuous infusion is being increased to 4 mg/min. With careful observation the patient may reveal evidence of minor central nervous symptoms such as changes in mentation, speech and paresthesias. Serious complications such as convulsions can be averted by altering or stopping the infusion when these minor symptoms are recognized. Since the San Pedro Peninsula Hospital adopted the use of infusion pumps for all lidocaine infusions (over 10 years ago) we have never had a convulsion. Furthermore, since the first toxic symptoms observed during lidocaine treatment are almost always mild to moderate central nervous system effects (37), careful observation of the patient essentially precludes the occurrence of cardiovascular toxicity. It has been our practice to withhold lidocaine until a pacemaker has been inserted in those patients with a complete heart block with either a junctional or infranodal pacemaker. Although exit block or slowing of the junctional pacemaker has been reported in patients with an acute inferior infarction (38), we have not observed this. One patient in our series developed slowing of an infranodal pacemaker but a pacemaker had been inserted and complications were averted.

The method of giving lidocaine as multiple boluses and continuous infusion has the advantage over a computerized program of being simpler, as well as being safe and effective. It is based on giving the least amount of medication that is necessary to control premature ventricular beats. In our series of 1500 consecutive acute myocardial infarctions, 57% required only the loading boluses of 125 mg and a 2 mg/min infusion.

**Factors Influencing the Selection of the Duration of Infusion.** It is generally accepted that frequent and complex ventricular arrhythmias should be treated, particularly in the first 24 hours after an AMI. The decision regarding the duration of therapy is easily justified because the incidence of ventricular fibrillation decreases logarithmically with time following the acute event. Approximately 90% of the patients who will develop primary ventricular fibrillation do so within the first 24 hours of an acute myocardial infarction (39). For this reason infusions longer than 24 hours are not usually needed unless the patient continues to exhibit complex premature ventricular contractions or a new episode of chest pain occurs. Furthermore, lidocaine *may* continue to accumulate in AMI patients for much longer than classical kinetics suggest (4–7). Therefore, the risk to the patient must be weighed against the potential benefit (39).

**Prophylactic Lidocaine.** In many coronary care units throughout the country the prophylactic administration of lidocaine to every patient suspected of having a myocardial infarction has become a standard procedure. If lidocaine is being used prophylactically (in the absence of arrhythmias), suppression of arrhythmias obviously cannot be used to determine efficacy. Therefore, we have developed the following guidelines.

To initiate therapy, the following safe and effective method has been used by us for the past 10 years. A 75 mg bolus (50 mg/min) is given at the time the patient is seen in the emergency room and this is followed by a second bolus of 50 mg in five minutes. A maintenance infusion, as discussed earlier, should be continued for 24 to 30 hours. This method of administering prophylactic lidocaine to all patients suspected of having a myocardial infarction has been used in over 4,000 patients at the San Pedro Peninsula Hospital with only occasional transient central nervous side effects and no toxic cardiovascular effects.

By stopping the infusion as soon as possible after 24 hours, problems of lidocaine accumulation have been averted. While the dosing guidelines proposed by Dr. Rodman are quite sufficient for most patients, the guidelines suggested above should accomplish the same goal. Practical guidelines that are available to the clinician based on present knowledge of lidocaine kinetics may be as useful as more sophisticated approaches.

**Tapering of Lidocaine Infusion.** After the decision to stop lidocaine treatment has been made, the physician must choose to abruptly discontinue treatment *or* to gradually decrease the infusion rate (i.e., to taper). It appears that only one study has compared the rate of recurrence of ventricular arrhythmias observed using these two techniques. In this study 29 patients admitted to a coronary care unit for suspected myocardial infarction were started on lidocaine for ventricular arrhythmia (i.e., frequent premature ventricular contractions greater than six per minute, ventricular tachycardia or ventricular fibrillation). Patients who had evidence of congestive heart failure, liver disease or renal impairment, had received other antiarrhythmic medication or had ventricular arrhythmias not secondary to myocardial infarction were excluded. Lidocaine infusions of at least 24 hours duration were either abruptly discontinued without tapering or decreased by one-third of the original rate every hour until discontinued. Recurrence of arrhythmias, as defined by greater than one premature ventricular contraction every five minutes or any dysrhythmia such as ventricular tachycardia or multifocal premature ventricular contraction which required reinstitution of lidocaine, was determined by continuous holter monitoring. The average duration of the infusion for the tapered and non-tapered groups was 50 and 45 hours respectively and the duration of infusion did not correlate with the recurrence of ventricular arrhythmias. Three of eleven patients in the tapered group and two of eighteen in the non-tapered group had recurrent arrhythmias requiring reinstitution of lidocaine or other antiarrhythmic drugs. If one assumes that the anitarrhythmic effects of lidocaine correlate with its plasma concentrations as well as considering the long half-life of lidocaine after prolonged infusion (4–7), the absence of any significant difference in the rate of recurrence of arrhythmias is not surprising. Clearly, a larger and more detailed study of this problem is warranted.

Supported in part by Grant GM-20852 from the Institute of General Medical Sciences, National Institutes of Health.

# REFERENCES

1. Tucker GT, Boas RA: Pharmacokinetic aspects of intravenous regional anesthesia. Anesthesiology 1971; 34:538–549.
2. Boyes RN, Scott DB, Jebson PJ, Godman MJ, Julian DG: Pharmacokinetics of lidocaine in man. Clin Pharmacol Ther 1971; 12:105–116.
3. Thompson PD, Melmon KL, Richardson JA, Cohn K, Steinbrumm W, Cudihee R, Rowland M: Lidocaine pharmacokinetics in advanced heart failure, liver disease, and renal failure in humans. Ann Int Med 1973; 78:499–508.
4. Prescott LF, Adjepon-Yamoah KK, Talbot RG: Impaired lignocaine metabolism in patients with myocardial infarction and cardiac failure. Brit Med J 1976; 1:939–941.
5. LeLorier J, Grenon D, Latour Y, Caille G, Dumont G, Brosseau A, Solignac A: Pharmacokinetics of lidocaine after prolonged intravenous infusions in uncomplicated myocardial infarction. Ann Int Med 1977; 87:700–702.
6. Sawyer DR, Ludden TM, Lutonsky RN, Crawford MH: Unpredictability of lidocaine kinetics in patients with cardiac arrhythmias. Clin Pharmacol Ther 1980; 27:284 (Abstract).
7. Lalka D, Slaughter RL, Goldreyer BN, Cannon DS, Halton DJ, Wyman MG: Lidocaine pharmacokinetics and metabolism in acute myocardial infarction patients. Clin Res 1980; 28:239A (Abstract).

8. Winkle RA, Glantz SA, Harrison DC: Pharmacologic therapy of ventricular arrhythmias. Am J Cardiol 1975; 36:629–642.

9. Wyman MG, Lalka D, Hammersmith L, Cannon DS, Goldreyer BN: Multiple bolus technique for lidocaine administration during the first hours of an acute myocardial infarction. Am J Cardiol 1978; 41:313–317.

10. Shnider SM, Way EL: The kinetics of transfer of lidocaine (Xylocaine) across the human placenta. Anesthesiology 1968; 29:944–950.

11. Tucker GT, Boyes RN, Bridenbaugh PO, Moore DC: Binding of anilidetype local anesthesics in human plasma. I. Relationships between binding, physicochemical properties, and anesthetic activity. Ibid. 1979; 33:287–302.

12. McNamara PJ, Slaughter RL, Pieper JA, Wyman MG, Lalka D: Factors influencing the serum free fraction of lidocaine in man. Clin Pharmacol Ther 1980; 27:271 (Abstract).

13. McNamara PJ, Slaughter RL, Visco JP, Elwood CM, Siegel JH, Lalka D: Effect of smoking on the binding of lidocaine to human serum proteins. J Pharm Sci 1980; 69:749–751.

14. Tucker GT, Wiklund L, Wahlen AB, Mather LE: Hepatic clearance of local anesthetics in man. J Pharmacokin Biopharm 1977; 5:111–122.

15. Vyden JK, Mandel WJ, Hayakawa H, Nagasawa K, Groseth-Dittrick M: The effect of lidocaine on peripheral hemodynamics. J Clin Pharmacol 1975; 15:506–510.

16. Lalka D, Manion CV, Berlin A, Baer DT, Dodd B, Meyer MB: Dose dependent pharmacokinetics of lidocaine in volunteers. Clin Pharmacol Ther 1976; 19:110 (Abstract).

17. Bending MR, Bennett PN, Rowland M, Steiner J: Lignocaine pharmacokinetics in man: dose and time studies. Brit J Clin Pharmacol 1976; 3:956P (Abstract).

18. LeLorier J, Moisan R, Gagne J, Caille J: Effect of the duration of infusion on the disposition of lidocaine in dogs. J Pharmacol Exp Ther 1977; 203:507–511.

19. Vicuna N, Lalka D, Burrow SR, McLean AJ, du Souich P, McNay JL: Dose-dependent pharmacokinetic behavior of lidocaine in the conscious dog. Res Commun Chem Pathol Pharmacol 1978; 22:485–491.

20. Sawinski VJ, Rapp GW: Interaction of human serum proteins with local anesthetic agents. J Dent Res 1963; 42:1429–1438.

21. Burney RG, BiFazio CA, Foster JA: Effect of pH on protein binding of lidocaine. Anesth Analg 1978; 57:478–480.

22. Stargel WW, Roe CR, Routledge PA, Shand DG: Importance of blood-collection tubes in plasma lidocaine determinations. Clin Chem 1979; 25:617–619.

23. Piafsky KM, Knoppert D: Binding of local anesthetics to $\alpha_1$ acid glycoprotein. Clin Res 1979; 26:836A.

24. Piafsky KM, Borga O, Cederlof IO, Johansson G, Sjoqvist F: Increased plasma protein binding of propranolol and chlorpromazine mediated by disease-induced elevations of plasma $\alpha_1$ acid glycoprotein. New Engl J Med 1978; 299:1435–1439.

25. Wood M, Shand DG, Wood AJJ: Propranolol binding in plasma during cardiopulmonary bypass. Anesthesiology 1979; 51:512–516.

26. Fremstad D, Bergerud K, Haffner JFW, Lunde PKM: Increased plasma binding of quinidine after surgery: A preliminary report. Eur J Clin Pharmacol 1976; 10:441–444.

27. Piafsky KM, Borga O: Plasma protein binding of basic drugs II. Importance of $\alpha_1$ acid glycoprotein for interindividual variation. Clin Pharmacol Ther 1977; 22:545–549.

28. Hollinshead AC, Chuang CY, Cooper EH, Catalona WJ: Interrelationship of prealbumin and $\alpha_1$ acid glycoprotein in cancer patient sera. Cancer 1977; 40:2993–2998.

29. Smith ER, Duce BR: The acute anti-arrhythmic and toxic effects in mice and dogs of 2-ethylamino-2, 6-acetoxylidine (L-86) a metabolite of lidocaine. J Pharmacol Exp Ther 1971; 179:580–585.
30. Blumer J, Strong JM, Atkinson AJ: The convulsant potency of lidocaine and its N-dealkylated metabolites. Ibid. 1973; 186:31–36.
31. Strong JM, Mayfield DE, Atkinson AJ, Burris BC, Raymon F, Webster LT: Pharmacological activity, metabolism, and pharmacokinetics of glycinexylidide. Clin Pharmacol Ther 1976; 17:184–194.
32. Strong JM, Mayfield DE, Atkinson AJ, Burris BC, Raymon F, Webster LT: The pharmacological activity, metabolism, and pharmacokinetics of glycinexylidide. Clin Pharmacol Ther 1975; 17:184–194.
33. Nelson SD, Garland WA, Breck GD, Trager WF: Quantification of lidocaine and several metabolites utilizing chemical-ionization mass spectroscopy and stable isotope labeling. J Pharm Sci 1977; 66:1180–1190.
34. Wyman MG, Hammersmith L: Comprehensive treatment plan for the prevention of primary ventricular fibrillation in acute myocardial infarction. Am J Cardiol 1974; 33:661–667.
35. Lie KI, Wellens HJ, van Capolle FJ, Durrer D: Lidocaine in the prevention of primary ventricular fibrillation. A double-blind randomized study of 212 consecutive patients. N Engl J Med 1974; 291:1324–1326.
36. Aps C, Bell JA, Jenkins BS, Poole-Wilson PA, Reynolds F: Logical approach to lignocaine therapy. Brit Med J 1975; 1:13–15.
37. Pfeifer JH, Greenblatt DF, Koch-Weser J: Clinical use and toxicity of intravenous lidocaine: A report from the Boston Collaborative Drug Surveillance Program. Am Heart J 1976; 92:168–173.
38. Kuo CS, Reddy CP: Effect of lidocaine on the rate of atrioventricular junctional escape pacemakers. Am J Cardiol 1980; 45:451 (Abstract).
39. Goldman L, Batsford WP: Risk-benefit stratification as a guide to lidocaine prophylaxis of primary ventricular fibrillation in acute myocardial infarction: An analytic review. Yale J Biol Med 1979; 52:455–466.
40. Fredericks DS, Boersma RB: Lidocaine infusions: Effect of duration and method of discontinuation on recurrence of arrhythmias and pharmacokinetic variables. Am J Hosp Pharm 1979; 36:778–781.

# 12

# Procainamide

John J. Lima, Pharm.D.

## INTRODUCTION/BACKGROUND

Of the antiarrhythmic agents in current use, procainamide (PA) is one of the most effective for the treatment of a variety of atrial and ventricular arrhythmias. Procainamide is probably the most commonly used of the agents which are available parenterally and orally. The use of PA as an intravenous bolus or rapid intravenous infusion fell into disfavor soon after it was marketed in 1951 because of a number of adverse reactions including hypotension, tachycardia, atrioventricular block, and myocardial depression (1–3). More recently, however, it has been demonstrated that PA may be used safely and effectively if given in a series of short infusions (4), or as a loading infusion followed immediately by a slower maintenance infusion (5). The oral use of PA to suppress ventricular dysrhythmic activity in select patients is severely limited in part by its short half-life, which necessitates administration of the drug every 3 or 4 hours. The emergence of PA-induced systemic lupus erythematosus, which can occur within three months of treatment, further limits its long-term use. Neither of these limitations apply, however, when the drug is used to control dysrhythmic activity in hospitalized patients. Consequently, the drug is commonly used intravenously in patients with potentially life-threatening ventricular arrhythmias who do not tolerate or respond to lidocaine. Likewise, it is common for PA to be given orally to less acutely ill patients, or to those patients who have responded to intravenous PA, and in whom for various reasons, the infusion is terminated.

The dosing of PA, relative to that of the other antiarrhythmic agents in current use, is probably the most difficult to individualize. Consequently, serum concentrations should be frequently and intensively monitored in most, if not all patients receiving the drug. It shares with other routinely monitored drugs those criteria which necessitate

frequent monitoring of blood or serum levels. It has a narrow therapeutic range, 4 to 10 µg/ml (6), and interpatient variability in the
drug's disposition kinetics is considerable. In addition, the N-acetylated PA metabolite, NAPA, achieves serum concentrations which
approach or exceed serum concentrations of the parent compound at
steady-state. NAPA is nearly or equally as active as PA and is currently under intensive investigation as an antiarrhythmic in its own
right (7,8). When patients receive PA by any route of administration
for a period of time exceeding 12 to 24 hours, they are receiving two
drugs, each with different pharmacokinetic profiles. Consequently,
serum concentrations of both drugs need to be monitored frequently.
The decisions one has to make relative to PA dosing include what
route of administration, how much to administer, and when to monitor
serum concentrations of the drug and its metabolite. These decisions
require an understanding of the drug's pharmacokinetic disposition.

## Absorption

Despite the fact that PA is one of the oldest antiarrhythmic drugs
in current use, its absorption characteristics, particularly in patients,
have not been intensively studied. In one study which compared
plasma concentrations following oral and intravenous doses of PA in
11 healthy young volunteers, 83% of PA was systemically available
when administered as PA HCl capsules (Pronestyl®), and the absorption half-life averaged about 20 minutes (9). Based on these data, and
assuming an average elimination half-life ($t\frac{1}{2}_\beta$) of about 3 hours, peak
concentrations occur about 75 minutes after the administration of an
oral dose of PA in healthy, young subjects. An entirely different picture
emerges, however, in older patients receiving the drug orally. For
example, three blood samples were obtained during one dosing interval at steady-state from each of 31 typical cardiac patients receiving
PA HCl capsules orally. The samples were drawn at the time the dose
of PA was given, and at 1 and 2 hours following the dose when the
dosing interval was 3 hours, at 1.5 and 3 hours following the dose
when the interval was 4 hours, at 2 and 4 hours during a dosing
interval of 6 hours duration, and at 3 and 6 hours during a dosing
interval of 8 hours (unpublished data). The highest serum concentrations of PA were contained in the samples drawn at the time PA was
given in 8 of the 31 patients. These data suggest that the absorption
of PA from the gut is delayed in many patients relative to healthy
volunteers. Similar findings were reported by Koch-Weser (10). The
factors responsible for the delayed rate of absorption of orally administered PA in some patients is unknown but may include the presence

of disease states, particularly congestive heart failure, delayed gastric emptying, and drug-drug interactions. Food apparently does not alter the rate and extent of absorption of an oral dose of PA (11). In addition to absorption rate, the systemic availability of PA may be reduced in patients (12).

For these reasons, it is wise to intensively monitor serum concentrations during one dosing interval at steady-state. Because serum concentrations of PA following oral doses are so unpredictable, the parenteral route is preferred, particularly during the initial, most critical period of treatment. Intramuscular doses are more rapidly and completely absorbed than oral doses (10). The intravenous route is the most advantageous and will be discussed later.

## Distribution

When PA is given intravenously as a bolus, the resulting serum concentrations decline biexponentially as shown in Figure 1. If drug distribution is related to blood flow, the initial, rapid decline in serum concentrations of PA reflects its distribution to highly perfused organs and tissues such as the liver and kidney. This group of tissues can be conceived kinetically as part of the central compartment volume, $V_c$. PA concentrations in poorly perfused tissue such as muscle and fat will increase, reach a maximum and begin to decline during the distributive phase. When equilibrium is achieved between tissues and fluids comprising the $V_c$ and those of poorly perfused tissues, serum concentrations of PA decline monoexponentially. These poorly perfused tissues may be conceived as part of a tissue or peripheral compartment volume, $V_t$. The sum of the $V_c$ and $V_t$ is equal to $V_{ss}$, which is the proportionality constant relating the amount of PA in the body to its concentration in plasma at steady-state. A fourth pharmacokinetic volume for PA, the apparent volume of distribution $V_{d\beta}$, relates the amount of PA in the body to its concentration in plasma during the post-distributive phase. Table 1 lists these volumes of distribution for PA obtained from various pharmacokinetic studies. Based on these data, the ratio of $V_c/V_{ss}$ ranges from 0.24 to 0.3. Consequently, since only a small fraction of PA in plasma is bound to plasma protein (about 15%), 70 to 75% of the total amount of PA in the body at steady-state is stored in the tissue compartment.

Several aspects of PA's distribution are clinically relevant. When serum or plasma concentrations of drugs are monitored, the assumption is often made that these reflect drug concentrations in the "biophase," or the site at which the drug is acting. In an elegant study of

| TABLE 1. | VOLUMES OF DISTRIBUTION FOR PROCAINAMIDE | | | | | |
|---|---|---|---|---|---|---|
| | Number and Type of Subject | Age | $V_c$ L/kg | $V_{ss}$ L/kg | $V_{d\beta}$ L/kg | $V_t$ L/kg |
| Galleazzi et al (13) | 4 normals | * | 0.5 | 2.4 | 2.8 | 1.9 |
| Manion et al (9) | 11 normals | 22 | 0.8 | 2.7 | 2.7 | 1.9 |
| Gibson et al (15) | 4 normal | 33 | 0.83 | 1.9 | * | 1.1 |
| | 4 anephric | 52 | 0.63 | 1.7 | * | 1.1 |
| Lima et al (14) | 21 patients | 61 | 0.58 | 2.4 | 2.6 | 1.8 |

*not reported

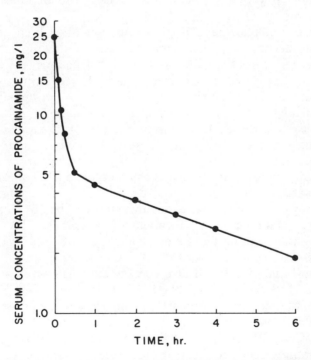

FIGURE 1. Serum concentrations of procainamide at various times following an intravenous bolus of 1 gm of the base (equivalent to 1.18 gm of procainamide HCl). Simulations were based on the pharmacokinetics of procainamide from reference 14.

the pharmacokinetics and pharmacodynamics of PA, Galeazzi et al (13) showed that prolongation of the QT interval induced by PA was delayed relative to its concentration in plasma and, further, that this index of PA's pharmacodynamics paralleled salivary concentrations. Serum concentrations of PA were adequately described by a two-compartment open model. These data suggest that PA's biophase resides in a compartment (reflected by salivary concentrations) distinguishable from the central compartment, at least with respect to prolongation of the QT interval. The authors correctly concluded that the concept of an effective plasma concentration for PA is meaningful only when it is associated with efficacy after attainment of equilibrium. If the antiarrhythmic effects of PA are delayed relative to its concentration in plasma, such a delay may be important in designing loading dose schedules. The delay, if it exists, is not clinically relevant when equilibrium has been achieved following a dose. At equilibrium, serum concentrations of PA parallel concentrations at the biophase, presumably in the myocardium.

The number of pharmacokinetic compartments which adequately describe the decline in plasma concentrations following intravenous administration is partly dependent on the frequency of sampling, particularly during the distribution phase. For example, failure to obtain serum levels earlier than 30 minutes in the example illustrated in Figure 1 may result in the assumption of a one-compartment open model to describe the decline in serum concentrations of PA. Under these conditions, about 15% of the total area under the serum concentration-time curve is missed. This results in an apparent clearance which is 15% higher than the true body clearance ($Cl_B$) of PA, and the measured serum concentration at steady-state ($C_{ss}$) following multiple oral doses or a constant intravenous infusion will be 15% higher than the predicted value based on this apparent clearance of PA. The error incurred by the assumption of a one-compartment open model to predict steady-state concentrations of PA following chronic dosing is relatively small and of little clinical consequence. However, serum concentrations of PA for a period shortly after administration of the drug may be two to three times higher than those predicted based on a one-compartment model (Figure 2). Failure to consider the distribution characteristics of PA is the most likely reason the intravenous use of the drug rapidly fell into disfavor soon after it became available for clinical use in 1951. It was common practice to administer bolus doses of 500 to 1000 mg or more of PA to patients with life-threatening ventricular arrhythmias (1–3). This often resulted in troublesome and dangerous side effects including severe episodes of hypotension, tachycardia, atrioventricular block, and myocardial depression. Toxic lev-

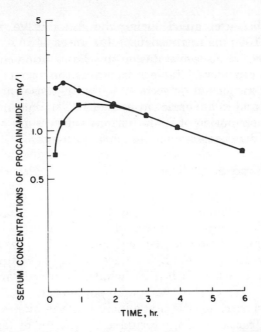

FIGURE 2A.  Comparison of serum concentrations at various times following an oral dose of 500 mg procainamide HCl according to a one (■) and a two (●) compartment open model. Simulations were based on data from reference 9.

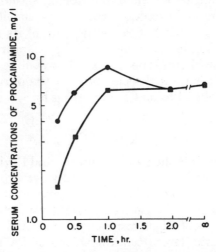

FIGURE 2B.  Comparison of serum concentrations at various times following an infusion of 14.5 mg/kg over one hour and a maintenance infusion of 2.4 mg/kg/hour of procainamide HCl according to a one (■) and a two (●) compartment model. Simulations were based on data from reference 43.

els were probably obtained during the distributive phase following these 500 to 1000 mg intravenous bolus doses of PA.

The influence of disease states on the distribution characteristics of PA should be considered. Table 1 compares the various PA volumes of distributions in normal subjects (9,13) with those in typical cardiac patients (14) and in anephric patients (15). The data indicate that the volumes of distribution of PA in normal subjects are similar to those in typical cardiac patients and anephric patients.

## Metabolism and Excretion

The metabolic fate of PA is complex and not completely known. Approximately one-half of the drug that reaches the systemic circulation in normal subjects appears in the urine unchanged (14,16,17). The remaining fraction is cleared non-renally, presumably by the liver. Much of the non-renal clearance of PA is accounted for by acetylation. This is accomplished by hepatic N-acetyltransferase, which is bimodally distributed in the human population (18,19), and possibly by enzymes in extrahepatic tissue including the kidney (20) and blood (21). A small fraction of PA in serum is eliminated by largely unknown metabolic pathways, which include hydrolysis to PABA (17,22). The metabolic and excretory pathways of PA and its N-acetylated metabolite, NAPA, are summarized in Figure 3. Because NAPA is cardioactive, it must be considered when monitoring serum concentrations of PA. Its metabolism and excretion will also be considered.

The body clearance ($Cl_B$) of PA is the sum of its renal ($Cl_R$), acetylation ($Cl_A$), and metabolic or hepatic ($Cl_H$) clearances (assuming no extrahepatic metabolism). The $Cl_A$ of PA probably comprises a large fraction of $Cl_H$ but is treated separately for the purpose of discussion. The $C_{ss}$ of PA is related to its $Cl_B$ according to:

$$C_{ss} = \frac{1}{Cl_R + Cl_A + Cl_H} \times \frac{D}{\tau}$$

where D is the dose, $\tau$ is the dosing interval and $D/\tau$ is the dose rate (or $FD/\tau$ when given orally). It is clear that any perturbation in the physiological processes which determine each component of $Cl_B$ will change $C_{ss}$. Assessment of how disease states might perturb each of the physiologic determinants of $Cl_B$ is necessary to select the dose of the drug which will maintain serum concentrations of PA in its therapeutic range.

**Renal Elimination.** The renal clearance ($Cl_R$) of PA in subjects with normal renal function is two to three times creatinine clearance, indicating that the drug is actively secreted by the kidney (18). Since

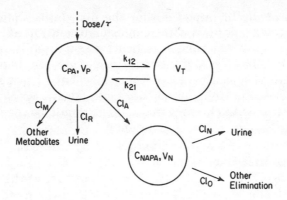

FIGURE 3. Pharmacokinetic model summarizing the disposition characteristics of procainamide and NAPA, where $k_{12}$ and $k_{21}$ are the intercompartmental rate constants. Serum or plasma concentrations of procainamide ($C_{PA}$) are cleared from its central volume of distribution ($V_c$ or $V_P$) by metabolic ($Cl_M$), renal ($Cl_R$), and acetylation ($Cl_A$) clearances. Serum or plasma concentrations of NAPA ($C_{NAPA}$) are cleared from its volume of distribution ($V_N$) by renal ($Cl_N$) and non-renal ($Cl_Q$) clearances. From reference 19.

the $Cl_R$ of PA does not change significantly under conditions of acid and alkali loads, it may be concluded that tubular reabsorption is not an important mechanism in its renal elimination (16).

Since the $Cl_R$ of PA comprises approximately one-half of its $Cl_B$ in normal subjects, it is not surprising that $C_{ss}$ of PA normalized for dosage is higher in patients with renal impairment than in patients with no renal impairment. The biological half-life of PA ($t\frac{1}{2}$) is also prolonged in patients with renal impairment. For example, the mean $t\frac{1}{2}_\beta$ of PA in patients with renal impairment (serum creatinine > 1.4 mg/dl or BUN > 25 mg/dl) was 11.3 hours, while the $t\frac{1}{2}_\beta$ in patients with no renal impairment averaged 4.45 hours (p < 0.005) (14). For these reasons, doses of PA must be decreased in patients with renal impairment.

Renal impairment may also depress the non-renal elimination of PA. In a study of the kinetics of PA and NAPA, Gibson et al compared the pharmacokinetics of both compounds in normal subjects and in functionally anephric patients of slow and fast acetylator phenotypes (15). Both renal and non-renal clearances of PA were depressed in the functionally anephric patients, while no differences in $V_{ss}$ between the two groups were evident. The authors concluded that the acetylation clearance as well as other non-renal clearances were slowed. In contrast, Lima et al (14) reported that the acetylation clearance of PA was unaffected in patients with renal impairment. Renal impairment in the Lima study was related to heart disease, while renal impairment in the Gibson study was due to chronic renal failure. Thus, differences in the patient populations may have accounted for this disparity. The potentially slower non-renal clearance of PA, particularly in patients with chronic renal failure, should be considered when determining PA doses in such patients.

In contrast to PA, NAPA is almost entirely cleared by the kidneys, and its renal clearance is normally 1.2 to 1.8 times the creatinine clearance (23). The $Cl_B$ of NAPA is less than that of the parent compound by a factor of two to four, and the $t\frac{1}{2}_B$ of the metabolite is two to three times longer than that of PA in normal subjects or in patients without renal impairment (8,23,24). Depending on the degree of renal impairment, acetylator status, and dose of PA, serum concentrations of NAPA may accumulate to dangerously high levels (25) and the ratio of NAPA/PA serum concentrations at steady-state may equal or exceed 2.4 (14). In such patients the half-life of NAPA may exceed 40 hours, which is markedly longer than the normal values of 6 to 10 hours (25). Because of this, the appropriate dosing of PA, particularly in patients with renal impairment, is very difficult. Consequently, the disease status of the patients, particularly renal function, must be carefully assessed during treatment with PA, and serum concentrations of both PA and NAPA must be intensively monitored.

**Acetylation.** The acetylation of PA is bimodally distributed in humans, with slow and fast acetylator phenotypes being equally distributed in the North American population (26). Normally, the ratio of NAPA/PA (N/P) serum concentrations at steady-state averages about 0.6 in slow acetylators, while the N/P ratio in fast acetylators averages about 1 to 1.2 (18). The acetylation clearance and $Cl_B$ of PA in fast acetylators is higher as compared to slow acetylators (5,15,16). Consequently, steady-state serum concentrations of PA are lower and its half-life shorter in fast acetylators as compared to slow acetylators (5,14). These relationships are illustrated in Figure 4.

Reidenberg et al demonstrated that steady-state N/P ratios in patients without renal impairment may be employed to distinguish between slow and fast acetylators (18). Because $Cl_R/Cl_B$ of NAPA is almost two times higher than the corresponding value for PA, N/P ratios cannot be used to phenotype patients with renal impairment. This is because steady-state serum concentrations of NAPA are disproportionately higher than concentrations of PA in renally impaired patients. Consequently, slow acetylators with renal impairment may

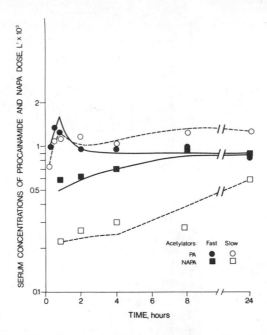

FIGURE 4. Mean serum concentrations of procainamide (circles) and NAPA (squares) normalized for dose at various times during the intravenous administration of a loading dose infused over one hour followed by a maintenance infusion in slow (open symbols) and fast (closed symbols) acetylators. The symbols are measured data points, and the lines were computer fitted. Published with permission, reference 43.

be mis-phenotyped as fast acetylators based on N/P ratios at steady-state.

To solve this problem, Lima and Jusko (19) derived an expression for the acetylation clearance of PA which is independent of renal function. By calculating the ratio of the urinary excretion rate of NAPA at steady-state and the steady-state serum concentration of PA, the apparent acetylation clearance of PA ($Cl_{ap}$), which estimates the $Cl_A$ of PA, is obtained. Figure 5 compares the various indices of PA acetylation with $Cl_{ap}$ values in patients. Of the indices compared, only $Cl_{ap}$ was bimodally distributed; values of 80 ml/min or less were slow acetylators, while $Cl_{ap}$ values of 120 ml/min or higher were fast (19).

The relationships between acetylator phenotype, renal function and steady-state N/P ratios are illustrated in Figure 6. No renal impairment was evident in patients LA and AM. The steady-state N/P ratios were 0.5 and 1.2 respectively and the former was phenotyped as a

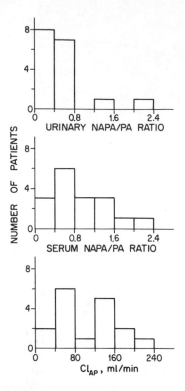

FIGURE 5.  Frequency distribution of procainamide treated patients according to three indices of acetylation phenotype. Published with permission, reference 19.

slow acetylator, while patient AM was a fast acetylator. The N/P ratios in patients JG and EW were 1.5 and 2.0 respectively, suggesting that both were fast acetylators. Both patients, however, had renal impairment, and subsequent analysis of the data in these patients (14) indicated that JG was a slow acetylator. His N/P ratio was elevated because of renal impairment.

Knowledge of the acetylator phenotype of patients receiving PA is useful because slow acetylators may be at greater risk of developing PA-induced systemic lupus erythematosus (SLE) (27,28). In a prospective study of the relationship between acetylator phenotype and PA-induced SLE, Woosley et al reported that the duration of therapy required to induce the disease was 12 months in 14 slow acetylators compared to 48 months in fast acetylators (28). These investigators further reported that the duration of therapy required to produce antinuclear antibodies was shorter and the total dose smaller in slow

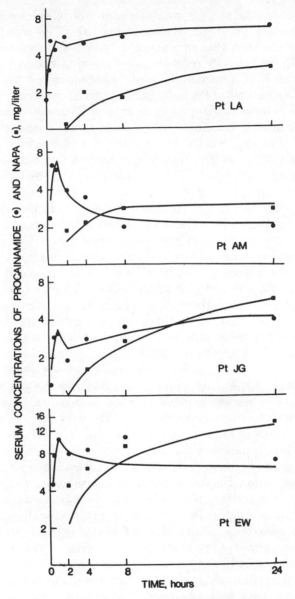

FIGURE 6. Serum concentrations of procainamide (●) and NAPA (■) at various times during the intravenous administration of loading doses infused over one hour followed by maintenance infusions in slow and fast acetylators with no renal impairment (LA and AM respectively) and in slow and fast acetylators with renal impairment (patients JG and EW respectively). The lines are computer fitted while the symbols are measured values. Published with permission, reference 14.

acetylators compared to fast acetylators. Similar results were reported by Henningsen et al in an earlier study (27). The results of these studies indicate that the emergence of signs and symptoms of PA-induced SLE are not only related to acetylator phenotype, but to dose and the duration of treatment as well. Whether or not the emergence of signs and symptoms of PA-induced SLE can be delayed or eliminated by carefully individualizing the dose rate of PA remains unknown.

Symptoms of SLE associated with PA are rarely encountered during the first three or four weeks of treatment in patients who receive the drug for the first time (29). However, if long-term treatment with PA is indicated, the patient should be made aware of the symptoms and instructed to promptly report these to his physician. Clinically, arthritis, pleuritis, fever, and pulmonary infiltrate hallmark the onset of PA-induced SLE (29). These are often accompanied by anemia, leukopenia, proteinuria, and positive antinuclear antibodies. LE cells are almost always present while skin changes, which are present in 75% of patients with the idiopathic form, appear in about 20% of the patients with PA-induced SLE (29,30). Renal changes are evident in about 50% of patients with idiopathic SLE but appear to be absent in the drug-induced form (29,30). However, recent evidence suggests that there are renal changes similar to lupus nephritis which are associated with PA administration (31,32). Perhaps a renal component has been absent in PA-induced SLE because other symptoms prompted discontinuance of the drug, thereby eliminating the opportunity for renal changes to become evident. In most patients, all clinical manifestations clear in days or weeks after PA is stopped, but in a few these have persisted for years (29).

The acetylation pathway for several drugs has been reported to be capacity-limited (33,34,35), and there is some evidence which suggests that the acetylation clearance of PA is saturable as well (36). Saturation of PA acetylation, if it exists, may not be readily evident by examining the decline in PA serum concentrations following a single intravenous dose, because the $Cl_A/Cl_B$ fraction is moderate, averaging 0.2 to 0.30 in normal subjects and patients without renal impairment (14,24). Neither is it likely to pose a major problem when altering the dose of PA in an individual patient. Assessment of acetylator phenotype, however, may be confounded. For example, as the PA dose is increased, its $Cl_A$ decreases. Hence, the steady-state N/P ratio (as well as $Cl_{ap}$ value) at the higher dose is less than it was at lower doses, and fast acetylators may be misclassified as intermediate or slow acetylators.

Saturation of the acetylation pathway could account for the disproportionately high fraction of patients who were classified as slow acetylators in our studies of PA infusions (5) as compared with a similar group of patients who were receiving oral PA (unpublished data). The total dose of PA HCl administered intravenously to 39 patients during the first 24 hours of treatment averaged 5 gm. Eighteen of 27 patients phenotyped (67%) were slow acetylators, seven (26%) were fast and two were classified as intermediate (5). In contrast, the dose of PA HCl administered orally to 31 patients averaged 2.5 gm. Thirteen of the 31 patients (42%) were classified as slow acetylators, 13 as fast acetylators, and five were intermediate.

Drugs which are substrates for acetylation may be expected to compete with PA when given simultaneously, and thus pose the potential for major drug-drug interactions. Hydralazine is often used in cardiac patients and has been reported to interact with PA in animal studies (37). However, when given to normal subjects simultaneously, no interaction between PA and hydralazine was evident (38); therefore no alteration in PA dosing is necessary when hydralazine is administered concurrently.

**Other Aspects of Metabolism.** The non-renal clearance of PA, including acetylation, comprises a major fraction of the $Cl_B$. The metabolism of PA may therefore be expected to be depressed in patients with various types of liver disease. The disposition of PA in patients with liver disease has not been studied extensively. In one study, DuSouich and Frill reported that acetylation and hydrolysis of PA was impaired in patients with chronic liver disease (22). Further investigation is needed to determine the extent that serum concentrations of PA are affected by liver disease and whether or not the dosage of PA needs to be altered. The end products of the metabolic pathways of PA, other than acetylation, are largely unknown. This aspect of PA's disposition has assumed greater importance since Freemen et al (39) reported that a hydroxylated metabolite may be the stimulus for PA-induced SLE. If this is the case, the $Cl_H$ of PA would presumably be larger in slow acetylators, who are at greater risk than fast acetylators. This relationship was not evident in the study reported by Lima et al (14). The mechanism responsible for PA-induced SLE is unknown but is associated with either PA, its non-acetylated metabolite, or some other factor related to acetylator phenotype.

**Congestive Failure.** There are no prospective studies of the metabolic disposition of PA in patients with congestive heart failure. Lima et al (5) reported that the $C_{ss}$ of PA, normalized for dose in four patients with pulmonary edema, was almost twice as high as the corresponding value in 19 patients with little or no evidence of severe congestive heart failure. Although Lalka et al (40) reported that the average $Cl_B$ of PA in patients following an acute myocardial infarction was decreased relative to normal subjects, the patient with the most severe degree of congestive failure had the highest $Cl_B$, exceeding 1000 ml/min. Since PA is often given to patients with varying degrees of congestive failure, it is important that its disposition be studied under these conditions. Until such time that this information is available, it seems prudent to alter the dose of PA in patients with congestive heart failure.

## CONCENTRATION VERSUS RESPONSE AND TOXICITY

The therapeutic serum concentration range of PA is difficult to assess because of the presence of NAPA. Koch-Weser reported that serum concentrations of PA between 4 and 8 µg/ml were therapeutic, while those above 8 or 10 µg/ml were associated with minor signs of toxicity including gastrointestinal disturbances, weakness, malaise, decreases in mean arterial pressure of less than 20%, and prolongation of ECG intervals of 10 to 30% (6,41). PA serum concentrations of 12 µg/ml or higher were associated with more severe hypotension and conduction disturbances, appearance of major new ventricular arrhythmias, and cardiac arrest. Plasma samples were obtained from these patients during the post-distributive phase following oral or parenteral doses of PA. It is likely that serum levels of NAPA, at least in some of these patients, had sufficient time to accumulate, particularly in patients with renal impairment. Consequently, conclusions about the relation of PA serum concentrations to clinical effects must be guarded, since therapeutic as well as toxic effects attributed solely to PA were probably due to the sum of both compounds.

In a recent study, 34 patients who were resistant to conventional doses of lidocaine were treated with PA according to a pharmacokinetically designed two-infusion method (5). Patient response to PA was graded on a scale of 0 (no response) to 4 (complete abolishment of ventricular arrhythmias). The relationship between steady-state PA concentrations and response is summarized in Figure 7. Dangerous ventricular arrhythmias were completely abolished within 30 minutes after the start of the loading infusion in the responders. Consequently, the effects seen in most, if not all of the responders were due to PA, since NAPA levels did not have sufficient time to accumulate. The mean serum PA concentration at steady-state was about 7 µg/ml in responders [1–4] and was higher than the corresponding value of about 4 µg/ml in the non-responders [0]. More importantly, 15 of 23 patients with steady-state levels of 8 µg/ml or less responded to PA treatment, while virtually all of the 10 patients who had steady-state levels higher than 8 µg/ml responded. Moreover, no signs of toxicity

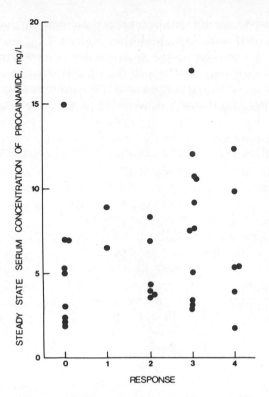

FIGURE 7.   Relation between antiarrhythmic response and steady-state serum concentrations of procainamide. Published with permission, reference 5.

were evident in 9 of the 10 patients with levels of PA higher than 8 µg/ml, the upper limit of the therapeutic range for PA reported by Koch-Weser (41). One patient who exhibited minor signs of PA toxicity (nausea, vomiting and malaise) achieved a steady-state serum level of 17 µg/ml. However, this patient also had a serum NAPA concentration of 20 µg/ml. Five patients had combined PA and NAPA steady-state serum concentrations of 21 to 25 µg/ml with no apparent signs of toxicity. These data suggest that the therapeutic range for PA is wider than 4 to 10 µg/ml and that patients can safely tolerate combined PA and NAPA concentrations of 25 to 30 µg/ml.

In addition to PA and NAPA levels, several indices of PA response, including the duration of ECG intervals and the appearance of minor signs of toxicity, may be assessed to roughly estimate the body load of drug. This is particularly important when PA is administered intravenously by the two-infusion method (see section on Infusions) or in the absence of PA and NAPA blood level data. Reliable measurements of ECG interval duration from rhythm strips at paper speeds of 50 mm/sec or higher should be obtained prior to and during treatment. During this time the patient should be carefully observed for clinical signs of toxicity, i.e., nausea and vomiting, profuse sweating, malaise, hypotension (decreases in mean arterial pressure of greater than 20 to 25% relative to baseline), and bradycardia. Complete abolishment or substantial reduction in the frequency of dysrhythmic activity and the absence of clinical and ECG evidence of PA toxicity are indicative of safe and effective body loads of PA. Appearance of one or more of the clinical signs of PA toxicity or PA-induced increases in PR, QRS, and QT intervals of greater than 0.2, 0.1, and 0.43 seconds respectively should be accompanied by a decrease in dosage.

If the arrhythmia is not well controlled during the first hour or two after infusion of the loading dose, the maintenance infusion may be increased 25%. ECG strips should be frequently monitored, and the patient should be carefully observed for signs of toxicity during this time. This procedure may be repeated every 3 or 4 hours until the arrhythmia is controlled, or until clinical or ECG signs of toxicity are observed. Of course, blood levels of PA and NAPA should also be frequently monitored, if available.


## CLINICAL APPLICATION OF PHARMACOKINETIC DATA

### Oral Dosing

PA is often given orally to hospitalized patients to suppress minor ventricular dysrhythmic activity. It is also commonly given to patients following a successful course of treatment with lidocaine. It is often asked whether the maintenance infusion of lidocaine should be tapered, or be discontinued when PA treatment is begun. Unfortunately, this aspect of antiarrhythmic therapy has not been studied. The following recommendations are therefore empirical but are based in part on the known pharmacokinetics of both lidocaine and PA. Twice the oral maintenance dose of PA HCl should be administered initially as a loading dose. The maintenance infusion of lidocaine is decreased 25% when the second dose of PA is given, and this procedure is repeated so that the lidocaine infusion is discontinued at the end of the fourth PA dosage interval. The frequency of dysrhythmic activity should be closely monitored during this time, and adjustment in the procedure should be made accordingly. If intravenous PA is initiated according to the two-infusion technique described below, the infusion of lidocaine may be discontinued when the loading infusion of PA is begun.

## Procainamide Infusions

PA can be used intravenously to treat life-threatening ventricular arrhythmias in patients who fail to respond to, or who cannot tolerate lidocaine. Its success largely depends on rapid achievement and maintenance of therapeutic serum concentrations. The safest and easiest way to achieve this goal is to give PA as a loading infusion $(K_0^L)$ followed by a maintenance infusion $(K_0^M)$ according to the guidelines suggested by Wagner (42) and applied to PA by Lima and Jusko (43). The maintenance infusion required to achieve $C_{ss}$ is:

$$K_0^M = C_{ss} Cl_B \qquad \text{(Eq. 1)}$$

The loading infusion of PA is:

$$K_0^L = \frac{K_0^M}{(1 - e^{-\beta t_i})} \qquad \text{(Eq. 2)}$$

where $t_i$ is the duration of time during which the loading infusion is given. The maximum serum concentration $(C_{max})$ of PA obtained by Equation 2 depends on the dose and the duration of the infusion. Table 2 compares $C_{max}$ values for PA obtained at various infusion rates and shows that a loading dose of about 1400 mg given over one hour achieves a safe $C_{max}$ of PA of about 8 µg/ml, assuming the following values: $Cl_B = 49$ L/hr, $\beta = 0.24$ hr$^{-1}$, $C_{ss}$ for PA = 5 µg/ml (43).

TABLE 2.   MAXIMUM SERUM CONCENTRATIONS
OF PROCAINAMIDE AT VARIOUS INFUSION RATES

| Duration (min) | Loading infusion rate, PA HCl (mg/min) | Loading dose, PA HCl (mg) | Maximum PA serum conc. (µg/ml) |
|---|---|---|---|
| 1 | 1227 | 1227 | 28.1 |
| 2 | 614 | 1228 | 26.6 |
| 5 | 247 | 1237 | 23.0 |
| 10 | 125 | 1250 | 18.6 |
| 15 | 84 | 1262 | 15.6 |
| 30 | 43 | 1300 | 10.9 |
| 60 | 23 | 1377 | 7.92 |
| 120 | 12.8 | 1542 | 6.33 |

The nomogram (Figure 8) for dosing PA was based on pharmaco-kinetic studies of slow and fast acetylators with varying degrees of renal and cardiac impairments (5,14). The loading infusion consists of 17 mg/kg of PA HCl intravenously over one hour to patients with normal or moderately impaired renal and/or cardiac function. The loading dose is added to 100 ml D5W and the solution is infused at a rate of 100 ml/hour. Placing a straightedge vertically from the appropriate body weight down to the last horizontal line of the nomogram indicates that patients with severe cardiac or renal impairment should receive a loading dose of 14 mg/kg infused over one hour. The maintenance infusion consists of 2.8 mg/kg of PA HCl per hour in patients with no apparent renal or cardiac impairment. This rate is reduced by one third in moderately impaired patients, and by two thirds in severely impaired patients. Since the maintenance infusion in the nomogram is expressed in mg of PA HCl per hour, this value is multiplied by 24 hours to obtain the total daily dose. The total daily dose is added to 500 ml D5W and infused at a rate of about 20 ml/hour. The following example should be illustrative.

The rhythm strip of a 175 lb, 60-year-old male who recently had an acute myocardial infarction shows frequent PVC's (6/min). He has received, in addition to multiple boluses, infusions of lidocaine ranging between 1 and 4 mg/min during the past 24 hours. The attending physician decided to use PA intravenously. Physical examination of the patient reveals basilar rales, and laboratory results from that day report a BUN of 30 mg/dl and a serum creatinine of 2.0 mg/dl. A straightedge is placed from the 175 lb point of the top horizontal line labeled body weight down to the horizontal line for moderately impaired. The loading dose at the upper part of the horizontal line indicates that this patient should receive about 1350 mg of PA HCl over one hour. PA HCl is commercially available for intravenous use in concentrations of 100 and 500 mg/ml. A volume of 2.7 ml of intravenous solution containing 500 mg of PA HCl/ml is added to 100 ml D5W and infused at 100 ml/hour. The rate of administration for the maintenance infusion is found on the bottom part of the horizontal line and is about 160 mg/hour, or about 3.8 gm of PA HCl for the 24 hour period. Consequently, 38 ml of intravenous solution containing 100 mg of PA HCl/ml, or 7.6 ml of 500 mg/ml PA HCl, is added to 500 ml D5W and infused at a rate of about 20 ml/hour. Because of bag over-fill and because either 38 or 7.6 ml of intravenous solution is added, the total volume of the solution to be administered to the patient exceeds 500 ml, and occasionally may approach 600 ml. Consequently, there will be some volume remaining at the end of 24 hours

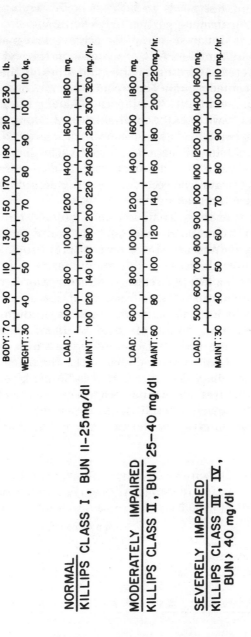

FIGURE 8. Nomogram for dosing procainamide according to the two-infusion method. Load = loading dose of procainamide HCl infused over 1 hour. Maint = maintenance infusion of procainamide HCl in mg/hour.

423

and the $C_{ss}$ achieved will be less than estimated. This is not usually clinically important but needs to be considered when determining pharmacokinetic parameters, particularly clearance.

The nomogram is designed to rapidly achieve and maintain a PA $C_{ss}$ of about 4 to 8 μg/ml. The PA $C_{max}$ achieved at the end of a loading infusion administered according to the guidelines of the nomogram should average about 8 μg/ml. Therapeutic serum concentrations of PA are usually achieved 15 to 30 minutes following the loading infusion, and steady-state is usually obtained 1 to 2 hours following the maintenance infusion. Steady-state concentrations of NAPA in patients with no renal impairment are usually obtained in 12 to 24 hours. The dose of PA HCl and various serum concentrations of PA and NAPA in 35 patients who received the drug according to the two-infusion method are included in Table 3.

The nomogram should be considered as a guide. The $Cl_B$ of PA in patients may vary from 200 to over 1000 ml/min depending on acetylator phenotype and disease states present (14). In our experience, when alterations were necessary, the maintenance infusion was increased because of inadequate response. Rarely was it necessary to decrease the maintenance infusion because of suspected PA toxicity. Because the $Cl_B$ of PA in an occasional patient is high, or because some patients require $C_{ss}$ values of 10 to 15 μg/ml for adequate response (5), or both, the dose of PA administered may be relatively high and may exceed recommended doses (41). For example, the currently recommended daily dose of PA HCl is 50 mg/kg/day. We have given some patients over twice this recommended dose and encountered no signs of PA toxicity. Based on our experience, it appears that PA is a safe drug when given by the two-infusion method.

TABLE 3. DOSAGE AND STEADY-STATE SERUM CONCENTRATIONS
OF PROCAINAMIDE AND N-ACETYLPROCAINAMIDE
WITH THE TWO-INFUSION METHOD*

| | Dosage** (mg/kg body weight) | Serum Concentration (μg/ml) | | |
| | | Procainamide | | NAPA Steady State |
| | | Peak | Steady State | |
|---|---|---|---|---|
| Mean ± SD | 64.4 ± 14.8 | 7.1 ± 2.8 | 6.5 ± 3.8 | 5.7 ± 4.6 |
| Range | 39.4 – 102 | 2.1 – 13.2 | 1.7 – 17 | 1.1 – 20 |

* In 35 patients
** Total dosage, including the loading dose, of procainamide hydrochloride administered during the first 24 hours of treatment. SD = standard deviation.

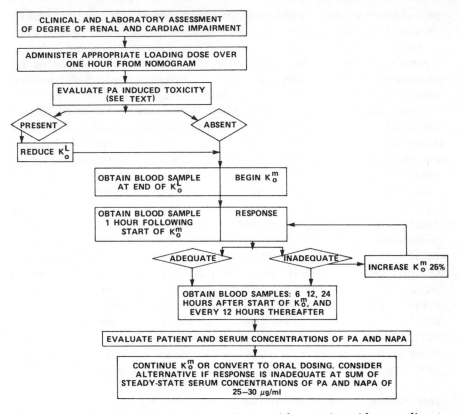

FIGURE 9. Algorithm for treating patients with procainamide according to the two-infusion technique.

Despite its apparent safety, the administration of PA according to the two-infusion technique has been associated with some side effects (5). These may be potentially serious, particularly in patients who are hemodynamically compromised because of the drug's cardiac depressant action (44). PA-induced hypotension is common in many patients treated with the two-infusion method. If hypotension occurs, it is certain to occur during the time the loading dose is infused and is usually mild, averaging about 10% decline in mean arterial pressure. Therefore, blood pressure should be monitored every 5 to 10 minutes during the loading infusion. Decreases in mean arterial pressure of greater than 20 to 25% should be accompanied by a decrease in the infusion to a rate which can be tolerated. We have seen this degree of hypotension in only one patient. To what extent the loading infusion should be decreased in unknown and probably varies from patient to patient. Unfortunately, PA-induced hypotension was not predictable; it was unrelated to disease state, the pretreatment mean arterial pressure, or the serum concentration of PA (5). For these reasons, all patients must be carefully monitored for hypotension as well as other signs of toxicity, especially during the loading infusion.

If the patient fails to respond adequately early during the maintenance infusion, the infusion rate may be increased by 25%. Any further increases in the maintenance infusion should be guided by clinical assessment of the patient and by serum levels of the drug and its metabolite. Since NAPA levels are increasing with time during the maintenance infusion of PA and contributing more and more antiarrhythmic effect, excessive increases in the maintenance infusion should be avioded. If patients fail to respond adequately to PA serum concentrations of 12 to 15 µg/ml, or to combined PA and NAPA serum concentrations of 25 µg/ml at steady-state, other alternatives should be considered. Combined PA and NAPA serum levels of 30 µg/ml or higher should be avoided. We have rarely encountered patients with levels in this range who failed to respond adequately. It should be noted that all the patients treated by the two-infusion method (5) failed to respond to conventional doses of lidocaine. Whether or not these patients comprise a subgroup of "resistant patients" who require more PA than "non-resistant patients" is not known.

### Conversion from Intravenous to Oral Dosing

Patients are often converted to oral PA after one or two days of intravenous treatment. The oral dose may be determined by assessing the relationship between response and the steady-state serum concentration of PA and NAPA observed during the maintenance infusion. The daily dose of PA required to maintain a $C_{ss}$ of PA may be calculated by:

$$\text{Dose} = \frac{C_{ss} \times Cl_B \times 24}{F} \qquad \text{(Eq. 3)}$$

where F is the bioavailability factor and may be assumed to be 0.83. The $Cl_B$ of PA may be easily determined by:

$$Cl_B = \frac{K_0^M}{C_{ss}} \qquad \text{(Eq. 4)}$$

where $K_0^M$ is the maintenance infusion, and $C_{ss}$ is the steady-state serum concentration of PA. For one reason or another, many patients may require less oral PA to suppress or control dysrhythmic activity than required with the two-infusion method. One possible explanation is the presence of NAPA. For example, assume a patient responds well to PA 30 minutes after the beginning of the loading infusion and at a PA serum concentration of 6 µg/ml. During this time NAPA has not had sufficient time to accumulate to pharmacologically active serum levels. At the end of the first day of treatment, steady-state serum concentrations of PA and NAPA of 6 and 7.2 µg/ml are achieved with a maintenance infusion of 180 mg of PA/hour. According to Equations 3 and 4, the daily dose of oral PA required to maintain an average $C_{ss}$ of 6 µg/ml is about 5.2 gm, which is equivalent to about 6.1 gm of PA HCl (5.2 ÷ 0.85) or 6 gm/day. Since NAPA is also active, the dose of PA may be decreased to take advantage of its antiarrhythmic activity as well. The minimum therapeutic steady-state serum concentrations of the sum of PA and NAPA is probably about 10 µg/ml (Dr. A. Atkinson, personal communication). The daily dose of PA required to maintain this sum value of 10 µg/ml or some other desired sum value may be determined by:

$$\text{Dose} = \frac{C^*_{ss} \times Cl_B \times 24}{F} \tag{Eq. 5}$$

where $C^*_{ss}$ is the steady-state serum concentration of PA required to maintain the desired sum of the two compounds in serum at steady-state. This may be obtained by the following:

$$C^*_{ss} = \frac{C_{ss} \times C^{des}_{sum}}{C^{obs}_{sum}} \tag{Eq. 6}$$

where $C_{ss}$ is the steady-state serum concentration of PA obtained during the maintenance infusion, $C^{des}_{sum}$ is the desired sum of PA and NAPA at steady-state, and $C^{obs}_{sum}$ is the sum of PA and NAPA steady-state serum concentrations observed during the maintenance infusion.

To illustrate, consider the example previously discussed, assuming that the desired sum of both compounds at steady-state is 10 µg/ml. Twenty four hours following the initiation of PA treatment by the two-infusion method:

$$
\begin{aligned}
K^M_0 &= 180 \text{ mg/hour} \\
\text{PA } C_{ss} &= 6 \text{ mg/L} \\
\text{NAPA } C_{ss} &= 7.2 \text{ mg/L} \\
Cl_B &= 30 \text{ L/hour}
\end{aligned}
$$

From Equation 6:

$$C^*_{ss} = \frac{6 \times 10}{6 + 7.2}$$

From Equation 5:

$$Dose = \frac{4.5 \times 30 \times 24}{0.83}$$

Thus, the total daily dose of PA HCl for this patient is about 4.0 gm. These equations for converting patients from intravenous to oral PA are valid providing the steady-state ratio of NAPA/PA is constant and independent of the dose of PA given.

Because the elimination half-life of PA cannot be easily determined from steady-state plasma level determinations obtained during a maintenance infusion, the optimal dosing interval for a given patient is difficult to predict. The elimination half-life of PA in typical patients without renal failure is slightly prolonged relative to the 2 to 4 hours reported in normal subjects. The absorption half-life of PA in some patients may be slightly prolonged as well, thereby prolonging its effective elimination half-life. Consequently, the dosing interval in patients with no renal impairment should not initially exceed 4 hours. If the patient remains stable during this period of time, further alterations in the dose and dosing interval may be attempted. In renal impairment, the optimal dosing interval may range between 6 and 12 hours (or more), depending on the degree of impairment.

## Sample Collection

Blood samples should be obtained through an intravenous catheter at the end of the loading infusion and two hours following the beginning of the maintenance infusion. This is to ensure that the $C_{max}$ at the end of the loading infusion is higher than the serum concentration of PA two hours following the maintenance infusion, and further, to document that this latter value is not excessively high. Failure to achieve either of these conditions may indicate that the patient's PA $Cl_B$ is lower, and the elimination half-life is more prolonged than expected based on clinical assessment prior to treatment. Consequently, the $C_{ss}$ of PA may be much higher, more time may be required to achieve steady-state, and the maintenance infusion may need to be decreased to a rate designated for patients with moderate or severe renal or cardiac impairment. In addition, blood samples should be obtained between 6 and 12 hours following beginning of the maintenance infusion, and at the end of 24 hours. Steady-state conditions for PA are usually obtained 1 to 2 hours following the start of the maintenance infusion, while 12 to 24 hours are required for NAPA (43). More time is required to achieve steady-state serum concentration of NAPA in patients with severe renal impairment. Once steady-state has been achieved for both compounds, a timed urine sample may be collected, and the patients $Cl_{ap}$ value determined. Steady-state N/P ratios may be used to phenotype patients with no renal impairment, thereby eliminating the need for urine collection. However, many patients have slightly elevated values for serum creatinine or BUN, and this may confound the assessment of acetylator phenotype. In this regard, the determination of $Cl_{ap}$ is a more reliable index of acetylator phenotype.

In patients taking PA orally, blood samples should be obtained when steady-state conditions are obtained. Normally, this is achieved at the end of two full days of treatment, but more time is required in patients with renal impairment. These time requirements, of course, do not apply when oral dosing is instituted immediately after intravenous treatment. Ideally, three blood samples during one dosing interval should be collected: the first at the time the dose of PA is given, and the others at equally spaced time intervals thereafter. Important inferences regarding absorption and elimination may be made, and excellent estimates of the average steady-state serum concentrations of PA and NAPA are afforded by simply calculating the average of three determinations, or by determining the ratio of the area under the plasma concentration time curve and $\tau$, the dosing interval. In the case where only two blood samples are obtained, these should be drawn at the end of the dosing interval and 2 hours following the dose. Analysis of one blood sample, even if drawn at the end of the dosing interval, may be very misleading because of the unpredictable rate of PA absorption in some patients. Therefore, decisions regarding PA dosing based on the analysis of one blood sample should be avoided.

## ASSAY METHODS

The number of assays available for the quantitation of PA and its N-acetylated metabolite in serum, urine, and other tissues reflects the remarkable advances made in drug assay technology during the past decade. In general, these include nonspecific assays such as spectrophotometry (SP) and spectrofluorophotometry (SPF), and specific drug assay methods such as chromatographic and competitive binding assays. The usefulness of the nonspecific assays for PA is limited because these fail to easily detect NAPA (41,45). In addition, large and variable blank values limit analytical sensitivity of many drugs, including PA. Because of these limitations, the newer, specific chromatographic and competitive binding assays are preferred, and are rapidly replacing the older SP and SPF methods in research and clinical laboratories.

TABLE 4.  COMPARISON OF ASSAY METHODS
FOR PROCAINAMIDE AND NAPA

| Analytical Method (References) | Limit of Sensitivity | Assayable Samples | | | Minimum Sample Volume Required | Analysis Time | Comments |
|---|---|---|---|---|---|---|---|
| | | Plasma/Serum | Urine | Saliva | | | |
| SP (45) | 3 | 3 | 3 | 3 | 3 | 3 | NAPA not assayable simultaneously |
| SPF (41) | 3 | 3 | 3 | 3 | 3 | 3 | NAPA not assayable simultaneously |
| HPLC (49–57) | 1 | 1 | 1 | 1 | 1 | 1 | |
| GC (16,47,58,59) | 1 | 1 | 1 | 1 | 1 | 1 | |
| TLC (18,60,61) | 1 | 1 | 1 | 1 | 1 | 1 | |
| EMIT | 3 | 1 | 5 | 5 | 1 | 1 | Separate test for NAPA available |
| RIA (62) | 3 | 1 | 5 | 5 | 2 | 1 | Does not measure NAPA |

*Arbitrary Ranking Scale of 1 (Excellent) to 5 (Poor) with a score of 3 being average or nominal.

Although the usefulness and importance of the nonspecific methods for quantitating PA are waning, consideration of these methods, particularly the SPF method, is extremely important and relevant. The SPF method was employed by Koch-Weser and Klein (41) in early studies to estimate the therapeutic range of PA. In later studies, the SPF method, and therefore the PA therapeutic range reported by Koch-Weser and Klein, was criticized because of reports which suggested that NAPA is hydrolyzed to PA during the back extraction step in 1N HCl (46,47). For example, Gibson et al reported that a considerable fraction of NAPA was hydrolyzed to PA when left in 1N HCl for 45 minutes or longer (46). It was later shown by Mutusik and Gibson (48) that the hydrolysis of NAPA is delayed when 0.1N HCl is used. If significant degrees of hydrolysis occurred during the analysis

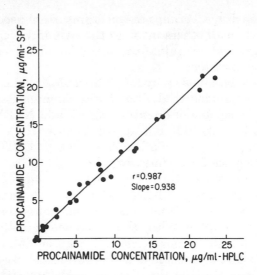

FIGURE 10. Relation between serum concentrations of procainamide analyzed by the spectrophotofluorometric (SPF) method and high performance liquid chromatography (HPLC). Published with permission, reference 49.

of serum samples obtained from the patients comprising Koch-Weser and Klein's study, the pharmacokinetics of PA as well as therapeutic and toxic concentrations reported by these investigators are questionable. More recent pharmacokinetic (14) and concentration-response (5) studies of PA, in which specific analytical assays were used, suggest that NAPA hydrolysis was not a problem in Koch-Weser and Klein's study. In addition, it is evident from data in Figure 10 that little hydrolysis of NAPA to PA occurs when serum concentrations of PA are analyzed according to the SPF method.

The specific chromatographic assays for the simultaneous quantitation of PA and NAPA, include high-performance liquid chromatography (HPLC) (49–57), gas chromatography (GC) (16,47,58,59), and thin layer chromatography (TLC) (18,60,61). While all of these specific methods are suited to a research lab, the HPLC assays are probably better suited to a clinical laboratory than are the others. This is due, in part, to the more tedious and time consuming aspects which characterize the GC and TLC methods relative to the HPLC methods. Most, if not all, of the HPLC assays for PA and NAPA share the common properties of speed, specificity, reproducibility, and sensitivity. The advantages of a given HPLC method which make it more attractive relative to others include small sample volume, chromatography time, cost, simplicity of the extraction procedure, and freedom from interfering drugs. Perhaps the most important aspect of an HPLC method relative to all others involves the ease in which other antiarrhythmic drugs, such as quinidine, disopyramide, lidocaine and propranolol are quantitated.

The competive bindings assay for PA include enzyme multiplication immunoassay technique (EMIT) and radioimmunoassay (RIA). The EMIT system is capable of quantitating PA and NAPA, whereas the RIA measures PA only (62). Because of its speed, lack of preparatory procedures, simplicity and small sample volume, EMIT appears to be the method of choice for quantitating PA and NAPA, particularly in a clinical laboratory. Non-linearity at low and high serum concentrations and the potential problems associated with quantitating drug concentrations in tissues other than serum, limits the usefulness of EMIT in the research lab. While the difference in cost between HPLC and an EMIT system is negligible, the cost of EMIT kits is much higher than the cost associated with continuous use of the HPLC. Moreover, the potential for quantitating a wider variety of drugs and other compounds is greater with HPLC as compared to EMIT. Table 4 compares several analytical variables of the assay methods available for monitoring PA and NAPA in patients. The choice as to which method to employ for quantitating serum levels of PA and NAPA depends on the volume of samples quantitated per unit of time, the number and variety of drugs monitored in patients, and the orientation of the laboratory.

## REFERENCES

1. Stearns NS, Callahan EJ, Eillis LB: Value and hazard of intravenous procainamide therapy. JAMA 1952; 184:360–364.
2. Berry K, Garrett EL, Bellet S: The use of pronestyl in treatment of ectopic rhythms. Am J Med 1951; 11:431–441.
3. Epstein MA: Ventricular standstill during intravenous procainamide treatment of ventricular tachycardia. Am Heart J 1953; 45:898–907.
4. Giardina EG, Heissenbuttel RH, Bigger JT: Intermittent intravenous procainamide to treat ventricular arrhythmias. Ann Intern Med 1973; 78:183–193.
5. Lima JJ, Goldfarb AL, Conti DR, Bascomb BL, Benedetti GM, Jusko WJ: Safety and efficacy of procainamide infusion. Am J Cardiol 1979; 43:98–105.
6. Koch-Weser J: Correlation of serum concentrations and pharmacological effects of antiarrhythmic drugs. In, Proceedings of the 5th International Congress of Pharmacology. San Francisco, 1972; 69–85.
7. Lee WK, Strong JM, Kehoe RF, Dutcher JS, Atkinson AJ: Antiarrhythmic efficacy of N-acetyl procainamide in patients with premature ventricular contractions. Clin Pharmacol Ther 1977; 19:508–514.

8. Atkinson AJ, Lee WK, Quinn ML, Kuschner W, Nevin JM, Strong JM: Dose-ranging trial of N-acetyl procainamide in patients with premature ventricular contractions. Clin Pharmacol Ther 1977; 21:575–587.

9. Manion CV, Lalka D, Baer DT, Meyer MB: Absorption kinetics of procainamide in humans. J Pharm Sci 1977; 66:981–984.

10. Koch-Weser J: Pharmacokinetics of procainamide in man. Ann NY Acad Sci 1971; 179:370–382.

11. McKnight WD, Murphy ML: The effect of food on procainamide absorption. Southern Med J 1976; 69:851–854.

12. Koch-Weser J: Clinical application of the pharmacokinetics of procainamide. Cardiovascular Clinics 1974; 6:63–75.

13. Galeazzi R, Benet LZ, Sheiner LB: Relationship between the pharmacokinetics and pharmacodynamics of procainamide. Clin Pharmacol Ther 1976; 10:278–289.

14. Lima JJ, Conti DR, Goldfarb AL, Tilstone WJ, Golden LH, Jusko WJ: Clinical pharmacokinetics of procainamide infusions in relation to acetylator phenotype. J Pharmacokinet Biopharm 1977; 7:69–85.

15. Gibson TP, Atkinson AJ, Matusik E, Nelson LD, Briggs WA: Kinetics of procainamide and N-acetylprocainamide in renal failure. Kidney Int 1977; 12:422–429.

16. Galeazzi RL, Sheiner LB, Lockwood T, Benet LZ: The renal elimination of procainamide. Clin Pharmacol Ther 1976; 19:55–62.

17. Giardina EG, Dreyfuss J, Bigger JT, Show JM, Schreiber EC: Metabolism of procainamide in normal and cardiac subjects. Clin Pharmacol Ther 1976; 19:339–351.

18. Reidenberg MM, Drayer DE, Levy M, Warner H: Polymorphic acetylation of procainamide in man. Clin Pharmacol Ther 1975; 17:722–730.

19. Lima JJ, Jusko WJ: Determination of procainamide acetylator status. Clin Pharmacol Ther 1978; 23:25–29.

20. Litterst CL, Mimnaugh EG, Reagan RL, Gram TE: Comparison of *in vitro* drug metabolism of lung, liver, and kidney of several common laboratory species. Drug Met Dis 1975; 3:259–265.

21. Drayer DE, Strong JM, Jones B, Sandler A, Reidenberg MM: *In vitro* acetylation of drugs by human blood cells. Drug Met Dis 1974; 2:499–505.

22. DuSouich P, Frill S: Patterns of acetylation of procainamide and procainamide-derived p-aminobenzoic acid in man. Eur J Clin Pharmacol 1976; 9:433–438.

23. Strong JM, Dutcher JS, Lee W, Atkinson AJ: Pharmacokinetics in man of the N-acetylated metabolite of procainamide. J Pharmacokinet Biopharm 1975; 3:223–234.

24. Dutcher JS, Strong JM, Lucas SV, Lee WK, Atkinson AJ: Procainamide and N-acetylprocainamide kinetics investigated simultaneously with stable isotope methodology. Clin Pharmacol Ther 1977; 22:447–457.

25. Drayer DE, Lowenthal DT, Woosley RL, Nies AS, Schwartz A, Reidenberg MM: Cumulation of N-acetylprocainamide, an active metabolite of procainamide, in patients with impaired renal function. Clin Pharmacol Ther 1977; 22:63–69.

26. Lunde PKM, Frislie K, Aansteen V: Disease and acetylation polymorphism. Drugs 1976; 182–197.

27. Henningsen NC, Cederberg A, Hanson A, Johansson BW: Effects of long-term treatment with procainamide. Acta Med Scand 1975; 198:472–482.

28. Woosley RL, Drayer DE, Reidenberg MM, Nies AS, Curr KJ, Oates JA: Effect of acetylator phenotype on the rate at which procainamide induces antinuclear antibodies and the lupus syndrome. N Engl J Med 1978; 298:1157–1159.

29. Dubois EL: Procainamide induction of a systemic lupus erythematosus syndrome. Medicine 1969; 48:217–228.

30. Heltne CE: Drug-induced systemic lupus erythematosus. West Virginia Med J 1977; 73:101–104.
31. Levo Y, Pick AI, Avidor I, Ben-bassat M: Clinicopathological study of a patient with procainamide-induced systemic lupus erythematosus. Ann Rheum Dis 1976; 35:181–185.
32. Whittle TS, Ainsworth SK: Procainamide-induced systemic lupus erythematosus. Arch Path Lab Med 1976; 100:469–474.
33. Ellard GA, Gammon PT: Pharmacokinetics of isoniazid metabolism in man. J Pharmacokinet Biopharm 1976; 4:83–113.
34. Olson W, Micelli J, Weber W: Dose-dependent changes in sulfamethazine kinetics in rapid and slow isoniazid acetylators. Clin Pharmacol Ther 1978; 23:204–211.
35. Talseth T: Kinetics of hydralazine elimination. Clin Pharmacol Ther 1977; 21:715–720.
36. Graffner C: Elimination rate of N-acetylprocainamide after a single intravenous dose of procainamide hydrochloride in man. J Pharmacokin Biopharm 1975; 3:69–76.
37. Schneck DW, Sprouse JS, Hayes AH, Shiroff RA: The effect of hydralazine and other drugs on the kinetics of procainamide acetylation by rat liver and kidney N-acetyltransferase. J Pharmacol Exp Ther 1978; 204:212–213.
38. Schneck DW, Sprouse JS, Miller K, Vary JE, DeWitt FO, Hayes AH: Plasma levels of free and acid-labile hydralazine: Effects of multiple dosing and of procainamide. Clin Pharmacol Ther 1978; 24:714–719.
39. Freeman RW, Woosley RL, Oates JA, Harbison RD: Evidence for the biotransformation of procainamide to a reactive metabolite. Toxicol App Pharmacol 1979; 50:9–16.
40. Lalka D, Wyman MG, Goldreyer BN, Ludden TM, Cannom DS: Procainamide accumulation kinetics in the immediate postmyocardial infarction period. J Clin Pharmacol 1978; 397–401.
41. Koch-Weser J, Klein SW: Procainamide dosage schedules, plasma concentrations, and clinical effects. JAMA 1971; 215:1454–1460.
42. Wagner JG: A safe method for rapidly achieving plasma concentration plateaus. Clin Pharmacol Ther 1974; 16:691–700.
43. Lima JJ, Jusko WJ: Pharmacokinetic approach to intravenous procainamide therapy. Eur J Clin Pharmacol 1978; 13:303–308.
44. Geleris P, Boudoulas H, Schaal SF, Lewis RP, Lima JJ: Effect of procainamide on left ventricular performance in patients with primary myocardial disease. Eur J Clin Pharmacol 1979; submitted for publication.
45. Mark JC, Kayden HJ, Steel JM: The physiological disposition and cardiac effects of procainamide. J Pharmacol Exp Ther 1951; 102:5–15.
46. Gibson TP, Lowenthal DT, Nelson HA, Briggs WA: Elimination of procainamide in end stage renal failure. Clin Pharmacol Ther 1975; 17:321–329.
47. Simons KJ, Levy RH, Cutler RE, Graham T, Lindner C, and Lindner A: The pharmacokinetics of procainamide in normal subjects using a specific gas chromatograph assay. Res Commun Chem Pathol Pharmacol 1975; 11:173.
48. Matusik E, Gibson TP: Fluorometric assay for N-acetylprocainamide. Clin Chem 1975; 21:1899–1902.
49. Lima JJ, Jusko WJ: Micromethod for procainamide and its acetylated metabolite by high performance liquid chromatography. In g. l. Hawkj (ed.), *Liquid Chromatography Symposium I: Biological/Biomedical Applications of Liquid Chromatography*, Dekker, New York, 1978.

50. Carr K, Woosley RL, Oates JA: Simultaneous quantitation of procainamide and N-acetylprocainamide with high performance liquid chromatography. J Chrom 1976; 129:363.

51. Dutcher JS, Strong JM: Determination of procainamide and N-acetylprocainamide concentration by high pressure liquid chromatography. Clin Chem 1977; 23:1318.

52. Shurkur LR, Powers JL, Marques RA, et. al: Measurement of procainamide and N-acetylprocainamide in plasma or serum by high performance liquid chromatography. Clin Chem 1977; 23:636.

53. Rocco RM, Abbott DC, Geise RW, Karger BL: Analysis for procainamide and N-acetylprocainamide in plasma or serum by high performance liquid chromatography. Clin Chem 1977; 23:705.

54. Weddle OH, Mason WD: Rapid determination of procainamide and its N-acetyl derivative in human plasma by high pressure liquid chromatography. J Pharm Sci 1977; 66:874.

55. Tilstone WJ, Lawson DH, Campbell W, Hutton I, Lawrie DV: The pharmacokinetics of slow-release procainamide. Eur J Clin Pharmacol 1978; 14:261–256.

56. Gadalla MAF, Peng GW, Chiou WL: Rapid and micro high-pressure liquid chromatographic method for simultaneous determination of procainamide and N-acetylprocainamide in plasma. J Pharm Sci 1978; 67:869–871.

57. Butterfield AG, Cooper JK, Midha KK: Simultaneous determination of procainamide and N-acetylprocainamide in plasma by high-performance liquid chromatography. J Pharm Sci 1978; 67:839–842.

58. Atkinson AJ, Parker M, Strong J: Rapid gas chromatographic measurement of plasma procainamide concentration. Clin Chem 1972; 18:643–646.

59. Gibson TP, Matusik E, Nelson HA, Wilkinson J, Briggs WA: Acetylation of procainamide in man and its relationship to isonicotinic acid hydrazide acetylation phenotype. Clin Pharmacol Ther 1975; 17:395–399.

60. Wesley-Hadzija B, Mattocks AM: Quantitative thin-layer chromatographic method for the determination of procainamide and its major metabolite in plasma. J Chromatag 1977; 143:307–313.

61. Gupta RN, Eng F, Lewis D: Fluorescence photometric quantitation of procainamide and N-acetylprocainamide in plasma after separation by thin-layer chromatography. Anal Chem 1978; 50:197–199.

62. Mojaverian P, Chase GD: Radioimmunoassay for procainamide in human serum. Abstracts. APhA Acad Pharm Sci 1979; 9:22.

# 13

# Quinidine

Clarence T. Ueda, Pharm.D., Ph.D.

## INTRODUCTION/BACKGROUND

Quinidine is a naturally occurring alkaloid which is widely used to treat cardiac arrhythmias. It is given orally and parenterally in the form of the sulfate, gluconate or polygalacturonate salt to control both ventricular and supraventricular rhythm disorders. The drug has a low therapeutic index (1–9) and the therapeutic and toxic effects have been shown to be related to quinidine concentrations in the serum and plasma (1,2,4,8,10,11).

Patient response to treatment with quinidine, particularly after oral ingestion which is the most common mode of administration, is known to vary markedly (8,12,13). This is due in part to the large patient-to-patient variation in quinidine bioavailability, distribution and elimination that have been seen with the drug (14–20). It is also undoubtedly related to the methods by which the drug is used. In order to obtain the most effective and efficient antiarrhythmic response with quinidine, drug therapy programs which monitor therapy on an individual patient basis should be developed.

## Absorption

Quinidine sulfate, gluconate and polygalacturonate are all given by mouth in solid dosage forms. For intramuscular and intravenous administration, quinidine gluconate is used almost exclusively. Following oral administration, the absolute bioavailability (F) of quinidine is about 70% of the ingested dose but may vary widely between patients (15,16,19). F has been shown in these studies to range from 0.45 to 1.0. The remaining drug appears to be cleared pre-systemically by the liver (15,16,19) which would be consistent with the observation that less than 5% of a given dose is detectable in the feces after oral administration (12,21).

Quinidine is a weakly basic drug. Optimal quinidine absorption from the gastrointestinal tract therefore occurs from the small intestine. With conventional quinidine sulfate tablets and capsules, peak plasma drug concentrations are reached in 1 to 3 hours after the dose (1,12,22–27). Quinidine gluconate is formulated as slow or sustained-release preparations, so the absorption of quinidine from these products is usually slower and protracted. The availability of quinidine from all of these preparations, however, appears to be comparable (24–26). At this time, there are insufficient data to comment on the bioavailability characteristics of the enteric-coated quinidine sulfate (Quinidex® Extentabs®) and polygalacturonate (Cardioquin®) drug products.

Plasma quinidine concentrations are generally higher and appear earlier when the drug is administered on an empty stomach (28,29). It is therefore reasonable to assume that quinidine absorption would be suppressed if the drug is given with meals. Furthermore, with the possible exception of aluminum hydroxide gel (26), the absorption of oral quinidine might also be adversely affected by the various antacid and antidiarrheal preparations that are given concomitantly to combat the side effect of quinidine-induced diarrhea (30).

In patients with congestive heart failure (31,32), the rate of oral quinidine absorption is depressed, probably as a result of a reduction in splanchnic blood flow rate. The extent of quinidine absorption, however, is not affected in the heart failure patient. (Ueda, C.T. and Dzindzio, B.S., unpublished data).

Intramuscular quinidine therapy has been employed for many years in patients requiring a rapid drug response and/or those who were unable to tolerate the drug orally. It was commonly believed that this mode of administration provided optimal drug absorption characteristics and antiarrhythmic response. Recent evidence shows that the rate and pattern of quinidine absorption after an intramuscular injection may be erratic and unpredictable with incomplete absorption of the administered dose (16). Protraction of quinidine absorption for over 4 hours has also been seen following intramuscular injections of quinidine gluconate (24). These observations are probably related to precipitation of drug at the injection site. Both quinidine base and its salt forms have low water solubility properties. This aspect would also explain the intense pain and muscle damage that are reported following injection of this drug.

Mason et al (24) observed no difference between the rate of quinidine absorption when given by intramuscular injection and the rate of oral absorption from conventional tablets and capsules and an aqueous solution. They did show, however, that the availability of quinidine is greater after an intramuscular injection.

## Distribution

Quinidine distribution in the body is rapid and primarily extravascular. It is described by a two-compartment open pharmacokinetic model with a half-life for the α, or distribution, phase of about 7 minutes and an overall volume of distribution ($V_B$) of 3 L/kg (14,16,17,19,20). The central compartment volume, $V_c$, is approximately 0.9 L/kg (14,16,20).

In the congestive heart failure patient, $V_c$ and $V_B$ are reduced from that seen in cardiac patients without heart failure (17,20,32). A 30 to 40% reduction in $V_c$ and $V_B$ has been observed in a group of patients with Class III heart failure (20). As a result, plasma quinidine concentrations are generally higher in the heart failure patient when unadjusted drug dosage regimens are employed (Figure 1). It is not presently known whether the magnitude of this change varies with the severity of the failing heart.

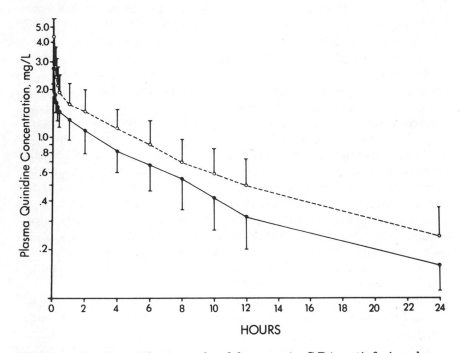

FIGURE 1.  Semilogarithmic graphs of the mean (± S.D.) postinfusion plasma quinidine concentrations obtained in congestive heart failure (O) and control cardiac patients (●) after a 22-minute zero-order infusion of quinidine gluconate. From Ueda and Dzindzio (20).

In the plasma concentration range generally considered to be therapeutic for quinidine, 2 to 5 µg/ml (6,7), quinidine binding to plasma proteins is moderate in terms of both the affinity and extent of the interaction. Approximately 70 to 80% of the drug is bound to these plasma constituents (primarily albumin) with an apparent association constant of $10^4$ $M^{-1}$ (33–38). Quinidine plasma protein binding is diminished in patients with liver disease (39–42). The binding of quinidine in plasma of patients with poor renal function (36,39) and hyperlipoproteinemia (43), on the other hand, is not altered.

On the basis of results obtained in healthy volunteers (44), $V_B$ and unbound plasma quinidine fractions do not appear to change with age. However, the apparent volume of distribution may be increased in patients with cirrhosis (42).

Quinidine readily diffuses into the red blood cell. Hughes et al (45) found a value of 0.82 for the red cell/plasma partition ratio.

Quinidine also distributes into the saliva with marked intra- and inter-patient variations in the ratio of saliva-to-serum quinidine (46–48). Therefore, the use of saliva quinidine levels as a reliable noninvasive method to monitor plasma or serum quinidine concentrations will require close scrutiny.

### Metabolism

The major route of quinidine elimination from the body appears to be via metabolism in the liver since renal excretion of intact drug accounts for only 10 to 20% of a given dose (14,15,17,20). The mean value for the elimination half-life of quinidine is 6 to 7 hours (7,14–20). However, this value, as well as the values for the other quinidine disposition constants, is known to vary considerably between patients (7,14–20). Ochs et al (44) report that the elimination half-life of quinidine is greater in the elderly (greater than 60 years) person when compared to the younger (less than 35 years) subject. It has also been suggested that patients with cirrhosis have a significantly longer quinidine half-life of 9 hours (42). The elimination half-life does not appear to be altered in patients with congestive heart failure (7,17,20,32) or poor renal function (7,49).

Total body quinidine clearance is about 4.5 ml/min/kg with wide patient-to-patient variations in this parameter (14,17,19,20). The clearance rate of quinidine is reduced in patients with congestive heart failure (17,20) and the elderly subject (44) as a result of a decrease in $V_B$ and an increase in half-life of the drug, respectively. Clearance does not appear to be altered in patients with liver or renal dysfunction.

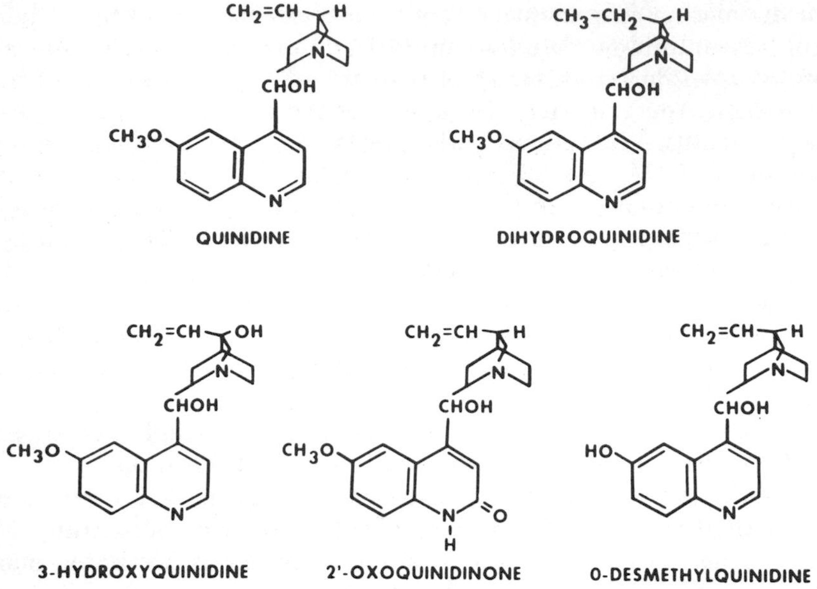

FIGURE 2. Structures of quinidine, dihydroquinidine and various metabolites.

Quinidine metabolites (Figure 2) that have been identified include 3-hydroxyquinidine, 2'-oxoquinidinone, and o-desmethylquinidine (50–53). Palmer et al (54) have suggested the existence of other unidentified hydroxylated metabolites as well as conjugated drug species. Additionally, the existence of a quinidine-N-oxide metabolite (55,56) and a lactic acid conjugate (57) have been proposed. The relative contribution of each biotransformation pathway to the overall removal of quinidine by drug metabolism is not presently known. The 3-hydroxyquinidine and 2'-oxoquinidinone metabolites are generally considered the principal end products of drug metabolism. Approximately 1 to 2% of a quinidine dose is converted to the o-demethylated derivative (53).

On a qualitative basis, there is little doubt that some of the metabolites of quinidine possess antiarrhythmic activity. Quantification of this activity, particularly as it relates to effectiveness in man, is much more difficult to ascertain. In various animal preparations, 3-hydroxyquinidine, 2'-oxoquinidinone, and o-desmethylquinidine have been all shown to suppress arrhythmias induced by different methods (53,58). Quinidine and the 2'-oxo metabolite appear to be equipotent when tested by two different antiarrhythmic screening methods (53).

These reports (53,58) suggest that the antiarrhythmic potencies of 3-hydroxy and o-desmethyl quinidine derivatives may be equal to or less than that of quinidine. The activities of the remaining metabolites are not known.

### Excretion

The excretion of quinidine by the kidneys accounts for 10 to 20% of an administered dose (14,15,17,20). Renal excretion occurs by glomerular filtration and is dependent upon the pH of the urine. Renal quinidine clearance has been shown to diminish with increasing urine pH (59,60). Drug clearance by the kidneys is lower in the elderly person and is positively correlated with creatinine clearance (44).

With the exception of the report that 1 to 2% of a quinidine dose is excreted in the urine as o-desmethylquinidine (53), the renal excretion characteristics of the other metabolites are not known.

## CONCENTRATION VERSUS RESPONSE AND TOXICITY

### Therapeutic Concentrations

From plasma and serum quinidine concentration-activity relationships (1,2,4,8,10,11), it is widely recognized that the antiarrhythmic effects of quinidine are achieved within a relatively narrow range of drug concentrations. For this reason, the determination of quinidine concentrations in plasma or serum has been advocated as a means to obtain the most efficient and effective response with the drug.

To effectively use plasma or serum quinidine concentration measurements, a knowledge of the drug assay procedure is required. This is because measured quinidine concentrations are dependent on the analytical method used. That is, if the same samples are analyzed by methods that differ in their specificity and/or sensitivity for quinidine, the reported concentrations for the drug will be different. Thus, because of this dependency, therapeutic plasma or serum quinidine concentrations vary with the drug analysis method.

Quinidine concentrations that are determined with a relatively nonspecific drug assay method such as the protein precipitation procedure (61), described in the Assay Methods section, will be higher than the true intact drug levels. With these methods, the therapeutic range for quinidine is generally higher and wider than the ranges determined with a more specific procedure. Quinidine concentrations of about 3 to 8 µg/ml are considered therapeutic when analyzed with these methods (1,2,5,56).

As assay specificity for quinidine improves, therapeutic effects with the drug are associated with lower plasma or serum concentrations. With the double extraction procedure of Cramer and Isaksson (62) which is considerably more specific for quinidine than the protein precipitation method, antiarrhythmic effects are achieved when the plasma or serum quinidine concentrations are between 2.3 and 5 μg/ml (6,7).

Although the therapeutic plasma and serum concentration range for quinidine is generally assumed to be lowest when determined with assay methods that are specific for quinidine, e.g., thin layer or high performance liquid chromatographic methods, it remains to be established if this is indeed the case. In a multiple dose quinidine study (Dzindzio, B.S., Vosik, W.M., and Ueda, C.T., unpublished data) with 24 hour Holter monitoring, antiarrhythmic effects were observed with steady-state serum quinidine concentrations as low as 0.8 to 0.9 μg/ml. Therapeutic effects without overt side reactions were detected with drug concentrations that ranged up to 3 μg/ml. These observations are in agreement with the results of Drayer et al (53) in which, using a specific high performance liquid chromatographic quinidine assay method, antiarrhythmic activity was achieved with serum quinidine concentrations of about 2 to 2.5 μg/ml. Therefore, it appears that therapeutic effects can be expected when the quinidine concentrations that are determined with a specific assay method are within a 1 to 3–3.5 μg/ml range.

At present, it is not known to what extent active quinidine metabolites contribute to the overall antiarrhythmic and/or side-toxic effects that are seen after the administration of quinidine. It has been suggested that the concentrations of these drug species in plasma and serum should also be determined since methods are available for their detection (63). Until more definitive information such as their precise antiarrhythmic activity or the extent to which they exist in the plasma or serum is known, however, the determination of quinidine and dihydroquinidine concentrations remain the most reliable and useful pieces of available information. The antiarrhythmic (111–114) and pharmacokinetic (115,116) properties of dihydroquinidine are similar to quinidine.

## Toxic Concentrations

Two adverse conditions are relatively common with quinidine. They are gastrointestinal side effects (primarily quinidine-induced diarrhea) and hypersensitivity to the drug. Patients have been known to discontinue the drug because of intolerable nausea, diarrhea, and/or vomiting. Because of a potential hypersensitivity reaction to the drug, a small test dose is recommended prior to initiation of the full quinidine treatment program. These effects, however, are generally not related to the concentrations of quinidine in the plasma or serum.

Toxic quinidine reactions such as cinchonism or arrhythmias, like side effects, vary extensively between patients. These differences are due to many factors including patient differences in physical status (64) and the route and rate by which the drug is given (2,64,65). Reports (66–68) exist in which patients have survived plasma and serum quinidine concentrations in excess of 20 μg/ml. However, most studies (1,2,4,66,67,69,70) suggest that regardless of the quinidine assay method used, plasma or serum quinidine concentrations above 10 μg/ml will almost assuredly produce toxic drug effects and may even be fatal.

In perhaps the most exhaustive study designed to delineate the relationship between serum quinidine concentrations and response, Sokolow and Ball (2) showed with 177 patients using the single extraction assay procedure described in the Assay Methods section that the incidence of important myocardial toxicity was only 1.6% when the drug concentrations were less than 6 μg/ml. Myocardial toxicity was never noted below 3 μg/ml, the lower limit of the therapeutic range. The incidence of toxicity increased to 12% with quinidine concentrations between 6 and 8 μg/ml, 30% at levels between 8 and 10 μg/ml, 45% at 12 to 13 μg/ml, and 65% when quinidine concentrations exceeded 14 μg/ml. Although this toxicity information was obtained with a single assay procedure, it does serve as a reasonable guideline upon which extrapolations to the remaining analytical methods can be made.

## CLINICAL APPLICATION OF PHARMACOKINETIC DATA

### Dosing

Quinidine pharmacokinetics vary widely between patients (14–20). As a result, interpatient requirements for quinidine can be substantially different. The following dosing recommendations are regimens that can be employed when initiating quinidine therapy. Adjustments in these dosing schedules might be necessary once steady-state conditions have been achieved and the patient's arrhythmia status has been re-evaluated. This is addressed in a later section.

Quinidine is most commonly given by mouth in the form of the sulfate, gluconate or polygalacturonate salt for chronic antiarrhythmic therapy. These quinidine salts contain 83, 62 and 60% of active drug, respectively. In initiating oral quinidine therapy, it is desirable to use conventional tablets and capsules containing the sulfate salt. Quinidine gluconate is manufactured as a prolonged-action dosage form which is known to have a higher potential for bioavailability problems. This form is associated with a lower incidence of gastrointestinal side effects, however, and might therefore be considered for patients who are not able to tolerate quinidine sulfate tablets and capsules. Once control of the arrhythmia has been achieved with quinidine sulfate together with knowledge of the quinidine concentrations at which this occurs, it would be appropriate at that time to consider a change to a longer acting quinidine preparation.

The daily dosage requirements for quinidine can be estimated from the following relationship:

$$\text{Daily Dosage} = \frac{(\overline{C})(Cl)(1440)}{F} \qquad \text{(Eq. 1)}$$

where $\overline{C}$ is the average plasma or serum quinidine concentration desired at steady-state, Cl is the total body drug clearance rate in ml/min/kg, and F is the bioavailability factor. The constant 1440 is the number of minutes in a day.

A treatment schedule with quinidine should achieve an average steady-state plasma (or serum) drug concentration of 1.5 µg/ml using a specific drug assay method. From Equation 1, the daily dosage requirement to reach this level would be:

$$\text{Daily Dosage} = \frac{(1.5 \ \mu g/ml)(4.5 \ ml/min/kg)(1440 \ min/day)}{0.70}$$

$$= \frac{9.72 \ mg/kg/day}{0.70} \simeq 14 \ mg/kg/day \text{ of free base}$$

This corresponds to a daily dosage with quinidine sulfate of 17 mg/kg/day [(14 mg/kg/day)/0.83] which is given in divided doses, e.g., every 6 hours. For a 70 kg patient, this represents 300 mg every 6 hours which is in agreement with the generally recommended dosages for this drug. With quinidine gluconate, the daily dosage requirement is (14 mg/kg/day)/0.62 or 23 mg/kg/day in divided doses, e.g., every 8 hours.

In younger patients (< 30 years) in whom Cl might be more rapid (44), larger daily doses may be required to obtain a $\overline{C}$ for quinidine of 1.5 µg/ml.

On a given dosage regimen, Equation 2 can be used to provide a reasonable estimate of the average quinidine concentration at steady-state or total body clearance when $\overline{C}$ can be assessed.

$$\overline{C} = \frac{(F)(Dose)}{(Cl)(\tau)}$$

(Eq. 2)

where F and Cl were previously defined and $\tau$ is the dosing interval.

In addition to patient-to-patient differences in quinidine disposition kinetics, oral drug availability may vary quite widely due to pre-systemic clearance of quinidine by the liver (15,16,19). This first-pass effect has been shown to account for the removal of from 5 to 55% of an orally administered quinidine dose. Major discrepancies that may be seen between the computed or predicted and observed quinidine concentrations in the plasma and serum are probably due to patient variations in disposition kinetics or first-pass effect or both. The variability in Cl between patients is greater than the variation in F. Both are, however, reasonably constant for a given patient.

At present, the only disease states where an adjustment in the quinidine dosage regimen would seem to be warranted are in patients with congestive heart failure or cirrhosis. In congestive heart failure patients, as a result of a diminished apparent volume for drug distribution, quinidine clearance is approximately 70% of the clearance rate of non-heart failure cardiac patients (20). This reduced clearance would lead to an elevation in plasma or serum quinidine concentrations. The congestive heart failure patient also absorbs the drug from the gastrointestinal tract at a slower rate (31,32) which has a lowering effect on the concentrations of drug in the plasma. As recently shown by Halkin et al (71), these divergent effects appear to offset each other to such an extent that the differences in drug concentrations between the two patient populations are not as pronounced as might be anticipated from clearance measurements alone. Thus, although no adjustments in the quinidine dosing regimens appear to be necessary with a congestive heart failure patient, the dosing of these patients should be approached conservatively.

Kessler et al (42) reported an increase in the elimination half-life of quinidine to 9 hours with no change in total body clearance in cirrhotics. A modification in quinidine dosage regimen as described in a previous chapter might be considered in patients with cirrhosis.

In acute situations, quinidine can be given by intramuscular injection or intravenous infusion. Intramuscular quinidine administration is associated with a great deal of pain and discomfort together with substantial increases in serum creatine phosphokinase levels (16). It is used largely by this route in emergency situations because of earlier findings (72–75) which suggested that intravenous quinidine was hazardous. Recent evidence (64,65) has shown, however, that intravenous quinidine is safe and effective when given by *slow* infusion and that this mode of parenteral administration might be the more desirable of the two methods.

For intravenous infusion, a quinidine gluconate dose of 5 to 8 mg/kg diluted in 40 ml of 5% dextrose in water and infused at a constant rate over 20 to 25 minutes has been shown to be a safe and effective method for giving quinidine (65). Using this procedure, peak plasma quinidine concentrations of about 3 to 4 µg/ml have been observed at the time of cessation of drug input. However, because of the two-compartment disposition characteristics of quinidine and the extremely short half-life of the α-phase, these plasma drug concentrations fall off rapidly to therapeutic levels after termination of the infusion as shown in Figure 1.

In patients with congestive heart failure, higher plasma quinidine concentrations are generally achieved with an infused dose of quinidine gluconate of 5 to 8 mg/kg when compared to non-heart failure cardiac patients (Figure 1). This is due to the diminished clearance rate of quinidine in these patients. Therefore, based on clearance measurements, a 25% reduction in the quinidine dose or 3.75 to 6 mg/kg of quinidine gluconate would appear to be an appropriate dose for infusion in the congestive heart failure patient.

In a single study (76), milligram for milligram, an intramuscular dose of quinidine gluconate produced serum quinidine concentrations at steady-state that were similar to the levels reached with the same dose of quinidine sulfate given orally.

## Blood Sampling

The absorption of quinidine from skeletal muscle and the gastrointestinal tract can be both erratic and highly variable. For these reasons, there is an inherently high degree of uncertainty associated with any attempt that is made to obtain the value of the peak or maximum plasma (or serum) quinidine concentration after a given dose. The lack of reliability of such a determination makes it impractical to try to obtain maximum drug concentration values.

Pre-dose or minimum quinidine concentration determinations, on the other hand, provide accurate and reliable assessments of the plasma drug levels in the preceding dosing interval. Because these concentrations are intimately related to the therapeutic range of the drug, they provide a meaningful expression of antiarrhythmic efficacy. One principal reason to monitor plasma or serum quinidine concentrations is to ensure that therapeutic drug concentrations have been achieved in patients not responding to drug treatment.

## Algorithm

It is widely recognized that when standard quinidine dosages (e.g., 200 mg every 6 hours) are used, patient-to-patient variations in plasma or serum quinidine concentrations can be extensive. With such regimens, Halkin et al (71) calculated between-individual coefficients of variation in serum drug concentration of 20 to 60% using results of their own study and other investigators (7,10,17). The mean coefficient of variation for within-patient differences in serum quinidine concentrations at steady-state, on the other hand, was only 18% (71). These observations show the value of individualized patient dosing with quinidine.

Interpatient plasma or serum quinidine concentration differences are reduced when the dosage is adjusted for body weight, i.e., mg/kg. This is perhaps a key to a successful treatment program with the drug. Other factors such as the coexistence of congestive heart failure, cirrhosis and patient age must also be considered when designing the quinidine dosage regimen.

The algorithm shown in Figure 3 provides a rational approach for treating arrhythmias with quinidine. Using mean patient data obtained with specific drug assays, it is appropriate to initiate quinidine therapy with a drug dosage regimen of 14 mg/kg/day of quinidine base in divided doses. With this dosage, the predicted or expected value of $\bar{C}$ would be 1.5 µg/ml and should produce quinidine concentrations that are within the therapeutic drug concentration range. The use of nonspecific quinidine assays results only in a difference in the reported value for the quinidine concentration. With these methods, the range of therapeutic drug concentrations is elevated as previously discussed. In the congestive heart failure and young adult cardiac patient, it is not unlikely for $\bar{C}$ to be higher and lower, respectively, than the levels seen in the average cardiac patient with this dosage regimen due to differences in drug clearance (20,32,44).

After a minimum of two to three days on this dosage regimen and the drug is tolerated by the patient, the status of the arrhythmia should be re-evaluated and blood sample(s) collected to obtain an estimate of $\bar{C}$. With standard quinidine sulfate tablets and capsules and an every six hour dosing schedule, this would be at approximately 4 hours post dose, i.e., midway between the maximum and minimum plasma or serum drug concentrations in the dosing interval. For quinidine gluconate given every 8 hours, it would be at about 5 to 6 hours post dose. If the arrhythmia is controlled and no adverse effects related to the drug are observed, quinidine administration should be continued on this dosing schedule.

ALGORITHM FOR THE TREATMENT OF ARRHYTHMIAS WITH QUINIDINE

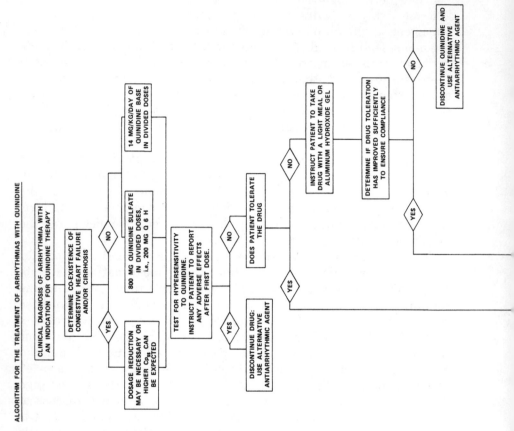

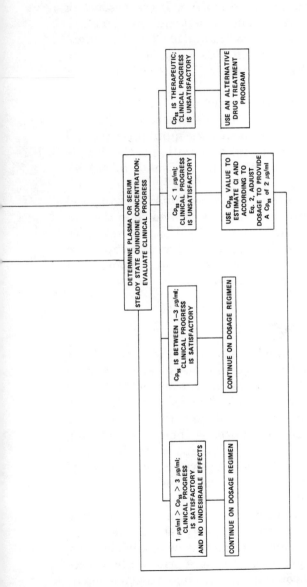

FIGURE 3.   Algorithm for the treatment of arrhythmias with quinidine.

In the absence of an antiarrhythmic effect with this quinidine dosing regimen, when it has been determined that the patient was compliant, the estimated value of $\bar{C}$ provides important information regarding whether therapeutic drug concentrations have been achieved and if there is a need to further increase the quinidine dosage in an attempt to control the arrhythmia with this drug. If the absence of arrhythmia control is felt to be due to an inadequate quinidine dosage, the $\bar{C}$ estimate is used to provide an approximation of Cl in the patient with Equation 2. With this same equation, this value is then used to determine the new quinidine dosage based on the desired plasma or serum quinidine concentrations.

If therapeutic quinidine concentrations have been reached without any apparent control of the arrhythmia, the likelihood of achieving an antiarrhythmic effect by further increasing the quinidine dose and not producing adverse effects requiring discontinuation of the drug is probably remote. In these cases, it would be advisable to use an alternate antiarrhythmic agent.

Gastrointestinal side effects are the chief complaints following oral administration. Quinidine gluconate is better tolerated than the sulfate salt, probably as a result of the effects of the dosage form. Thus, in patients who are not able to tolerate quinidine sulfate, a comparable daily dose of the gluconate salt should be used before abandoning attempts to control the arrhythmia with quinidine.

## ASSAY METHODS

Over the years, a number of quinidine assay methods have been developed and used to assess the levels of quinidine in various biological samples. The majority of these methods fall into one of the following major drug assay categories: spectroscopic (fluorescence, ultraviolet and visible) or chromatographic (gas, liquid, and thin layer). The principal difference between these procedures is their specificity for quinidine. In general, most of the commonly used methods do not separate quinidine from dihydroquinidine (a known impurity in drug-grade quinidine, Figure 2) and drug metabolites and are therefore nonspecific. This is particularly the case for the fluorometric quinidine assay procedures that are described below and which are the ones that are most commonly employed in clinical pathology laboratories.

The assay specificity for quinidine is improved when the method includes an extraction and/or separation procedure prior to the detection step. In this manner, extraneous endogenous and exogenous substances such as drug metabolites that would normally interfere with the quinidine determination are effectively removed or, at least, minimized. The most specific quinidine assays incorporate both an extraction and chromatographic separation procedure in the assay method.

## Spectroscopic Assay Methods

**Fluorometric.** Quinidine possesses native fluorescence. Fluorometric assay methods for quinidine are therefore quite common since fluorescence spectroscopy is a highly sensitive analytical tool. In general, these methods are reasonably rapid, easy to perform, and readily detect sub-microgram per milliliter concentrations of quinidine in plasma, serum, and urine. Halogen ions quench the fluorescence of quinidine (77) which results in a loss in sensitivity. Quinidine fluoresces maximally in an acidic pH (77) at excitation and emission wavelength maxima of 350 and 450 nm, respectively.

While simplicity is the major advantage of fluorometric quinidine assay methods, the principal shortcoming of fluorometric procedures is their lack of specificity for quinidine. None of these methods is able to differentiate quinidine from dihydroquinidine in a given sample. In addition, the removal or separation of quinidine metabolites from intact drug is never complete with these methods and the extent of metabolite inclusion is variable and highly dependent on the extraction procedure that is used (56,62,78–83). Quinidine concentrations determined by these methods will therefore always be an overestimate of the true drug concentration.

The major pieces of equipment that are needed to perform a fluorometric quinidine assay are a fluorometer, high speed centrifuge, and mixing or shaking device. The availability of a chart recorder would be convenient. Fluorometers vary quite extensively in price. Analytical models, which are the most expensive, afford greater sensitivity and accuracy and are probably most appropriate for research purposes. A less expensive fluorometer would adequately serve the needs of routine day-to-day quinidine concentration determinations since the drug has a high fluorescence property (i.e., quantum yield) and the lower limit of sensitivity with these instruments is well below the quinidine concentrations that would be normally encountered in clinical practice.

The simplest, but least specific, fluorometric quinidine assay procedure is the *protein precipitation method* (61). With this method, serum or plasma proteins are precipitated with a 20% metaphosphoric acid solution and, after centrifugation, the resultant supernatant liquid, which should be clear, is read directly in a cuvette with a suitable fluorometer. Standard quinidine solutions of known concentrations are used to determine the concentration of drug in the unknown sample.

Although simple and rapid, the protein precipitation method has an inherently high degree of nonspecificity. Quinidine metabolites, which are present to varying extents and known to fluoresce, are included in the quinidine determination. Additionally, the presence of native substances, particularly chloride ions, in the plasma supernates quench the fluorescence of quinidine (77).

Trichloroacetic acid has also been used as the protein-precipitating agent. When this protein precipitant is used, the intensity of quinidine fluorescence is reduced and the quenching effects appear to be greater when compared with metaphosphoric acid (79).

In an attempt to improve the assay specificity for quinidine, various *extraction procedures* have been developed (16,62,78,79,81,82,84,85). With these methods, the biological sample (approximately 1 ml) is alkalinized, usually with sodium hydroxide, and the drug is extracted from the aqueous phase with a suitable organic solvent. In an alkaline media, quinidine exists almost entirely in its undissociated, lipid soluble form, the drug species that readily partitions into non-polar solvents. Direct fluorescence measurements can be made on an aliquot of this extract after it has been acidified (62,78,84). Alternatively, the organic solvent extract can be re-extracted with sulfuric acid which is then read fluorometrically (16,62,79,81,82,84). These single and double extraction procedures, respectively, significantly improve the specificity and therefore reliability of the quinidine determination.

A comparison of the single extraction method with the protein precipitation procedure has shown that the latter assay method consistently yields higher values for quinidine when the same serum samples are analyzed by both methods (78). These differences can be attributed to the presence of greater amounts of quinidine metabolites in the protein-free plasma supernates.

Ethylene dichloride (62,78) and benzene (62,79,81,84,85) are the most commonly used extracting solvents for quinidine. Both solvents have been clearly shown to extract dihydroquinidine and small amounts of quinidine metabolites (62,81,84,85). However, benzene removes smaller amounts of these latter fluorescing quinidine derivatives (80,81). For this reason, benzene is the solvent of choice for the extraction of quinidine from biological samples. Other extraction solvents that have been used to assay for quinidine include chloroform (54,80,86), toluene (16,87) and a 1:1 amyl alcohol-benzene mixture (80,85).

The most widely used fluorometric quinidine assay is the *double-extraction method* of Cramer and Isaksson (62). A simple re-extraction of the organic solvent extract with sulfuric acid significantly improves the specificity of the assay procedure for quinidine. In this procedure, after extracting the sample (serum, plasma, or urine) with benzene, an aliquot of the clear benzene extract is re-extracted with 0.1 N sulfuric acid. Using standard quinidine samples that are prepared in the same manner, the fluorescence of an aliquot of the sulfuric acid extract is used to assess the concentration of quinidine in the unknown sample.

It has been reported (88) that aqueous alkaline washes of the benzene extract with 0.1 N sodium hydroxide prior to re-extraction with sulfuric acid removes a significant fraction of the benzene-extractable quinidine metabolites.

With the additional extraction step(s), these methods require more time than the simpler protein precipitation procedure. However, the improved specificity for quinidine that is obtained with the extraction methods significantly outweighs any savings in time that might be gained by using the simpler procedure. The extraction methods have the added advantage that they can be used to determine quinidine concentrations in urine and virtually any other biological sample.

**Ultraviolet and Colorimetric.** Quinidine determination by ultraviolet spectroscopy (89) and colorimetry (90) are available but have been largely replaced by more specific and sensitive methods. The ultraviolet spectrophotometric assay is virtually identical to the double extraction fluorometric procedure of Cramer and Isaksson (62) in terms of preparation of the sample. In this procedure, the absorbance of quinidine in 0.1 N sulfuric acid is determined with a suitable spectrophotometer. The colorimetric technique is based on ion-pair extraction of quinidine into ethylene dichloride or chloroform with methyl orange (90). With this method quinidine concentrations are estimated by determining the percent transmission of the resultant colored solutions in a colorimeter or spectrophotometer.

## Chromatographic Assay Methods

These methods were developed in response to a need for a quinidine assay with improved specificity and sensitivity and which could be performed in a shorter length of time. In general, they are methods that can be used with all biological materials without resorting to any special wash or clean-up procedure as previously discussed. With these assays, the drug (and metabolites) is isolated from the biological sample by solvent extraction and/or separation on a chromatographic column or plate. The limiting factor with these assay methods may be the availability of the appropriate instrumentation.

**Gas-Liquid Chromatography.** Although the available gas-liquid chromatographic quinidine assays (91–93) do not separate dihydroquinidine from quinidine, they readily separate these substances from drug metabolites. These procedures are therefore quite specific for intact drug. Additionally, they are very sensitive. With the method of Midha and Charette (91), described below, the lower limit of detectability is 0.05 μg/ml of plasma or blood. The time required for the performance of a quinidine determination with these methods as well as the costs are comparable to the extraction procedures.

The major instrumentation and equipment needs to perform a quinidine analysis by gas-liquid chromatography are a gas chromatograph equipped with a flame-ionization (91,92) or nitrogen-specific (93) detector and recorder or integrator, centrifuge, and mixing or shaking device. The availability of a multiposition evaporating apparatus would significantly reduce the analysis time. A single column gas chromatograph that is designed to operate isocratically is comparable in price with other analytical instruments such as the fluorometer or spectrophotometer. For routine usage, the costs that are incurred for the purchase of columns and gases can potentially be quite significant depending upon the rate of use.

The method of Midha and Charette (91), which involves the derivatization of quinidine with trimethylanilinium hydroxide, is representative of quinidine analysis by gas-liquid chromatography.

**High Performance Liquid Chromatography.** Quinidine analysis by high performance liquid chromatography is specific, sensitive, efficient and rapid. Methods are available for the assay of quinidine, dihydroquinidine, and the principal quinidine metabolites in various biological materials (17,63,94–103). The time required for the performance of a liquid chromatographic quinidine determination varies with the method. Direct on-column injection of the unknown sample requires less time than a procedure that includes an extraction step in the quinidine determination.

A liquid chromatographic system is relatively expensive when compared with a fluorometer or gas chromatograph. The cost of a fluorescence detector alone can be as much as the latter instruments themselves. Additionally, liquid chromatographic columns and solvents are generally more expensive than the columns and gases used in gas chromatographic procedures.

The major instrumentation and equipment needs include a liquid chromatograph or comparable components (i.e., solvent pump(s) and injector) with an ultraviolet or fluorescence detector, recorder and/or integrator, high speed centrifuge, and a mixing or shaking device. A fluorescence detector is the more sensitive of the two types of detectors. It is also more expensive.

Powers and Sadee (97) have described a procedure in which a protein-free serum sample is injected directly onto an alkyl phenyl reverse-phase liquid chromatographic column. With this procedure, the lower limit of sensitivity for quinidine is 0.3 µg/ml. Quinidine metabolites and dihydroquinidine are not determined with this method.

Using various extraction and chromatographic conditions, liquid chromatographic procedures are available that are capable of quantitating quinidine, dihydroquinidine, 2'-oxoquinidinone, 3-hydroxyquinidine, o-desmethylquinidine, and/or quinidine-N-oxide in essentially all biological materials (63,94,101,103). With these methods, a sample size of 1 ml or less is required and their drug and metabolite content are extracted with a suitable organic solvent(s) prior to injection onto a liquid chromatographic column and quantitation with a fluorescence or ultraviolet detector. Sensitivity limits with these procedures range from 5 to 100 ng/ml and depend on the nature of the biological sample. The retention times of quinidine, dihydroquinidine, and drug metabolites range up to 15 to 35 minutes depending on the method used. These retention values coupled with the time required for the extraction step prolong the overall analysis time with these methods.

Other high performance liquid chromatographic methods (95–100,102) are available for the determination of quinidine and/or dihydroquinidine alone.

**Thin Layer Chromatography.** Several quinidine assay procedures separate quinidine from dihydroquinidine and drug metabolites by thin layer chromatography (15,80,104–106) and quantitate the drug (and dihydroquinidine) by measuring the fluorescence of the isolated drug. This procedure requires the following major pieces of instrumentation and equipment: fluorometer with recorder and/or integrator, centrifuge, and mixer or shaker. Direct fluorometric determination of quinidine on the thin layer plate requires a plate-scanning device which adds significantly to the cost for instrumentation.

Steyn and Hundt (104) and Christiansen (105) have described microanalytical methods for the determination of quinidine using 10 and 50 µl plasma or serum samples, respectively, and direct application and on-plate (silica gel) analysis of protein-free drug samples.

The more common thin layer chromatographic procedures (15,80,106) involve extraction of a 0.5 to 1 ml biological sample with benzene or dichloromethane before separation on a thin layer plate. The isolated quinidine (and dihydroquinidine) can be read directly on the plate with a thin layer plate scanner (106) or removed by scraping and read in a fluorometer after elution of the drug from the silica gel with 0.1 N sulfuric acid (15,80). Although these methods are specific for quinidine and are reasonably sensitive (approximately 0.1 μg/ml), they generally require a greater amount of care in the handling and preparation of the assay sample and they are time-consuming. These limitations can be major deterrents to routine clinical use of these methods. Direct fluorescence measurements of quinidine on the thin layer plates improves the precision of this method.

## Other Assay Methods

Several other types of assay methods have been used to estimate quinidine levels in various biological specimens. They include an extraction procedure with chloroform and subsequent quantitation via titration with bromine water (107) and a nephelometric procedure (108) in which the turbidity of a suspension of quinidine silicotungstate is measured. In addition to their lack of specificity for quinidine, these methods are less sensitive than the previously described procedures.

A sensitive and specific method for the determination of quinidine is by chemical ionization-mass spectrometry (109). The instrument costs for this system are high and its use requires a highly trained operator. For these reasons, this method is not suited for the average laboratory.

A new enzyme immunoassay (EMIT®—Enzyme Mulitiplied Immunoassay Technique) for quinidine has been recently developed for the determination of quinidine in plasma and serum (110). This method is based on the direct relationship between changes in glucose-6-phosphate dehydrogenase activity, which can be measured spectrophotometrically, and the concentration of quinidine in plasma or serum. The method requires a sample size of 50 μl and is sensitive down to a quinidine concentration of 0.5 μg/ml. With this assay procedure, it is not possible to differentiate between quinidine and dihydroquinidine. The principal advantages of the EMIT assay for quinidine are convenience and rapidity with which a quinidine determination can be made.

## Summary and Ranking of the Methods

Table 1 summarizes the relative advantages and disadvantages of the various methods that are available for the determination of quinidine in biological materials. The type of quinidine assay procedure that should be employed is highly dependent upon the requirements

TABLE 1. COMPARISON OF THE RELATIVE ADVANTAGES AND DISADVANTAGES OF THE VARIOUS QUINIDINE ASSAY METHODS*

| Analysis Method | Specificity for Quinidine | Sensitivity | Metabolite Analysis | Dihydroquinidine Analysis | Assayable Samples | | | | Minimum Sample Volume | Analysis Time | Analysis Cost | Instrument and Equipment Costs | Specialized Operator Training |
|---|---|---|---|---|---|---|---|---|---|---|---|---|---|
| | | | | | Plasma/Serum | Urine | Saliva | Others | | | | | |
| *SPECTROSCOPIC* | | | | | | | | | | | | | |
| *Fluorometric* | | | | | | | | | | | | | |
| Protein Precipitation | 5 | 3 | No | No | X | | X | | 3 | 2 | 3 | 3 | None |
| Single Extraction | 4 | 3 | No | No | X | X | X | | 3 | 2 | 3 | 3 | None |
| Double Extraction | 3 | 3 | No | No | X | X | X | X | 3 | 3 | 3 | 3 | None |
| *Ultraviolet* | 3 | 3 | No | No | X | X | X | X | 3 | 3 | 3 | 3 | None |
| *Colorimetric* | 4 | 4 | No | No | X | X | X | ? | 3 | 3 | 3 | 3 | None |
| *CHROMATOGRAPHIC* | | | | | | | | | | | | | |
| *Gas-Liquid* | 2 | 2 | No | No | X | X | X | X | 2 | 2 | 2–3 | 3 | None |
| *Liquid* | 1 | 2 | Yes | Yes | X | X | X | X | 2 | 2 | 2–3 | 4 | None |
| *Thin-Layer* | 1 | 2 | Possible | Yes | X | X | X | X | 3 | 4 | 3 | 3–4 | Some |
| *OTHERS* | | | | | | | | | | | | | |
| *Titration* | 5 | 5 | No | No | X | ? | ? | ? | 5 | 5 | 2 | 2 | None |
| *Nephelometric* | 5 | 5 | No | No | X | ? | ? | ? | 5 | 2 | 2 | 2 | None |
| *Mass Spectrometry* | 1 | 1 | ? | No | X | ? | ? | ? | 3 | 3 | 5 | 5 | Yes |
| *EMIT^R* | 2 | 3 | No | No | X | ? | ? | | 1 | 1 | 2–4† | 3 | None |

* Arbitrary Ranking Scale of 1 (Excellent) to 5 (Poor) with a score of 3 being average or nominal.

† Analytical costs decrease as sample numbers per run increase.

of the determination. Pharmacokinetic studies with quinidine require a much higher degree of specificity and sensitivity for the drug than are required for routine clinical drug monitoring. The reverse situation would be true in terms of the analysis time required for a quinidine determination. Instrument and equipment availability, analysis costs, and other factors will also enter into the decision of which quinidine assay to use. For these reasons, the analytical method of choice for quinidine will vary with each laboratory.

In terms of specificity, sensitivity, efficiency, and rapidity of the assay procedure, quinidine analysis by high pressure liquid chromatography is versatile and can be readily adapted to various needs. The method is applicable for routine clinical drug determinations as well as for research purposes, the major active drug metabolites can be quantitated, and the procedure is easily performed by a laboratory technician with a minimal amount of supervision once established in the laboratory.

## ACKNOWLEDGMENTS

I am extremely grateful to Dr. Barry S. Dzindzio and Dr. Bill J. Cady for their suggestions and comments and to Mrs. Donna M. Earnshaw for her excellent secretarial assistance during the entire period that this chapter was being prepared.

## REFERENCES

1. Sokolow M, Edgar AL: Blood quinidine concentrations as a guide in the treatment of cardiac arrhythmias. Circulation 1950; 1:576–592.
2. Sokolow M, Ball RE: Factors influencing conversion of chronic atrial fibrillation with special reference to serum quinidine concentration. Circulation 1956; 14:568–583.
3. Koch-Weser J: Serum drug concentrations as therapeutic guides. N Engl J Med 1972; 287:227–231.
4. Koch-Weser J: Correlation of serum concentrations and pharmacologic effects of antiarrhythmic drugs. In: Pharmacology and the future of man. Proc 5th Int Congr Pharmacol. San Francisco, Karger, Basel, 1973; 3:69–85.
5. Bellet S: Clinical Disorders of the Heart Beat. 3rd ed. Philadelphia: Lea & Febiger, 1971; 980–1007.
6. Warner H: Therapy of common arrhythmias. Med Clin N Am 1974; 58:995–1017.
7. Kessler KM, Lowenthal DT, Warner H, Gibson T, Briggs W, Reidenberg MM: Quinidine elimination in patients with congestive heart failure or poor renal function. N Engl J Med 1974; 290:706–709.
8. Gaughan CE, Lown B, Lanigan J, Voukydis P, Besser HW: Acute oral testing for determining antiarrhythmic drug efficacy I: Quinidine. Am J Cardiol 1976; 38:677–684.
9. Woosley RL, Shand DG: Pharmacokinetics of antiarrhythmic drugs. Am J Cardiol 1978; 41:986–995.
10. Heissenbuttel RH, Bigger JT: The effect of oral quinidine on intraventricular conduction in man: Correlation of plasma quinidine with changes in QRS duration. Am Heart J 1970; 80:453–462.

11. Fieldman A, Beebe RD, Chow MSS: The effect of quinidine sulfate on QRS duration and QT and systolic time intervals in man. J Clin Pharmacol 1977; 17:134–139.
12. Yount EH, Rosenblum M: Studies of plasma quinidine levels in relation to therapeutic effect and toxic manifestations. South Med J 1950; 43:324–329.
13. Weisman SA: Review and evaluation of quinidine therapy for auricular fibrillation. JAMA 1953; 152:496–499.
14. Ueda CT, Hirschfeld DS, Scheinman MM, Rowland M, Williamson BJ, Dzindzio BS: Disposition kinetics of quinidine. Clin Pharmacol Ther 1976; 19:30–36.
15. Ueda CT, Williamson BJ, Dzindzio BS: Absolute quinidine bioavailability. Clin Pharmacol Ther 1976; 20:260–265.
16. Greenblatt DJ, Pfeifer HJ, Ochs HR, et al: Pharmacokinetics of quinidine in humans after intravenous, intramuscular and oral administration. J Pharmacol Exp Ther 1977; 202:365–378.
17. Conrad KA, Molk BL, Chidsey CA: Pharmacokinetic studies of quinidine in patients with arrhythmia. Circulation 1977; 55:1–7.
18. Ochs HR, Greenblatt DJ, Woo E, Franke K, Pfeifer HJ, Smith TW: Single and multiple dose pharmacokinetics of oral quinidine sulfate and gluconate. Am J Cardiol 1978; 41:770–777.
19. Guentert TW, Holford NHG, Coates PE, Upton RA, Riegelman S: Quinidine pharmacokinetics in man: choice of a disposition model and absolute bioavailability studies. J Pharmacok Biopharm 1979; 7:315–330.
20. Ueda CT, Dzindzio BS: Quinidine kinetics in congestive heart failure. Clin Pharmacol Ther 1978; 23:158–164.
21. Houston AB, Perry WF: The plasma concentration of quinidine after oral administration and its effect on auricular fibrillation. Can Med Assoc J 1950; 36:56–60.
22. Hamfelt A, Malers E: Determination of quinidine concentration in serum in the control of quinidine therapy. Acta Soc Med Ups 1963; 68:181–191.
23. Goldberg WM, Chakrabarti SG: The relationship of dosage schedule to the blood level of quinidine, using all available quinidine preparations. Can Med Assoc J 1964; 91:991–996.
24. Mason WD, Covinsky JO, Valentine JL, Kelly KL, Weddle OH, Martz BL: Comparative plasma concentrations of quinidine following administration of one intramuscular and three oral formulations to 13 human subjects. J Pharm Sci 1976; 65:1325–1329.
25. Strum JD, Colaizzi JL, Jaffe JM, Martineau PC, Poust RI: Comparative bioavailability of four commercial quinidine sulfate tablets. J Pharm Sci 1977; 66:539–542.
26. Romankiewicz JA, Reidenberg M, Drayer D, Franklin JE. The noninterference of aluminum hydroxide gel with quinidine sulfate absorption: an approach to control quinidine-induced diarrhea. Am Heart J 1978; 96:518–520.
27. Covinsky JO, Russo J, Kelly KL, Cashman J, Amick EN, Mason WD: Relative bioavailability of quinidine gluconate and quinidine sulfate in healthy volunteers. J Clin Pharmacol 1979; 19:261–269.
28. Hiatt EP: Plasma concentrations following the oral administration of single doses of the principal alkaloids of cinchona bark. J Pharmacol Exp Ther 1944; 81:160–163.
29. Ditlefsen EML: Concentrations of quinidine in blood following oral, parenteral and rectal administration. Acta Med Scand 1953; 146:81–92.
30. Remon JP, Van Severen R, Braeckman P: Interaction entre antiarythmiques, antiacides et antidiarrhéiques III. Influence d'antiacides et d'antidiarrhéiques sur la résorption in vitro de sels de quinidine. Pharm Acta Helv 1979; 54:19–22.
31. Anonymous: The pharmacokinetics and bioavailability of drugs in disease states. NIH Guide for Contracts and Grants 1976; 8:39–42.

32. Crouthamel WG: The effect of congestive heart failure on quinidine pharmacokinetics. Am Heart J 1975; 90:335–339.
33. Conn HL, Luchi RJ: Ionic influences of quinidine-albumin interaction. J Pharmacol Exp Ther 1961; 133:76–83.
34. Conn HL, Luchi RJ: Some quantitative aspects of the binding of quinidine and related quinoline compounds by human serum albumin. J Clin Invest 1961; 40:509–516.
35. Koch-Weser J: Correlation of plasma levels of antiarrhythmic drugs with their pharmacologic effects. In: Symposium: Basis of drug therapy in man. 5th Int Congr Pharmacol. San Francisco 1972; 56–57.
36. Skuterud B, Enger E, Halvorsen S, Jacobsen S, Lunde PKM: Serum protein binding of quinidine and diphenylhydantoin in healthy human volunteers and in patients with chronic renal failure. In: Symposium: Basis of drug therapy in man. 5th Int Congr Pharmacol. San Francisco 1972; 79–80.
37. Ueda CT, Makoid MC: Quinidine and dihydroquinidine interactions in human plasma. J Pharm Sci 1979; 68:448–450.
38. Woo E, Greenblatt DJ: Pharmacokinetic and clinical implications of quinidine protein binding. J Pharm Sci 1979; 68:466–470.
39. Reidenberg MM, Affrime M: Influence of disease on binding of drugs to plasma proteins. Ann N Y Acad Sci 1973; 226:115–126.
40. Affrime M, Reidenberg MM: The protein binding of some drugs in plasma from patients with alcoholic liver disease. Europ J Clin Pharmacol 1975; 8:267–269.
41. Perez-Mateo M, Erill S: Protein binding of salicylate and quinidine in plasma from patients with renal failure, chronic liver disease and chronic respiratory insufficiency. Europ J Clin Pharmacol 1977; 11:225–231.
42. Kessler KM, Humphries WC, Black M, Spann JF: Quinidine pharmacokinetics in patients with cirrhosis or receiving propranolol. Am Heart J 1978; 96:627–635.
43. Kates RE, Sokoloski TD, Comstock TJ: Binding of quinidine to plasma proteins in normal subjects and in patients with hyperlipoproteinemias. Clin Pharmacol Ther 1978; 23:30–35.
44. Ochs HR, Greenblatt DJ, Woo E, Smith TW: Reduced quinidine clearance in elderly persons. Am J Cardiol 1978; 42:481–485.
45. Hughes IE, Ilett KF, Jellett LB: The distribution of quinidine in human blood. Br J Clin Pharmacol 1975; 2:521–525.
46. Jaffe JM, Strum JD, Martineau PC, Colaizzi JL: Relationship between quinidine plasma and saliva levels in humans. J Pharm Sci 1975; 64:2028–2029.
47. Coates P, Riegelman S: Salivary excretion of quinidine. Abstract, APhA, Acad Pharm Sci 1978; 8(1):127.
48. Ueda CT, Beckmann PJ, Dzindzio BS: Saliva/plasma quinidine ratio after repeated drug administration. Abstract, APhA, Acad Pharm Sci 1979; 9(2):81.
49. Levy R, Sellers A, Mandel WJ, Okun R: Quinidine pharmacokinetics in anephric and normal subjects. Clin Res 1976; 24:85A.
50. Carroll FI, Smith D, Wall ME, Moreland CG: Carbon-13 magnetic resonance study. Structure of the metabolites of orally administered quinidine in humans. J Med Chem 1974; 17:985–987.
51. Beerman B, Leander K, Lindstrom B: The metabolism of quinidine in man: structure of a main metabolite. Acta Chem Scand B 1976; 30:465.
52. Drayer DE, Cook CE, Reidenberg MM: Active quinidine metabolites. Clin Res 1976; 24:623A.
53. Drayer DE, Lowenthal DT, Restivo KM, Schwartz A, Cook CE, Reidenberg MM: Steady-state serum levels of quinidine and active metabolites in cardiac patients with varying degrees of renal function. Clin Pharmacol Ther 1978; 24:31–39.

54. Palmer KH, Martin B, Baggett B, Wall ME: The metabolic fate of orally administered quinidine gluconate in humans. Biochem Pharmacol 1969; 18:1845–1860.
55. Guentert TW, Coates PE, Riegelman S: Isolation and identification of a new quinidine metabolite. Abstract, APhA, Acad Pharm Sci 1978; 8(1):137.
56. Guentert TW, Upton RA, Holford NHG, Riegelman S: Divergence in pharmacokinetic parameters of quinidine obtained by specific and nonspecific assay methods. J Pharmacok Biopharm 1979; 7:303–311.
57. Leferink JG, Maes RAA, Sunshine I, Forney RB: A novel quinidine metabolism in a suicide case with quinidine sulphate detected by gas chromatography—mass spectrometry. J Anal Tox 1977; 1:62–65.
58. Nwangwu PU, Holcslaw TL, Rosenberg H, Small LD, Stohs SJ: The antiarrhythmic activities of 6'-hydroxycinchonine, 6'-benzyloxycinchonine and 6'-allyloxycinchonine compared with quinidine in mice. J Pharm Pharmacol 1979; 31:488–489.
59. Conn HL, Luchi RJ: Some cellular and metabolic considerations relating to the action of quinidine as a prototype antiarrhythmic agent. Am J Med 1964; 37:685–699.
60. Gerhardt RE, Knouss RF, Thyrum PT, Luchi RJ, Morris JJ: Quinidine excretion in aciduria and alkaluria. Ann Intern Med 1969; 71:927–933.
61. Brodie BB, Udenfriend S: The estimation of quinidine in human plasma with a note on the estimation of quinidine. J Pharmacol Exp Ther 1943; 78:154–158.
62. Cramer G, Isaksson B: Quantitative determination of quinidine in plasma. Scand J Clin Lab Invest 1963; 15:553–556.
63. Guentert TW, Coates PE, Upton RA, Combs DL, Riegelman S: Determination of quinidine and its major metabolites by high-performance liquid chromatography. J Chromatogr 1976; 162:59–70.
64. Woo E, Greenblatt DJ: A reevaluation of intravenous quinidine. Am Heart J 1978; 96:829–832.
65. Hirschfeld DS, Ueda CT, Rowland M, Scheinman MM: Clinical and electrophysiological effects of intravenous quinidine in man. Br Heart J 1977; 39:309–316.
66. Kalmansohn RW, Sampson JJ: Studies of plasma quinidine content II. Relation to toxic manifestations and therapeutic effect. Circulation 1950; 1:569–575.
67. Ditlefsen EML, Knutsen B: Quinidine treatment in chronic auricular fibrillation I. Conversion to sinus rhythm, related to quinidine serum concentration. Acta Med Scand 1956; 156:1–14.
68. Bailey DJ: Cardiotoxic effects of quinidine and their treatment. Arch Intern Med 1960; 105:13–22.
69. Kalmansohn RW, Sampson JJ: Studies of plasma quinidine content in relation to single dose administration, toxic manifestations and therapeutic effect. Am J Med 1949; 6:393–394.
70. Ditlefsen EML: Concentrations of quinidine in blood following oral, parenteral and rectal administration. Acta Med Scand 1953; 146:81–92.
71. Halkin H, Vered Z, Millman P, Rabinowitz B, Neufeld HN: Steady-state serum quinidine concentration: role in prophylactic therapy following acute myocardial infarction. Isr J Med Sci 1979; 15:583–587.
72. Hepburn J, Kykert HE: Use of quinidine sulfate intravenously in ventricular tachycardia. Am Heart J 1937; 14:620–623.
73. Chapman DW: Observations on two patients with paroxysmal ventricular tachycardia treated by the intravenous administration of quinidine lactate. Am Heart J 1945; 30:276–283.
74. Armbrust CA, Levine S: Paroxysmal ventricular tachycardia: A study of 107 cases. Circulation 1950; 1:28–40.

75. Acierno LJ, Gubner R: Utility and limitations of intravenous quinidine in arrhythmias. Am Heart J 1951; 41:733–741.
76. Griggs DE, Stevens HG, Hadley GG: Therapeutic use of quinidine. Med Clin N Am 1952; 26:1025–1034.
77. Udenfriend S: *Fluorescence Assay in Biology and Medicine.* New York: Academic Press, 1962.
78. Edgar AL, Sokolow M: Experiences with the photofluorometric determination of quinidine in blood. J Lab Clin Med 1950; 36:478–484.
79. Gelfman N, Seligson D: Quinidine. Am J Clin Path 1961; 36:390–392.
80. Hartel G, Korhonen A: Thin-layer chromatography for the quantitative separation of quinidine and quinidine metabolites from biological fluids and tissues. J Chromatogr 1968; 37:70–75.
81. Hartel G, Harjanne A: Comparison of two methods for quinidine determination and chromatographic analysis of the difference. Clin Chim Acta 1969; 23:289–294.
82. Byrne-Quinn E, Wing AJ: Maintenance of sinus rhythm after DC reversion of atrial fibrillation: A double-blind controlled trial of long-acting quinidine bisulphate. Br Heart J 1970; 32:370–376.
83. Ueda CT, Ballard BE, Rowland M: Concentration-time effects on quinidine disposition kinetics in rhesus monkeys. J Pharmacol Exp Ther 1977; 200:459–468.
84. Brodie BB, Udenfriend S, Dill W, Downing G: The estimation of basic organic compounds in biological material II. Estimation of fluorescent compounds. J Biol Chem 1947; 168:311–318.
85. Brodie BB, Udenfriend S, Baer JE: The estimation of basic organic compounds in biological material I. General principles. J Biol Chem 1947; 168:299–309.
86. Archer HE, Weitzman D, Kay HL: Control of quinidine dosage. Br Heart J 1955; 17:534–540.
87. Abramson FP, Yago KB, Feuillan P: Observations on methods of assaying, and the value of monitoring plasma quinidine concentrations. Res Commun Chem Path Pharmacol 1979; 23:631–634.
88. Armand J, Badinand A: Dosage de la quinidine (ou de la quinine) dans les milieux biologiques. Ann Biol Clin 1972; 30:599–604.
89. Josephson ES, Udenfriend S, Brodie BB: The estimation of basic organic compounds in biological material VI. Estimation by ultraviolet spectrophotometry. J Biol Chem 1947; 168:341–344.
90. Brodie BB, Udenfriend S: The estimation of basic organic compounds and a technique for the appraisal of specificity: Application to the cinchona alkaloids. J Biol Chem 1945; 158:705–714.
91. Midha KK, Charette C: GLC determination of quinidine from plasma and whole blood. J Pharm Sci 1974; 63:1244–1247.
92. Valentine JL, Driscoll P, Hamburg EL, Thompson ED: GLC determination of quinidines in human plasma. J Pharm Sci 1976; 65:96–98.
93. Moulin MA, Kinsun H: A gas-liquid chromatographic method for the quantitative determination of quinidine in blood. Clin Chim Acta 1977; 75:491–495.
94. Drayer DE, Restivo K, Reidenberg MM: Specific determination of quinidine and (3S)-3-hydroxyquinidine in human serum by high-pressure liquid chromatography. J Lab Clin Med 1977; 90:816–822.
95. Crouthamel WG, Kowarski B, Narang PK: Specific serum quinidine assay by high-performance liquid chromatography. Clin Chem 1977; 23:2030–2033.
96. Achari RG, Baldridge JL, Koziol TR, Yu L: Rapid determination of quinidine in human plasma by high-performance liquid chromatography. J Chomatogr Sci 1978; 16:271–273.
97. Powers JL, Sadee W: Determination of quinidine by high-performance liquid chromatography. Clin Chem 1978; 24:299–302.

98. Peat MA, Jennison TA: High-performance liquid chromatography of quinidine in plasma, with use of a microparticulate silica column. Clin Chem 1978; 24:2166–2168.

99. Sved S, McGilveray IJ, Beaudoin N: The estimation of quinidine in human plasma by ion pair extraction and high-performance liquid chromatography. J Chromatogr 1978; 145:437–444.

100. Kates RE, McKennon DW, Comstock TJ: Rapid high-pressure liquid chromatographic determination of quinidine and dihydroquinidine in plasma samples. J Pharm Sci 1978; 67:269–270.

101. Bonora MR, Guentert TW, Upton RA, Riegelman S: Determination of quinidine and metabolites in urine by reverse-phase high-pressure liquid chromatography. Clin Chim Acta 1979; 91:277–284.

102. Kline BJ, Turner VA, Barr WH: Determination of quinidine and dihydroquinidine in plasma by high performance liquid chromatography. Anal Chem 1979; 51:449–451.

103. Weidner N, Ladenson JH, Larson L, Kessler G, McDonald JM: A high-pressure liquid chromatography method for serum quinidine and (3S)-3-hydroxyquinidine. Clin Chem Acta 1979; 91:7–13.

104. Steyn JM, Hundt HKL: A thin-layer chromatographic method for the quantitative determination of quinidine in human serum. J Chromatogr 1975; 111:463–465.

105. Christiansen J: Quantitative *in situ* thin-layer chromatography of quinidine and salicylic acid in capillary blood. J Chromatogr 1976; 123:57–63.

106. Wesley-Hadzija B, Mattocks AM: Specific thin-layer chromatographic method for the determination of quinidine in biological fluids. J Chromatogr 1977; 144:223–230.

107. Weiss S, Hatcher RA: III. Studies on quinidine: J Pharmacol Exp Ther 1927; 30:335–345.

108. Kyker GC, Webb BD, Andrews JC: The estimation of small amounts of quinine in blood and other biological materials. J Biol Chem 1941; 139:551–567.

109. Garland WA, Trager WF: Direct (non-chromatographic) quantification of drugs and their metabolites from human plasma utilizing chemical ionization mass spectrometry and stable isotope labeling: Quinidine and lidocaine. Biomed Mass Spec 1974; 1:124–129.

110. Syva: Emit^R-cad^R: for in vitro diagnostic use: for use in the quantitative enzyme immunoassay of quinidine in serum or plasma. Product information booklet. Palo Alto, CA: Syva, 1979.

111. Lewis T: The value of quinidine in cases of auricular fibrillation and methods of studying the clinical reaction. Am J Med Sci 1922; 163:781–794.

112. Lewis T, Drury AN, Wedd AM, Iliescu CC: Observations upon the action of certain drugs upon fibrillation of the auricles. Heart 1922; 9:207–267.

113. Alexander F, Gold H, Katz LN, Levy RL, Scott R, White PD: The relative value of synthetic quinidine, dihydroquinidine, commercial quinidine, and quinine in the control of cardiac arrhythmias. J Pharmacol Exp Ther 1947; 90:191–201.

114. Model W, Shane SJ, Dayrit C, Gold H: Relative potencies of various cinchona alkaloids in patients with auricular fibrillation. Fed Proc 1949; 8:320–321.

115. Ueda CT, Williamson BJ, Dzindzio BS: Disposition kinetics of dihydroquinidine following quinidine administration. Res Commun Chem Path Pharmacol 1976; 14:215–225.

116. Ueda CT, Dzindzio BS: Pharmacokinetics of dihydroquinidine in congestive heart failure patients after intravenous quinidine administration. Eur J Clin Pharmacol 1979; 16:101–105.

# 14

# Propranolol

Philip A. Routledge, M.D.
David G. Shand, M.B., Ph.D.

## INTRODUCTION/BACKGROUND

Since its discovery in 1964, propranolol has been widely used in therapeutics despite the subsequent introduction of several other beta-adrenergic blocking drugs. With the exception of metoprolol (which is now available for use in hypertension), it is presently the only beta-blocker available for prescription in the United States.

Propranolol as prescribed is a racemic mixture of equal parts of d- and l-isomers. The d-isomer does not possess beta-blocking activity, although it does share with the l-isomer some non-specific properties such as membrane stabilizing action. In the following discussion, unless otherwise specified, we will refer to the properties of the racemic mixture since the drug is both administered and measured in body fluids in this form.

### Absorption

Propranolol absorption is normally rapid and complete (1). The mean time to attainment of peak concentrations is approximately 2 hours (healthy fasting individuals) (1,2,3,4,5). Peak plasma concentrations may be achieved more rapidly in hyperthyroid patients and those with coeliac or Crohn's disease, and more slowly in hypothyroid patients (6,7). Food does not appear to affect the time taken to achieve peak concentrations after oral administration and the half-life of gastric emptying does not correlate with this time (8,9).

As with many other drugs which are avidly extracted by the liver, bioavailability is less than 100%, despite complete absorption from the gut. It is also dose-dependent, being lower at small doses. After a single 80 mg oral dose, bioavailability was 22% in six healthy volunteers but rose to 35% after continuous administration of 80 mg t.i.d.

for seven doses (10). It has been reported that concomitant administration of food increases the bioavailability of orally administered propranolol (8) although other workers have been unable to confirm this observation (11,12).

## Distribution

Propranolol is a lipophilic, basic compound (pk = 10.42) which is widely distributed throughout the body. The calculated volume of distribution of roughly 300 liters indicates that some tissues may have higher concentration of the drug than the corresponding blood concentration. Indeed, very high concentrations of propranolol have been shown in human brain at post-mortem (13) as well as in the lungs, liver, kidneys, heart and brains of animals (13,14). Propranolol is distributed within physiological fluids such as breast milk (15) and cerebrospinal fluid (16). However, the concentrations seen in breast milk are insufficient to expose breast-fed infants to therapeutic quantities of the drug (17). At physiological temperature (37°C) propranolol is bound to the extent of approximately 80 to 90% in human plasma. Since binding to human serum albumin solution (4.5 gm/dl) is only about 44% at therapeutic concentrations (18), other proteins are involved in the plasma binding of this drug. Alpha-1-acid glycoprotein, a constituent of normal plasma, has recently been shown to directly bind propranolol in plasma (19). Variation in the concentration of this protein is probably responsible for much of the variation in plasma propranolol binding (20,21) in health and disease. Lipoproteins appear to be a minor site of propranolol binding and this phenomenon is likely to be due to partitioning rather than to formation of a drug-protein complex (21).

The distribution of propranolol into tissues is determined partly by the extent of plasma protein binding, and the two are negatively correlated even over the normal range of distribution volume (22). Uptake of propranolol by red cells also appears to be determined principally by the degree of plasma protein binding, indicating that the affinity of red cells for propranolol is relatively constant (23).

## Metabolism and Excretion

One of the first studies of propranolol metabolism in man indicated that propranolol was essentially completely eliminated by metabolism, only 1 to 4% of a single radiolabelled dose being excreted as parent drug in the urine and feces (1). After repeated oral doses, unchanged propranolol accounts for 0.15 to 1.5% of the total elimination (24) which appears to be confined to the liver (25) and involves the cytochrome P450 system. The four major pathways described to date are o-dealkylation, side chain oxidation, glucuronic acid conjugation and ring oxidation.

The ring-hydroxylated metabolite, 4-OH propranolol, appears to have β-adrenoreceptor blocking potency equal to the parent compound (26). It is found in plasma only after oral administration (1) and is said to be present in concentrations equal to unchanged propranolol at or below oral doses of 160 mg daily (27). At larger doses, the ratio of 4-OH propranolol to propranolol decreases rapidly. Saturation of this pathway occurs even at small doses, and probably contributes to the non-linear bioavailability of parent drug with increasing oral propranolol dose. Other ring hydroxylated metabolites have been identified in plasma and urine, mainly as glucuronic and sulphate conjugates, and although they may also be products of other active metabolites, their biological significance is presently unknown (28). o-Dealkylation and side chain oxidation produce several other metabolites, of which one, naphthoxylactic acid, accounted for 20% of total urinary metabolites after oral administration of a single intravenous dose (1,29) and 40% of total urinary metabolites after a single intravenous dose (1).

Propranolol is also conjugated with glucuronic acid (24,27). Although plasma propranolol glucuronide concentrations are also non-linearly related to propranolol dose, they are linearly related to plasma propranolol concentrations. The plasma propranolol glucuronide concentration is approximately six times greater than the concentration of parent drug at doses of oral propranolol between 40 and 320 mg daily. Propranolol glucuronide accounts for 2.5 to 25% of the total urine recovery of metabolites (24).

Both 4-OH propranolol and its glucuronide conjugate are also excreted in the urine. The percentage of administered propranolol excreted as the 4-OH metabolite decreases with increasing propranolol dose, from approximately 8.5% after 20 mg, to 4% after 360 mg as a single oral dose (29).

Other metabolites, e.g., propranolol glycol, N-deisopropylpropranolol and naphthoxyacetic acid together account for less than 1.5% of the urinary recovery of metabolites after single oral propranolol doses ranging from 20 to 360 mg (29). Since total recovery of propranolol metabolites in this study was less than 45%, major urinary metabolite(s) of propranolol still remain unidentified (29).

Propranolol is rapidly eliminated from plasma and concentrations after intravenous administration can be described with a two-compartment open model. The terminal half-life ($t\frac{1}{2}_\beta$) is approximately 2 hours (30,31). Plasma clearance is therefore approximately 0.8 liters/minute (whole blood clearance approximately 1.0 liter/min). After oral administration $t\frac{1}{2}_\beta$, is approximately 4 hours and apparent oral blood clearance, because of the marked presystemic effect, is 5.3 liters/min (10), after a single dose (Figure 1).

The apparent half-life of the active metabolite 4-OH propranolol was 3 hours at steady-state in 23 patients receiving oral propranolol in doses ranging from 40 to 960 mg daily. This was reported to be identical with the half-life of the parent compound in these same individuals (27).

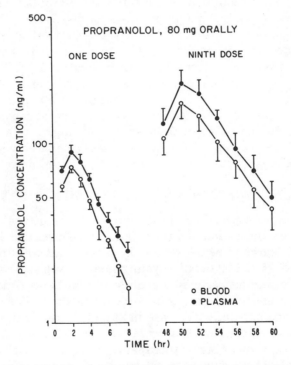

FIGURE 1. Blood and plasma propranolol concentrations following the oral administration of a single 80 mg dose and following the ninth dose during chronic administration of 80 mg every 6 hours. Each point represents the mean ± SE in six subjects (From Evans and Shand: Clin Pharmacol Ther 1973; 14: 487–493, with permission).

**Effects of Disease, Age, and Other Drugs**

Marked changes in propranolol disposition occur in a variety of diseases (Tables 1 and 2). In cirrhosis, reduced intrinsic clearance and/or mesenteric shunting are accompanied by decreased plasma binding (32). In patients with chronic renal failure, intrinsic clearance is diminished in those patients not receiving regular hemodialysis (33). The situation in thyroid disease is less clear although systemic clearance may be increased in hyperthyroid patients (34). Intrinsic clearance of propranolol may also be diminished in poorly nourished patients (35).

Factors other than disease may also alter the pharmacokinetics of propranolol. The elderly have diminished intrinsic and systemic clearances of propranolol (5,36,37). Smoking may also increase the intrinsic clearance of propranolol although it is possible that this effect is attenuated in older subjects (37). Finally the administration of other drugs may cause alterations in propranolol disposition. The lipolytic agent halofenate appeared to cause a significant fall in plasma propranolol concentration associated with a decrease in beta-blockade (38). In contrast, the concomitant administration of chlorpromazine was associated with an increase in plasma propranolol concentrations, probably due to a fall in intrinsic clearance (39). Increased blood propranolol concentration associated with decreased sensitivity to isoproterenol was noted when propranolol (40 mg) was administered orally together with oral furosemide (25 mg) compared with propranolol alone. The mechanism of this interaction is unknown (40).

## CONCENTRATION VERSUS RESPONSE AND TOXICITY

Despite its wide use, little is known of the relationship between propranolol concentration and therapeutic response. It is known that a very high degree of beta-blockade is obtained at total plasma concentrations of 75 to 100 ng/ml in young healthy subjects (41) and that patients with angina pectoris appear to obtain benefit at concentrations which produce a degree of beta-blockade above 65% of the maximum (42). The maximum decrease in essential tremor in six patients also occured at plasma levels at or below about 100 ng/ml (43,44). In other diseases, a meaningful therapeutic range has not yet been established. It has been suggested, for example, that some patients with ventricular arrythmias (45) or low renin hypertension (46) may require plasma concentrations greater than those necessary to produce maximum beta-blockade (i.e., approximately 100 ng/ml). In some of the patients studied by Woosley and co-workers, however, ventricular

## TABLE 1. FACTORS WHICH MAY INCREASE PLASMA PROPRANOLOL CONCENTRATIONS

|  | Probable Mechanism | Reference(s) |
|---|---|---|
| Chronic oral dosing | Decreased intrinsic clearance | 10 |
| Increasing age | Decreased hepatic intrinsic clearance (orally administered drug). Reduced liver blood flow (intravenously administered drug) | 36,37 |
| Hypothermia (during surgery) | ? Drug redistribution (? decreased tissue binding) | 89 |
| Crohn's disease | ? Drug redistribution | 90 |
| Celiac disease | ? Increased plasma protein binding | 90,91 |
| Chronic renal failure | ? Decreased hepatic intrinsic clearance | 33 |
| Chlorpromazine | Decreased hepatic intrinsic clearance | 39 |
| Furosemide | Unknown | 40 |
| Malnutrition | ? Diminished hepatic intrinsic clearance | 35 |
| Chronic cirrhosis | Diminished intrinsic hepatic clearance (and reduced liver blood flow) | 32 |

## TABLE 2. FACTORS WHICH MAY DECREASE PLASMA PROPRANOLOL CONCENTRATIONS

|  | Mechanism | Reference(s) |
|---|---|---|
| Hyperthyroidism | Increased systemic clearance (? increased liver blood flow) | 34 |
| Smoking | Increased hepatic intrinsic clearance | 37 |
| Halofenate | ? Increased hepatic intrinsic clearance | 38 |
| Some commercial collecting tubes | An *in-vitro* artifact caused by redistribution of propranolol between blood and plasma secondary to reduced drug binding | 58 |

premature beats previously controlled at plasma propranolol concentrations below 100 ng/ml reappeared when plasma concentrations were raised by increasing the dose (45). It is difficult to determine whether this effect was caused by non-homogeneity of the disease classification, or variation in sensitivity at a receptor level. It has been shown that the elderly are less responsive to equivalent free plasma propranolol concentrations than younger individuals (47) and it is possible that sensitivity may also vary in different diseases.

The major adverse effects of propranolol are precipitation of cardiac failure in patients critically dependent on sympathetic drive to maintain an adequate cardiac output and precipitation of asthma in susceptible individuals. Since cardiac failure often occurs early in the course of treatment of low doses of propranolol, toxic concentrations in these subjects are those which would be considered therapeutic in other individuals. Similarly, asthma may also occur with only small propranolol doses and presumably at low plasma drug concentrations. With the exception of heart failure and bronchospasm, the therapeutic ratio is high and little dose-related toxicity occurs. Other reported adverse effects are central nervous systemic disturbances such as vivid dreams, hallucinations and occasionally psychosis, all of which appear more frequently with high doses (48). In acute poisoning with large doses of propranolol, seizures and intraventricular conduction defects have been described (49).

The contribution of the active metabolite 4-OH propranolol to the effect of propranolol is still unclear. It is known that 4-OH propranolol has beta-blocking potency equal to the parent compound in animals (26). It is present during chronic oral administration of propranolol (27). The plasma levels of 4-OH propranolol in 17 hypertensive patients receiving chronic oral therapy with propranolol were related to the plasma propranolol concentrations ($r = 0.911, p < 0.005$). The ratio of the 4-OH metabolite to parent compound was low, however, (mean 0.127, range 0.057 to 0.241) suggesting that the contribution of 4-OH propranolol to the total drug effect may be relatively small during chronic oral therapy (50).

## CLINICAL APPLICATION OF PHARMACOKINETIC DATA

### Dosing

Since orally administered propranolol is subject to a high and variable degree of presystemic extraction, plasma levels of the drug after administration of equivalent doses may vary widely (30,50,51,52). The smallest variation reported to date was threefold at steady-state at

TABLE 3. APPROXIMATE PEAK (2 HOUR) PLASMA CONCENTRATION ACHIEVED AT STEADY-STATE AT VARYING ORAL PROPRANOLOL DOSES*

| Daily oral dose of propranolol (mg), 6 hourly dosage schedule | Peak plasma propranolol concentration (ng/ml) |
|---|---|
| < 120 | <45 |
| 120 | 45 |
| 160 | 65 |
| 240 | 155 |
| 400 | 330 |
| 560 | 510 |
| 720 | 590 |
| 960 | 950 |

*Based on the data of Walle et al, 1978, ref 12.

the 40 mg dose level and decreasing linearly with dose to a 1.3-fold variation at doses greater than 600 mg daily (12), but this was much less variation than reported in the other studies (about ten-fold).

The clearance of intravenously administered propranolol, like many efficiently cleared compounds, is chiefly dependent on liver blood flow (53). Since this varies only twofold in normal subjects (30), it is not surprising that variation in clearance after intravenous administration is much smaller (1.6 to 2-fold) (54) than after oral administration. Systemic plasma clearance of propranolol also appears to be reduced in the elderly compared to young subjects (36). For these reasons, it is not possible to predict with a great degree of accuracy the plasma propranolol concentration achieved by a given oral dose of the drug although the accuracy will be greater when propranolol is given intravenously.

**Oral Administration.** The following information based on the data of Walle et al (12) will for the reasons mentioned earlier serve at best as a rough guide to the plasma concentration of propranolol obtained at steady-state at varying oral doses of propranolol up to 960 mg per day (Table 3). Although peak (2 hour) concentrations are given, it was shown that the trough concentration at a 6 hourly dosage interval was very close to 50% of the peak concentration (12).

**Intravenous Administration.** Intravenous administration is the route of choice for rapid achievement and maintenance of effective plasma propranolol concentrations. Therefore, in clinical situations where it has been practicable, intravenous infusion of propranolol has been used with success. As mentioned, this route of administration is also associated with a smaller degree of variation between subjects in plasma clearance of propranolol. Infusion has been performed both by stepwise (31) and two step infusion techniques (55,56). The latter technique is a rapid and safe method to achieve plasma concentration plateaus (57) and is to be recommended.

The final infusion rate $(I_2)$ of the two step infusion required to achieve the desired plasma propranolol concentration (C) is calculated using the relationship

$$I_2 = C \times Cl \qquad \text{(Eq. 1)}$$

where Cl is an average estimate of the systemic plasma clearance of propranolol (e.g. approximately 0.8 L/min).

The rate of initial infusion $(I_1)$ is then calculated using the relationship

$$\frac{I_1}{I_2} \simeq 0.5 + 1.443 \ (t\tfrac{1}{2}/t_i) \qquad \text{(Eq. 2)}$$

where $t\frac{1}{2}$ is the half-life of disappearance from the plasma and $t_1$ the length of time the initial infusion was administered (51). Thus for propranolol, $I_1/I_2$ is approximately 10 when the initial infusion rate is used for a period of 20 minutes. Thus, a "plateau" concentration of 37 ng/ml was achieved within minutes using an initial infusion $(I_1)$ of 385 µg/kg/min for 25 minutes followed by an infusion $(I_2)$ of 38.5 µg/kg/min (55).

**Percentage of Propranolol Unbound in Plasma.** Propranolol is only one of a small group of drugs in which the unbound plasma concentration of drug has been directly shown to correlate more closely with drug effect than the total plasma concentration (56). The percentage of propranolol unbound in plasma may vary as much as two-fold in normal individuals (22,20,21) and even more in patients with certain diseases (20); a similar variation may be seen in the unbound plasma concentration in individuals showing the same total plasma propranolol concentration. Measurement of the unbound percentage of the drug is time consuming and normally requires a radiolabelled ligand. It is therefore unsuitable for routine clinical use. Following the observation of Piafsky et al (20) that the unbound percentage of propranolol at 37°C was inversely related to the concentration of $\alpha_1$ acid glycoprotein (AAG) in plasma (r = −0.77, p < 0.001), we re-examined this relationship at a higher propranolol concentration (88 rather than 8.8 ng/ml) using plasma from 24 normal subjects and measured immediately without freezing of samples (Figure 2). The close relationship between the binding ratio (molar ratio of bound to unbound drug) of propranolol and the AAG concentration (r = 0.956, p < 0.001) indicates that over 90% of the variation in binding of

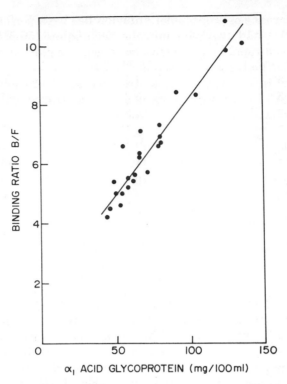

FIGURE 2.   Relationship between the binding ratio of propranolol (88 ng/ml) in plasma and AAG concentration measured by radial immunodiffusion (Behring Diagnostics).

propranolol is associated with differences in AAG concentration in plasma. A similar though weaker relationship ($r = 0.849$) was observed in 21 healthy male subjects, when binding was measured at 4°C on stored serum (21). The closeness of the relationship is such that AAG concentration may be a valuable predictor of the percentage of propranolol unbound in plasma at least in healthy individuals. Table 4 indicates the mean percentage of propranolol unbound in plasma, together with the range of values based on the 95% confidence limits of the regression line, at varying AAG concentrations. This relationship uses the equations

$$F\% = \frac{100}{(B/F) + 1}$$  (Eq. 3)

and

$$\frac{B}{F} = 0.0654\alpha + 1.7244$$  (Eq. 4)

TABLE 4. PERCENTAGE OF PROPRANOLOL UNBOUND IN PLASMA AT VARYING $\alpha_1$ ACID GLYCOPROTEIN CONCENTRATIONS*

| AAG concentration (mg/100 ml) | Mean percentage unbound (%) | Range (%) |
|---|---|---|
| 45 | 17.6 | 16.6 – 18.8 |
| 55 | 15.8 | 15.1 – 16.6 |
| 65 | 14.3 | 13.9 – 14.9 |
| 75 | 13.1 | 12.7 – 13.5 |
| 85 | 12.1 | 11.7 – 12.5 |
| 95 | 11.2 | 10.8 – 11.6 |
| 105 | 10.4 | 10.0 – 10.8 |
| 120 | 9.5 | 9.1 – 9.9 |
| 135 | 8.7 | 8.2 – 9.1 |

*See text for further details.

where F% = the percentage of propranolol unbound in plasma, $\alpha$ = the plasma AAG concentration and B/F = the binding ratio (molar ratio of bound to unbound drug) in plasma. This relationship will need further validation for the effect of disease states before being used to calculate the percentage of propranolol unbound in sick patients. Although propranolol binding appears to show little concentration dependence over the range of propranolol concentrations seen during therapy, it must also be remembered that the relationship was determined at one specific propranolol concentration (88 ng/ml).

## When to Obtain Blood Levels

Because of the marked variation between individuals in response to propranolol even at the same plasma propranolol concentration, and because of a lack of concentration-related toxicity, monitoring of plasma concentrations is of modest value except as a research tool. In two clinical situations plasma concentration monitoring may be of some value, however. If large doses are being prescribed with little apparent benefit, low plasma concentrations (< 10–20 ng/ml) will indicate poor compliance, particularly if they fail to rise at all when the dosage is further increased.

It is also likely that patients whose angina pectoris does not respond with trough plasma propranolol concentrations greater than 100 ng/ml will fail to respond to further increases in daily dosage. In other disease situations, it need only be remembered that great variability

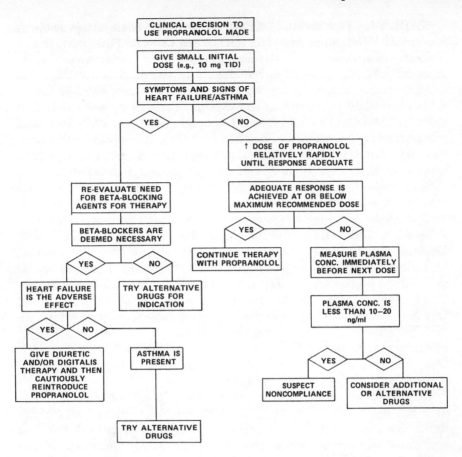

FIGURE 3. Algorithm for the clinical use of propranolol.

in dose requirements exists so that doses should be titrated against clinical endpoints such as control of hypertension or arrhythmias (Figure 3).

## ASSAY METHODS

Since collection and storage techniques may markedly affect the plasma concentrations of propranolol and 4-OH propranolol, it is necessary to discuss these methods before considering assay techniques.

### Collection and Storage of Samples

Spuriously low plasma concentrations have been observed when blood was collected into some types of commercial collecting tubes, not only with propranolol (58) but with other basic drugs such as meperidine (59), quinidine (60), and lidocaine (61). This is caused by leaching of a plasticizer with marked affinity for propranolol binding sites on AAG from the rubber stopper into the plasma (62). The displaced drug is taken up by red cells to form a new equilibrium in which less drug is present in the plasma. For this reason, we collect samples into silanized all-glass tubes or glass tubes with teflon-lined screw caps, which do not affect drug binding (unpublished observations). It has been shown that plastic syringes do not lower plasma propranolol concentrations compared with glass syringes (58).

Spuriously low plasma propranolol concentrations were also reported when blood was collected through a commercial type of "butterfly" needle although the phenomenon could not be reproduced with subsequent indwelling cannulae from the same manufacturer (58). Because of potential problems, however, we recommend that samples be collected by direct venipuncture unless the effect of the particular cannula on propranolol concentrations has been previously evaluated.

It has been shown that the injection of as little as 50 units of heparin intravenously could decrease the ability of plasma to bind added radiolabelled propranolol by approximately 30% (63). This is an indirect effect probably due to the release of non-esterified fatty acids. It is therefore important to avoid the use of heparin if repeated samples are collected through suitable cannulae.

4-OH propranolol is stable in plasma for at least one week if frozen (64) but is relatively unstable at room temperature unless antioxidants are added (65). In sera supplemented with propranolol no loss was detected after storage at room temperature for one week (66), at 4°C for four weeks (10), or at −20°C for four weeks (67).

## Assay Techniques

As with many other compounds, propranolol has a characteristic UV absorption spectrum so that quantitation may be obtained by this means (68). However, propranolol is one of a small number of drugs which has native fluorescence properties, and most of the assay methods which have been developed employ this property. When gas chromatography has been used, derivatization and subsequent electron capture detection or mass fragmentography have been used.

**Non-Chromatographic Methods.** The first and most widely used method for measurement of propranolol in blood or plasma is that of Black et al (69) as modified by Shand and coworkers (30). This method uses organic extraction from alkalinized plasma and subsequent back-extraction into acid, in which fluorescence is measured.

Further modifications have been published (70,71). The major problem with these non-chromatographic methods, however, has been the high and variable extent of background fluorescence which have even been seen in plasma from patients not receiving propranolol, despite meticulous acid washing of all glassware (51). Thus, although good correspondence was obtained between plasma propranolol levels measured both by HPLC method of Wood et al (10) and the Shand method, this was true only when the subject's plasma before propranolol therapy was available to prepare standard samples. In routine clinical samples poorer correlation was obtained between the two methods (10).

Kraml and Robinson (72) have therefore scanned the fluorescence of samples prepared by the method of Shand et al (30) using a spectrophotofluorometer. By this technique they were able to identify interference due to solvent or chemical contamination or the presence of other fluorescent materials or drugs. They also confirmed that recovery using the Shand method was good as well as reproducible and specific. Of six metabolites examined, only N-deisopropyl propranolol produced significant fluorescence under the conditions of the assay but it is unlikely to be present in biological fluids in concentrations sufficient to interfere substantially with propranolol estimations (73). By measuring fluorescence at two different wavelengths Rao and co-workers (74) claimed to be able to measure propranolol and 4-OH propranolol in the same sample.

**Chromatographic Methods.** Because of the potential problems with non-chromatographic methods, many workers have employed chromatographic techniques to separate propranolol from its metabolites and other compounds.

*Thin Layer Chromatography (TLC).* Thin layer chromatography has been combined with direct fluorescence scanning of propranolol and its metabolites on the TLC plate (75,76). With the initial method, plates were sprayed with citric acid solution to achieve maximum fluorescence and had to be scanned while still wet, a factor which may result in variation if delays occur during the measurement (Garceau and co-workers using 50/50 propylene glycol/water). Another TLC method uses direct scanning by spectrodensitometry of propranolol absorbance only on the TLC plate and was claimed to be sensitive (68). Recently, sequential thin layer chromatography has been used to measure propranolol and seven of its possible metabolites (77), but the method appears to be more useful as a method to study propranolol metabolism than for analysis of the parent compound. None of these TLC methods uses an internal standard and the time taken for development of the TLC plate and subsequent quantitations is longer than

TABLE 5. COMPARISON OF THE RELATIVE ADVANTAGES AND DISADVANTAGES OF THE VARIOUS PROPRANOLOL ASSAY METHODS*

| Analytical Method | Specificity for propranolol | Limit of sensitivity | Metabolite Analysis | Assayable Samples | | Minimum Sample Volume Required | Analysis Time | Analysis Costs | | |
|---|---|---|---|---|---|---|---|---|---|---|
| | | | | Plasma/Serum | Urine | | | Estimated Reagent and Tech. Cost Per Assay | Initial Equipment Costs | Specialized Operator Training |
| H.P.L.C. | 1 | 1 | Yes | Yes | Yes | 1 ml | 3 | 3 | 4 | 3 |
| GC | 1 | 1 | No | Yes | Yes | 1 ml | 4 | 3 | 4 | 3 |
| TLC | 1 | 2 | Yes | Yes | Yes | 1 ml | 4 | 3 | 3 | 3 |
| Fluorometer | 2 | 3 | No | Yes | Yes | 2–4 ml | 2 | 2 | 2 | 2 |
| GC (mass fragment) | 1 | 1 | Yes | Yes | Yes | 1 ml | 5 | 4 | 5 | 5 |
| Radioimmunoassay | 1 | 1 | No | Yes | No | 1 ml | 3 | 3 | 4 | 3 |
| Radioreceptor assay | 1 | 1 | No | Yes | No | 0.2 ml | 3 | 3 | 4 | 4 |

* Arbitrary Ranking Scale of 1 (Excellent) to 5 (Poor) with a score of 3 being average or nominal.

the separation and analysis times using high performance liquid chromatography.

*High Performance Liquid Chromatography (HPLC).* The first report of the use of HPLC-fluorescence detection of propranolol and 4 hydroxy propranolol (78) was followed by several other publications. This method used normal phase chromatography, as distinct from reversed phase HPLC, and therefore required much larger volumes of organic solvents. No internal standard was used and there was no back-extraction into acid (a process which often results in cleaner chromatograms). No details were given of chromatograms measuring propranolol and 4-OH propranolol in patients. The method was subsequently modified to increase sensitivity (79), but otherwise was subject to the same criticisms and was not used to measure 4-OH propranolol by these authors.

A reversed phase HPLC method for propranolol (10) with an internal standard and requiring 4 ml of plasma similarly does not contain a back-extraction step but requires the often time consuming drying down of the organic solvent under nitrogen. A more sensitive reversed phase method which also measures 4-OH propranolol and does involve back-extraction into acid unfortunately only shows a patient chromatogram after oral dosage when no 4-OH propranolol is expected to be present (80). We have been unable to satisfactorily separate 4-OH propranolol from the solvent front on the chromatogram using this method for analysis of samples of patients receiving propranolol orally.

Schneck and co-workers have developed another reversed phase HPLC method which uses pronethalol as an internal standard and measures propranolol glycol as well as propranolol and 4-OH propranolol in plasma. It has also been used to measure six metabolites in urine (29). Back-extraction is not used so that drying down of organic solvent is necessary and non-specific peaks are present on the chromatograms. The results obtained by measurement of propranolol and 4-OH propranolol in six subjects indicate that this method is relatively specific and sensitive, although 3 ml of plasma are required for analysis. The possibility of interference with the assay by other drugs was not tested.

Taburet and co-workers have combined reversed-phase HPLC with paired-ion techniques to obtain better retention on column and separation of 4-OH propranolol (61). Separate injections at different detector settings and the use of two different internal standards were necessary to measure the concentrations of the two compounds, however, and drying-down of organic solvent was also necessary. Only triamterene, quinidine, and possibly prazosin caused interference with the assay.

Finally, a reversed-phase HPLC assay which incorporates an internal standard and a back-extraction clean-up step to measure only propranolol has recently been published (81).

*Gas Chromatography (GC).* A GC method for propranolol determination using electron capture detection was shown to be sensitive and specific (82). Other methods were also devised (83,84). All of these methods are time consuming and require derivatization reactions. Walle and co-workers have combined GC with mass-fragmentography to measure propranolol and 4-OH propranolol (85), but such methods are also time consuming and require expensive equipment (mass spectrometer). Recently, GC and electron capture detection of derivatized enantiomers of propranolol have been performed (86). Although still time consuming, this method may allow accurate quantitation of propranolol enantiomers in man, which has been possible previously using radioimmunoassay techniques.

**Radioimmunoassays and Radioreceptor Assays.** A sensitive and stereospecific radioimmunoassay for propranolol has been developed (87) but the antisera are not presently widely available. An alternative approach is based upon competition between the radiolabeled β-adrenergic inhibitor [$^{125}$I] iodohydroxybenzylpindolol and propranolol for specific beta receptor sites in turkey erythrocyte membranes. This method is very sensitive (0.25 ng/ml plasma) and specific for the active l-isomer but does require an initial outlay for a relatively expensive piece of equipment, a gamma counter (88). The methods presently available for measurement of plasma propranolol are listed together with their respective advantages and disadvantages, in Table 5. We feel that HPLC combines speed and sensitivity with specificity and is the method of choice. In terms of measurement of the parent compound we have found the methods of Nation et al (80), Wood et al (10) and Taburet et al (61) to give satisfactory results but have had no personal experience using the other methods.

## REFERENCES

1. Paterson JW, Conolly ME, Dollery CT, Hayes A and Cooper RG: The pharmacodynamics and metabolism of propranolol in man. Pharmacologia Clinica 1970; 2:127–133.
2. Lowenthal DT, Briggs WA, Gibson TP, Nelson H and Cirksena WJ: Pharmacokinetics of oral propranolol in chronic renal disease. Clin Pharmacol Therap 1974; 16:761–769.
3. Parsons RL, Kaye CM, Raymond K, Trounce JR and Turner P: Absorption of propranolol and practolol in coeliac disease. Gut 1976; 17:139–143.
4. Shand DG and Rangno RE: The disposition of propranolol. I. Elimination during oral absorption in man. Pharmacology 1972; 7:159–168.

5. Castleden CM, Kaye CM and Parsons RL: The effect of age on plasma levels of propranolol and practolol in man. Br J Clin Pharmacol 1975; 2:303–306.
6. Bell JM, Russell CJ, Nelson JK, Kelly JG and McDevitt DG: Studies of the effect of thyroid dysfunction on the elimination of β-adrenoceptor blocking drugs. Br J Clin Pharmacol 1977; 4:79–81.
7. Schneider RE, Babb J, Bishop H, Mitchard M and Hoare AM: Plasma levels of propranolol in treated patients with coeliac disease and patients with Crohn's disease. Br Med J 1977; 2:794–795.
8. Melander A, Danielson K, Schersten B and Wahlin E: Enhancement of the bioavailability of propranolol and metoprolol by food. Clin Pharmacol Ther 1977; 22:108–112.
9. Castleden CM, George CF, and Short MD: Contribution of individual differences in gastric emptying to variability in plasma propranolol concentrations. Br J Clin Pharmacol 1978; 5:121–122.
10. Wood AJJ, Carr K, Vestal RE, Belcher S, Wilkinson GR and Shand DG: Direct measurement of propranolol bioavailability during accumulation to steady-state. Br J Clin Pharmacol 1978; 6:345–350.
11. Vervloet E, Takx-kohlen BCMJ, Pluym BFM and Merkus FWHM: Blood/plasma concentration ratio of propranolol. Clin Pharmacol Ther 1978; 23:133.
12. Walle T, Conradi EC, Walle K, Fagan TC and Gaffney TE: The predictable relationship between plasma levels and dose during chronic propranolol therapy. Clin Pharmacol Ther 1978; 24:668–677.
13. Myers MG, Lewis PJ, Reid JL and Dollery CT: Brain concentration of propranolol in relation to hypertensive effect in the rabbit with observations on brain propranolol levels in man. J Pharmacol Exp Ther 1975; 192:327–335.
14. Hayes A, and Cooper RG: Studies on the absorption distribution and excretion of propranolol in various species. J Pharmacol Exp Ther 1971; 176:302–311.
15. Karlsberg B, Lundberg D and Aberg H: Excretion of propranolol in human breast milk. Acta Pharmacol Toxicol 1974; 34:222–223.
16. Taylor EA, Carrol D and Turner P: CSF/Plasma ratios of propranolol in man. Br J Clin Pharmacol 1978; 6:447.
17. Bauer JH, Pape B, Zajicek J and Groshong T: Propranolol in human plasma and breast milk. Am J Cardiol 1979; 43:860–862.
18. Barber HE, Hawksworth GM, Kitteringham NR, Petersen J, Petrie JC and Swann JM: Protein binding of atenolol and propranolol to human serum albumin and in human plasma. Br J Clin Pharmacol 1978; 446–447.
19. Scott BJ, Bradwell AR, Schneider RE and Bishop H: Propranolol binding to serum orosomucoid. Lancet 1979; 1:930.
20. Piafsky KM, Borga O, Odar-Cederlof I, Johnasson C and Sjoqvist F: Increased plasma protein binding of propranolol and chlorpromazine mediated by disease-induced elevations of plasma $\alpha_1$ acid glycoprotein. New Engl J Med 1978; 299:1435–1439.
21. Sager G, Nilsen OG, and Jacobsen S: Variable binding of propronolol in human serum. Biochem Pharmacol 1979; 28:905–911.
22. Evans GH, Nies AS and Shand DG: The disposition of propranolol. iii) Decreased half-life and volume of distribution as a result of plasma binding in man, monkey, dog and rat. J Pharmacol Exp Ther 1973; 186:114–122.
23. Jellet LB and Shand DG: Uptake of propranolol by washed human red cells. Pharmacologist 1973; 15:245.
24. Walle T, Conradi EC, Walle K and Gaffney TE: Steady-state plasma concentrations and urinary excretion of propranolol-o-glucuronide and propranolol in patients during chronic oral propranolol therapy. Fed Proceed 1976; 35:665.

25. Pessayre D, Lebrec D, Descatoire V, Peignoux M and Benhamou J: Mechanism for reduced drug clearance in patients with cirrhosis. Gastroenterology 1978; 74:566–571.

26. Fitzgerald JD and O'Donnell SR: Pharmacology of 4-hydroxy propranolol, a metabolite of propranolol. Br J Pharmacol 1971; 43:222–235.

27. Walle T, Conradi E, Walle K, Fagan T and Gaffney TE: Steady state kinetics of the active propranolol metabolite 4-hydroxypropranolol and its glucuronic acid conjugate in patients with hypertension and coronary artery disease. Clin Res 1977; 25:10A.

28. Walle T, Conradi EC, Walle K and Gaffney TE: O-methylated catechol-like metabolites of propranolol in man. Drug Metab Dispos 1978; 6:481–487.

29. Schneck DW, Pritchard JF and Hayes AH: Measurement propranolol, 4-hydroxypropranolol and propranolol glycol in human plasma. Res Comm Chem Path Pharmacol 1979; 24:3–12.

30. Shand DG, Nuckolls EM and Oates JA: Plasma propranolol levels in adults, with observations in four children. Clin Pharmacol Therap 1970; 11:112–120.

31. McAllister RG: Intravenous propranolol administration: A method for rapidly achieving and sustaining desired plasma levels. Clin Pharmacol Ther 1976; 20:517–523.

32. Wood AJJ, Kornhauser DM, Wilkinson GR, Shand DG and Branch RA: The influence of cirrhosis on steady-state blood concentrations of unbound propranolol after oral administration. Clin Pharmacokinet 1978; 3:478–487.

33. Bianchetti G, Graziani G, Brancaccio D, Morganti A, Leonetti G, Manfrin M, Sega R, Gomeni R, Ponticelli C and Morselli PL: Pharmacokinetics and effects of propranolol in terminal uremic patients and in patients undergoing regular dialysis treatment. Clin Pharmacokinet 1976; 1:373–384.

34. Rubenfeld S, Silverman VE, Welch KMA, Mallette LE, and Kohler PO: Variable plasma propranolol levels in thyrotoxicosis. New Engl J Med 1979; 300:353–354.

35. Obel ADK and Vere DW: Antipyrine and propranolol disposition in malnutrition. East Afr Med Jr 1978; 55:20–24.

36. Castleden CM and George CF: The effect of aging on the hepatic clearance of propranolol. Br J Clin Pharmacol 1979; 7:49–54.

37. Vestal RE, Wodd AJJ, Branch RA, Shand DG and Wilkinson GR: The effects of aging and cigarette smoking on propranolol's disposition in man. Clin Pharmacol Ther 1979; 18:8–15.

38. Huffman DH, Azarnoff DL, Shoeman DW and DuJovne CA: The interaction between halofenate and propranolol. Clin Pharmacol Ther 1976; 19:807–812.

39. Vestal RE, Kornhauser DM, Hollifield JW and Shand DG: Inhibition of propranolol metabolism by chlorpromazine. Clin Pharmacol Ther 1979; 25:19–24.

40. Chiariello M, Volpe M, Rengo F, Trimarco B, Violini R, Ricciardelli B and Condorelli M: Effect of furosemide on plasma concentration and β-blockade by propranolol. Clin Pharmacol Ther 1979; 26:433–436.

41. Coltart DJ and Shand DG: Plasma propranolol levels in the quantitative assessment of beta-adrenergic blockade in man. Br Med J 1970; 3:731–735.

42. Pine M, Favrot L, Smith S, McDonald K and Chidsey CA: Correlation of plasma propranolol concentration with therapeutic response in patients with angina pectoris. Circ 1975; 52:886–893.

43. McAllister RG, Markesbery WR, Ware RW and Howell SM: Suppression of essential tremor by propranolol: Correlation of effect with drug plasma levels and intensity of beta-adrenergic blockade. Annals of Neurology 1977; 1:160–166.

44. Jefferson D, Jenner P and Marsden CD: Relationship between plasma propranolol concentration and relief of essential tremor. J Neurol Neurosurg Psychiatr 1979; 42:831–837.
45. Woosley RL, Shand DG and Kornhauser DM: Suppression of chronic ventricular arrythmias with propranolol. Circ 1979; 60:819–824.
46. Hollifield JW, Sherman K, Zwagg RV and Shand DG: Proposed mechanisms of propranolol's antihypertensive effect in essential hypertension. New Engl J Med 1976; 295:68–73.
47. Vestal RE, Wood AJJ and Shand DG: Reduced β-adrenoceptor sensitivity in the elderly. Clin Pharmacol Ther 1979; 26:181–186.
48. Peters NL, Anderson KC, Reid PR and Taylor GJ: Acute mental status changes caused by propranolol. Johns Hopkins Medical Journal 1978; 143:163–164.
49. Buiumsohn A, Eisenberg ES, Jacob H, Rosen N, Bock J and Frishman WH: Seizures and intraventricular conduction defect in propranolol poisoning—report of 2 cases. Ann Intern Med 1979; 91:860.
50. Wong GL, Nation RL, Chiou RL, Win L and Mehta PK: Plasma concentrations of propranolol and 4-hydroxypropranolol during chronic oral propranolol therapy. Br J Clin Pharmacol 1979; 8:163.
51. Chidsey CA, Morselli P, Bianchetti G, Morganti A, Leonetti G and Zanchetti A: Studies of the absorption and removal of propranolol in hypertensive patients during therapy. Circ 1975; 52:313–318.
52. Vervloet E, Pluym BFM, Cilissen J, Kohlen K and Merkus FWHM: Propranolol serum levels during twenty four hours. Clin Pharmacol Ther 1977; 22:853–857.
53. Routledge PA and Shand DG: Presystemic drug elimination. Ann Rev Pharmacol Toxicol 1979; 19:447–468.
54. Evans GH and Shand DG: Disposition of propranolol. v. Drug accumulation and steady-state concentrations during chronic oral administration in man. Clin Pharmacol Ther 1973; 14:487–493.
55. Woosley RL and Shand DG: Pharmacokinetics of antiarrhythmic drugs. Am J Cardiol 1978; 41:986–995.
56. McDevitt, Frish-Holmberg M, Hollifield JW and Shand DG: Plasma binding and the affinity of propranolol for a beta-receptor in man. Clin Pharmacol Ther 1976; 20:152–157.
57. Wagner JG: A safe method for rapidly achieving plasma concentrations plateaus. Clin Pharmacol Ther 1974; 16:691–700.
58. Cotham RH and Shand DG: Spuriously low plasma propranolol concentrations resulting from blood collection methods. Clin Pharmacol Ther 1975; 18:535–538.
59. Wilkinson GR and Schenker S: Pharmacokinetics of meperidine in man. Clin Pharmacol Ther 1976; 20:120.
60. Fremstad D: Reduced binding of quinidine in plasma from Vacutainers. Clin Pharmacol Ther 1976; 20:120 (correspondence).
61. Stargel WW, Roe CR, Routledge PA and Shand DG: Importance of blood collection tubes in plasma lidocaine determinations. Clin Chem 1979; 25:617–619.
62. Borga O, Piafsky KM and Nilsen OG: Plasma protein binding of basic drugs. I. Selective displacement from $\alpha_1$-acid glycoprotein by tris (2 butoyethyl) phosphate. Clin Pharmacol Ther 1977; 22:539–544.
63. Wood M, Shand DG and Wood AJJ: Altered drug binding due to the use of indwelling heparinised canulae (heparin-lock) for sampling. Clin Pharmacol Therap 1979; 25:103–107.

64. Walle T, Morrison J, Walle K and Conradi E: Simultaneous determination of propranolol and 4-hydroxypropranolol in plasma by mass fragmentography. J Chromatogr 1975; 114:351–359.
65. Pritchard JF, Schneck DW and Hayes AH Jr: Determination of propranolol and six metabolites in human urine by high pressure liquid chromatography. J Chromatogr 1979; 162:47–58.
66. Kraml M and Robinson WT: Fluorimetry of propranolol and its glucuronide: applicability, specificity and limitations. Clin Chem 1978; 24:169–171.
67. Taburet A, Taylor AA, Mitchell JR, Rollins DE and Pool JL: Plasma concentrations of propranolol and 4-hydroxy propranolol in man measured by high pressure liquid chromatography. Life Sci 1979; 24:209–218.
68. Hadzijza BW and Mattocks AM: Quantitative TLC determination of propranolol in human plasma. J Pharm Sci 1978; 67:1307–1309.
69. Black JW, Duncan WAM and Shanks RG: Comparison of some properties of pronethalol and propranolol. Br J Pharmacol 1965; 25:577–591.
70. Ambler PK, Singh BN and Lever M: A simple and rapid fluorometric method for the estimation of 1-(2-hydroxy-3-isopropylaminopropoxy)-naphthalene hydrochloride, propranolol, in blood. Clin Chim Acta 1974; 54:373–375.
71. Offerhaus L and Van der Vecht JR: Improved fluorimetric assay of plasma propranolol. Br J Clin Pharmacol 1976; 3:1061–1064.
72. Kraml M and Robinson WT: Fluorimetry of propranolol and its glucuronide: applicability, specificity and limitations. Clin Chem 1978; 24:169–171.
73. Walle T and Gaffney TE: Propranolol metabolism in man and dog: Mass spectrometric identification of six new metabolites. J Pharmacol Exp Ther 1972; 182:83–92.
74. Rao PS, Quesada LC and Mueller HS: A simple micromethod for simultaneous determination of plasma propranolol and 4-hydroxypropranolol. Clin Chim Acta 1978; 88:355–361.
75. Schafer M, Geissler HE and Mutschler E: Fluorimetrische Bestimmung von propranolol und seines metabliten n-desisipropylpropranolol in plasma and urin durch direkte auswertung von dünnschichtchromatogrammen. J Chromatogr 1977; 143:607–613.
76. Garceau Y, Davis I and Hasegawa: Fluorometric TLC determination of free and conjugated propranolol, naphthoxylactic acid and p-hydroxy-propranolol in human plasma and urine. J Pharm Sci 1978; 67:826–831.
77. Abou-Donia MB, Bakry NM and Strauss HC: Sequential thin-layer chromatography of propranolol. J Chromatogr 1979; 172:463–467.
78. Mason WD, Amick EN and Weddle OH: Rapid determination of propranolol and 4-hydroxy-propranolol in plasma by high pressure liquid chromatography. Analytical Letters 1977; 10:515–521.
79. Mackichan J, Psyzczynski DR and Jusko WJ: Analysis and disposition of low dose oral propranolol. Res Comm Chem Path Pharmacol 1978; 20:531–538.
80. Nation RL, Peng GW and Chiou WL: High-pressure liquid chromatographic method for the simultaneous quantitative analysis of propranolol and 4-hydroxypropranolol in plasma. J Chromatogr 1978; 145:429–436.
81. Jatlow P, Bush W and Hochster H: Improved liquid-chromatographic determination of propranolol in plasma, with fluorescence detection. Clin Chem 1979; 25:777–779.
82. DiSalle E, Baker KM and Bareggi SR: A sensitive gas chromatographic method for the determination of propranolol in human plasma. J Chromatogr 1973; 84:347–353.

83. Walle T: GLC determinations of propranolol, other β-blocking drugs and metabolites in biological fluids and tissues. J Pharm Sci 1974; 63:1885–1891.

84. Kates RE and Jones LL: Rapid GLC determination of propranolol in human plasma samples. J Pharm Sci 1977; 66:1490–1492.

85. Walle T, Morrison J, Walle K and Conradi E: Simultaneous determination of propranolol and 4-hydroxypropranolol in plasma by mass fragmentography. J Chromatogr 1975; 114:351–359.

86. Caccia S, Guiso G, Ballabio M and DePonte P: Simultaneous determination of the propranolol of enantiomers in biological samples by gas-liquid chromatography. J Chromatog 1979; 172:457–462.

87. Kawashima K, Levy A and Spector S: Stereospecific radioimmunoassay for propranolol isomers. J Pharmacol Exp Ther 1976; 196:517–523.

88. Bilezikian JP, Gammon DE, Rochester CL and Shand DG: A radioreceptor assay for propranolol. Clin Pharmacol Ther 1979; 26:173–180.

89. McAllister RG, Bourne DW, Tan TG, Erickson JL, Wachtel CC and Todd EP: Effects of hypothermia on propranolol kinetics. Clin Pharmacol Ther 1979; 25:1–7.

90. Schneider RE, Babb J, Bishop H, Mitchard M and Hoare AM: Plasma levels of propranolol in treated patients with coeliac disease and patients with Crohn's disease. Br Med J 1976; 2:794–795.

91. Parsons RL, Kaye CM, Raymond K, Trounce JR and Turner P: Absorption of propranolol and practolol in coeliac disease. Gut 1976; 17:139–143.

# 15

# Salicylates

Sydney H. Dromgoole, Ph.D.
Daniel E. Furst, M.D.

## INTRODUCTION/BACKGROUND

Despite the widespread use of salicylates as antipyretic, analgesic and antiinflammatory agents for over 100 years, it was only after the elucidation of the complicated pharmacokinetics of salicylates that a more rational approach to therapy could be attained.

There are many different derivatives of salicylic acid commercially available. The structures of these derivatives are shown in Figure 1. The most important ester derivative of salicylic acid is acetylsalicylic acid or aspirin. Choline salicylate is the salt of the strongly basic choline ion and salicylic acid. Because of its hygroscopic nature, it is marketed in a liquid form (Arthropan®). Choline magnesium trisalicylate (Trilisate®) is a combination of choline salicylate and magnesium salicylate. Salicylsalicylic acid (Disalcid®) is a salicylate derivative which on hydrolysis produces two molecules of salicylate. Benorylate (4-(acetamido) phenyl-2-acetoxy-benzoate) is the paracetamol (acetominophen) ester of aspirin which is absorbed and broken down to its active constituents in the gastrointestinal tract. Diflunisal (2,4-difluoro-4-hydroxy-3-biphenylcarboxylic acid) is a derivative of salicylic acid which differs from aspirin in having a difluorophenyl group and lacks the acetyl groups. It is not, however, metabolized to salicylic acid. All the other salicylate derivatives are rapidly hydrolyzed to salicylic acid. They circulate in the blood in the ionized form, salicylate.

In this chapter, the words *salicylic acid* and *salicylate* will be used interchangeably while the term *salicylates* will refer to the group of drugs that produce salicylate *in vivo* (e.g. aspirin, sodium salicylate, Trilisate®).

## Absorption

Salicylic acid and its derivatives are absorbed rapidly from the stomach and intestine by passive diffusion of undissociated molecules (1). Absorption is usually complete within 2 to 4 hours and the rate of absorption is determined more by the physical characteristics of the particular formulation than by any other feature (2–6).

Salicylates exist in many dosage forms including tablets, suppositories, powders, suspensions and parenteral preparations. In general, salicylates are taken as tablets or capsules and as such must undergo a series of consecutive steps to be absorbed. Schematically, absorption from these dosage forms can be illustrated as follows:

$$\text{Tablet, capsule} \xrightarrow{\text{disintegration}} \text{granules} \xrightarrow{\text{dissolution}} \text{solution} \xrightarrow{\text{absorption}} \text{drug in blood}$$

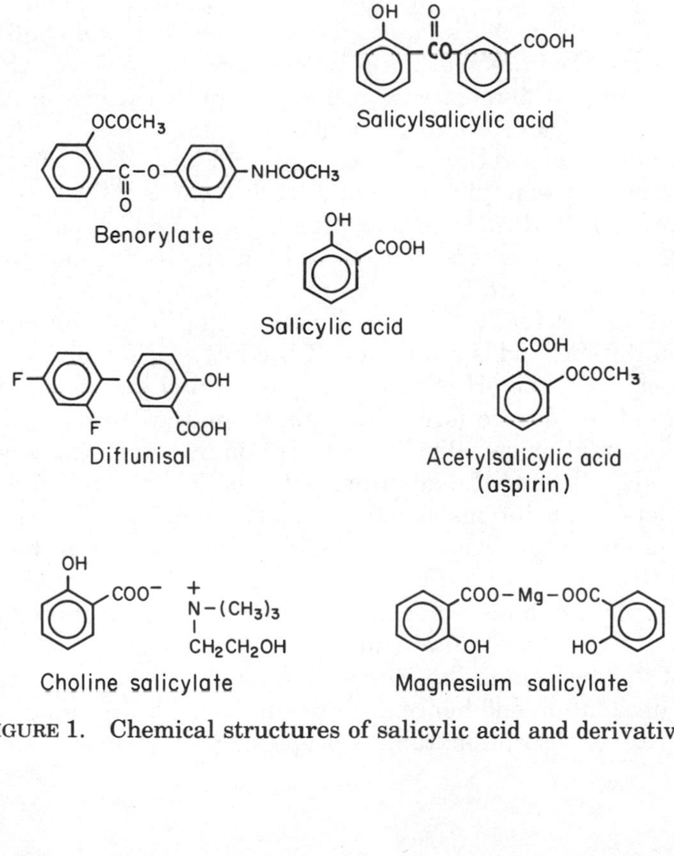

FIGURE 1.  Chemical structures of salicylic acid and derivatives.

The most desirable formulations must, therefore, achieve rapid tablet or capsule disintegration and subsequent rapid drug dissolution; however, in the formulation of drugs, ingredients or excipients are added (in addition to the active drug) to hold the tablet together during manufacture, shipping and storage. Thus, the resulting formulations depend on the balance between the ingredients that promote and those that inhibit disintegration. In addition, absorption should occur with minimal side effects at the site of absorption. Gastrointestinal intolerance to salicylates in some individuals is well documented (7–20). This problem has been reduced or eliminated by employing salicylate formulations with enteric coatings (21,22), buffers (23), suppositories (24,25), or chemically modifying the salicylate molecule (26–28). These formulations (e.g. salicylsalicylic acid) preferentially dissolve in the large surface area of the small intestine where the pH is neutral, rather than in the stomach where the pH is acidic. Optimum absorption of salicylates in the human stomach occurs in the pH range of 2.5 to 4.0 (29). This low pH of the stomach, as compared with the higher pH in the intestinal tract, favors gastric absorption of salicylates, and aspirin, salicylic acid, and choline salicylate are absorbed to some extent in the stomach. However, the small intestine is the optimum site for rapid absorption because of its much larger surface area (1). Stomach emptying time is also a critical determinant of the absorption rate of drugs, and large doses of salicylate may decrease the emptying time and lead to a decreased rate of drug absorption (30). Evidence to support this is found in patients with salicylate overdoses where there may be a significant amount of salicylates in the stomach 9 to 10 hours after an overdose (31).

Dissolution is usually the rate limiting step in the absorption of solid formulations and is a function of the intrinsic dissolution rate of the drug crystals, the pH of the environment and the physiochemical properties of the dosage form (32). Liberman and Woods studied the effect of formulation on salicylate absorption by measuring blood salicylate levels following the administration of "plain" and buffered aspirin tablets and solutions of sodium acetylsalicylate and aspirin (5). Most rapid absorption was obtained with solutions of both the sodium salt and the free acid; buffered aspirin gave a slower rise to peak levels and plain unbuffered aspirin was the slowest. Buffered aspirin formulations contain small amounts of antacids which probably raise the pH of the medium in the microenvironment of the tablet and thus increase dissolution and hence absorption. Particle size can also influence the rate of absorption; tablets prepared with 80 mesh aspirin are more rapidly absorbed than tablets made with coarser material (20 mesh). Peak salicylate levels were obtained 30 to 60 minutes after the administration of 80 mesh aspirin, while tablets made from 20 mesh aspirin produced peak salicylate levels in 2 hours (20).

The rate of absorption determines the time to peak blood levels, but it is the extent of absorption which determines the bioavailability of a drug. Strictly, bioavailability is defined as the availability of a drug at the actual site of action; however, this would require measurement of drug at a cellular level and direct measurement of bioavailability is not possible in human subjects. Instead, serum, blood or plasma concentrations are used. The chemical form of salicylate can influence its bioavailability. Levy and associates found that aluminum aspirin and aspirin anhydride were only about 80% and 60% respectively as bioavailable as aspirin itself (32,33). Cohen (34) reported that salicylsalicylic acid was only 77% as available as choline magnesium salicylate (as measured by area under the plasma salicylate-time curves). While this suggests incomplete absorption of salicylsalicylic acid, unpublished data from our laboratory indicate that absorption is complete and that the lower salicylate levels following salicylsalicylic acid administration may be caused by the formation of glucuronides of salicylsalicylic acid. Although the enteric coated formulations are more slowly absorbed than uncoated aspirin tablets, the bioavailability of the coated preparations is, in general, equivalent to uncoated (buffered or unbuffered) aspirin (21,22,35,36). However, erratic, delayed and incomplete absorption has been observed with some enteric coated formulations (37). Rectal suppositories have been used to circumvent the gastrointestinal irritation caused by oral administration of aspirin. The absorption half-life from suppositories is much longer (3 hours) than the oral absorption half-life of 15 to 30 minutes and such slow absorption may result in prolonged low subtherapeutic salicylate blood levels over the dosage interval (24). Gibaldi and Grundhofer (38) have shown that the bioavailability of aspirin from five commercially available suppositories was much less than orally administered aspirin. Four out of the five brands gave substantially slower absorption rates, with only about 20% of the aspirin being bioavailable from the suppositories. Bioavailability from suppositories increases markedly with retention time (24).

Absorption of salicylates can also be influenced by disease. Patients with coeliac disease absorb salicylates faster than normal subjects (39). It has been suggested that the difference is caused by changes in gastric emptying or altered small intestinal permeability.

## Distribution

The distribution of salicylates in the body is a reflection of the manner in which the drug is bound to albumin and equilibrates with the tissues. The protein bound salicylate molecules are pharmacologically inactive and as such cannot gain access to the sites of action or biotransformation and excretion. Only the free or unbound drug can leave the circulatory system and diffuse into the tissues. However, protein binding is reversible and the bound drug serves as a reservoir which is gradually depleted as the unbound drug is metabolized or excreted.

In general, the fraction of drug that is protein bound remains constant over the therapeutic range. However, with salicylates the amount bound to albumin decreases with increasing total salicylate concentration (40–50). At low therapeutic salicylate concentration in plasma (100 µg/ml) about 90% is bound, while at higher concentrations of salicylate (400 µg/ml), only 76% of the salicylate is bound (40). Consequently, more drug is available for distribution into the tissues and/or urinary excretion.

The binding of salicylates is also influenced by age (48,50,51) and disease (52–56). For example, low albumin concentrations in nephrotic syndrome, liver disease or protein losing enteropathy can change distribution, since less albumin is present to bind salicylate (55,56). Uremia may alter protein binding by affecting the affinity and/or number of binding sites (54). The clinical significance of the concentration-dependent protein binding of salicylates will be discussed later.

## Metabolism

Irrespective of the parent source of salicylic acid, once the drug is absorbed and rapidly hydrolyzed (in the bowel wall and liver) to salicylic acid, the metabolism and elimination is essentially that of salicylic acid. Consequently, blood and urinary concentrations of salicylic acid or salicylate are usually more meaningful than blood and urine concentrations of the parent source.

The metabolic and elimination pathways of salicylic acid are now well characterized (57–78). Salicylic acid (SA) is eliminated from the body 1) by renal excretion of salicylic acid; 2) by conjugation with glycine to form salicyluric acid (SU); 3) by conjugation with glucuronic acid to form salicyl phenolic glucuronide (SPG) and salicyl acyl glucuronide (SAG); 4) by oxidation to gentisic acid (GA); and 5) by the formation of gentisuric acid (GU) from either SU (via microsomal oxidation) or GA (via glycine conjugation).

The elimination pathways of salicylic acid involve two processes that are saturable and follow Michaelis-Menten type kinetics (SU and SPG) and three linear or first-order pathways, all acting in parallel (62,66,67). The kinetics of the minor elimination pathway of GU have not been characterized but will be assumed to be first-order for the purpose of this review. The elimination of salicylate from the body can, therefore, be described by the following differential equation:

$$\frac{dSA_{body}}{dt} = -(K_{SA} + K_{SAG} + K_{GA} + K_{GU})SA_{body} - \frac{V_{SPG}SA_{body}}{K_{M,SPG} + SA_{body}} - \frac{V_{SU}SA_{body}}{K_{M,SU} + SA_{body}}$$

(Eq. 1)

Where $K_{SA}$, $K_{SAG}$, $K_{GA}$ and $K_{GU}$ are the first-order elimination constants for SA, SAG, GA and GU. $K_{M,SPG}$ and $K_{M,SU}$ are the Michaelis constants for SPG and SU. $V_{SPG}$ and $V_{SU}$ are the theoretical maximal velocities of the formation of SPG and SU respectively. The predominant pathway for salicylic acid elimination is the conjugation with glycine and excretion as salicyluric acid. After a small dose of aspirin (300 mg or less) about 90% is excreted as salicyluric acid and SPG (73). However, after moderate doses, when the amount of salicylate in the body is more than about 600 mg, the maximum rate of formation of salicyluric acid and SPG is reached (72,73). As the capacities of these major pathways are approached, the linear pathways become more important in the elimination of salicylates. This means that the amount of salicylic acid in the body increases nonlinearly with increasing dosage. Consequently, the serum half-life of salicylate becomes longer with increasing dosage and the blood level of salicylate increases disproportionately as the salicylate dosage is increased. Thus, when the amount of salicylate increases from 250 mg (equivalent to one aspirin tablet) to 10 grams, the time required for the first 50% of the dose to be removed from the body increases from 3 to 20 hours. Recent evidence suggests that salicylate may induce its own metabolism by increasing the production of salicyluric acid (75), while evidence implicating induction of the other pathways is as yet speculative. Decreased formation of salicyluric acid has been noted in children with Down's Syndrome (77). The clinical application of various aspects of the pharmacokinetics of salicylate will be discussed later.

## Excretion

Non-protein bound or free salicylate is filtered across the renal glomerulus. Renal excretion of salicylate is the summation of glomerular filtration, active proximal tubular secretion, passive tubular secretion and passive tubular absorption (77). The excretion of salicylic acid is markedly pH dependent and as the urinary pH changes from 5 to 8, the renal clearance of free ionized salicylate increases from 2 to 3% of the amount excreted to more than 80% (78–79). This influence of urinary pH on the excretion of salicylic acid has been well known, and recent micropuncture studies in rats have indicated that the urine pH dependent enhancement of salicylate excretion appears to be due mainly to depressed reabsorption from (or enhanced excretion into) both parts of the proximal tubules and/or Henle's loop (80). Even at high pH, however, some reabsorption does occur, since the urine concentrating processes tend to increase the salicylate concentration in the tubules resulting in a concentration gradient from tubules to plasma and a passive diffusion of salicylic acid across the gradient.

There are several reports of circadian rhythms in the urinary excretion of salicylate, salicylate excretion being faster after the drug is ingested between 1900 and 2300 hours (81). This increased excretion may be in part related to the circadian changes in urinary pH (82) or the increased clearance of salicylate during bed rest or prolonged supination (83). Preliminary evidence also suggests that females excrete salicylate faster than males (84,85).

## CONCENTRATION versus RESPONSE and TOXICITY

Salicylate concentrations in the blood correlate with the pharmacological actions and adverse effects observed. Figure 2 shows the approximate relationship of plasma salicylate levels to pharmacodynamics and complications. These therapeutic plasma salicylate levels are only approximations, since the analgesic and antiinflammatory effects of salicylates (in patients) have thus far not been measured in a graded rather than an all or none manner (86). Salicylate serum levels of up to 100 µg/ml are required for effective analgesia (87); steady-state serum levels of 150 to 300 µg/ml are generally accepted as correlating with antiinflammatory effects and are, therefore, used for the treatment of rheumatoid arthritis (88). In the management of acute rheumatic fever, most authorities aim to achieve serum salicylate levels of 300 to 350 µg/ml (89). In adults, symptoms of intoxication can appear at serum salicylate levels of 300 µg/ml while higher levels are associated with more severe salicylate intoxication (90). Hoffman (91) has indicated that the toxic concentration for infants is 350 µg/ml and that marked hyperventilation may occur when the serum salicylate level is 450 µg/ml. From the above data, one can easily see that therapeutic concentrations of salicylates are frequently very close to those concentrations at which toxic manifestations may appear.

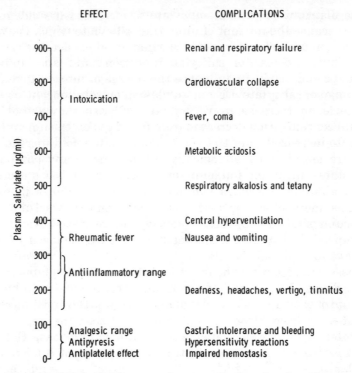

FIGURE 2.  Relationships between plasma salicylate levels, effects and complications.

Because of the unusual pharmacokinetics of salicylates, there are numerous exceptions and limitations to these therapeutic and toxic plasma concentrations. Firstly, the volume of distribution (V) increases with increasing dose. Levy et al (92) studied children who had ingested large doses of salicylate and found that the volume of distribution increased from 162 mg/kg to 345 ml/kg as the dose increased from 50 mg/kg to greater than 300 mg/kg. This change in V is an important factor to remember in the treatment of salicylate intoxication because it means that a given plasma concentration in an individual who ingests a large dose of salicylate reflects a much larger amount of drug in the body than the same plasma concentration in another individual who had taken a smaller dose of salicylate. This explains why some patients are clinically ill when overdosed, despite relatively low serum salicylate levels. One factor which contributes to the increased volume of distribution in salicylate intoxication is the pH of plasma. Studies in animals have shown that the tissue:

plasma distribution ratio of salicylate is increased in acidemia (93). This is because the amount of unionized salicylate which is available to cross membrane barriers doubles when blood pH decreases from 7.4 to 7.2. Thus, acidosis after salicylate ingestion could cause an increase in V and could markedly influence the degree of intoxication after an overdosage of salicylate. Decreased plasma protein concentrations can also cause an increase in V. Woislait (40) has shown that as the albumin concentration decreased from 5 to 2 gm/dl, the amount of free salicylate increased from 10 to 50%. This is a five-fold increase in the concentration of pharmacologically active drug. Many pathophysiological states, including inflammatory disease, can cause a decrease in plasma albumin concentrations as a result of changes in albumin synthesis, metabolism, or distribution between extravascular and intravascular sites (94,95). Consequently, the serum salicylate concentration needed to produce a therapeutic effect will be lower in subjects who have low albumin levels.

Disease can also alter the effect of diffusion of salicylates into joint spaces. Soren (96–98) studied the kinetics of salicylates in blood and joint fluid of patients and found that diffusion was the major mechanism for transport from blood to joint fluid, and that the appearance of salicylates in joints was related to the type of joint disease. Salicylates are transported from the blood stream into the joint fluid rapidly in articular diseases in which the inner part of the joint capsule is hyperemic and edematous. In contrast, salicylates diffuse much more slowly in diseases where there is hyperplasia of the synovial cover, extensive infiltrates in the subsynoviocytic tissue, and thickening of the synovial blood vessels.

The extent of drug-protein interaction can also be altered as a result of disease or drug induced conformational changes in the proteins. Reduced protein binding of salicylates in patients with renal disease has been demonstrated by Börga et al (54). The protein binding was considerably lower in uremic plasma at salicylate concentrations ranging from 14 to 1400 µg/ml. Scatchard binding plots indicated that the decreased binding was due to a marked decrease in the number and association constants of the primary set of binding sites. The decreased protein binding of salicylate in patients can, therefore, produce high unbound drug levels and cause a "potentiated" single dose pharmacological response.

Drug induced conformational changes in proteins can also affect the protein binding of drugs. The acetyl group of aspirin can become covalently attached to the lysine of albumin and cause a conformational change in the albumin tertiary structure, thus altering the latter's binding to other drugs (99–101). This acetylated albumin has a high affinity for phenylbutazone and a lower affinity for flufenamic acid (99). The full significance of this acetylation phenomenon is unknown, but it does contribute to the prolonged anti-platelet effect of aspirin. There is also some evidence to suggest that the amino-acid composition of albumin from arthritic patients is different than normals with respect to the phenylalanine and lysine residues (102). If this represents a real change in polypeptide composition (and not due to the binding of extraneous amino-acids), it is possible that the binding of anionic drugs such as salicylates may be affected (since the positively charged residues are potential binding sites on the albumin molecule).

Another area of significance is the competition for binding between salicylates and other chemicals. Aspirin is synergistic in its interaction with anticoagulants (103–107). Aspirin irreversibly acetylates platelets, interfering with all *in vitro* tests of platelet adhesiveness (103,104,106,107). Although this action of aspirin lasts the life of the platelet, other salicylates do not have the same *in vitro* effects (103). In larger doses, aspirin also affects prothrombin times and may affect bleeding times, particularly in the presence of factor VIII deficiency (103,106,107). This anticoagulant effect of aspirin can also cause increased bleeding in heparin treated patients (108).

The interactions of salicylates with other non-steroidal antiinflammatory drugs (NSAID's) is a subject of continuing dispute (109–120). In general, the area under the plasma concentration versus time curve (AUC) of NSAID's is decreased in man when the NSAID and aspirin are taken together. Thus, the AUC of naproxen is decreased by 15% (113), the AUC of fenoprofen is lessened by 46% (111), and the AUC of the active metabolite of sulindac is decreased by 25% (114). The cause of this decreased AUC is considered to be displacement of the NSAID from serum albumin and consequent increased clearance in some cases (112,113,115). However, no displacement of fenoprofen could be documented despite the decreased AUC (115), while there appeared to be increased binding of phenylbutazone to serum albumin when the albumin was pre-incubated with aspirin (117). Thus, the mechanism of the decreased AUC of fenoprofen has not been adequately explained. A pharmacokinetic study of the indomethacin-aspirin interaction demonstrated that the 20% decrease in the AUC of indomethacin during chronic aspirin therapy (1200 mg t.i.d.) was caused by suppression of the renal clearance, increased biliary clearance, decreased gastrointestinal absorption and enhancement of the enterohepatic circulation of indomethacin by aspirin. Concomitant chronic therapeutic dosages of indomethacin had no effect on salicylate accumulation with repetitive doses of aspirin (120). The clinical significance of these changes remains to be elucidated. Brooks et al observed no increase in the efficacy of aspirin when combined with indomethacin in the treatment of rheumatoid arthritis, while there was a trend toward increased toxicity (110). On the other hand, another study, although flawed, suggested some synergistic action between aspirin and naproxen (109).

The influence of corticosteroids on the elimination of salicylates is also important, since these drugs are often administered with salicylates to patients with severe rheumatoid arthritis. Corticosteroids appear to decrease the steady-state levels of salicylates during long term aspirin administration (121). Klinenberg and Miller suggested that this decrease is due to an increased renal clearance of salicylic acid, while Graham et al (122) have suggested that steroids induce the metabolism of salicylic acid, rather than increase its urinary excretion. The mode of action is, therefore, still unresolved.

## CLINICAL APPLICATION OF PHARMACOKINETIC DATA

Although the dosage regimen is the primary determinant of serum concentrations, interpatient differences in the relation between drug dosage and serum concentration are not surprising when one considers the number of different factors involved. As summarized in Figure 3, these include the bioavailability of the dosage form used, the various factors that affect absorption from the GI tract, distribution through the different compartments, and rates of metabolism and excretion. All of these determinants are subject to both individual and temporal variation due to genetic and environmental factors, consequences of disease, and concomitant administration of other drugs.

Individual variability in response to drugs is a crucial but often neglected fact of pharmacotherapeutics. Many drugs are still habitually prescribed in "usual" or "average" doses, and an inadequate dosage may be interpreted as inefficacy of the drug, while excessive dosages may be judged as intolerance. Such variability has been reported with salicylate therapy (123–127) and is in part due to the unusual and variable metabolism and elimination kinetics of salicylate. In addition, there is still considerable uncertainty among physicians concerning the optimum salicylate dosage for achievement of analgesic and/or antiinflammatory effects. For antiinflammatory effects, a reasonable and relatively conservative approach to individualized aspirin therapy is to initiate therapy with a daily aspirin dosage of 45 to 60 mg/kg, taken as 15 to 20 mg/kg every eight hours or 10 to 15 mg/kg every four hours during the day. It has been demonstrated by computer simulations (128) that there is considerable latitude with respect to the timing and size of the salicylate dose fractions, but the total daily dosage of salicylate is critical. It is, however, important to remember that because of the saturable kinetics of salicylate, steady-state will only be achieved after five to seven days and that it may be misleading to measure plasma salicylate levels prior to this time. After a week, blood samples should be obtained one to three hours after a dose for measurement of peak serum salicylate concentrations or, alternatively, just prior to the next dose of salicylate to measure the minimum drug level. Serum salicylate levels of 150 to 300 μg/ml are generally accepted as correlating with antiinflammatory effect (88).

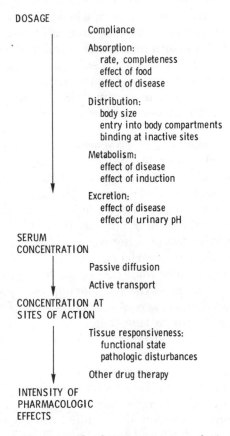

DOSAGE
　　Compliance

　　Absorption:
　　　rate, completeness
　　　effect of food
　　　effect of disease

　　Distribution:
　　　body size
　　　entry into body compartments
　　　binding at inactive sites

　　Metabolism:
　　　effect of disease
　　　effect of induction

　　Excretion:
　　　effect of disease
　　　effect of urinary pH

SERUM
CONCENTRATION
　　Passive diffusion

　　Active transport

CONCENTRATION AT
SITES OF ACTION
　　Tissue responsiveness:
　　　functional state
　　　pathologic disturbances

　　Other drug therapy

INTENSITY OF
PHARMACOLOGIC
EFFECTS

FIGURE 3.   Factors influencing the dosage-response relationship of drugs (Modified from reference 138)

Another important factor to remember for patients on chronic salicylate is that serum salicylate levels may decrease on long term therapy (129,130). This is not necessarily due to poor compliance (which has been reported in patients undergoing salicylate therapy) (131), but may be due to the induction of salicylate metabolism (75). For example, the average salicylic acid level in five normal volunteers after three weeks of 60 mg aspirin/kg/day was 48% less than that measured after seven days (129). This reinforces the fact that serum salicylate levels of patients on long term salicylate therapy should be measured occasionally to determine whether therapeutic concentrations are being maintained.

Low salicylate levels may also be observed in some patients who are receiving concomitant antacids to reduce or prevent salicylate induced dyspepsia (132–135). This is due to the alkalinizing effect of antacids on urine pH, which may result in a marked increase in the excretion of salicylic acid. Because of the easy availability of these antacids, physicians should check with patients regarding possible concomitant antacid therapy before increasing the salicylate dosage because of low serum salicylate levels. Conversely, patients whose salicylate dosage regimen has been adjusted to produce therapeutic salicylate levels while taking antacid may become intoxicated on withdrawal of the antacid.

In light of these comments, it is important to individualize salicylate dosages to the needs and tolerance of each patient; interindividual differences in metabolism and elimination kinetics are not taken into account in any standard dosage regimen. The ideal method is to titrate the dosage against a direct clinical effect. The onset of tinnitus has been used as such an indicator but has proved to be an unreliable guide in patients with pre-existing hearing loss. Mongan et al (136) noted that in 59 subjects experiencing tinnitus the serum salicylate level was invariably greater than 196 µg/ml (average, 304 µg/ml), but 15 of 22 patients with pre-existing hearing loss did not experience tinnitus, despite an average serum salicylate level of 431 µg/ml. Thus, the clinical adage, "push to tinnitus, then back off slightly" is not applicable in this group of patients. In addition, one report states that some patients on placebo reported tinnitus (137). Individualization of dosage can be achieved by monitoring serum concentrations of salicylate. However, serum salicylate levels per se should only be used in conjunction with the clinical assessment of the patient. The possibility of drug interactions (discussed above) must always be kept in mind, as must concomitant disease and patient age. Further, the dose-related and relatively complicated pharmacokinetics of the salicylates must be understood in order to obtain meaningful information from salicylate levels in serum (138).

## Therapeutic Nomogram for Salicylates

Despite interindividual differences in metabolism and elimination, an attempt has been made to use a nomogram to establish a working relationship between aspirin dosage schedules and steady-state serum salicylate levels in patients with rheumatoid arthritis (139). The nomogram was developed from the results of dose-serum salicylate level response curve in patients with rheumatoid arthritis. Thirty patients with rheumatoid arthritis (after initial screening for normal renal and hepatic function, and serum albumin levels > 3.5 gm/dl) received doses of aspirin (Ascriptin®) at fixed dose intervals for one week. The initial daily dosage of 50 mg/kg aspirin was administered in divided doses given four times a day. To minimize intersubject variation in the urinary excretion of salicylic acid, ammonium chloride or ascorbic acid was used to maintain a urine pH of 5.0 or lower during the last three days of each regimen. After five to seven days of salicylate therapy, steady-state serum salicylate levels were obtained just prior to the dose of aspirin and at 1, 2 and 3 hours after the dose, and an average steady-state serum salicylate level was obtained. These procedures were then repeated after increasing the dosage by 5 mg/kg/day for an additional five to seven days until a serum salicylate level between 200 to 300 µg/ml was attained. During this study, the administration of acetaminophen, all other non-steroidal antiinflammatory agents and corticosteroids in doses of greater than 10mg/day of prednisone (or its equivalent) were prohibited and patient compliance was monitored. A wide range of response of serum salicylate levels versus dosage was observed for all patients. Those patients who achieved serum salicylate concentration of at least 250 µg/ml at less than 55 mg/kg/day were designated Group A; Group B were those who required between 55 and 65 mg/kg/day; Group C were those who required between 65 and 118 mg/kg/day; Group D were those who required greater than 118 mg/kg/day. Least squares linear regression lines, calculated for Groups A through D are labeled I through IV respectively on Figure 4.

The applicability and reliability of the nomogram was tested prospectively to determine optimal aspirin dosage in an additional 30 patients (139). Eight patients achieved levels of 180 to 290 µg/ml with the initial 50 mg/kg dosage; 16 patients achieved salicylate levels of 185 to 280 µg/ml after the second week of therapy using doses predicted by the nomogram. Six patients failed to achieve satisfactory

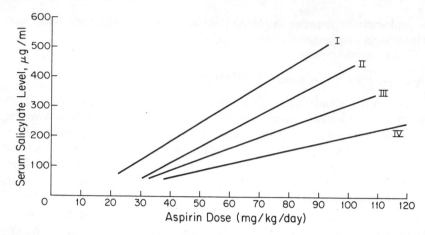

FIGURE 4. Serum salicylate level-aspirin dosage nomogram. Doses at which the nomogram lines intersect at 250 μg/ml. Line I: 50 mg/kg/day; Line II: 65 mg/kg/day; Line III: 83 mg/kg/day; Line IV: 118 mg/kg/day.

salicylate concentrations with the predicted dose, and noncompliance was suspected in these patients due to the inconsistent blood levels measured during the study period. None of the 30 patients developed toxic levels of salicylate.

On the basis of these preliminary studies it appears that the nomogram can help achieve optimal serum salicylate levels rapidly and without toxicity. Therapeutic levels were safely attained within two weeks by 80% of the patients. However, this approach depends on several important factors including good absorption of the salicylate preparation, urinary acidification to reduce salicylic acid excretion, and, most importantly, good patient compliance. Its applicability to a general population must, therefore, await further testing.

## Nomogram for Acute Intoxication

Initial attempts to correlate serum salicylate concentrations at the time of hospital admission with degree of intoxication and prognosis were unsatisfactory. A more reliable correlation was found between prognosis and an estimate of the probable concentration of drug shortly after the salicylate was ingested (140). This estimation requires use of the following formula:

$$\log C_0 = \log C + 0.015t \qquad \text{(Eq. 2)}$$

where $C_0$ is the peak salicylate level following the ingestion as determined by back extrapolation; C is the serum salicylate level at time t; t is the time interval in hours between salicylate ingestion and collection of the blood sample; and 0.015 is a factor to correct for the excretion of salicylate in the time between ingestion and hospitalization. When the amount of ingested drug is known, the "initial" serum salicylate level ($C_0$) can also be estimated as follows (141):

$$C_0(\mu g/ml) = \frac{\text{Salicylate Dose (mg)}}{\text{Total Body Water (70\% of body weight in gm)}} \times 1000 \quad \text{(Eq. 3)}$$

Using this equation, Done (140) derived the following correlations between $C_0$ and clinical severity. A value of $C_0$ between 500 and 800 µg/ml was associated with mild intoxication; 800 to 1100 µg/ml moderate intoxication; and 1100 to 1600 µg/ml severe intoxication. $C_0$ values greater than 1600 µg/ml correlated, in Done's estimation, with lethal doses of salicylate. However, concentrations of 1600 µg/ml or greater may not be lethal with the use of dialysis (140,144). Done's formulation applies only to cases of acute intoxication and does not pertain to therapeutic overdosage where chronic ingestion has taken place. The nomogram also has other limitations since it does not take into account continuing absorption of the salicylate, promotion of salicylate clearance by alkaline diuresis, changes in salicylate clearance in disease, the age of the patient (children clear salicylates more slowly than adults) and changes in the pH of the patient's blood (142–150). Systemic acidosis in salicylate intoxication can lead to severe poisoning in the face of relatively low blood salicylate levels. This is because as the pH decreases, the amount of unionized salicylate available for distribution into the tissues, including the CNS, is increased (93).

## Algorithm for the Monitoring of Salicylate Therapy

As we have pointed out, the major variation in the dose-effect relationship of salicylates is primarily due to individual differences in the absorption, distribution, metabolism and excretion processes. These processes are under the influence of genetic and environmental factors such as the effect of disease, urine and blood pH, and concomitant drug therapy.

The pharmacological response to salicylates is not directly quantifiable in the usual clinical situation, but in general, antiinflammatory therapy can be optimized by monitoring serum salicylate levels and adjusting the therapy to achieve steady-state serum salicylate levels of 150 to 300 µg/ml. If for any reason subtherapeutic salicylate levels (less than 150 µg/ml) are measured in patients undergoing antiinflammatory therapy with salicylates, the scheme outlined in Figure 5 should be followed to attempt to identify the source of the low serum

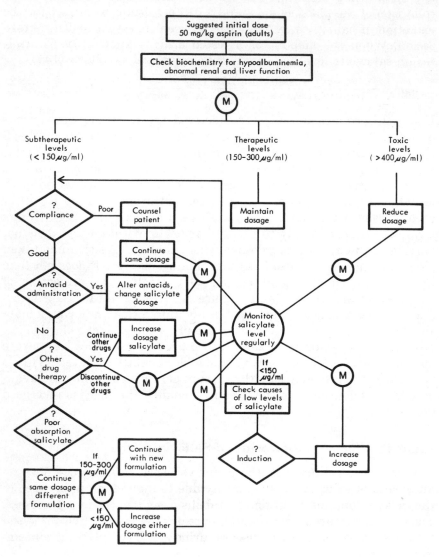

FIGURE 5. Diagrammatic approach to salicylate therapy by monitoring serum salicylate levels. (M)= measurement of salicylate level in plasma after five to seven days salicylate treatment on the calculated or adjusted dosing regimen.

salicylate levels. The objective of this diagrammatic approach to individualized therapy is the maintenance of therapeutic salicylate levels by regular monitoring. The only limitation of this approach is that since the pharmacological effect of salicylates (as well as many other drugs) may correlate with the unbound molecules and not the protein bound fraction (249), monitoring should involve measurement of unbound or free salicylate rather than total salicylate. This is because some patients may have apparently low serum concentrations of total salicylate while the concentration of free drug may be within the therapeutic range. Unfortunately, the therapeutic range of unbound salicylate concentrations has not been established. Nevertheless, as Levy has pointed out (250), it is better to monitor the total salicylate concentration than not to monitor at all. Several studies have indicated the possibility of monitoring salicylate therapy by measuring drug levels in saliva (202,251–253). There was some correlation between salicylate levels in saliva and the total ($r = 0.74$) and free salicylate ($r = 0.84$) levels in plasma. However, the use of salivary salicylate monitoring assumes no active secretion of salicylate in the saliva. Such secretion has not been observed with other acidic drugs (254,255). It, therefore, seems likely that after the therapeutic range has been determined, salicylate levels in saliva may provide a simple, non-invasive technique for monitoring salicylate therapy in patients with rheumatoid arthritis. Nevertheless, it should be remembered that the serum or saliva levels of salicylate should only be used in conjunction with the clinical assessment of the patient (92).

## ASSAY METHODS

Numerous methods are available for the qualitative and quantitative estimation of salicylate derivatives, salicylic acid and its metabolites in biological fluids and pharmaceutical preparations. These include various colorimetric, ultraviolet, fluorescent, gas-liquid chromatographic, thin layer and paper chromatographic, and high pressure liquid chromatographic techniques (151–240). Table 1 compares the relative advantages and disadvantages of these various assay methods.

### Comparison of Methods (See Table 1)

The choice of method for measuring salicylates depends on the nature of the biological fluid to be examined (since the relative concentrations of salicylic acid, its metabolites and parent source of salicylate vary with the biological matrix) and the type of instrumentation available to the analyst. In general, the colorimetric methods, al-

TABLE 1.  COMPARISON OF THE RELATIVE ADVANTAGES AND DISADVANTAGES OF THE VARIOUS SALICYLATE ASSAY METHODS

| Analysis Method | Specificity for Salicylate | Limit of Sensitivity (µg/ml) | Assayable Samples | | | Minimum Sample Volume in Microliters | Speed[1] | | Analysis Cost[2] | | Preference and Rank[3] | | | References |
|---|---|---|---|---|---|---|---|---|---|---|---|---|---|---|
| | | | Metabolite Analysis | Serum and Urine | Tissue and Other | | 1–10 | 10–100 | Estimated Reagents & Tech. | Equipment | Small | Large | Research | |
| I. Colorimetric | | | | | | | | | | | | | | |
| A. Ferric Salts | | 11 | | yes | | 200–1000 | 1 | 1 | 5 | 3 | 3 | 3 | 5 | (155) |
| B. Folin Ciocalteu Reagent | | 75 | | yes | | 200–2000 | 1 | 1 | 5 | 3 | 3 | 3 | 5 | (171, 172) |
| II. Ultraviolet | | 2.5 | yes | yes | yes | 300–2000 | 2 | 2 | 4 | 3 | 3 | 4 | 4 | (186–188) |
| III. Fluorometric | | 0.5–20 | yes | yes | yes | 10–2000 | 2 | 3 | 3 | 2 | 2 | 4 | 2 | (191–206) |
| IV. Paper and Thin Layer Chromatography (TLC) | yes | 0.001 | yes | yes | yes | 10–50 | 3 | 2 | 3 | 3 | 4 | 5 | 3 | (208–213) |
| V. Gas Liquid Chromatography (GLC) | yes | 0.2–2 | yes | yes | yes | 500–1000 | 3 | 4 | 2 | 1 | 2 | 2 | 2 | (198,227,226,229) |
| VI. High Pressure Liquid Chromatography (HPLC) | yes | 0.02–0.05 | yes | yes | yes | 3–1000 | 2 | 2 | 1 | 1 | 1 | 1 | 1 | (234–240) |

[1] Most rapid = 1
[2] Highest cost = 1
[3] Arbitrary ranking scale of 1 (excellent) to 5 (poor) with a score of 3 being average or nominal.

though not as sensitive and specific as the ultraviolet and fluorometric techniques, are sufficiently accurate to measure steady-state salicylate levels in plasma and total salicylates in urine. However, it is important to remember that if patients are taking other drugs that interfere with the colorimetric assay, a falsely high reading may be observed. The sensitive fluorometric techniques are ideal for measuring small amounts of salicylate in saliva and unbound salicylate in plasma. The various chromatographic assays can also be used to measure steady-state salicylate levels, but these assays require more sophisticated, expensive equipment. Chromatographic assays are usually employed to determine the concentrations of the metabolites of salicylic acid as well as salicylic acid or to characterize the rate of hydrolysis of the parent source of salicylate to salicylic acid (198,226,227).

To date, there is no single method available that can simultaneously measure directly the concentrations of all the metabolites of salicylic acid (gentisic acid, gentisuric acid, salicyluric acid, salicyl acyl glucuronide and salicyl phenolic glucuronide). The total glucuronides are determined indirectly by measuring the increase in salicylic acid levels after hydrolysis with β-glucuronidase (159) or acid (173) while salicyl acyl glucuronide can be determined after conversion to its hydroxamate (241). A direct method for the quantitation of the salicyl glucuronides would greatly enhance the understanding of the differences of salicylate metabolism in individuals; however, the development of such a method, in part, depends on the commercial availability of the glucuronides of salicylic acid for standardization. Salicyl phenolic glucuronides have been synthesized (242,243) but as yet, the successful synthesis of the acyl glucuronide has not been achieved (243,244), although it has been reportedly isolated from human urine (245).

The ingestion of aspirin can interfere with other biochemical assays commonly done in the laboratory (246–248); significant changes in chloride, total protein, calcium, cholesterol, uric acid, bilirubin and thyroxin have been observed in normal subjects on aspirin therapy. These abnormalities reverted towards normal on discontinuation of the drug (246). Hoeldtke reported that aspirin, salicylic acid, and an unidentified metabolite of salicylic acid interferes with the assay of homovanillic acid, which is used in the diagnosis of dopamine-secreting tumors (248).

## ACKNOWLEDGMENTS

The authors are indebted to the secretarial help of Lynn Miller and Evelyn Tackels in the typing and preparation of this manuscript.

## REFERENCES

1. Levy G: Biopharmaceutical aspects of the gastrointestinal absorption of salicylates. In: *Salicylates, An International Symposium.* Smith MJH & Smith P (eds) Churchill, London 1963:9–17.
2. Levy G: Comparison of dissolution and absorption rates of different commercial aspirin tablets. J Pharm Sci 1961; 50:388–392.
3. Leonards JR: The influence of solubility on the rate of gastrointestinal absorption of aspirin. Clin Pharmacol Ther 1963; 4:476–479.
4. Cooke AR, Hunt JN: Absorption of acetylsalicylic acid from unbuffered and buffered gastric contents. Am J Dig Dis 1970; 15:95–102.
5. Lieberman SV, Wood JH: Aspirin formulation and absorption rate II. Influence on serum levels of tablets, antacids and solutions. J Pharm Sci 1964; 53:1492–1496.
6. Levy G, Gumtow RH, Rutowski JM: The effect of dosage form upon the gastrointestinal absorption rate of salicylate. Canad Med J 1961; 85:414–419.
7. Alvarez AS, Summerskill WHJ: Gastrointestinal hemorrhage and salicylates. Lancet 1958; 2:920–925.
8. Keith JD, Ross A: Observations on salicylate therapy in rheumatic fever. Canad Med Assoc J 1945; 52:554–559.
9. Barager FD, Duthie JJR: Importance of aspirin as a cause of anemia and peptic ulcer in rheumatoid arthritis. Br Med J 1960; 1:1105–1106.
10. Gyory AZ, Steil JN: Effect of particle size on aspirin induced gastrointestinal bleeding. Lancet 1968; 2:300–301.
11. Mielants H, Veys EM, Verbruggen G, Schelstraete K: Salicylate induced gastrointestinal bleeding. Comparison between soluble buffered, enteric coated and intravenous administration. J Rheumatol 1979; 6:210–218.
12. Leonards JR, Levy G: Effect of pharmaceutical formulation on gastrointestinal bleeding from aspirin tablets. Arch Intern Med 1972; 129:457–460.
13. Arvidson B, Magnusson B, Solvell L, Magnusson A: Acetylsalicylic acid and gastrointestinal bleeding. Measurement of blood loss using a modified radioactive chronium method. Scand J Gastroenterol 1975; 10:155–160.
14. Leonards JR, Levy G: Gastrointestinal blood loss from aspirin and sodium salicylate tablets in man. Clin Pharmacol Ther 1973; 14:62–66.
15. Davenport AW: Salicylate damage to the gastric mucosal barrier. N Engl J Med 1967; 276:1307–1312.
16. Frenkel EP, McCall MS, Douglass CC, Eisenberg S: Fecal blood loss following aspirin and coated aspirin microspherule administration. J Clin Pharmacol 1968; 8:347–351.
17. Kuiper DH, Overholt BF, Fall DJ, Pollard HM: Gastroscopic findings and fecal blood loss following aspirin administration. Am J Dig Dis 1969; 14:761–769.
18. Ivey DJ, Morrison S, Gray C: Effect of intravenous salicylates on the gastric mucosal barrier in man. Am J Dig Dis 1972; 17:1055–1064.
19. Leonard JR, Levy G, Niemczura R: Gastrointestinal blood loss during prolonged aspirin administration. N Engl J Med 1973; 289:1020–1022.
20. Leonards JR, Levy G: The role of dosage form in aspirin-induced gastrointestinal bleeding. Clin Pharmacol Ther 1967; 8:400–408.
21. Leonards JR, Levy G: Absorption and metabolism of aspirin administered in enteric coated tablets. JAMA 1965; 193:99–104.
22. Canada AT, Little AH, Creighton EL: The bioavailability of enteric-coated acetylsalicylic acid: a comparison with buffered ASA in rheumatoid arthritis II. Curr Ther Res 1976; 19:544–556.

23. Leonards JR, Levy G: Reduction or prevention of aspirin-induced occult gastrointestinal blood loss in man. Clin Pharmacol Ther 1965; 10:571–575.

24. Nowak M, Brundhofer B, Gibaldi M: Rectal absorption from aspirin suppositories in children and adults. Pediatrics 1974; 54:23–26.

25. Parrott EJ: Salicylate absorption from rectal suppositories. J Pharm Sci 1971; 60:867–872.

26. Cohen A, Garber HE: Comparison of choline magnesium trisalicylate and acetylsalicylic acid in relation to fecal blood loss. Curr Ther Res 1978; 23:187–193.

27. Leonards JR: Absence of gastrointestinal bleeding following administration of salicylsalicylic acid. J Lab Clin Med 1969; 74:911–914.

28. Cohen A: Fecal blood loss and plasma salicylate study of salicylsalicylic acid and aspirin. J Clin Pharmacol 1979; 19:242–247.

29. Cohen LS: Clinical pharmacology of acetylsalicylic acid. Semin Thromb Hem 1976; 2:146–175.

30. Rushton DG: Discussion of the toxicity of salicylates In: *Salicylates,* Dixon A St. J, Smith MJH, Martin BK, Wood PHN (eds) Churchill, London 1963:253–254.

31. Matthew H, Mackintosh TF, Tompsett SH, Cameron JC: Gastric aspiration and lavage in acute poisoning. Br Med J 1966; 1:1333–1337.

32. Levy G, Gagliardi B: Gastrointestinal absorption of aspirin anhydride. J Pharm Sci 1963; 52:730–732.

33. Levy G, Sahli B: Comparison of the gastrointestinal absorption of aluminum acetylsalicylate and acetylsalicylic acid in man. J Pharm Sci 1962; 51:58–62.

34. Cohen A: A comparative blood salicylate study in two salicylate tablet formulations utilizing normal volunteers. Curr Ther Res 1978; 23:772–778.

35. Paull P, Day R, Graham G, Champion D: Single-dose evaluation of a new enteric-coated aspirin preparation. Med J Aust 1976; 1:617–619.

36. Baum J: Blood salicylate levels and clinical trials with a new form of enteric-coated aspirin: Studies in rheumatoid arthritis and degenerative joint diseases. J Clin Pharmacol 1970; 10:132–137.

37. Bogentoft C, Carsson I, Ekenved G, Magnusson A: Influence of food on the absorption of acetylsalicylic acid from enteric-coated dosage forms. Eur J Clin Pharmacol 1978; 14:351–355.

38. Gibaldi M, Grundhofer B: Bioavailability of aspirin from commercial suppositories. J Pharm Sci 1975; 64:1064–1066.

39. Parsins RL, Kaye CM, Raymond D: Pharmacokinetics of salicylate and indomethacin in coeliac disease. Eur J Clin Pharmacol 1973; 11:473–477.

40. Wosilait WD: Theoretical analysis of the binding of salicylate by human serum albumin. Eur J Clin Pharmacol 1976; 9:285–290.

41. Yacobi A, Levy G: Intraindividual relationships between serum protein binding of drugs in normal human subjects, patients with impaired renal function and rats. J Pharm Sci 1977; 66:1285–1288.

42. Kucera JL, Bullock FJ: The binding of salicylate to plasma protein from several animal species. J Pharm Pharmacol 1969; 21:293–296.

43. McArthur JN, Dawkins PD, Smith MJH: The binding of indomethacin, salicylate and phenobarbitone to human whole blood *in vitro.* J Pharm Pharmacol 1971; 23:32–36.

44. Sturman JA, Smith MJH: The binding of salicylates to plasma proteins from several animal species. J Pharm Pharmacol 1967; 19:621–622.

45. McArthur JN, Smith MJ: The determination of the binding of salicylate to serum proteins. J Pharm Pharmacol 1969; 21:589–594.

46. Kramer E, Routh JI: The binding of salicylic acid and acetylsalicylic acid to human serum albumin. Clin Biochem 1973; 6:98–105.
47. Zaroslinski JF, Keresztes-Nagy S, Mais RF, Oester YT: Effect of temperature on the binding of salicylate by human serum albumin. Biochem Pharmacol 1974; 23:1767–1776.
48. Windorfer A, Kuenzer W, Urbanek R: The influence of age on the activity of acetylsalicylic acid-esterase and protein salicylate binding. Eur J Clin Pharmacol 1974; 7:227–231.
49. Otagiri M, Perrin H: Circular dichroic investigations of the binding of salicylate and related compounds to human serum albumin. Biochem Pharmacol 1977; 26:283–288.
50. Windorfer A, Karitzky D, Gasteiger U, Stehr K: Investigations on salicylate protein binding in newborns and infants. Eur J Pediat 1978; 127:163–172.
51. Ganshorn A, Kurz H: Differences between the protein binding of newborns and adults and their importance for pharmacological action. Naunyn Schmiedebergs Arch Pharmacol 1968; 260:117–118.
52. Wallace S, Brodie MJ: Decreased drug binding in serum from patients with chronic hepatic disease. Eur J Clin Pharmacol 1976; 9:429–432.
53. Wallace S, Whiting B: Factors affecting drug binding in plasma of elderly patients. Brit J Clin Pharmacol 1976; 3:327–330.
54. Börga O, Cederlof IO, Ringberger VA, Norlin A: Protein binding of salicylate in uremic and normal plasma. Clin Pharmacol Ther 1976; 20:464–475.
55. Perez-Mateo M, Erill S: Protein binding of salicylate and quinidine in plasma from patients with renal failure, chronic liver disease and chronic respiratory insufficiency. Eur J Clin Pharmacol 1977; 11:225–231.
56. Steele WH, Boobis SW, Moore MR, Goldberg A, Brodie MJ, Summer DJ: Protein binding of salicylate in cutaneous hepatic porphyria. Eur J Clin Pharmacol 1978; 13:309–318.
57. Kapp EM, Coburn AF: Urinary metabolites of sodium salicylate. J Biol Chem 1942; 145:549–565.
58. Lester D, Lolli G, Greenberg LA: The fate of acetylsalicylic acid. J Pharm Exp Therap 1946; 87:329–342.
59. Roseman S, Dorfman A: The determination and metabolism of gentisic acid. J Biol Chem 1951; 192:105–114.
60. Cummings AJ, Martin BK: Factors influencing the plasma salicylate concentration and urinary salicylate excretion after oral dosage with aspirin. Biochem Pharmacol 1964; 13:767–776.
61. Hollister L, Levy G: Some aspects of salicylate distribution and metabolism in man. J Pharm Sci 1965; 54:1126–1129.
62. Levy G: Pharmacokinetics of salicylate elimination in man. J Pharm Sci 1965; 54:959–967.
63. Cummings AJ, Martin BK, Renton R: The elimination of salicylic acid in man: serum concentrations and urinary excretion rates. Brit J Pharmacol 1966; 26:461–467.
64. Rowland M, Riegelman S: Pharmacokinetics of acetylsalicylic acid and salicylic acid after intravenous administration in man. J Pharm Sci 1968; 57:1313–1319.
65. Boreham DR, Martin BK: The kinetics of elimination of salicylic acid and the formation of gentisic acid. Brit J Pharmacol 1969; 37:294–300.
66. Levy G, Vogel AW, Amsel LP: Capacity limited salicylurate formation during prolonged administration of aspirin to healthy human subjects. J Pharm Sci 1969; 58:503–504.

67. Levy G, Tsuchiya T: Salicylate accumulation kinetics in man. N Engl J Med 1972; 287:430–432.

68. Levy G, Tsuchiya T, Amsel LP: Limited capacity for salicyl phenolic glucuronide formation and its effect on the kinetics of salicylate elimination in man. Clin Pharmacol Ther 1972; 13:258–268.

69. Gibson T, Zaphiropoulos G, Grove J, Widdop B, Berry D: Kinetics of salicylate metabolism. Brit J Clin Pharmacol 1975; 2:233–238.

70. Levy G, Garrettson LK: Kinetics of salicylate elimination by newborn infants of mothers who ingested aspirin before delivery. Pediatrics 1974; 53:201–210.

71. Levy G, Procknal JA: Drug biotransformation interactions in man. I. Mutual inhibition in glucuronide formation of salicylic acid and salicylamide in man. J Pharm Sci 1968; 57:1330–1335.

72. Levy G, Amsel LP, Elliott HC: Kinetics of salicyluric acid elimination in man. J Pharm Sci 1969; 58:827–829.

73. Tsuchiya T, Levy G: Biotransformation of salicylic acid to its acyl and phenolic glucuronides in man. J Pharm Sci 1972; 61:800–801.

74. Gupta N, Sarkissian E, Paulus HE: Correlation of plateau serum salicylate level with rate of salicylate metabolism. Clin Pharmacol Ther 1975; 18:350–355.

75. Furst DE, Gupta N, Paulus HE: Salicylate metabolism in twins. Evidence suggesting a genetic influence and induction of salicylurate formation. J Clin Invest 1977; 60:32–42.

76. Wilson JT, Howell RL, Holladay MW, et al: Gentisuric acid: Metabolic formation in animals and identification as a metabolite of aspirin in man. Clin Pharmacol Ther 1978; 23:635–643.

77. Ebadi MS, Kugel RB: Alteration in metabolism of acetylsalicylic acid in children with Down's Syndrome: Decreased plasma binding and formation of salicyluric acid. Pediatric Res 1970; 4:187–193.

78. Smith PK, Gleason HL, Stoll CG: Studies on the pharmacology of salicylates. J Pharmacol Exp Ther 1946; 87:237–255.

79. MacPherson CR, Milne MD, Evans DM: The excretion of salicylate. Brit J Pharmacol 1955; 10:484–489.

80. Roch-Ramel F, Peters G: Micropuncture techniques as a tool in renal pharmacology. Ann Rev Pharmacol Toxicol 1979; 19:323–345.

81. Reinberg A, Clench J, Ghata J, et al: Circadian rhythms in the urinary excretion of salicylate (chronopharmacokinetics) in healthy adults. C R Acad Sci 1975; 280:1697–1699.

82. Ayres JW, Weidler DJ, Mackichan J, Wagner JG: Circadian rhythm of urinary pH in man with and without chronic antacid administration. Eur J Clin Pharmacol 1977; 12:415–420.

83. Levy G: Effect of bed rest on the distribution and elimination of drugs. J Pharm Sci 1967; 56:928–929.

84. Menguy R, Desbaillets L, Masters YF, Okabe S: Evidence for a sex-linked difference in aspirin metabolism. Nature 1972; 239:102–103.

85. Seahserova M, Sechser T, Raskova H, Jecna J, Elis J, Vanecek J: Sexual differences in the metabolism of salicylates. Arzneim Forsch 1975; 25:1581–1582.

86. Levy G: Pharmacokinetics of salicylates. Drug Metab Rev 1979; 9:3–19.

87. Ventafridda V, Martino G: Observations on the relationships between plasma concentration and analgesic activity of a soluble acetylsalicylic acid derivative after intravenous administration in man. Advances in Pain Research and Therapy 1976; 1:529–536.

88. Koch-Weser J: Serum drug concentrations as therapeutic guides. N Engl J Med 1972; 287:227–231.
89. Bywaters EGL: Rheumatic Fever (including chorea) in *Copeman's Textbook of the Rheumatic Diseases.* J T Scott (ed) Churchill, New York 1978:764–807.
90. Bencher KJ: Salicylate Intoxication. Drug Intell Clin Pharmacy 1975; 9:350–360.
91. Hoffman WS: Pitfalls of acetylsalicylic acid medication. Amer J Dis Child 1953; 85:58.
92. Levy G, Yaffe J: Relationship between dose and apparent volume of distribution of salicylate in children. Pediatrics 1974; 54:713–717.
93. Hill JB: Experimental salicylate poisoning: Observation of the effects of altering blood pH on tissue and plasma salicylate concentrations. Pediatrics 1971; 47:658–665.
94. Cockel R, Kendall MJ, Becker JF, Hawkins CF: Serum biochemical values in rheumatoid disease. Ann Rheum Dis 1971; 30:166–170.
95. Jusko WJ: Pharmacokinetics in disease states changing protein binding. In: *The Effect of Disease States on Drug Pharacokinetics.* Benet LZ (ed) American Pharmaceutical Assoc, Washington 1976:99–123.
96. Soren A: Kinetics of salicylates in blood and joint fluid. J Clin Pharmacol 1975; 15:173–177.
97. Soren A: Transport time for salicylates from blood to joint fluid—a test of histopathology of the synovial membrane. J Rheumatol 1975; 34:213–220.
98. Soren A: Transport of salicylates from blood to joint fluid. Wein Klin Wochenschr 1977; 89:599–602.
99. Farr RS, Reid PT, Minden P: Spontaneous and induced alterations in the anion binding properties of human albumin. J Clin Invest 1966; 45:1006.
100. Reid RT, Farr RS: Further evidence for albumin alterations in some patients with rheumatic disease. Arthritis Rheum 1964; 7:747–748.
101. Hawkins D, Pinckard RN, Farr RS: Acetylation of human serum albumin by acetylsalicylic acid. Science 1966; 160:780–781.
102. Denko CW, Purser DB, Johnson RM: Albumin amino acids in patients with rheumatoid arthritis. Arthritis Rheum 1970; 13:311–312.
103. Rothschild BM: Hematologic perturbations associated with salicylates. Clin Pharmacol Ther 1979; 26:145–152.
104. Evans G, Nishizawa EE, Packam MA, Mustard JF: The effect of acetylsalicylic acid (aspirin) on platelet function. Blood 1967; 30:550–555.
105. Moncada S, Vane JR: Unstable metabolites of arachidonic acid and their role in hemostasis and thrombosis. Brit Med Bull 1978; 34:129–135.
106. Vinazzer H, Putter J, Loew D: Influence of intravenously administered acetylsalicylic acid on platelet function. Haemostasis 1975; 4:12–22.
107. Loew D, Vinazzer H: Dose-dependent influence of acetylsalicylic acid on platelet function and plasmatin coagulation factors. Haemostasis 1976; 5:329–249.
108. Yett HS, Skillman JJ, Salzman EW: The hazards of aspirin plus heparin. N Engl J Med 1978; 298:1092.
109. Wilkens RF, Segre EJ: Combination therapy with naproxen and aspirin in rheumatoid arthritis. Arthritis Rheum 1976; 19:677–682.
110. Brooks PM, Walker JJ, Bell MA, Buchanan WW, Rhymer AR: Indomethacin-aspirin interaction a clinical appraisal. Br Med J 1975; 3:69–71.
111. Rubin A, Rodda BE, Warrick P, Gruber CM, Ridolfo AS: Interaction of aspirin and nonsteroidal antiinflammatory drugs in man. Arthritis Rheum 1973; 16:635–645.
112. Selley ML, Madsen BW, Thomas J: Protein binding of tolmetin. Clin Pharmacol Ther 1978; 24:694–705.
113. Segre EJ, Chaplin M, Forchielli E, Runkel R, Sevelius H: Naproxen aspirin interactions in man. Clin Pharmacol Ther 1974; 15:374–379.

114. IND submission to FDA, Feb 1979.
115. Rubin A, Warrick P, Wolen RI, Chernish SM, Ridolfo AS, Gruber CM Jr: Physiological disposition of fenoprofen in man III. J Pharmacol Exp Ther 1972; 183:449–457.
116. Moller PW: Antiinflammatory drugs and their interaction. NZ Med J 1973; 78:79.
117. Chignell CF, Starkweather DK: Optical studies of drug protein complexes. Mole Pharmacol 1971; 7:229–237.
118. Champion GD, Paulus HE, Morgan E, Okun R, Pearson CM, Sakissian E: The effect of aspirin on serum indomethacin. Clin Pharmacol Ther 1972; 13:239–244.
119. Lindqvist B, Jensen KM, Johansson G, Hansen T: Effect of concurrent administration of aspirin and indomethacin on serum concentrations. Clin Pharmacol Ther 1974; 15:247–252.
120. Kwan KC, Breault GO, Davis RL, et al: Effects of concomitant aspirin administration on the pharmacokinetics of indomethacin in man. J Pharmacokinet Biopharm 1978; 6:451–476.
121. Klinenberg JR, Miller F: Effect of corticosteroids on blood salicylate concentration. JAMA 1965; 194:601–604.
122. Graham GG, Champion GD, Day RO, Paull PD: Patterns of plasma concentrations and urinary excretion of salicylate in rheumatoid arthritis. Clin Pharmacol Ther 1978; 22:410–420.
123. Paulus HE, Siegel M, Mongan E, Okun R, Calabro JJ: Variations of serum concentrations and half-life of salicylate in patients with rheumatoid arthritis. Arthritis Rheum 1971; 14:527–531.
124. Champion GD, Day RO, Graham GG: Salicylate in rheumatoid arthritis. Clin Rheum Dis 1975; 1:245–265.
125. Barraclough DR, Muirden KD, Laby G: Salicylate therapy and drug interaction in rheumatoid arthritis. Aust NZ J Med 1975; 5:518–523.
126. Perez-Mateo M, Erill S, Cabezas R: Blood and saliva salicylate measurement in the monitoring of salicylate therapy. Int J Clin Pharmacol Biopharm 1977; 15:113–115.
127. Bardare M, Cislaughi GU, Mandelli M, Sereni F: Value of monitoring plasma salicylate levels in treating juvenile rheumatoid arthritis: Observations in 42 cases. Arch Dis Child 1978; 53:381–385.
128. Levy G, Giacomini KM: Rational aspirin dosage regimens. Clin Pharmacol Ther 1978; 23:247–252.
129. Muller IO, Hundt HKL, deKock AC: Decreased steady-state salicylic acid plasma levels associated with chronic aspirin ingestion. Curr Med Res Opin 1975; 3:417–422.
130. Day RO, Shen D, Azarnoff D: Decline of steady state serum salicylate in rheumatoid arthritics given high-dosage salicylate therapy. Clin Pharmacol Ther 1979; 25:220–221.
131. Gerstein HR, Gray RM, Ward JR: Patient compliance within the context of seeking medical care for arthritis. J Chron Disease 1973; 26:689–698.
132. Levy G, Leonards JR: Urine pH and salicylate therapy. JAMA 1971; 217:81.
133. Gibaldi M, Grundhofer B, Levy G: Effects of antacids on pH of urine. Clin Pharmacol Ther 1974; 16:520–525.
134. Gibaldi M, Grundhofer B, Levy G: Time course and dose dependence of antacid effect on urine pH. J Pharm Sci 1975; 64:2003–2004.
135. Levy G, Lampman T, Kamath BL: Decreased serum salicylate concentrations in children with rheumatic fever treated with antacid. N Engl J Med 1975; 293:323–325.
136. Mongan E, Kelly P, Nies K, Porter WW, Paulus HE: Tinnitus as an indication of therapeutic serum salicylate levels. JAMA 1973; 226:142–145.

137. Champion GD, Day RO, Paull RD et al: Clinical pharmacology and efficacy of benorylate in patients with RA. Aust NZ J Med 1978; 8:22–28.
138. Koch Weser J: The serum level approach to individualization of drug dosage. Eur J Clin Pharmacol 1975; 9:1–8.
139. Ross M, Mongan E, Paulus H: Salicylate nomogram. XIV International Congress of Rheumatology June-July, 1977 p. 118 (abst 470) San Francisco, California.
140. Done AK: Salicylate intoxication: Significance of measurements of salicylate in blood in cases of acute ingestion. Pediatrics 1960; 26:800–807.
141. Spector S: Management of acute aspirin poisoning in children. Quart Rev Pediat 1958; 13:179–187.
142. Done AK: Ontogenetic studies of salicylate intoxication. In: *Salicylates: An International Symposium.* Dixon A St. J, Martin BK, Smith MJH, Wood PHN (eds). Churchill, London 1965:260–266.
143. Buchanan N: Salicylate intoxication in infancy, a review. S Afr Med J 1975; 49:349–353.
144. Smith MJH: The metabolic basis of the major symptoms in acute salicylate intoxication. Clin Tox 1968; 1:387–407.
145. Melmon KL, Rowland M, Morrelli H: The clinical pharmacology of salicylates. Calif Med 1969; 110:410–422.
146. Brown GL, Wilson WP: Salicylate intoxication and the CNS with special reference to EEG findings. Dis Nerv Syst 1971; 32:135–140.
147. McCleave DJ, Havill J: A review of acute salicylate poisoning. Anesth Intensive Care 1974; 2:340–344.
148. Andersson RJ, Potts DE, Gabow PA, Rumack BH, Schrier RW: Unrecognized adult salicylate intoxication. Ann Intern Med 1976; 75:745–748.
149. Reimold EW, Worthen HG, Reilly TP Jr: Salicylate poisoning. Amer J Dis Children 1973; 125:668–674.
150. Chicoine L, Royer A: Salicylate intoxication in pediatrics. Appl Ther 1963; 5:238–240.
151. Harry FT, Mummery WR: The colorimetric estimation of salicylic acid in foodstuffs. Analyst 1905; 30:124–130.
152. Friderichsen C: Determination of salicylic acid in blood and its action on the heart. Arch Exp Path Pharm 1917; 80:285–288.
153. Brodie BB, Udenfriend S, Coburn AF: The determination of salicylic acid in plasma. J Pharm Exp Therap 1944; 80:114–117.
154. Tarnoky AL, Brews VAL: A simple estimation of salicylate in serum. J Clin Path 1950; 3:289–291.
155. Trinder P: Rapid determination of salicylate in biological fluids. Biochem J 1954; 57:301–303.
156. Routh JI, Paul WD, Arredondo E, Dryer RL: Semimicro method for the determination of salicylate levels in blood. Clin Chem 1956; 2:432–438.
157. Morgan AM, Truitt EB: Evaluation of acetylsalicylic acid esterase in aspirin in metabolism: Interspecies comparison. J Pharm Sci 1965; 54:1640–1645.
158. Furman M, Finberg L: A rapid method for estimation of salicylate in serum. Pediatrics 1967; 70:287–289.
159. Levy G, Procknal JA: Drug biotransformation interactions in man I. Mutual inhibition in glucuronide formation of salicylic acid and salicylamide in man. J Pharm Sci 1968; 57:1330–1335.
160. Hankiewicz J: Bestimmung von salizylsaure derivaten im urin. Zschr Inn Med 1970; 12:554–556.

161. Cid E, Delporte JP, Jaminet FR: Methode rapide de dosage des salicylates dans le sang. Pharm Acta Helv 1971; 46:737–741.
162. Chiou WL, Onyemelukwe I: Simple modified colorimetric method for total salicylate assay in urine after salicylate administration. J Pharm Sci 1974; 63:630–632.
163. Biber MZ, Rhodes CT: Modification of Trinders method for the assay of salicylates in biological fluids. Clin ChimActa 1974; 54:135–136.
164. Kim H, Skodon SB, Barnett RN: Performance of "kits" used for the clinical chemical analysis of salicylates in serum. Am J Clin Path 1974; 61:936–942.
165. Farid NA, Born GS, Kessler WV, Shaw SM, Lange WE: Improved colorimetric determination of salicylic acid and its metabolites in urine. Clin Chem 1975; 21:1167–1168.
166. Keller WJ: Method for the determination of salicylates in serum or plasma. Amer J Clin Path 1947; 17:415–417.
167. Burston GR: A simple method of estimating plasma salicylate levels. Scott Med J 1969; 14:55–56.
168. Smith PK, Gleason HL, Stoll CG, Ogorzalek: Studies in the pharmacology of salicylates. J Pharm Exper Ther 1946; 87:237–255.
169. Routh JI, Dryer RL: Salicylate. In: *Standard Methods of Clinical Chemistry*. New York Academic 1961; 3:194–199.
170. Weichselbaum TE, Shapiro IM: Rapid and simple method for determination of salicylic acid in small amounts of blood plasma. Am J Clin Path 1945; 9:42–44.
171. Smith MJH, Talbot JM: The estimation of plasma salicylate levels. Brit J Exp Path 1950; 31:65–70.
172. Smith MJH: Plasma salicylate concentrations after small doses of acetylsalicylic acid. J Pharm Pharmacol 1951; 3:409–414.
173. Tompsett SL: Metabolites of salicylic acid in urine. Quantitative determination. Clin Chem 1956; 2:166–169.
174. Muni IA, Leeling JL, Helms RJ, Johnson N, Bare JJ, Phillips BM: Improved colorimetric determination of aspirin and salicylic acid concentrations in human plasma. J Pharm Sci 1978; 67:289–291.
175. Moss DG: Micromethod for blood salicylate estimations. J Clin Pathol 1952; 5:208–211.
176. Mallick SMK, Rehmann A: Quantitative colorimetric determination of salicylates in blood. Ann Biochem Exp Med 1945; 5:97–100.
177. Reid J: Does sodium salicylate cure rheumatic fever. Quart J Med 1948; 17:139–151.
178. Sherman MC, Gross A: The detection of salicylic acid. J Ind Eng Chem 1911; 3:492–493.
179. Volterra M, Jacobs MD: A simple method for the determination of salicylates in blood. J Lab Clin Med 1947; 32:1282–1283.
180. Cotty VF, Ederma HM: Method for the direct measurement of acetylsalicylic acid in human blood. J Pharm Sci 1966; 55:837–839.
181. Sharma NN, Mehrotra RC: Cerate Oxidimetry. II. Oxidation of maleic, fumaric, benzoic, salicylic and phthalic acids. Anal Chim Acta 1954; 11:507–511.
182. Vogel AI: *Elementary Practical Organic Chemistry*. Longmans, Greens, London 1958; p. 518.
183. Accoyer P, Camelin A, Richard A: Determination of gentisic acid in biological fluids. Ann Pharm Francais 1949; 7:746–748.

184. Neuberger A, Alcaptonuria I: Estimation of homogentisic acid. Biochem J 1947; 41: 431–438.
185. Roseman S, Dorfman A: Determination and metabolism of gentisic acid. J Biol Chem 1951; 192:105–114.
186. Ungar G, Damgaard E, Wong WK: Determination of salicylic acid and related substances in serum by ultraviolet spectrophotometry. Proc Soc Exp Biol Med 1952; 80:45–47.
187. Stevenson GW: Rapid ultraviolet spectrophotometric determination of salicylate in blood. Anal Chem 1960; 32:1522–1525.
188. Routh JI, Shane NA, Arredondo EG, Paul WD: Method for the determination of acetylsalicylic acid in the blood. Clin Chem 1967; 13:734–743.
189. Williams LA, Linn RA, Zak B: Differential ultraviolet spectrophotometric determination of serum salicylates. J Lab Clin Med 1959; 53:156–162.
190. Clayton AW, Thiers RE: Direct spectrophotometric determination of salicylic acid, acetylsalicylic acid, salicylamide, caffeine and phenacetin in tablets or powders. J Pharm Sci 1966; 55:404–407.
191. Saltzmann A: Fluorophotometric method for the estimation of salicylate in blood. J Biol Chem 1948; 174:399–404.
192. Truitt EB, Morgan AM, Little JM: Determination of salicylic acid and two metabolites in plasma and urine using fluorimetry for directly measuring salicyluric acid. J Am Pharm Assoc 1955; 44:142–148.
193. Schachter D, Manis JG: Salicylate and salicyl conjugates: Fluorimetric estimation, biosynthesis and renal excretion in man. J Clin Invest 1958; 37:800–807.
194. Chirigos MA, Udenfriend S: A simple fluorometric procedure for determining salicylic acid in biologic tissues. J Lab Clin Med 1959; 54:769–772.
195. Lange WE, Bell SA: Fluorometric determination of acetylsalicylic acid and salicylic acid in blood. J Pharm Sci 1966; 55:386–389.
196. Verush SA, Hom FS, Miskel JJ: Spectrophotofluorimetric determination of salicylamide in blood serum and urine. J Pharm Sci 1971; 60:1092–1095.
197. Harris PA, Riegelman S: Acetylsalicylic acid hydrolysis in human blood and plasma I: Methodology and *in vitro* studies. J Pharm Sci 1967; 56:713–716.
198. Rowland M, Riegelman S: Determination of acetylsalicylic acid and salicylic acid in plasma. J Pharm Sci 1967; 56:717–720.
199. Putney JW, Borzelleca JF: A method for the determination of small quantities of salicylate metabolites in the presence of a great excess of salicylic acid. Arch Int Pharmacodyn 1970; 188:119–126.
200. Hill JB, Smith RM: An automated microfluorometric determination for salicylate in body fluids and tissue extracts. Biochem Med 1970; 4:24–35.
201. Øie S, Frislid D: A fluormetric method for direct determination for total salicylate in plasma. Pharm Acta Helva 1971; 46:632–636.
202. Graham G, Rowland M: Application of salivary salicylate data to biopharmaceutical studies of salicylates. J Pharm Sci 1972; 61:1219–1222.
203. Lever M, Powell JC: Simplified fluorometric determination of salicylate. Biochem Med 1973; 7:203–207.
204. Putter J: Quantitative bestimmung der haupt metaboliten der acetylsalizylsaure. 1. Mitterlung: Eine methode zur quantitativen bestimmung der salizylsaure und ihrer metaboliten; untersuchung bei gesunden. Arznei Forsch 1975; 25:941–944.
205. Baselt RC, Stewart CB: Rapid fluorometric analysis of unbound salicylate in whole blood. Res Comm Chem Path and Pharm 1976; 15:351–360.
206. Jacobs JC, Pesce M: Micromeasurement of plasma salicylate in arthritic children. Arthritis Rheum 1978; 21:129–132.

207. Thommes GA, Leninger E: Fluorometric determination of ortho- and meta-hydroxybenzoic acids in mixtures. Anal Chem 1958; 30:1361–1363.
208. Becher A, Miksch J, Rambacher P, Schafer A: Uber das verhalten des salicylamid im stoffwechsel des menschen. Klin Woshschr 1952; 30:913–917.
209. Bray HG, Thorpe WV, White K: The application of paper chromatography to metabolic studies of hydroxybenzoic acids and amides. Biochem J 1950; 46:271–275.
210. El-Darawy ZI, Wassel GM, Mobarak ZM: Direct estimation of micrograms of salicylates on paper chromatograms. Pharmazie 1973; 28:320–321.
211. Putter J, Daneels R: Qualitative chromatografischer nachweis der konjugate der salizyl-und salizylursaure in blutplasma und urin. Arznei-Forsch 1974; 24:1833–1834.
212. Christiansen J: Quantitative *in situ* thin layer chromatography of quinidine and salicylic acid in capillary blood. J Chromatog 1976; 123:57–63.
213. Chrastil J, Wilson JT: Quantitative estimation of salicylic acid and its metabolites by thin-layer densitometry. J Chromatog 1978; 152:183–189.
214. Hoffman AJ, Mitchell HF: Gas chromatographic analysis of acetylsalicylic acid, acetophenetidine and caffeine mixture in pharmaceutical tablet formulations. J Pharm Sci 1963; 52:305–306.
215. Nikelly JG: Gas chromatographic determination of acetylsalicylic acid. Anal Chem 1964; 36:2248–2250.
216. Dechene EB, Both LH, Gaughey MJ: Gas chromatographic analysis of acetylsalicylic acid phenacetin, caffeine and codeine in APC and codeine tablets. J Pharm Pharmacol 1969; 21:678–680.
217. Crippen RC, Freimuth HC: Determination of aspirin by gas chromatography. Anal Chem 1964; 36:273–275.
218. Morris CH, Christian JE, Landolt RR, Hansen WG: Gas liquid chromatography of salicylate metabolites. J Pharm Sci 1970; 59:270–271.
219. Watson JR, Crescuolo P, Matsui F: Rapid simultaneous determination of salicylic acid and aspirin by gas chromatography. I. Analysis of synthetic aspirin-salicylic acid mixtures of single-component aspirin tablets. J Pharm Sci 1971; 60:454–458.
220. Horii Z, Makita M, Takeda I, Tamura Y, Ohnishi Y: Gas chromatography of aromatic acids. Chem Pharm Bull 1965; 13:636–638.
221. Blakley ER: Gas chromatography of phenolic acids. Anal Biochem 1966; 15:350–354.
222. Rowland M, Riegelman S: Determination of acetylsalicylic acid and salicylic acid in plasma. J Pharm Sci 1967; 56:717–720.
223. Mamer OA, Crawhall JC, Tjoa SS: The identification of urinary acids by coupled gas chromatography-mass spectrometry. Clin Chim Acta 1971; 32:171–184.
224. Burkhard CA: Trimethylsilyl derivatives of hydroxy aromatic acids. J Org Chem 1957; 22:592–593.
225. Choby EG, Neuworth MB: Trimethylsilyl derivatives of salicylic acid. J Org Chem 1966; 31:632–634.
226. Rance MJ, Jordan BJ, Nichols JD: A simultaneous determination of acetylsalicylic acid, salicylic acid and salicylamide in plasma by gas liquid chromatography. J Pharm Pharmacol 1975; 27:425–429.
227. Thomas BIT, Solomonraj G, Coldwell BB: The estimation of acetylsalicylic acid and salicylate in biological fluids by gas-liquid chromatography. J Pharm Pharmacol 1973; 25:201–204.
228. Patel S, Perrin JH, Windheuser JJ: GLC analysis of aspirin from solid dosage forms. J Pharm Sci 1972; 61:1794–1796.

229. Walter LJ, Biggs DF, Coutts RT: Simultaneous GLC determination of salicylic acid and aspirin in plasma. J Pharm Sci 1974; 63:1754–1758.
230. Ali L: Determination of traces of salicylic acid in acetylsalicylic acid bulk, tablets and other preparations containing phenacetin and caffeine; simultaneous determination of salicylic acid and acetylsalicylic acid with additional components in pharmaceutical preparations. Chromatographia 1974; 7:655–658.
231. Tischio JP: Determination of salicylates by GLC. J Pharm Sci 1976; 65:1530–1533.
232. Nicholson JD: Derivative formation in the quantitative analysis of pharmaceuticals. The Analyst 1978; 103:1–28.
233. Horning MG, Knox KL, Dalgliesh CE, Horning EG: Gas liquid chromatography study and estimation of several urinary aromatic acids. Anal Biochem 1966; 17:244–257.
234. Cham EB, Johns D, Bochner F, Imhoff DM, Rowland M: Simultaneous liquid-chromatographic quantitation of salicylic acid, salicyluric acid and gentisic acid in plasma. Clin Chem 1979; 25:1420–1425.
235. Blair D, Rumack BH, Peterson RG: Analysis for salicylic acid in serum by high performance liquid chromatography. Clin Chem 1978; 24:1543–1544.
236. Peng GW, Gadalla MAF, Smith V, Peng A, Chiou WL: Simple and rapid high pressure liquid chromatographic simultaneous determination of aspirin, salicylic acid and salicyluric acid in plasma. J Pharm Sci 1978; 67:710–712.
237. Terweij-Groen CP, Vahlkamp T, Kraak JC: Rapid, direct determination of trace amounts of salicylic acid in deproteinized serum by means of high pressure liquid-liquid chromatography. J Chromatog 1978; 145:115–122.
238. Bekersky I, Boxenbaum HG, Whitson MH, Puglisi CV, Pocelinko R, Kaplan SA: Simultaneous determination of salicylic acid and salicyluric acid in urine and plasma by high pressure liquid chromatography. Anal Letts 1977; 10:539–550.
239. Lubran MM, Steen SN, Smith RL: Measurement of salicylsalicylic acid and salicylic acid in plasma by high pressure liquid chromatography. Ann Clin Lab Sci 1979; 9:501–510.
240. Cham BE, Bochmer F, Imhoff DM, Johns D, Rowland M: Simultaneous liquid chromatographic quantitation of salicylic acid, salicyluric acid and gentisic acid in urine. Clin Chem 1980; 26:111–114.
241. Schachter D: The chemical determination of acyl glucuronides and its application to studies on the metabolism of benzoate and salicylate in man. J Clin Invest 1957; 36:297–302.
242. Lunsford CD, Murphy RS: A synthesis of o-carboxyphenyl-β-D-glucopyranosiduric acids. J Org Chem 1956; 21:580–582.
243. Bollenback GN, Long JW, Benjamin DG, Lindqvist JA: The synthesis of aryl-D-glycopyranosiduric acids. J Am Chem Soc 1955; 77:3310–3315.
244. Tsukamoto H, Kato K, Tatsumi K: Metabolism of drugs XV. Isolation and paper chromatography of urinary glucuronide of salicylic acid in the rabbit. Pharm Bull (Japan) 1957; 5:570–572.
245. Robinson D, Williams RT: Glucuronides of salicylic acid. Biochem J 1965; 62:23.
246. Routh JI, Paul WD: Assessment of interference by aspirin with some assays commonly done in the clinical laboratory. Clin Chem 1976; 22:837–842.
247. Singh HP, Herbert MA, Gault MH: Effect of some drugs on clinical laboratory values as determined by the technicon SMA 12/60. Clin Chem 1972; 18:137–144.
248. Hoeldtke R: Effect of aspirin on the assay of homovanillic acid. Am J Clin Pathol 1972; 57:324–325.

249. Reynolds RC, Cluff LE: Interaction of serum and sodium salicylate: changes during acute infection and its influence on pharmacological activity. Bull Johns Hopkins Hosp 1960; 105:278–290.
250. Levy G: Clinical pharmacokinetics of aspirin. Pediatrics 1978; 62:867–872.
251. Borzelleca JF, Doyle CH: Excretion of drugs in the saliva. Salicylate, barbiturate, sulphonamide. J Oral Therap Pharmacol 1966; 3:104–111.
252. Borzelleca JF, Putney JW: A model for the movement of salicylate across the parotid epithelium. J Pharmacol Exp Ther 1970; 174:527–534.
253. Perez-Mateo M, Erill S, Cabezas R: Blood and saliva salicylate measurement in the monitoring of salicylate therapy. Int J Clin Pharmacol 1977; 15:113–115.
254. Killman SA, Thayssen JH: The permeability of the human parotid gland to a series of sulfonamide compounds, para-aminohippurate and inulin. Scand J Clin Lab Invest 1955; 7:86–91.
255. Rasmussen F: Salivary excretion of sulphonamides and barbiturates by cows and goats. Acta Pharmacol 1964; 21:11–19.

# 16

# Methotrexate

William E. Evans, Pharm.D.

## INTRODUCTION/BACKGROUND

Methotrexate (MTX, amethopterin, 4-amino-$N^{10}$-methyl pteroylglutamic acid) is an analogue of aminopterin, the folic acid antagonist introduced in 1948 by Farber for the treatment of acute leukemia. MTX is a weak acid with a $pK_a$ in the range of 4.8 to 5.5 (1) and differs from aminopterin by being methylated at the $N^{10}$ position. MTX exerts its cytotoxic effects by competitively inhibiting dihydrofolate reductase, the intracellular enzyme responsible for converting folic acid to reduced folate cofactors.

## Absorption

Despite the number of years that MTX has been used and the number of oral doses that have been given, relatively little is known about its absorption from the gastrointestinal tract. There have been several published studies describing the oral absorption of MTX; however, they either included a small number of patients, used a nonspecific assay or both. Nevertheless, these studies have provided the basis for current recommendations regarding oral dosing. The gastrointestinal absorption of MTX is considered to be dose dependent, with low dosages of MTX ($<30$ mg/m$^2$) reported to be well absorbed (2, 3) while the extent of absorption is reduced to 50 to 70% with doses in excess of 80 mg/m$^2$ (3). However, absorption characteristics at these higher dosages ($\geq 80$ mg/m$^2$) are based on observations in one patient administered 80 mg/m$^2$(3) and one patient given 10 mg/kg ($\sim$300 mg/m$^2$) (2). These data are also difficult to interpret because of the non-specific assay methods used.

The data regarding oral absorption at the lower dosages are based on a somewhat larger patient population, but do not necessarily indicate that the drug is completely absorbed. Re-evaluation of published data from two patients given 3 mg/m$^2$ (2), 28 patients given 15

518

mg/m$^2$ (4,5) and seven patients given 30 mg/m$^2$ (3) indicates that the percentage of absorption was 83%, 57 to 69% and 47% respectively. Most of these studies also used non-specific assays, making precise interpretations difficult. In two patients given 3 mg/m$^2$, ≤ 9% of the administered dose was recovered in a three day stool collection while 39% of the dose was recovered in the stool following 10 mg/kg ($\sim$300 mg/m$^2$) given to one patient. In a study (3) where chromatographic analysis was used, approximately 47% of the administered dose (30 mg/m$^2$) was recovered in feces as MTX and 35% as a metabolite, while 6% was recovered as metabolite after the same dosage given intravenously. This suggests that metabolism occurs during the absorption process from the gastrointestinal tract, which is supported by the studies of Valerino (6), who reported that MTX is metabolized by intestinal bacteria to 4-amino-4-deoxy-N$^{10}$-methylpteroic acid (DAMPA). The intestinal metabolite (DAMPA) has about 1/200th the affinity of MTX for dihydrofolate reductase (DHFR), the target enzyme. This metabolite is also produced during enterohepatic circulation of systemically administered MTX (6). In children given oral MTX in dosages of 20, 30 and 40 mg/m$^2$ every 6 hours for four doses, we found significantly higher MTX concentrations following 30 or 40 mg/m$^2$ versus 20 mg/m$^2$, but no significant difference between 30 and 40 mg/m$^2$ (7). Animal studies (8) support the dose dependent nature of MTX absorption, with the process being best described using Michaelis-Menten kinetics with Km and Vmax values of $1.5 \times 10^{-5}$ M and $4.8 \times 10^{-7}$ M/min, respectively. There is also substantial variability in the time of peak concentrations following oral doses (7,9), and the rate of absorption has been reported (5) to decline during a six week course of therapy.

The administration of a four drug regimen of oral non-absorbable antibiotics has been reported (5) to reduce the oral absorption of MTX (15 mg/m$^2$) from 69% to 44%, while similar findings have also been described following pretreatment with oral neomycin alone (10). This is apparently the result of malabsorption secondary to the oral antibiotics. However, Shen and Azarnoff (10) report that pretreatment with systemic kanamycin leads to a substantial increase in the plasma level and recovery of intact MTX after oral administration, presumably due to reduction in MTX metabolism by gut bacteria.

## Distribution

Following intravenous administration, MTX distributes within an initial volume approximating 18% (0.18 L/kg) of body weight (11) and exhibits a steady-state volume of approximately 75 to 80% of body weight (2,12). Methotrexate is approximately 50% bound to plasma proteins (1,2,3), primarily albumin, at serum concentrations ranging from $10^{-6}$ M to $10^{-3}$ M, (0.5 to 50 μg/ml). Other protein-bound organic acids such as salicylates, sulfonamides and para aminohippurate can displace MTX from protein binding sites (1,13). The clinical significance of these drug-drug interactions is difficult to assess, since many of these organic acids may also competitively inhibit renal tubular secretion of MTX (1).

In animals (14) and man (15) the highest tissue/plasma equilibrium distribution ratios are reported for the kidney and liver, followed by the gastrointestinal tract and muscle. The gastrointestinal tract is apparently an important site of distribution and metabolism of both orally and intravenously administered methotrexate. Zaharko (14) and Bischoff (15) in studies of MTX disposition in lower animals and man reported the persistence of higher MTX concentrations in gut lumen of the small intestine when compared to liver, kidney, muscle or plasma. Their model predictions in mouse and man indicated that higher plasma levels in man are due to less rapid clearances by the kidney and bile and a longer residence time in the human small intestine. Methotrexate in the gastrointestinal tract may either be reabsorbed by a saturable process, excreted in the feces, or taken up and metabolized by bacteria in the large intestine. The differences between man and smaller animals in the persistence of MTX in the gastrointestinal tract, and the rate and extent of metabolism by gut bacteria are due in part to differences in transit time in the small and large intestine (14). Decreased GI transit rate secondary to complete or partial gastrointestinal obstruction has been described as a potential mechanism for delayed total body clearance of MTX in man (16,17).

Following the administration of high doses of MTX, distribution of MTX into pleural fluid or ascites may also have a substantial influence on MTX total body clearance (18,19). The presence of a pleural effusion resulted in a significant increase in the terminal phase half-life in a patient extensively evaluated with and without a pleural effusion (19). The presence of a pleural effusion resulted in significant decreases in the disposition rate constant and the $K_{21}$ intercompartment distribution rate constant of a two-compartment first-order kinetic model. Beginning six hours after the high-dose methotrexate (HDMTX) infusion, MTX concentrations in pleural fluid were always greater than the simultaneous serum concentrations. These data support the hypothesis that patients with ascites or pleural effusions are at increased risk for developing toxicity following HDMTX because of delayed MTX clearance. The maximum concentration of MTX in pleural effusions and ascitic fluid is only about 10% of the maximum serum concentration, but declines more slowly with an eventual pleural fluid/serum equilibrium ratio of approximately 10. This makes the influence of pleural effusions or ascites most significant when high doses (>50 mg/kg) of MTX are given. When such high doses are given in patients with "third spaces," MTX accumulated in these extravascular compartments acts as a source of "sustained release" and delays total body clearance of MTX. Such patients are at greater risk of having potentially cytotoxic MTX concentrations beyond the usual duration of leucovorin rescue. Although the effect of pleural effusion on the decline in serum concentrations may not be evident until 24 to 30 hours after the dose, serum concentrations at this time are still approximately 100-fold greater than the minimum concentration required for inhibition of DNA synthesis ($\sim 10^{-8}$ M).

An important consideration in the distribution of MTX is the process of membrane transport, since the effects of MTX are dependent upon an intracellular concentration sufficient to inhibit dihydrofolate reductase activity. The mechanism of membrane transport of MTX has been extensively studied and reviewed by Goldman and associates (20). Simplistically, intracellular transport can occur by two processes: simple transmembrane diffusion and a carrier-mediated active transport process. At relatively low extracellular MTX concentrations (i.e. $10^{-6}$ M), the active transport process predominates. This active transport process follows Michaelis-Menten kinetics, with the rate of influx proceeding at half the maximum transport velocity when extracellular concentrations are approximately $5 \times 10^{-6}$ M (19). This Michaelis constant is similar to values reported for naturally occurring reduced folates. Following the intravenous administration of high doses of MTX ($\geq$100 mg/kg), serum concentrations in the ranges of $10^{-4}$ to $10^{-3}$ M are achieved. At these concentrations, the active transport process is saturated and passive diffusion becomes a major pathway by which effective intracellular concentrations can be achieved. This may be of particular importance in the treatment of malignant diseases which have an acquired or *de novo* resistance to MTX due to a reduced active transport process. Additionally, since MTX and reduced folates (i.e. leucovorin) share the same active transport process, high extracellular MTX concentrations can reduce or inhibit the intracellular transport of leucovorin (21). Thus, leucovorin "rescue" following HDMTX is a competitive rescue, despite its non-competitive biochemical mechanism of circumventing the inhibition of DHFR with reduced folates. When MTX serum concentrations are $\sim 10^{-7}$ M, MTX effects can be rescued with equimolar serum concentrations of leucovorin, while $10^{-3}$ M concentrations of leucovorin may be required when MTX concentrations are $10^{-5}$ M (21).

Using L1210 leukemia cells in-vitro, Zager et al (22) reported that transmembrane influx and efflux of MTX may also be affected by other drugs, including vincristine, corticosteroids, asparaginase and cephalothin. Using Ehrlich ascites tumor cells, Fyfe and Goldman (23) further characterized this interaction, demonstrating that $1 \times 10^{-5}$ M vincristine (VCR) slowed the efflux of MTX. It was initially proposed that the inhibition of MTX efflux by vincristine could be exploited clinically to produce higher intracellular concentrations of MTX. However, more recent studies using human leukemia cells (24) indicate that VCR concentrations of $1 \times 10^{-5}$ M and $1 \times 10^{-7}$ M enhance the intracellular accumulation of MTX by 54% and 33%, respectively. More important, however, was their observation that if VCR-incubated cells were washed free of VCR and resuspended in VCR-free media, the inhibition of MTX efflux is lost. Thus, VCR must be present (in sufficient concentrations) for enhancement of MTX intracellular accumulation to be observed. Owellen and coworkers first reported on the pharmacokinetics of VCR in man in 1976 (25,26). Their studies demonstrated that the peak concentrations of VCR achieved after bolus intravenous administration of dosages tolerated clinically were approximately $1 \times 10^{-7}$ M. Moreover, these concentrations were very short-lived with a $t\frac{1}{2}_{alpha}$ of 3.37 ± 0.72 minutes and a $t\frac{1}{2}_{beta}$ of 155 ± 18 minutes. More recently, Warren and coworkers (27) failed to demonstrate a significant enhancement of intracellular MTX accumulation in human lymphoblastoid cells when the clinically achievable VCR concentration of $1 \times 10^{-7}$ M was used. This was noted for extracellular MTX concentrations achieved after either conventional or high-dose MTX administration.

The blood-cerebrospinal fluid (CSF) barrier is relatively impermeable to MTX (2,28,29) and CSF concentrations following intravenous administration of MTX are dose dependent. Animal studies indicate that the brain:serum ratio for MTX after low dosages (10 mg/kg) is small (i.e. 0.11) (30,31). In humans, CSF MTX concentrations have been reported to range from $10^{-7}$ M after a 24-hour infusion of 500 mg/m$^2$ to greater than $10^{-5}$ M following 7500 mg/m$^2$ given as an intravenous bolus (32,33). The distribution of MTX from plasma into CSF is apparently slow, with two recent reports demonstrating that peak CSF concentrations are reached only toward the end of 24-hour infusions of 500 or 1000 mg/m$^2$ (34,35). Studies conducted in a small number of patients indicate that lumbar CSF and brain extracellular fluid concentrations are similar following intravenous high-dose MTX administration (36). This is not the case when MTX is given intrathecally into the lumbar CSF, since MTX distribution into ventricular CSF is variable and unpredictable following intrathecal administration.

Ionizing radiation has been shown to alter the permeability of the blood-brain barrier to MTX, although these changes may vary from one region of the brain to another and from one species to another. Griffin and associates (30) reported that no MTX was detectable in brains of unirradiated mice following 100 mg/kg intraperitoneal MTX, while detectable MTX levels were present after 2000 rads cranial irradiation, but not after 500, 1000 or 1500 rads. These findings are consistent with the suggestions of previous clinical investigators that MTX-related leukoencephalopathy is most often a result of combined therapy with cranial irradiation and systemic MTX, based on the postulate that radiation alters the integrity of the blood-brain barrier, allowing MTX to diffuse more easily into the white matter (2,37,38).

## Metabolism

As previously stated, MTX is metabolized by intestinal bacteria to 4-amino-4-deoxy-$N^{10}$-methylpteroic acid (DAMPA) and other minor metabolites (6). The DAMPA metabolite has about 1/200th the affinity of MTX for the target enzyme, DHFR (6).

Another potentially important metabolite of MTX is its oxidation (aldelhyde oxidase) product, 7-hydroxy methotrexate (7-OH MTX) (39). This metabolite is reported to constitute 1 to 11% of the administered dose recovered in a cumulative 24-hour urine collection following high-dose intravenous MTX. Because 7-OH MTX is about two orders of magnitude less effective as an inhibitor of DHFR (40) and because it represents such a small percentage of the total dose found in the urine, it was initially considered to be a relatively unimportant metabolite. However, more recent studies (41) report serum concentrations of 7-OH MTX exceeding concurrent serum concentrations of the parent drug, following high-dose (200 mg/kg) intravenous administration of MTX. This finding (which has recently been confirmed) coupled with the fact that 7-OH MTX is three- to five-fold less water soluble than MTX (39) makes this a potentially important metabolite, since the urine concentrations may exceed the solubility of the parent compound and metabolite (42). The aqueous solubility of MTX is pH dependent, and can be reduced from 10 mg/ml to 1 mg/ml by reducing the pH from 6.9 to 5.7 (42). MTX urine concentrations exceeding 5 mg/ml ($10^{-2}$ M) have been reported (42), and urine pH's less than 6.0 are frequently observed following high doses of MTX (without urinary alkalinization). Thus, intratubular precipitation leading to obstructive nephropathy has been suggested as one mechanism of MTX renal toxicity (43). For these reasons, alkalinization of the urine prior to and following high-dose MTX infusions has become standard practice.

Animal studies have shown that MTX may be converted to mono- and diglutamate forms *in vivo* (44). Whitehead and coworkers (45) have reported that MTX monoglutamate was formed immediately after administration and then disappeared with a half-life of 6.5 days. Poly-γ-glutamates have been reported in red blood cells of a patient being treated with MTX (44). The fact that poly-γ-glutamates can be converted back to MTX by hydrolase enzymes suggests that they may serve as an intracellular reservoir for MTX. However, their presence in human tissues and the pharmacological importance of the glutamate metabolites remain to be determined.

## Excretion

Renal excretion is the major route of methotrexate elimination, constituting greater than 80% of total body elimination (42,46–49). Estimates of MTX clearance in adults with normal renal function yield values of about 110 ml/min/$m^2$ (1). MTX clearance in these patients exceeded glomerular filtration rate (inulin clearance) by 6 to 49%, suggesting active tubular secretion. Following intravenous infusion of high doses of MTX, greater than 40% of the administered dose has been recovered unchanged in urine within 6 hours and 90% within 24 hours (2,46,50,51). However, these values are somewhat greater than those described by Isacoff et al (52) who reported only 60% cumulative urinary recovery following 64 high-dose infusions. The reason for these discrepancies may involve the specificity of the assays used, although this does not explain all of the observed differences. Cumulative 24-hour urinary recovery of lower intravenous doses of MTX (0.1 to 10 mg/kg) is reported to be 58 to 92% (median 78%). As previously stated, urinary recovery following oral administration is lower and dose dependent, reflecting gut metabolism and the incompleteness of absorption.

Net renal clearance of MTX has been reported to decrease from $78 \pm 5$ ml/min when serum concentrations range from $10^{-7}$ to $10^{-5}$ M, to 25 to 50 ml/min at serum levels ranging from $10^{-6}$ M to $10^{-3}$ M (53). The low net renal clearance at lower serum levels suggests extensive tubular reabsorption of MTX, while the decreasing renal clearance at higher serum concentrations indicates that tubular secretion of MTX may be saturated at concentrations attained clinically. Renal tubular secretion of MTX can be competitively inhibited by other organic acids such as salicylates and sulfonamides (1), and can be totally blocked by probenecid (54). However, the reduction in total body clearance due to saturation of the active tubular secretory process or competitive inhibition by organic acids is seldom clinically significant.

The time course of MTX disappearance from plasma following high-dose intravenous infusions is essentially biexponential (16,17,42,52,55). Mean half-lives for the initial phase have been reported to range from 1.5 to 3.5 hours (42,49,50), while the terminal phase half-life is around 8 to 15 hours in patients with normal total body clearance. Many of the early studies reporting half-lives were not designed as pharmacokinetic studies, and the reported initial-phase half-lives represent the rate of decline in serum concentrations (during the first 24 hours) and not $t\frac{1}{2}_{alpha}$ (alpha/0.693). However, Isacoff and coworkers (52) fit serum concentrations following 172 high-dose infusions to a biexponential equation and calculated parameters of a two-compartment model, yielding a $t\frac{1}{2}_{alpha}$ of 1.8 ± 0.5 hours. These values are similar to those reported by Stoller et al (42) who also used a biexponential model. No significant differences in kinetic parameters were observed at dosages ranging from 50 to 200 mg/kg (52). The early distribution half-life observed after IV bolus administration (11,49) is usually not observed following IV infusions, since distribution in the central compartment essentially occurs during administration. The terminal phase half-life of 27 hours reported by Huffman et al (49) is longer than reported by other investigators and is most likely a result of the non-specific assay which measured total radioactivity of both MTX and metabolites (56). Importantly, the terminal phase half-life appears to correlate best with toxicity (12), as will be discussed later in detail.

There are currently data (57) which suggest that the pharmacokinetics of HDMTX may be significantly different in children. Wang and coworkers (57) recently reported significantly lower 6 and 24 hour serum MTX concentrations in children ≤ 10 years of age compared to adults. Pharmacokinetic parameters derived from a very small number of subjects (three children and six adults) indicated a shorter $t\frac{1}{2}_{alpha}$ and larger Vd in children. Urinary recovery of MTX in children was also greater during the infusion when compared to adults. However, there was considerable overlap in serum concentrations in both age groups at all time points and absolutely no difference at 48 and 72 hours post-infusion. Moreover, the significant differences in concentrations at 6 hours may not be clinically important. It seems reasonable for children with creatinine clearances greater than adults to excrete MTX more rapidly; however, these potential age-related differences remain to be clearly defined.

Because the large amount of MTX excreted in urine (after high doses) may exceed the 2 mM solubility at pH 5.5, vigorous hydration and urinary alkalinization have been recommended to prevent MTX precipitation and nephrotoxicity. The use of vigorous intravenous hydration ($>100$ ml/m$^2$/hour) does not appear to alter the plasma disposition curve of MTX when compared to the same patients given maintenance IV hydration ($\sim$40 ml/m$^2$/hour). (58) The maintenance of urinary pH 7 (using oral sodium bicarbonate) for 12 hours before and 48 hours after high-dose MTX significantly reduces the risk of renal toxicity (33) and is currently recommended for all patients (59,60).

Active biliary secretion of MTX probably occurs (53,61), but is a relatively minor excretory pathway. The total amount recovered in the gastrointestinal tract following intravenous administration is less than 10% of the administered dose (49,53,62). Shen and coworkers (53) have reported bile-plasma concentration ratios ranging from 63 to 145 in six cancer patients. The contribution enterohepatic circulation makes to the long terminal half-life of MTX remains undefined. However, this relatively minor excretory pathway ($<10$% fecal excretion) may become clinically important when impaired (i.e. GI obstruction) (16,17).

## Intrathecal Methotrexate

Intrathecal (IT) administration of MTX is currently a standard component of preventive CNS therapy for childhood acute lymphocytic leukemia. Intrathecal MTX is also frequently used to treat active CNS involvement of leukemia, lymphoma and other responsive malignancies. The disposition of IT MTX in the cerebrospinal fluid (CSF) is difficult to assess because of the need for repeated lumbar punctures to obtain serial CSF samples from individual patients. For this reason, very few studies report pharmacokinetic parameters derived from serial CSF concentrations. Assessment of MTX CSF disposition is further complicated by the uneven distribution of IT MTX between lumbar and ventricular CSF, and the intrinsic difficulties in obtaining ventricular CSF samples. Despite these limitations, some potentially useful information about the CSF disposition of IT MTX is available.

Bleyer and coworkers (63) measured lumbar CSF MTX concentrations in 76 patients given IT MTX, with serial samples assessed in five of these patients. All patients were given the same dosage of 12 mg/m$^2$, in an injection volume of 12 ml/m$^2$ up to a maximum of 18 ml. None of these patients had evidence of active CNS disease. When the lumbar CSF MTX concentrations measured at various times (12 to 96 hours) after an IT dose (for 76 patients) were collectively used to simulate CSF disposition, a biphasic disappearance curve was produced. Half-lives of 4.5 hours and 14 hours were estimated during the intervals of 4 to 36 and 48 to 96 hours after the injection, respectively. These two half-life values were similar to values estimated from serial concentrations measured in one patient with chronic meningeal leukemia. Concurrent MTX concentrations in plasma (resulting from the IT dose) reached a peak of about $10^{-7}$ M between 3 and 12 hours after the IT injection, and declined in parallel with the CSF concentrations. The terminal CSF half-life of MTX appears to be longer (64) in patients with active meningeal leukemia, which is consistent with previous observations that CSF MTX concentrations and the likelihood of neurotoxicity are greater in patients with active meningeal leukemia and/or meningeal carcinomatosis (28,65). The disappearance of MTX from lumbar CSF is apparently dependent upon a number of physiologic processes including: [1] bulk flow removal via normal pathways of CSF absorption, [2] bulk flow distribution within the subarachnoid and ventricular CSF, [3] diffusion throughout the ECF of the brain parenchyma and spinal cord, [4] diffusion from the ECF into the capillaries of the brain and spinal cord and [5] absorption from ventricular fluid by the energy-dependent transport process of the choroid plexus (66). It has been hypothesized that delayed clearance of MTX from the CSF of patients with active meningeal disease is due to impairment of bulk flow removal of MTX. The rate of decline in MTX CSF concentrations can also be prolonged by either probenecid (67) or vincristine (68).

The dose of intrathecal MTX is usually based on the patient's body surface area (12 mg/m²). However, the CNS volume of children older than 3 years approaches that of adults, while body surface area does not plateau at adult levels until 16 to 20 years of age. Thus, CSF concentrations of MTX after IT administration of 12 mg/m² are generally higher as age increases from 3 to 20 years (64). This may partially explain the increased risk of neurotoxicity in older patients given IT MTX (65). It has been proposed that all patients greater than 3 years of age be given the same dose of MTX (12 mg) and not a dosage based on body surface area (64). The clinical use of CSF MTX concentrations to modify therapy will be discussed later in greater detail.

Methotrexate may also be given intraventricularly, and at least one study (28) has indicated that the distribution of methotrexate in CSF is more reliable when the drug is administered intraventricularly via an indwelling intraventricular subcutaneous reservoir compared to intrathecal administration. However, the distribution of intrathecal MTX in this study was sufficient to achieve therapeutic levels in the ventricular CSF and may have been significantly better had the volume of the intrathecal preparation been larger. Rieselbach et al (69) reported that the volume of the injected solution is an important factor in attaining widespread distribution following intrathecal administration. When the volume of injected solution is ~10% of the estimated cerebrospinal fluid volume, adequate distribution is obtained only at the level of the basal cisterns; whereas when the volume is approximately 25% of the estimated CSF, distribution is obtained throughout the cerebral subarachnoid space and ventricular system (28). Although subarachnoid and ventricular distribution of methotrexate may not be critical when cranial irradiation is given concomitantly for CNS prophylaxis, good cerebrospinal fluid distribution is essential if methotrexate alone is employed for the treatment or prophylaxis of CNS leukemia.

## CONCENTRATION versus RESPONSE and TOXICITY

### Therapeutic Concentrations

The cytotoxic effects of MTX are a result of its competitive inhibition of the intracellular enzyme dihydrofolate reductase (DHFR). The $K_i$ for this inhibition has not been precisely defined, although estimates of $10^{-10}$ M have been made (70). Extensive studies by Goldman (71, 72) and others have demonstrated that a free intracellular MTX concentrations in excess of that required to saturate the tight binding sites on DHFR are necessary for maximal suppression of DNA synthesis. It appears that only a small fraction of uninhibited DHFR is sufficient to maintain reduced folate pools adequate to sustain DNA synthesis (71), thus necessitating intracellular concentrations of free MTX in excess of DHFR to maintain inhibition of the biochemical pathway. There is no feasible means by which intracellular MTX concentrations can be routinely measured in clinical specimens. While the relationship between extracellular and intracellular MTX concentrations has been determined for several experimental tumors (73–76) and for intestinal mucosa (75) it remains to be clearly established for most tissues. Since extracellular drug is in rapid exchange with intracellular free drug in sensitive cells, it seems reasonable that extracellular drug concentrations might relate to intracellular drug effects.

Animal studies have indicated that the inhibition of DNA synthesis in tumor cells, bone marrow and intestinal epithelium requires the presence of a serum concentration of free MTX specific for each tissue

(75). The inhibition of DNA synthesis in mouse bone marrow is virtually complete with plasma MTX concentrations above ~$10^{-8}$ M, whereas intestinal epithelium shows similar inhibition at MTX levels above 5 × $10^{-9}$ M. Subsequent studies using an infusion device to maintain constant serum concentrations demonstrated the partial inhibition of DNA synthesis at levels of 2 × $10^{-8}$ M and more complete inhibition of intestinal mucosa at this concentration (76,77). Similar findings have been reported in humans, where resumption of DNA synthesis did not occur until serum concentrations were 2 × $10^{-8}$ M or below (78). Pinedo and Chabner (79) have shown that at MTX concentrations >$10^{-8}$ M the cytotoxic effects are a function of both drug concentration and duration of exposure. Their data demonstrated that exposure to extracellular concentration of 5 × $10^{-8}$ M for 72 hours produces the same effect as exposure to $10^{-5}$ M for 12 hours. It therefore seems reasonable to assume that extracellular concentrations less than $10^{-8}$ M are not likely to produce pharmacologic or toxicologic effects. Although the absolute threshold appears to be organ dependent and a function of duration of exposure to suprathreshold concentrations, the precise relation between serum concentrations and pharmacologic effects remains to be precisely defined in human experiments.

## Toxic Concentrations—Intravenous Methotrexate

When MTX is given in low dosages (≤50 mg/m²) either orally or parenterally, peak serum concentrations are generally in the range of $10^{-6}$ M. When these dosages are given on a weekly basis they usually do not require leucovorin "rescue," although individual patient tolerance may vary and necessitate either an upward or downward dosage modification. At present, there are no clear guidelines by which the likelihood of toxicity (mucositis, marrow suppression) can be predicted from measurement of serum concentrations at this dosage level. However, patients with delayed MTX clearance are generally at a greater risk for toxicity (17) if dosage modifications are not made.

More extensive data are available regarding potentially toxic serum (or plasma) concentrations of MTX following high-dose MTX (>50 mg/kg) with leucovorin rescue (LR). The rationale for monitoring serum MTX concentrations in patients given HDMTX with LR is based on at least two principles: [1] delayed clearance of MTX may result in cytotoxic concentrations being sustained beyond the usual duration of leucovorin rescue (72 to 96 hours) and [2] high extracellular concentrations of MTX may competitively inhibit intracellular transport of leucovorin (21) and thereby reduce its effectiveness as a "rescue" agent. Thus, the two major concerns are that rescue will be inadequate because leucovorin is either discontinued too early in patients who sustain cytotoxic MTX concentrations for long periods after rescue is terminated, or that the leucovorin dosage is too low to overcome inhibition of intracellular transport due to high extracellular MTX concentrations. These two reasons for inadequate "rescue" often can be overcome by either extending the duration and/or escalating the dosage of leucovorin rescue. Alterations in leucovorin rescue must be made expediently in those patients at increased risk, since the effects of MTX may not be readily reversible if adequate leucovorin rescue is delayed for more than 42–48 hours (80–82). Conversely, an escalated dose and duration of leucovorin rescue should be avoided in those patients not at high risk, since recent studies (83) have demonstrated that progressive increases in leucovorin dosage on any schedule may reduce both the toxicity and antitumor effects of MTX.

The need for methods to monitor patients given HDMTX with leucovorin rescue became obvious when a nationwide survey conducted prior to 1977 revealed a 6% incidence of *mortality* secondary to HDMTX (84). Another report (60) indicated that severe morbidity also occurs in an equal number of patients, making the risk of significant complications (mucositis, GI desquamation, leukopenia, anemia, thrombocytopenia, renal and hepatic dysfunction) greater than 10%. Efforts were therefore made to identify factors which predisposed to toxicity (60,85) and to establish guidelines which reduce the risk of morbidity and mortality.

Pharmacokinetic monitoring of MTX has evolved as a standard approach for prospective identification of patients at high risk for toxicity. There is general agreement that patients with delayed plasma clearance and/or elevated MTX concentrations are at greater risk for toxicity. However, there is no consensus among investigators regarding the exact criteria to be used in identifying such patients. The following criteria have been proposed for patients administered HDMTX as a relatively short intravenous infusion ($< 6$ hours). Tattersal et al (86) reported that patients with a serum concentration $>5 \times 10^{-7}$ M at 48 hours are likely to encounter severe myelosuppression. Isacoff et al (87) initially reported that patients with serum levels $>5 \times 10^{-6}$ M at 24 hours were at increased risk for toxicity. More recently these investigators have reported (88) that patients with a 24 hour level $>10^{-5}$ M or a 48 hour concentration $>5 \times 10^{-7}$ M are at increased risk for toxicity. Nirenberg et al (89) reported that patients with a 24 hour serum concentration $>10^{-5}$ M, a 48 hour level $>10^{-6}$ M and a 72 hour concentration $>10^{-7}$ M were at high risk for toxicity. However,

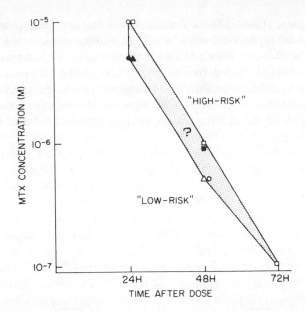

FIGURE 1. Composite plot of serum MTX concentrations which have been proposed as values identifying patients at "high-risk" to develop toxicity from high-dose MTX if conventional low-dose leucovorin is given. Concentrations (LOG) are plotted against time from the end of a six-hour infusion. Data have been obtained from studies of (△) Tattersal[86], (●) Isacoff[87], (○) Isacoff[88], (□) Nirenberg[89], (■) Stollar[90], and (▲) Evans[16].

continued low dose leucovorin rescue did not prevent clinical toxicity in the patients identified at high risk. Stoller et al (90) suggest that patients with a 48 hour serum concentration $>9 \times 10^{-7}$ M and evidence of delayed clearance beyond 48 hours are at high risk for toxicity with conventional rescue. Evans et al (16) reported that patients with a 24 hour serum concentration $<5 \times 10^{-6}$ M, a half-life for decline in serum concentrations less than 3.5 hours during this interval and no evidence of clinical features associated with delayed MTX clearance (i.e. renal dysfunction, pleural effusions, ascites, GI obstruction) are at low risk for toxicity with conventional low-dose leucovorin rescue.

When these criteria are evaluated collectively as shown in Figure 1, there is relatively good agreement among investigators. Only a narrow range of serum concentrations exists between the high and low risk groups, which is surprisingly good considering that the MTX dosages ranged from 0.75 to 20 gm/m$^2$ in these studies. In addition, at least four different assay procedures were used to measure MTX serum concentration in these six studies. Clinical application of these criteria, whether derived from a single study or from the collective data, should only be used to establish a relative risk for toxicity. As stated by several of these investigators (16,17,90), the rate of decline in serum concentrations should be used in conjunction with the absolute concentration to establish the risk of toxicity. This requires measurement of serial samples as will be described later in greater detail.

The exact criteria described above cannot be applied to patients who receive HDMTX as a prolonged intravenous infusion (i.e. 24 to 42 hour infusions). Criteria for these patients have not been as completely established, although the general principles are similar (91). When moderate to high dose MTX is infused over 24 to 42 hours, leucovorin rescue is being initiated much later than conventional rescue following shorter infusions. Leucovorin rescue may also be delayed 24 to 30 hours after short (6 hour) HDMTX infusions. When rescue is delayed in this manner, MTX serum concentrations must be promptly monitored to ensure that the initial doses of leucovorin are adequate to initiate rescue.

## Toxic Concentrations—Intrathecal Methotrexate

Three general types of clinical manifestations of neurotoxicity have been reported to follow the use of intrathecal MTX; meningeal irritation, transient or permanent paresis, and encephalopathy. The signs, symptoms and proposed pathogenesis of each have been reviewed elsewhere in detail (92). A number of potential mechanisms by which IT MTX may cause neurotoxicity have been proposed and include: high concentrations of MTX in CSF, toxic preservatives in IT MTX solutions, and unphysiologic IT MTX solutions. None of these possible causes has been conclusively substantiated. However, neurotoxicity continues to occur in some patients despite the current use of preservative-free MTX in physiologic solutions. Moreover, Bleyer and coworkers (64,65) have reported that CSF MTX concentrations are significantly higher in patients who develop neurotoxicity compared to those who do not. In his initial report (65), mean CSF MTX concentrations were 13.8 times higher in five neurotoxic patients when compared to 20 asymptomatic patients at 48 hours after a dose. Patients developing neurotoxicity were significantly older than nontoxic patients, and four of five toxic patients had overt meningeal leukemia at the time of therapy. In a subsequent study (65) of 47 patients, CSF MTX concentrations measured from 48 to 192 hours post-dose were consistently higher in 10 toxic patients when compared to nontoxic patients. This study also demonstrated that CSF MTX concentrations correlated directly with age (over the range of 3 to 26 years) when all patients were given the standard dosage of 12 mg/m$^2$/dose. This is consistent with the fact that CSF volume increases rapidly to adult levels by the age of about 3 years, and then increases very little thereafter despite a continual increase in body surface area (65).

## CLINICAL APPLICATION OF PHARMACOKINETIC DATA

### Intrathecal Methotrexate

As shown in Figure 2, the data by Bleyer et al (65) indicate that MTX concentrations measured in lumbar CSF from 2 to 8 days after an IT dose may correlate with both response and toxicity. The inherent difficulties in obtaining CSF samples limit the usefulness of this approach to monitoring intrathecal MTX therapy. We currently use CSF MTX concentrations only in patients who are at increased risk for neurotoxicity because of acute meningeal disease or in patients who exhibit signs or symptoms of MTX neurotoxicity temporally related to intrathecal MTX therapy. In patients receiving several doses of IT MTX, MTX concentrations in CSF withdrawn in the process of intrathecal administration may be useful in adjusting the interval between subsequent IT doses (Figure 3).

Following intrathecal MTX administration, potentially cytotoxic serum concentrations of MTX ($10^{-7}$ M) may result and persist for 24 to 48 hours (28). This may result in systemic effects of MTX following intrathecal administration and has led some clinicians to administer low doses of leucovorin to prevent any systemic effect. However, the administration of leucovorin is usually not necessary and may be detrimental, since 5-methyltetrahydrofolate (a leucovorin metabolite) readily enters the CSF. This reduced folate metabolite is active as a rescue agent and may thereby diminish the CNS activity of IT MTX. Therefore, when leucovorin is given following IT MTX, it should probably be delayed for 24 to 36 hours after the IT dose to minimize the potential for any compromise in the intrathecal therapy.

### Intravenous Methotrexate

The use of serial MTX serum concentrations to identify patients at high risk for toxicity following high-dose MTX (HDMTX) infusions is probably the best defined and most clinically important application of MTX pharmacokinetic data. Although there is speculation that MTX serum concentrations may correlate with clinical response in patients

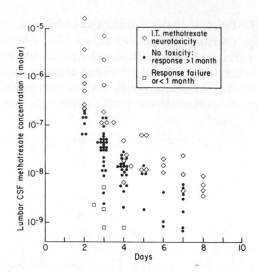

FIGURE 2.  CSF-antifolate concentration after intrathecal MTX (12 mg/m² of BSA). ◇ = patients with neurotoxic reactions to intrathecal MTX, □ = patients who failed to achieve CNS remission or who had a meningeal relapse within 1 month after therapy, and ● = patients who had neither neurotoxic reactions nor early CNS relapse. (Reproduced with permission from Bleyer WA: Cancer Treat Rep 61:1419–1425, 1977, Reference 64)

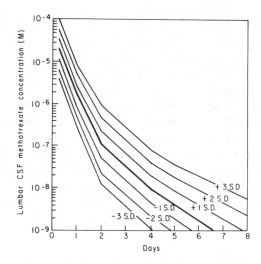

FIGURE 3.  Cerebrospinal-fluid methotrexate concentration as a therapeutic guide to intrathecal methotrexate therapy. Dosage should be adjusted to bring the lumbar cerebrospinal-fluid methotrexate concentration into the range depicted. (Reproduced with permission from Bleyer WA: Cancer Treat Rev 4:87–101, 1977, Reference 99)

534

treated with HDMTX-LR (94), statistically valid and clinically useful criteria defining "therapeutic" concentrations for selected diseases are not currently available. The fact that a clear relation between a given serum concentration and the likelihood of clinical response does not exist is not surprising when one considers the number of factors which may influence tumor response to MTX (i.e. membrane transport, dihydrofolate reductase levels and binding characteristics, tissue (tumor) distribution of drug, dosage, duration, route and schedule of leucovorin rescue, previous or concurrent anticancer therapy, etc.). However, pharmacokinetic monitoring has had an impact on patients given HDMTX-LR by reducing the number of drug-related deaths (16,90). At our institution, the number of drug-related deaths has decreased from approximately 5% of treated patients (prior to prospective pharmacokinetic monitoring) to no drug-related deaths since the program was initiated in 1976 (16). Similar reduction in drug-related toxicity has been reported by other investigators (95). The absolute impact of pharmacokinetic monitoring is difficult to assess, since the importance of adequate hydration and urinary alkalinization has been recognized and given greater attention during this time period as well. However, delayed clearance of MTX may occur following HDMTX given to patients with none of the high-risk clinical features such as dehydration, aciduria, renal dysfunction and pleural effusion or ascites (60). These patients may be prospectively identified by monitoring MTX serum concentrations, and toxicity may be diminished or prevented by altering the leucovorin rescue. The criteria which have been proposed by several investigators are summarized above (see Toxic Concentrations). Regardless of the exact criteria used, there are two features which should be assessed in all patients given HDMTX: [1] What are the serum concentrations at selected times (24, 48, 72 hours) following the HDMTX dose and how do they relate to published criteria regarding the risk of toxicity (Figure 1)? [2] How rapidly are the serum concentrations of MTX declining and what is the likelihood of concentrations remaining above levels which can be "rescued" by conventional low-dose leucovorin? Clearly, a single MTX serum concentration at any point in time cannot be used according to any published criteria, with absolute confidence. Stoller et al (90) reported that the rate of decline in serum concentrations was slower in patients who developed toxicity when compared to a group of patients who had similarly elevated MTX serum concentrations at 48 hours but did not develop toxicity. Unfortunately, the identification of high-risk patients cannot be safely delayed beyond 48 hours post-dose, since the effects of MTX may not be reversible if effective leucovorin rescue is delayed for more than 42 to 48 hours (80–82). For this reason, we have developed criteria which allow potentially high-risk patients to be identified within 24 to 36 hours post-dose (16). Our criteria (16) utilize the rate of decline in serum concentrations during the first 24 hours post-infusion and the serum concentration at 24 hours. Patients who have a half-life for decline in serum concentrations <3.5 hours and a 24 hour serum concentration $\leqslant 5 \times 10^{-6}$ M are considered at low risk for toxicity. These patients receive the standard low-dose leucovorin rescue for 72 hours. Patients who do not meet these criteria are considered at greater risk for toxicity and pharmacokinetic monitoring is continued to regulate the dose and duration of leucovorin rescue. These guidelines have allowed the administration of over 300 doses of HDMTX to patients at St. Jude Children's Research Hospital without severe toxicity, since being initiated in 1976.

The dosage of leucovorin given to patients with delayed MTX clearance must be adjusted to an appropriate level dependent upon the serum concentrations of MTX. As described in detail by Pinedo et al (21), MTX and leucovorin share the same intracellular transport mechanisms. When extracellular MTX concentrations are high relative to leucovorin concentrations, "rescue" may not be achieved because of inadequate intracellular transport of leucovorin. Previous studies (21) have demonstrated that the effects of MTX can be completely reversed by equimolar concentrations of leucovorin when extracellular MTX concentrations are $\leqslant 10^{-7}$ M. The effects of $10^{-5}$ M MTX were reversed by $10^{-3}$ M leucovorin while rescue of the toxic effects of $10^{-4}$ M MTX by $10^{-3}$ M leucovorin was not observed. Thus, leucovorin doses must be escalated to achieve serum concentrations relative to the serum concentration of MTX.

The pharmacokinetics of leucovorin have not been extensively studied in man. Limited data (96) obtained in fifteen healthy adult volunteers indicate that peak l-5-formyltetrahydrofolate (citrovorum factor) serum concentrations of $\sim 10^{-8}$ M are achieved following oral doses of 15 mg. Equivalent intramuscular doses produced peak concentrations of $\sim 5 \times 10^{-7}$ M. These studies reported peak serum concentrations of 5-methyltetrahydrofolate (a reduced folate metabolite) of $\sim 5 \times 10^{-7}$ M following oral doses and $10^{-6}$ M following intramuscular doses. Thus, the serum concentrations of total reduced folates were $<10^{-6}$ M following oral doses and $\sim 2 \times 10^{-6}$ M following IM doses of 15 mg calcium leucovorin (d,l-formyl tetrahydrofolate). The observed differences in metabolite concentrations following oral and intramuscular administration are consistent with previous studies in man (97).

Assuming a linear increase in serum concentration proportional to an increase in dosage, and estimating the dose of 15 mg to adults to be equivalent to ~10mg/m², a calcium leucovorin dosage of 100 mg/m² should yield peak concentrations of about $10^{-5}$ M and 1000 mg/m² should yield peak concentrations of ~$10^{-4}$ M. These estimated serum concentrations of reduced folates are consistent with those reported by Mehta et al (96,98) and the leucovorin dosage guidelines of Bleyer (99) (Figure 4).

Serum concentrations of both of these reduced folates decline rapidly, with a half-life of approximately 0.7 hours for citrovorum factor and 2.2 hours for 5-methyltetrahydrofolate. Thus, doses of leucovorin should be given at frequent intervals (2 to 3 hours) or by continuous infusion for patients with high MTX serum concentrations and should be continued until MTX serum concentrations approach $10^{-8}$ M (16). However, it is important to reserve escalated doses of leucovorin for only those patients at high risk for toxicity, since progressive increases in the leucovorin dosage on any schedule may not only reduce toxicity but also compromise the antitumor effect (83).

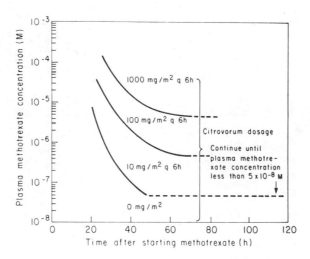

FIGURE 4. Plasma methotrexate concentration as a therapeutic guide to high-dose methotrexate therapy with citrovorum-factor rescue. (Reproduced with permission from Bleyer WA: Cancer Treat Rev 4:87–101, 1977, Reference 99)

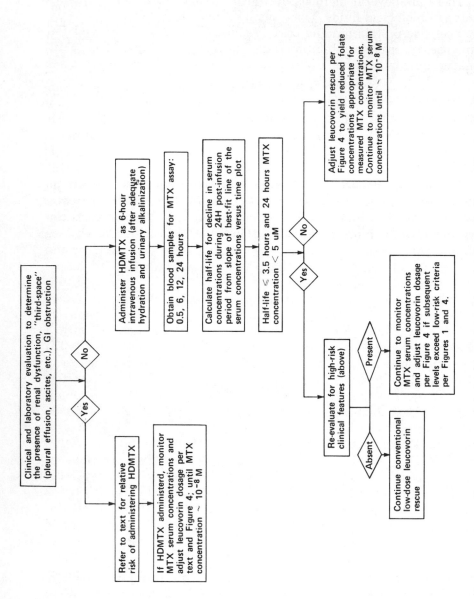

FIGURE 5. Algorithm for pharmacokinetic monitoring of high-dose methotrexate.

## ASSAY METHODS

There are several methods by which methotrexate can be quantitated in biological fluids. These methods include radioimmune assay, competitive protein binding assay, radioenzymatic assay, enzyme immunoassay, enzyme inhibition assay, and high-pressure liquid chromatography with either UV or fluorescence detection. However, these assays differ with regards to specificity, sensitivity, length of procedure, sample preparation, cost and ability to detect metabolites. No procedure is clearly superior in all respects and the relative advantages and disadvantages of each will be briefly reviewed.

### Enzyme Immunoassay (EMIT®)

The homogeneous enzyme immunoassay for MTX (100) is based on the same principles and procedures as other EMIT assays for anticonvulsants, theophylline, lidocaine and gentamicin. The reagents are available in kit-form from Syva Corporation, Palo Alto, CA. Precise timing and pipetting is facilitated by an interfaced timer-printer and an automated pipetter diluter. The assay requires only 50 μl of sample and can detect concentrations as low as $1 \times 10^{-7}$ M without modification of the standard procedures. The coefficient of variation (%) for within-run and between-run precision is about 5%. The procedure is rapid, with a "turnaround" time of 5 to 30 minutes. The specificity of this method appears to be comparable to the radioimmune assay (Diagnostic Biochemistry, San Diego, CA) and the radioenzymatic assay (New England Enzyme Center, Boston, MA) with regards to interference by the 7-OH metabolite (101). This method does not allow quantitation of metabolites, although this is probably not clinically important at present. Preliminary data (unpublished observations) suggest that the DAMPA metabolite may cross-react with the RIA (~100%) and EMIT (~100%) procedures significantly more than the radioenzymatic assay (~20%). However, a recent comparative study (102) evaluating results of clinical serum samples obtained within 24 hours after high-dose 6-hour IV infusions of MTX demonstrated no significant difference using EMIT, REA, RIA and HPLC. The advantages of this method are the rapid turnaround time, the low cost and versatility of necessary equipment, the stability of the standard curve and reagents, and the small volume of patient sample required. The major limitation at present is the inability to detect concentrations less than $1 \times 10^{-7}$ M, and the potential nonspecificity with regards to the DAMPA metabolite. However, precise manipulation of the initial dilution techniques has permitted accurate and reproducible quantitation of concentrations as low as $3 \times 10^{-8}$ M in our laboratory and significant interference with DAMPA metabolites apparently does not occur within 24 hours following high-dose IV MTX administration. The accuracy of this assay and RIA for measuring low concentrations following IV or oral administration remains to be defined. The advantages of this assay make it the currently recommended method for routine clinical monitoring of high-dose IV methotrexate. Each 100 tube kit costs $175 and will yield 40 to 50 results (in duplicate) with routine clinical use.

### Radioenzymatic Assay

This assay, previously described in detail by Myers et al (103), employs competitive binding of unlabeled and $^{125}$I-labeled MTX to the enzyme dihydrofolate reductase derived from *Lactobacillus casei*. The assay is commercially available in kit-form from New England Enzyme Center (Boston, MA) and requires a gamma counter as the major equipment investment. The assay requires 300 μl of patient serum, 2 to 4 hours to complete, and precise manual timing and pipetting. The enzyme and reagents have a shelf-life of 30 to 60 days, and a new standard curve must be performed daily. The advantage of this method is that it can quantitate as little as $1 \times 10^{-8}$ M of MTX. By using dihydrofolate reductase as the binding protein, any affinity of the MTX metabolites should be proportional to their relative activity against the target enzyme. The aminopteroic acid metabolite does not substantially interfere with the assay (101). Each 100 tube kit costs $90 and will yield 20 to 40 results (in duplicate) with routine use.

### Radioimmune Assay

A radioimmune assay utilizing $^{125}$I-methotrexate as the radioactive hapten is commercially available from Diagnostic Biochemistry Inc. (San Diego, CA). Like the radioenzymatic assay described above, this assay requires a gamma counter, and precise timing and pipetting. The procedure requires 200 μl of patient serum to assay in duplicate, and approximately 2 to 3 hours for completion. The commercially available kit has a shelf-life of 30 to 60 days, and a new standard curve must be run daily. There is apparently more cross-reactivity with MTX metabolites (i.e. DAMPA, 7-OH MTX) for this assay when compared to the radioenzymatic method (101). The difference between results by this method and the other methods is probably not of any clinical significance when high concentrations are being measured following high-dose MTX (102). However, significant interference may

TABLE 1. COMPARISON OF THE RELATIVE ADVANTAGES AND DISADVANTAGES OF THE VARIOUS METHOTREXATE ASSAY METHODS

| Analytical Method(†) | Specificity for Methotrexate* | Limit of sensitivity | Assayable Samples | | | | | Minimum Sample Volume Required | Speed | | Analysis Costs** | | Specialized Operator Training*** | Preference & Rank**** | | | Comments |
|---|---|---|---|---|---|---|---|---|---|---|---|---|---|---|---|---|---|
| | | | Metabolite Analysis | Plasma/Serum | Urine | Saliva | CSF | | 1-10 Samples | 10-100 Samples | Estimated Reagent and Tech. Cost Per Assay | Initial Equipment Costs | | Small Service | Large Service | Research | |
| HPLC | 1 | $10^{-7}$M $5\times10^{-8}$M | Yes | Yes | Yes | Yes | Yes | 1 ml for $10^{-8}$ | 2 Hr | >2 Hr | 3 | 5 | 5 | 4 | 3 | 1 | UV Detection |
| EMIT | 3 | $5\times10^{-8}$M | No | Yes | Yes | ? | Yes | 50 μl | 5 Min | 1-2 Min/Sample | 4 | 3 | 2 | 2 | 3 | 4 | Syva Co. |
| RIA | 3 | $10^{-8}$M | No | Yes | Yes | Yes | Yes | 100 μl | 2 Hr | 2 Hr | 4 | 5 | 3 | 3 | 3 | 4 | Diagnostic Biochemistry |
| REA | 2 | $10^{-8}$M | No | Yes | Yes | Yes | Yes | 300 μl | 2 Hr | 2 Hr | 4 | 5 | 3.5 | 3 | 3 | 3 | New England Enzyme |
| ENZYME | 2-3 | $2\times10^{-8}$M | No | Yes | ? | ? | Yes | 20-50 μl | 5 Min | 1-2 Min/Sample | 3 | 3 | 4 | 4 | 3 | 3 | |

* Arbitrary Ranking Scale of 1 (Excellent) to 5 (Poor).
** 1 = least expense
*** 1 = least training
**** 1 = preferred method
† (HPLC, high pressure liquid chromatography; EMIT, enzyme immunoassay; RIA, radioimmunoassay; REA, radioenzymatic assay; ENZYME, enzyme inhibition.

541

occur when low ($10^{-8}$ to $10^{-7}$ M) concentrations are being measured at later times after high-dose therapy or after oral administration, when metabolite concentrations may approach or exceed concentrations of the parent compound. Each 100 tube kit costs $75 and will yield 20 to 40 results (in duplicate) with routine clinical use.

### High-Pressure Liquid Chromatography (HPLC)

Several procedures for quantitating MTX and metabolites in biological fluids by HPLC have been published (104–106). The methods of Watson et al (104) and Wisnicki et al (106) utilize an ultraviolet detector at 315 nm and 254 nm, respectively. The reported sensitivity for both MTX and 7-OH MTX is $1 \times 10^{-7}$ M. The method of Watson et al (104) utilizes a strong anion exchange column for separation, while the Wisnicki method (106) uses a μ-Bondapak $C_{18}$ reverse-phase column for separation of urine samples and a strong anion exchange column for aqueous solutions. The total retention time for all compounds was about 12 minutes for the method of Watson et al (104). Plasma samples must also be extracted prior to analysis. The method of Watson appears to be useful for analysis of patient serum, while the method of Wisnicki was only evaluated for analysis of MTX solutions and urine. Nelson and coworkers (105) have reported an HPLC procedure which utilizes a fluorescence detector to quantitate MTX in human plasma. This procedure requires the oxidation of MTX to a fluorescent product by a five minute incubation with potassium permanganate. Separation from other fluorescent materials in plasma is then accomplished by a reversed-phase column and detection performed with excitation at 275 nm and emission cutoff at 410 nm. This procedure detected down to $2 \times 10^{-8}$ M of MTX in plasma. However, no attempt was made to separate and quantitate MTX metabolites (7-OH MTX, DAMPA) and the possible conversion of MTX and its metabolites to fluorescent compounds that are not separated chromatographically from the parent compound would substantially compromise the specificity of this procedure. If this is the case, post-column derivitization may be required to maintain the specificity while improving the sensitivity with fluorescent procedures.

### Enzyme Inhibition Assay

The enzyme inhibition assay, as described by Falk et al (107), is based on inhibition by MTX of the enzyme dihydrofolate reductase (DHRF) derived from *Lactobacillus casei*. The change in absorbance of a mixture of NADPH, DHFR and standards or unknowns is monitored over 120 seconds with a microsample spectrophotometer at 340 nm. The change in absorbance decreases linearly over the concentration range of $2 \times 10^{-8}$ M to $3 \times 10^{-7}$ M. Within-run precision is reported to be $\pm 5\%$ (CV) and day-to-day variation is ~18%. Disadvantages of this assay are that it is not commercially available in kit form, the reaction mixture (NADPH, DHFR) must be prepared fresh each day, and other inhibitors of bacterial DHFR (trimethoprim) may interfere with the assay. Most of the reagents needed for this assay, including NADPH and DHFR, are commercially available.

## Miscellaneous Assay Procedures

Several other methods for quantitating MTX in biological fluids have been published, but are rarely used. These include fluorometric (108), microbiological (109), and direct ligand-binding (110) methods.

## REFERENCES

1. Liegler DG, Henderson ES, Hahn MA and Oliverio VT: The effect of organic acids on renal clearance of methotrexate in man. Clin Pharmacol Ther 1969; 10:849–857.
2. Henderson E, Adamson R and Oliverio VT: The metabolic fate of tritiated methotrexate II, Absorption and excretion in man. Cancer Res 1965; 25:1018–1024.
3. Wan K, Huffman DH, Azarnoff DL et al: Effect of route of administration and effusion on methotrexate pharmacokinetics. Cancer Res. 1974; 34:3487–3491.
4. Freeman-Narrod M, Gerstley BJ, Engstrom PF et al: Comparison of serum concentrations of methotrexate after various routes of administration. Cancer 1975; 36:1619–1624.
5. Cohen MH, Creaven PJ, Fossieck BF et al: Effect of oral prophylactic broad spectrum nonabsorbable antibiotics on the gastrointestinal absorption of nutrients and methotrexate in small cell bronchogenic carcinoma patients. Cancer 1976; 38:1556–1559.
6. Valerino DM, John DG, Zaharko DS and Oliverio VT: Studies of the metabolism of methotrexate by intestinal flora-I. Identification and study of biological properties of the metabolite 4-amino-4-deoxy-N10-methylpteroic acid. Biochem Pharmacol 1972; 21:821–831.
7. Evans WE and Rivera G: Pharmacokinetic studies of high dose oral methotrexate in children with acute lymphocytic leukemia. Proc Amer Assoc Cancer Res 1979; 20:266 (abstract).
8. Chungi VS, Bourne DWA and Dittert LW: Drug absorption VIII: Kinetics of GI absorption of methotrexate. J Pharm Sci 1978; 67:560–561.
9. Freeman-Narrod: The pharmacology of methotrexate: in Porter and Willshaw (eds) *Methotrexate in the Treatment of Cancer*, p. 17–21. Williams and Wilkins, Baltimore 1962.
10. Shen DD and Azarnoff DL: Clinical pharmacokinetics of methotrexate. Clin Pharmacokin 1978; 3:1–13.
11. Lerne PR, Creaven PJ, Allen LM and Berman M: Kinetic model for the disposition and metabolism of moderate and high-dose methotrexate (NSC-740) in man. Cancer Chemother Rep 1975; 59:811–817.

12. Pratt CB, Howarth C, Evans WE et al: High-dose methotrexate used alone and in combination for measurable primary or metastatic osteosarcoma. Cancer Treat Rep 1980; 64:11–20.
13. Mandel MS: The synergistic effect of salicylates on methotrexate toxicity. Plast Reconstr Surg 1976; 57:733–737.
14. Zaharko DS, Dedrick RL, Bischoff KB et al: Methotrexate tissue distribution: Prediction by a mathematical model. J Natl Cancer Inst 1971; 46:775–784.
15. Bischoff KB, Dedrick RL, Zaharko DS and Longsheth JA: Methotrexate pharmacokinetics. J Pharm Sci 1971; 60:1128–1133.
16. Evans WE, Pratt CB, Taylor RH, Barker LF and Crom, WR: Pharmacokinetic monitoring of high-dose methotrexate: early recognition of high-risk patients. Cancer Chemother Pharmacol 1979; 3:161–166.
17. Evans WE, Tsiatis A, Crom, WR et al: Pharmacokinetic simulation of gastrointestinal obstruction as a mechanism of delayed clearance of high dose methotrexate. Proc Amer Coll Clin Pharmacol, Clin Research, 1980.
18. Tattersall MHN, Parker LM, Pitman SW et al: Clinical pharmacology of high-dose methotrexate (NSC-740) Cancer Chemother Rep 1975; 6 (part 3):25–29.
19. Evans WE and Pratt CB: Effect of pleural effusion of high-dose methotrexate kinetics. Clin Pharmacol Ther 1978; 23:68–72.
20. Goldman ID: Membrane transport of methotrexate (NSC-740) and other folate compounds. Relevance to rescue protocols. Cancer Chemother Rep 1975; (part 3), 6:63–72.
21. Pinedo HM, Zaharko DS, Bull JM and Chabner BA: The reversal of methotrexate cytotoxicity to mouse bone marrow cells by leucovorin and nucleosides. Cancer Res 1976; 36:4418–4424.
22. Zager RF, Frisby SA and Oliverio VT: The effects of antibiotics and cancer chemotherapy agents on cellular transport and antitumor activity of methotrexate in L1210 murine leukemia. Cancer Res 1973; 33:1670–1676.
23. Fyfe MF and Goldman ID: Characteristics of the vincristine-induced augmentation of methotrexate uptake in Ehrlich ascites tumor cells. J Biol Chem 1973; 248:5067–5073.
24. Bender RA, Bleyer WA, Frisby SA et al: Alteration of methotrexate uptake in human leukemia cells by other agents. Cancer Res 1975; 35:1305–1306.
25. Owellen RJ and Hains FD: Clinical pharmacokinetics of vincristine and vindesine as determined by radioimmunoassay (abstract). Proc Am Assoc Cancer Res 17:102 1976.
26. Owellen RJ, Root MA and Hains FD: Pharmacokinetics of vindesine and vincristine in humans. Cancer Res 1977; 37:2603–2607.
27. Warren RD, Nichols AP and Bender RA: The effect of vincristine on methotrexate uptake and inhibition of DNA synthesis by human lymphoblastoid cells. Cancer Res 1977; 37:2993–2997.
28. Shapiro WR, Young DF and Mehta BM: Methotrexate distribution in cerebrospinal fluid after intravenous, ventricular and lumbar injections. N Engl J Med 1975; 293:161–166.
29. Ushio Y, Kayakawa J and Morgami H: Uptake of trititated methotrexate by mouse brain tumors after intravenous or intrathecal administration. J Neurosurg 1974; 40:706–716.
30. Griffin TW, Rasey JS and Bleyer WA: The effect of photon irradiation on blood-brain barrier permeability to methotrexate in mice. Cancer 1977; 40:1109–1111.
31. Mellott LB: Physiochemical considerations and pharmacokinetic behavior in delivery of drugs to the central nervous system. Cancer Treat Rep 1977; 61:527–531.

32. Freeman AI, Wang JJ, Sinks LF: High-dose methotrexate in acute lymphocytic leukemia. Cancer Treat Rep 1977; 61:727–731.
33. Pitman SW and Frei E: Weekly methotrexate-calcium leucovorin rescue: Effect of alkalinization on nephrotoxicity; pharmacokinetics in the CNS; and use in CNS non-Hodgkin's lymphoma. Cancer Treat Rep 1977; 61:695–701.
34. Bratlid D and Moe PJ: Pharmacokinetics of high-dose methotrexate treatment in children. Europ J Clin Pharmacol 1978; 14:143–147.
35. Tejada F, Radomski JL, Greenhawt M and Zubrod CG: Methotrexate CSF levels during high dose methotrexate-leucovorin therapy. Proc Am Assoc Cancer Res 1977; 18:363.
36. Rosen G, Ghavimi F, Nirenberg A et al: High-dose methotrexate with citrovorum factor rescue for the treatment of central nervous system tumors in children. Cancer Treat Rep 1977; 61:681–690.
37. Fusner JE, Poplack DG, Pizzo PA and Di Chiro G: Leukoencephalopathy following chemotherapy for rhabdomyosarcoma: Reversibility of cerebral changes demonstrated by computed tomography. J Pediatr 1977; 91:77–79.
38. Price RA and Jamieson PA: The central nervous system in childhood leukemia. Cancer 1975; 35:306–318.
39. Jacobs SA, Stoller RG, Chabner BA and Johns DG: 7-hydroxymethotrexate as a urinary metabolite in human subjects and rhesus monkeys receiving high dose methotrexate. J Clinical Invest 1976; 57:534–538.
40. Johns DG and Loo TL: Metabolite of 4-amino-4-deoxy-N$^{10}$methyl pteroylglutamic acid (methotrexate). J Pharm Sci 1967; 56:356–359.
41. Wang YM, Howell SK, Smith RG et al: Effect of metabolism on pharmacokinetics and toxicity of high dose methotrexate therapy in children. Proc Amer Soc Clin Oncol 1979; 20:334.
42. Stoller RG, Jacobs SA, Drake JC, Lutz RJ and Chabner BA: Pharmacokinetics of high-dose methotrexate (NSC-740). Cancer Chemother Rep 1975; (part 3), 6:19–24.
43. Frei F III: Methotrexate revisited. Med Pediatr Oncol 1976; 2:227–241.
44. Baugh CM, Krumdieck CL and Nair MG: Polygammaglutamyl metabolites of methotrexate. Biochemical and Biophysical Research Communications 1973; 52:27–34.
45. Whitehead VM, Perrault MM and Stelener S: Tissue-specific synthesis of methotrexate polyglutamates in the rat. Cancer Res 1975; 35:2985–2990.
46. Pratt CB, Robert D, Shanks EC and Warmath EL: Clinical trials and pharmacokinetics of intermittent high-dose methotrexate "leucovorin rescue" for children with malignant tumors. Cancer Res 1974; 34:3326–3331.
47. Freeman MV: The fluorometric measurement of the absorption, distribution and excretion of single doses of 4-amino-10-methyl-pteroylglytamic acid (amethopterin) in man. J Pharmacol Exp Ther 1958; 122:154–162.
48. Zurek WZ, Ojima Y, Anderson LL, Collins GJ, Oberfield RA and Sullivan RD: Pharmacologic studies of methotrexate in man. Gyn Obst 1968; 126:331–338.
49. Huffman DH, Wan SH, Azarnoff DL and Hoogstraten B: Pharmacokinetics of methotrexate. Clin Pharmacol Ther 1973; 14:572–579.
50. Pratt CB, Roberts O, Shanks F and Warmath FI: Response, toxicity and pharmacokinetics of high-dose methotrexate (NSC-740) with citrovorum factor (NSC-3500) rescue for children with osteosarcoma and other malignant tumors. Cancer Chemother Rep 1975; 6:13–18.
51. Wang Y, Lantin E and Sutow WW: Methotrexate in blood, urine and cerebrospinal fluid of children receiving high doses by infusion. Clin Chem 1976; 22:1053–1056.

52. Isacoff WH, Morrison PF, Aroesty J et al: Pharmacokinetics of high-dose methotrexate with citrovorum factor rescue. Cancer Treat Rep 1977; 61:1665–1674.

53. Shen DD and Azarnoff DL: Clinical pharmacokinetics of methotrexate. Clin Pharmacokin 1978; 3:1–13.

54. Bourke RS, Cheda G, Bremer A, Watanabe O and Tower DB: Inhibition of renal tubular transport of methotrexate by probenicid. Cancer Res 1975; 35:110–116.

55. Reich SD, Bachur NR, Goebel RH et al: A pharmacokinetic model for high-dose methotrexate infusions in man. J Pharmacokin Biopharm 1977; 5:421–433.

56. Calvert AH, Bondy PK and Hamap KR: Some observations on the human pharmacology of methotrexate. Cancer Treat Rep 1977; 61:1647–1656.

57. Wang YM, Sutow WW, Romsdahl MM et al: Age-related pharmacokinetics of high-dose methotrexate in patients with osteosarcoma. Cancer Treat Rep 1979; 63:405–410.

58. Romolo JL, Goldberg NH, Hande KR et al: Effect of hydration on plasma-methotrexate levels. Cancer Treat Rep 1977; 61:1393–1396.

59. Bleyer WA: Clinical pharmacology of methotrexate. Cancer 1978; 41:36–51.

60. Chan H, Evans WE and Pratt CB: Recovery from toxicity associated with high-dose methotrexate: prognostic factors. Cancer Treat Rep 1977; 61:797–804.

61. Strum WB and Liem HH: Hepatic uptake intracellular protein binding and biliary excretion of amethopterin. Biochem Pharmacol 1977; 26:1235–1240.

62. Creaven PJ, Hansen HH, Alford DA and Allen LM: Methotrexate in liver and bile after intravenous dosage in man. Brit J Cancer 1973; 28:589–591.

63. Bleyer WA and Dedrick RL: Clinical pharmacology of intrathecal methotrexate I. Pharmacokinetics in non-toxic patients after lumbar injection. Cancer Treat Rep 1977; 61:703–708.

64. Bleyer WA: Clinical pharmacology of intrathecal methotrexate. II. An improved dosage schedule derived from age-related pharmacokinetics. Cancer Treat Rep 1977; 61:1419–1425.

65. Bleyer WA, Drake JC and Chabner BA: Pharmacokinetics and neurotoxicity of intrathecal methotrexate therapy. N Engl J Med 1973; 289:770–773.

66. Rubin R, Owens E, Rall D: Transport of methotrexate by choroid plexus. Cancer Res 1968; 28:689–694.

67. Spector R: Inhibition of methotrexate transport from cerebrospinal fluid by probenecid. Cancer Treat Rep 1976; 60:913–916.

68. Tejada F and Zubrod CG: Vincristine effect on methotrexate cerebrospinal fluid concentration. Cancer Treat Rep 1979; 63:143–145.

69. Rieselbach RE et al: Subarachnoid distribution of drugs after lumbar injection. N Engl J Med 1962; 267:1273.

70. Werkheiser WC: Specific binding of 4-amino folic acid analogues by folic acid reductase. J Biol Chem 1961; 2236:888–893.

71. Goldman D: Analysis of the cytotoxic determinants for methotrexate: A role for free intracellular drug. Cancer Chemother Rep 1975; (part 3) 6:51–61.

72. Goldman D: Effects of methotrexate on cellular metabolism: Some critical elements in the drug-cell interaction. Cancer Treat Rep 1977; 61:549–558.

73. Sirotnak FF: Further evidence for a basis of selective activity and relative responsiveness during antifolate therapy of murine tumors. Cancer Res 1975; 35:1737–1744.

74. Goldman D, Gupha V, White JC et al: Exchangeable intracellular methotrexate levels in the presence and absence of vincristine at extracellular drug concentra-

tions relevant to those achieved in high-dose methotrexate-folinic acid rescue protocols. Cancer Res 1976; 36:276–279.

75. Chabner BA and Young RC: Threshold methotrexate concentrations for in-vivo inhibition of DNA synthesis in normal and tumorous target tissues. J Clin Invest 1973; 52:1804–1811.

76. Zaharko DS, Dedrick RL, Peale AL, Drake JC and Lutz RJ: Relative toxicity of methotrexate in several tissues of mice bearing lewis lung carcinoma. J Pharm Exp Ther 1974; 189:585–592.

77. Zaharko DS, Fung WP and Yang KH: Relative biochemical aspects of low and high doses of methotrexate in mice. Cancer Res 1977; 37:1602–1607.

78. Young RC and Chabner BA: An in-vivo method for monitoring differential effects of chemotherapy on target tissue in animals and man: Correlation with plasma pharmacokinetics. Cancer Res 1973; 52:92a.

79. Pinedo HM and Chabner BA: Role of drug concentration, duration of exposure and endogenous metabolites in determining methotrexate cytotoxicity. Cancer Treat Rep 1977; 61:709–715.

80. Levitt M, Mosher MS and Deconti RC: Improved therapeutic index of methotrexate with "leucovorin rescue". Cancer Res 1973; 33:1729–1734.

81. Bertino JR: Techniques in cancer chemotherapy. Use of leucovorin and other rescue agents after methotrexate treatment. Semin Oncol 1977; 4:203–216.

82. Goldie JH, Price LA, and Harrap KR: Methotrexate toxicity: Correlation with duration of administration, plasma levels, dose and excretion pattern. Eur J Cancer 1972; 8:409–414.

83. Sirotnak FM, Moccio DM and Dorick DM: Optimization of high-dose methotrexate and leucovorin rescue therapy in L1210 leukemia and sarcoma 180 murine tumor models. Cancer Res 1978; 38:345–353.

84. Von Hoff DD, Penta JS, Helman LJ et al: Incidence of drug-related deaths secondary to high-dose methotrexate and citrovorum factor administration. Cancer Treat Rep 1977; 61:745–748.

85. Jaffe N and Traggis D: Toxicity of high-dose methotrexate (NSC-740) and citrovorum factor (NSC-3590) in osteogenic sarcoma. Cancer Chemother Rep 1975; (part 3), 6:31–36.

86. Tattersall MHN, Parker LM, Pitman SW and Frei E: Clinical pharmacology of high-dose methotrexate. Cancer Treat Rep 1975; (part 3) 6:25–29.

87. Isacoff WH, Townsend CT, Eilber FR et al: High-dose methotrexate therapy of solid tumors: observations relating to clinical toxicity. Med Pediatr Oncol 1976; 2:319–325.

88. Isacoff WH, Morrison PF, Aroesty J et al: Pharmacokinetics of high-dose methotrexate with citrovorum factor rescue. Cancer Treat Rep 1977; 61:1665–1674.

89. Nirenberg A, Mosende C, Mehta BM, Gisolfi AL and Rosen G: High dose methotrexate with CF rescue: Predictive value of serum methotrexate concentrations and corrective measures to avert toxicity. Cancer Treat Rep 1977; 61:779–783.

90. Stoller RC, Hande KR, Jacobs SA, Rosenberg SA and Chabner BA: Use of plasma pharmacokinetics to predict and prevent methotrexate toxicity. N Engl J Med 1977; 297:630–634.

91. Cohen HJ and Jaffe N: Pharmacokinetics and clinical studies of 24-h infusions of high-dose methotrexate. Cancer Chemother Pharmacol 1978; 1:61–64.

92. Pochedly C: Neurotoxicity due to CNS therapy for leukemia. Med Pediatr Oncol 1977; 3:101–115.

93. Ettinger LJ, Freeman AI and Creaven PJ: Intrathecal methotrexate overdose without neurotoxicity. Cancer 1978; 41:1270–1273.
94. Jurrgens H, Kosloff C, Nirenberg A et al: Clinical and pharmacokinetic prognostic factors in the response of primary osteogenic sarcoma to preoperative chemotherapy. (High dose methotrexate with citrovorum factor rescue). Proc. Symposium on Sarcoma of Soft Tissue and Bone in Childhood, Orlando, FL, 1979.
95. Rosen G, Nirenberg A et al: Osteogenic sarcoma: Three year disease free survival in excess of 80% with combination chemotherapy including effective high dose methotrexate with citrovorum factor rescue. Proc. Symposium on Sarcoma of Soft Tissue and Bone in Childhood, Orlando, FL., 1979.
96. Mehta BM, Gisolfi AL, Hutchinson DJ et al: Serum distribution of citrovorum factor and 5-methyltetrahydrofolate following oral and IM administration of calcium leucovorin in normal adults. Cancer Treat Rep 1978; 62:345–350.
97. Nixon PF and Bertino JR: Effective absorption and utilization of oral formyltetrahydrofolate in man. N Engl J Med 1972; 286:175–179.
98. Mehta BM, Rosen G and Hutchinson DJ: Serum distribution of 5-methyltetrahydrofolate following high dose methotrexate-leucovorin rescue regimen in osteogenic sarcoma. Proc Amer Assoc Cancer Res 1979; 20:127.
99. Bleyer WA: Methotrexate clinical pharmacology, current status and therapeutic guidelines. Cancer Treat Rev 1977; 4:87–101.
100. Gushaw JB and Miller JG: Homogeneous enzyme immunoassay for methotrexate in serum. Clin Chem 1978; 24:1032.
101. Donehower RC, Hande KR, Drake JC and Chabner BA: Presence of 2,4-diamino-$N^{10}$-methylpteroic acid after high-dose methotrexate. Clin Pharmacol Ther 1979; 26:63–72.
102. Buice RG, Evans WE, Nicholas CA et al: Evaluation of the enzyme mediated immunoassay (EMIT), radioenzyme assay (REA) and radioimmunoassay (RIA) of methotrexate using HPLC as a standard. Clin Chem 1980 (In Press).
103. Myers C, Kippman M, Eliot H and Chabner B: Competitive protein binding assay for methotrexate. Proc Natl Acad Sci 1975; 72:3683–3686.
104. Watson E, Cohen JL and Chan KK: High pressure liquid chromatographic determination of methotrexate and its major metabolite, 7-hydroxymethotrexate, in human plasma. Cancer Treat Rep 1978; 62:381–387.
105. Nelson JA, Harris BA, Decker WJ and Fargutar D: Analysis of methotrexate in human plasma by high-pressure liquid chromatography with fluorescence detection. Cancer Res 1977; 37:3970–3973.
106. Wisnicki JL, Tong WP and Ludlum DB: Analysis of methotrexate and 7-hydroxymethotrexate by high-pressure liquid chromatography. Cancer Treat Rep 1978; 62:529–532.
107. Falk LC, Clark DR, Kalman SM et al: Enzymatic assay for methotrexate in serum and cerebrospinal fluid. Clin Chem 1976; 22:785–788.
108. Freeman MV: A fluorometric method for the measurement of a 4-amino-10-methylpteroylglutamic acid (amethopterin) in plasma. J Pharmacol Exp Ther 1957; 120:1–7.
109. Noble WC, White PM and Baker H: Assay of therapeutic doses of MTX in body fluids of patients with psoriasis. J Invest Dermatol 1975; 64:69–74.
110. Arons E, Rothenberg SP, da Costa M et al: A direct ligand-binding radioassay for the measurement of methotrexate in tissues and biological fluids. Cancer Res 1975; 35:2033–2037.

# 17

# Tricyclic Antidepressants

C. Lindsay DeVane, Pharm.D.

## INTRODUCTION/BACKGROUND

Several classes of drugs are useful in the pharmacologic treatment of depression, a mental illness characterized by varying degrees of morbidity, worldwide distribution, and requiring a large expenditure of health care resources. The tricyclic antidepressants (tricyclics) ameliorate various symptoms of depression and are unrivaled as primary drugs used in its treatment. Current research suggests that the term "depression" may in time become as vague a description of a single disease entity as "infection" once was (1). The tricyclics have been found to be generally beneficial in study groups with a variety of patient characteristics (2), but efficacy is less than 100% in any single group. This situation demands optimal dosing for the best therapeutic outcome.

Until recently, questions of dosing received little attention. As assay methodology advanced, large variability in plasma concentrations among patients taking similar doses of tricyclics was revealed (3,4). Answers to questions of optimal dosing have been sought in pharmacokinetic research. This chapter will review our progress and suggest areas from which useful knowledge may be forthcoming.

The name "tricyclic" derives from the three-ring structure shared by this group of drugs. Seven tricyclics are available by prescription in the United States, and the structures of six are shown in Figure 1. Trimipramine (not shown) has a structure identical to that of imipramine except for an additional methyl group in its side chain. The tricyclics can be subclassed into dibenzazepines, dibenzocycloheptadienes, and a dibenzoxepin according to differences in bridging between their benzyl rings. This classification is rarely heard as all seven drugs possess similar physicochemical and pharmacologic properties. For example, as aliphatic amines, these compounds all have pKa values of 8.4 or greater and are therefore highly ionized at pH

7.4. They share antihistaminic and anticholinergic properties and inhibit the reuptake of norepinephrine into adrenergic nerves through a saturable, energy-dependent, active transport system known as the "amine pump". A similar action relates to inhibition of neuronal reuptake of 5-hydroxytryptamine (serotonin). The importance of structure-activity relationships and the neurotransmitter reuptake predominantly inhibited by each tricyclic has been discussed in relation to the "amine hypothesis of depression" (5,6) and is fully reviewed elsewhere (7).

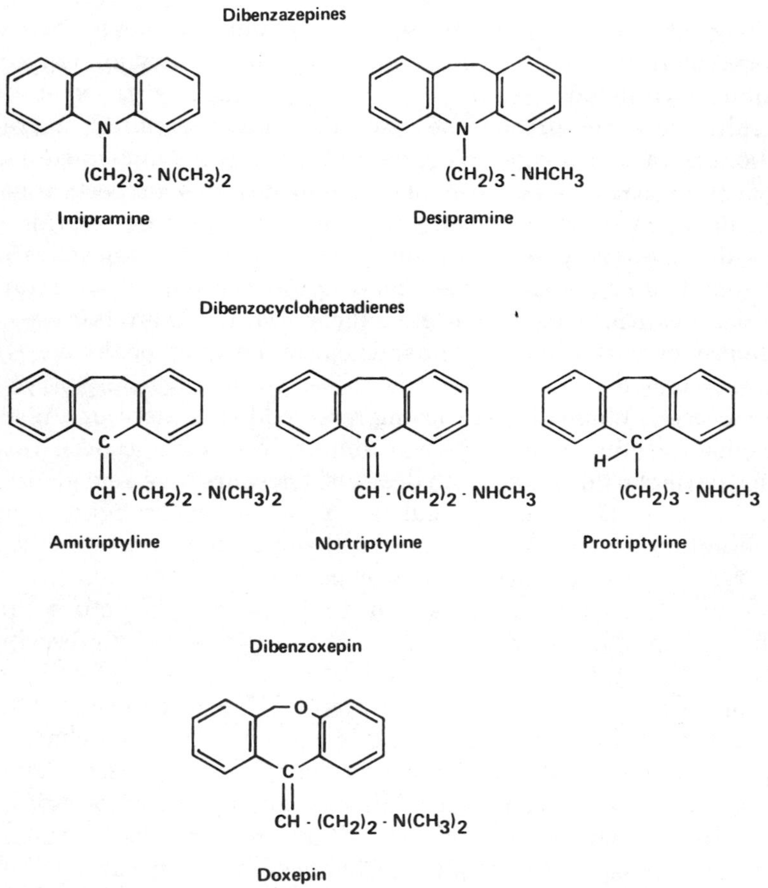

FIGURE 1. Tricyclic antidepressants available in the United States.

## Absorption

The pharmacokinetic properties of the tricyclics are summarized in Table 1. Trimipramine, for which detailed information is not yet available, should possess pharmacokinetic properties similar to imipramine. The tricyclics are rapidly absorbed when taken orally with peak concentrations usually occurring 2 to 6 hours after the dose. An exception is protriptyline, as peak concentrations may not be reached for 12 hours after an oral dose (8). There have been no studies which have specifically examined the influence of food on tricyclic absorption, but in the fasting state, absorption appears complete as suggested by nearly identical urinary recovery of nortriptyline metabolites following oral and intramuscular administration (9), and equal recovery of radioactivity in the urine following oral and intravenous doses of radiolabeled nortriptyline (10) and imipramine (11). Only 2% of an oral radioactive dose of protriptyline was excreted in the feces in a 10-day collection period (12).

Despite the evidence for complete oral absorption, the systemic availability of tricyclics is low. Comparison of area under the concentration-time curve for oral and intravenous doses in the same subjects indicates an availability of drug between 30 and 70% (10,11). This phenomenon is termed the "first pass effect" and is explained by the fact that all the absorbed drug in the portal vein must pass through the liver where it can be metabolized before reaching the systemic circulation (13). This is compatible with earlier and higher metabolite concentrations from oral compared to parenteral administration. Differences in metabolite-parent drug ratios may assume importance in dosing as some metabolites formed during the first pass of tricyclics are active as antidepressants and will be discussed below.

## Distribution

Tricyclics are highly lipophilic compounds which distribute widely in the body. Steady-state volumes of distribution may be as large as 60 L/kg (Table 1), so most of an ingested dose will thus be present in body tissues and fluids other than plasma. Linnoila et al (14) found a strong positive correlation between drug concentration in plasma and erythrocytes, but with six-fold interindividual variation. Imipramine, desipramine, and probably the other tricyclics pass into breast milk, and women who require tricyclic therapy are advised not to breast feed (15). Animal studies indicate that tricyclics concentrate in cerebral and cardiac tissue (16,17), and doxepin has a special affinity for the eye (18). Post-mortem toxicological examinations of brain tissue from overdosed human patients have revealed microgram per gram amounts of imipramine and its metabolites compared to nanogram per milliliter concentrations in plasma (19).

Distribution is closely related to protein binding. It was earlier assumed that tricyclics were highly bound to plasma proteins, principally albumin, with little intersubject variation (20). Recent reports have focused on the importance of binding to erythrocytes and proteins other than albumin in plasma (21,22). The binding of imipramine is higher in plasma of hyperlipoproteinemic patients and correlates well to plasma cholesterol and triglyceride concentrations (23). Alpha-1-acid glycoprotein (AGP) concentrations have been shown to negatively correlate to individual differences in the free fraction of imipramine in healthy volunteers (21). AGP concentrations may be altered in short and long-term inflammation, malignancy, and hepatic and renal disease (24,25). The plasma protein binding of tricyclics may therefore vary widely in patients with these conditions, and has not been systematically studied. Also, tricyclic binding in depressed psychiatric patients has not been thoroughly studied in relation to the concentration of AGP.

Protein binding differences among patients will exert an influence on the free fraction of drug available to the receptor site and has been suggested to account for part of the variability in response to treatment (26). This raises the question of whether clinical studies should correlate free or total plasma tricyclic concentrations to clinical effect. Most previous surveys have measured free plus bound tricyclic concentration. Recently, Potter et al (27) found that the concentration of imipramine in cerebrospinal fluid, which is an indirect estimate of free drug *in vivo,* was closely correlated to imipramine concentration in plasma at steady-state. This observation leads to the conclusion that measurement of total tricyclic plasma concentration is usually an adequate reflection of free drug available to bind to brain receptor sites. This issue will likely remain controversial as the methodology used in protein binding studies greatly influences the results (28).

## Metabolism

Tricyclics are cleared from the body primarily by hepatic biotransformation (29). Figure 2 illustrates the major metabolic pathways in man of imipramine, which has been the most thoroughly studied tricyclic. The pathways of quantitative importance are demethylation to the active secondary amine, desmethylimipramine (desipramine), aromatic hydroxylation of imipramine and desipramine at the 2-carbon position, and glucuronide conjugation followed by excretion in the

TABLE 1. PHARMACOKINETIC PROPERTIES OF TRICYCLIC ANTIDEPRESSANTS

| Drugs | Percent Bioavailable | t½, hr[a] | $V_D$, L/kg[b] | $Cl_M$, ml/min[c] | Fraction[d] Bound | References |
|---|---|---|---|---|---|---|
| Imipramine | 29–77 | 8–28 | 9.3–23 | 700–1700 | .63–.96 | 11,20,27,43,139,161 |
| Desipramine | 33–51[e] | 12–28 | 24–60 | 1300–2800 | .73–.92 | 20,130,139,140 |
| Amitriptyline | 30–60[e] | 9–46 | 6.4–36 | 320–630 | .92–.97 | 20,139,141–143 |
| Nortriptyline | 46–70 | 18–56 | 15–23 | 290–1330 | .87–.93 | 20,130,139,144–146,161 |
| Doxepin | 13–45[e] | 8–25 | 9–33 | 690–1020 | — | 131 |
| Protriptyline | 75–90[e] | 54–198 | 15–31 | 140–390 | .90–.94 | 8,20,147 |

[a] t½ = Biologic half-life
[b] $V_D$ = Volume of distribution, either in the steady-state or during the slowest phase of elimination
[c] $Cl_M$ = Plasma clearance
[d] Fraction bound to human plasma proteins
[e] Calculated, using an average hepatic blood flow

553

urine. When imipramine is administered orally, 2-hydroxylated imipramine (2-OH-IMI), desipramine (DMI), and 2-hydroxylated desipramine (2-OH-DMI) rapidly appear in plasma due to their formation
during the first pass through the liver (unpublished observations).
The time course of these metabolites in plasma following a single oral
dose of imipramine can be seen in Figure 3. Minor pathways of imipramine metabolism include dealkylation of the entire side chain to
form imidodibenzyl, further demethylation of desipramine to the primary amine, didesmethylimipramine, and hydroxylation at the 10-
carbon position. N-oxidation, by which imipramine-N-oxide is formed,
occurs as a reversible reaction. Other metabolic transformations occur
and unidentified radioactivity is excreted in the urine after an oral
dose of radiolabeled imipramine. This extensive metabolism results in
less than 5% of an oral imipramine dose excreted unchanged in the
urine (30).

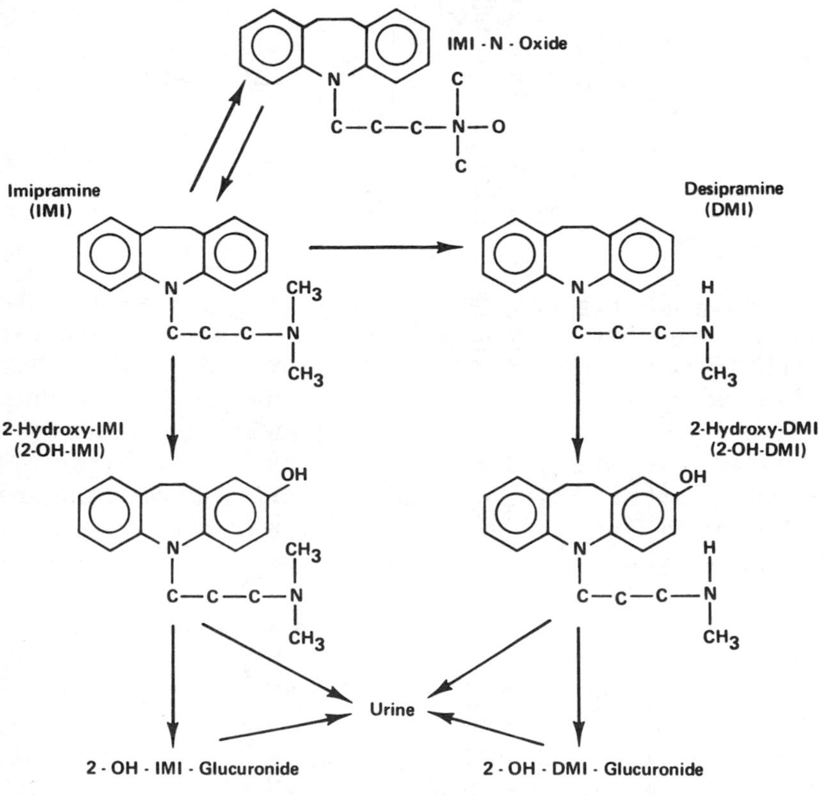

FIGURE 2.  Major pathways of imipramine metabolism in man.

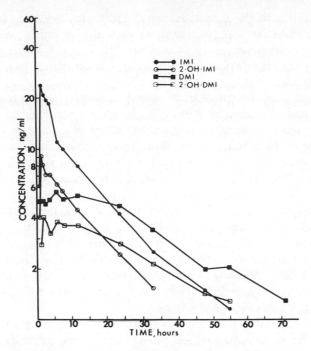

FIGURE 3. Plasma concentrations of imipramine and its major metabolites (see text) following a single 50 mg oral dose.

The metabolism of the other tricyclics is similar to that of imipramine. Amitriptyline, also a tertiary amine, is demethylated to a secondary amine metabolite, nortriptyline. In contrast to the aromatic hydroxylation of the dibenzazepines, the dibenzocycloheptadienes (amitriptyline, nortriptyline, protriptyline) preferentially undergo aliphatic hydroxylation, at the 10-carbon position. These hydroxylated metabolites are also efficiently conjugated and excreted in the urine (31). Doxepin undergoes demethylation to its secondary amine metabolite, desmethyldoxepin, and further conversion to analogous imipramine metabolites (18).

The site of tricyclic metabolism appears to be exclusively in the liver. An early study found imipramine to be demethylated by lower gastrointestinal contents which were obtained from autopsied humans (32). This finding suggests that pre-systemic metabolism could occur before drug reaches the liver. More recently, Dencker et al (33) studied imipramine absorption and metabolism in man by portal vein catheterization and could find no evidence for demethylation of imipra-

mine occurring in the intestinal wall. However, evidence for enterohepatic circulation of imipramine and desipramine was found.
Metabolism which occurs at sites other than in the liver, such as in
the pulmonary circulation, is so small by comparison it can be considered negligible.

Studies of tricyclic metabolism have demonstrated cytochrome P-
450 catalyzed biotransformation (34). Based on response to metabolic
inhibitors used in rat liver preparations, Perel et al (35) concluded
that the demethylation, N-oxidation, and aromatic hydroxylation reactions are independent pathways. This implies that variability in the
rate of tricyclic metabolism may occur from either inhibition or stimulation of several microsomal enzyme systems.

The rates of tricyclic metabolism vary widely, both among drugs
and patients. It can be appreciated (Table 1) that half-lives vary from
less than 12 hours to greater than 190 hours. A large variability in
plasma concentration, more than a 30-fold difference, has been documented in studies of patients taking similar doses of the same tricyclic.
The milligram per kilogram daily dose is thus not a reliable guide to
steady-state plasma concentrations.

Active metabolites are important for this class of drugs. Table 2
indicates the metabolites which have documented or suspected antidepressant activity in man. The ratio of parent tricyclic to its active
metabolite varies widely. The ratio at steady-state of imipramine to
desipramine has been reported to vary from 0.07 to 5.5 with mean
values of 0.47 and 0.70 reported in two studies (36,37). Thus, administration of imipramine results in a greater proportion of desipramine
in plasma at steady-state for the majority of patients. The amitrip-
tyline-nortriptyline ratio, calculated from concentrations reported in
the two largest amitriptyline studies (38,97) are 0.83 and 1.16. One
reason for these larger values is that amitriptyline may not be demethylated as effectively as imipramine. The implication of variable
demethylation is that total pharmacologic effect can vary between
patients with identical total drug plus metabolite concentration, but
having different proportions of parent drug-active metabolites. This
is because each active metabolite inhibits neurotransmitter re-uptake
to a different degree than its parent compound. These differences may
assume clinical importance if depressive subtypes of patients are identified that respond preferentially to inhibition of either serotonin or
norepinephrine reuptake (39).

The metabolism of tricyclics appears to proceed by linear pharmacokinetics in the usual dosage range. Support for this statement comes
from studies predicting steady-state concentrations of nortriptyline

TABLE 2.  ACTIVE METABOLITES OF TRICYCLIC ANTIDEPRESSANTS

| Administered Drug | Active Metabolites |
| --- | --- |
| Imipramine | 2-hydroxy imipramine<br>desipramine<br>2-hydroxy desipramine |
| Desipramine | 2-hydroxy desipramine |
| Amitriptyline | nortriptyline<br>10-hydroxy nortriptyline |
| Nortriptyline | 10-hydroxy nortriptyline |
| Doxepin | desmethyldoxepin<br>(cis & trans isomers) |

and imipramine from single doses (40–43). A recent study of imipramine metabolism in the perfused liver preparation suggests that saturation of desipramine metabolism can occur in rats (44), but at concentrations generally not achieved in humans. Evidence for nonlinear metabolism in man is limited. In a case report where high doses of desipramine were used to treat a recalcitrant patient, a 14-fold increase in plasma concentration resulted from less than a 4-fold increase in dosage (45). This report is suggestive of metabolic saturation; however, it is unlikely that 500 mg doses, as was used to treat this patient, will be widely utilized in the absence of plasma concentration monitoring. Nevertheless, saturation of tricyclic metabolic pathways may occur in situations of inadvertent or intentional overdosage, and long observation periods are recommended for these patients.

## Factors Influencing Plasma Concentration

Good agreement was found within monozygotic (identical) but not in dizygotic (fraternal) twins in the half-life and volume of distribution of nortriptyline (46), indicating that tricyclic disposition is influenced by common genetic factors. Nies et al (47) found a significant age associated increase in steady-state plasma concentrations of the tertiary amines imipramine and amitriptyline, but not with the secondary amines desipramine and nortriptyline in patients older than 65. Ziegler and Biggs (48) found no dependence of the steady-state of amitriptyline or nortriptyline on age, but their study divided patients into groups older and younger than 40. Reanalyzed data (49) from a Danish study (50) confirms an age associated increase in steady-state concentrations of imipramine, but this factor alone may not explain the subtle differences in antidepressant response associated with aging (51). The effects of aging on the plasma concentrations of the other tricyclics have not been reported.

Black patients have been reported to achieve significantly higher nortriptyline plasma concentrations than white patients (48). Although black patients may respond more rapidly to tricyclic antidepressant effects than white (52), any firm conclusion regarding race related differences in tricyclic disposition awaits further documentation. The same is true for sex. Females show a differential response from males, such as the improvement produced by addition of thyroid hormone during antidepressant therapy (53,63), but there are no clear demonstrable differences between the sexes in tricyclic pharmacokinetics (48).

Tobacco smoking has been reported to markedly diminsh plasma concentrations of imipramine and desipramine (54), but does not affect nortriptyline (55). This inconsistency may be related to the differences in the major biotransformation pathways involved with these drugs. There are no data available for the other tricyclics but, generally, tobacco smoking can be expected to have either no effect or to stimulate metabolism, as there are no documented instances of metabolic inhibition of drugs in man from smoking tobacco (56).

Tricyclic disposition has not been systematically studied in regard to specific disease states. The higher steady-state plasma concentrations and slower clearance of nortriptyline in depressed patients (57) compared to normal volunteers (10,46,58) raises a pertinent question of how applicable pharmacokinetic data derived from normals reflects tricyclic disposition in depressed patients. As tricyclic clearance may be dependent upon hepatic blood flow, the possibility of reduced clearance in "retarded" depressed patients, whose psychomotor activity (and possibly hepatic blood flow) is reduced, makes this a reasonable research question. Hepatic disease is expected to alter the clearance of tricyclics, but this has not yet been reported. In patients with alcoholic liver disease, acute intoxication should inhibit metabolism while chronic ingestion of alcohol may cause a proliferation of enzymes within the endoplasmic reticulum and increase metabolism.

Other drugs alter tricyclic metabolism. Most phenothiazines and haloperidol cause an inhibition of tricyclic metabolism resulting in an increase in tricyclic plasma concentration (59). This effect is dose related and unpredictable. The same effect is produced by methylphenidate (60). Barbiturates predictably increase tricyclic metabolism while benzodiazepines, fortunately, have no effect (61).

TABLE 3. FACTORS REPORTED TO AFFECT TRICYCLIC
ANTIDEPRESSANT PLASMA CONCENTRATION

| Lower | No Effect | Raise |
|---|---|---|
| Barbiturates | Benzodiazepines | Aging |
| Smoking | Fluphenazine | Methylphenidate |
| Chloral Hydrate | L-triiodothyronine | Chloramphenicol |
| Trihexyphenidyl | | Haloperidol |
| Acidic Urine pH | | Phenothiazines |
| | | Weight Loss |
| | | Basic Urine pH |

In summary, the metabolism of tricyclics is remarkably variable
among patients, and is subject to perturbation by social and environmental influences. Some factors known to influence tricyclic plasma
concentrations are listed in Table 3.

## CONCENTRATION VERSUS RESPONSE AND TOXICITY

Since the first account of imipramine's clinical effects in 1958 (62),
it was recognized that tricyclics have a delayed onset of therapeutic
effects, and that all patients treated do not benefit. Efforts to increase
the onset of beneficial effects and increase efficacy have included
concomitant administration of thyroid hormones (53,63), and methylphenidate (60), once daily therapy (64,65), high dose therapy (66),
intramuscular therapy (67), and now, plasma concentration monitoring (68,69). Despite the extensive clinical use of these drugs, the
number of studies relating plasma concentration to clinical effects is
sparce. The bulk of published concentration effect studies for tricyclics
concern the antidepressant effect in adults. There are some data relating plasma concentration to toxicity and side effects, but little data
for enuresis and childhood psychiatric disorders, where tricyclics are
increasingly used.

### Research Methodology for Antidepressant Effect

The studies relating plasma concentration to antidepressant effect
can be divided into those in which a relationship was found and those
in which no simple relationship was found (Table 4). The apparent
conflict in findings can be criticized on the basis of patient selection,

differences in design of trials, sample handling, and assay methodology. These studies have recently been comprehensively reviewed (70) and a brief summary will be given here. One study will be examined to illustrate design methodology as clinicians will be continually faced with evaluating the results of future studies.

A representative example of well designed research for correlating plasma concentration to antidepressant effect is the multi-center trial of Reisby and Gram et al (50,71). Of primary consideration is patient inclusion and exclusion criteria. Low reliabilities have generally been reported for psychiatrists' categorization of their patients (72). This is due to differences in training, experience, and clinical orientation. As all statistical tests assume homogeniety among subjects in the treatment group, the extent to which investigators go to assemble a homogenous group will increase the probability of finding the true relationship between plasma concentration and effect. It is appropriate to use rating scales such as the Beck depression inventory (73) and the Hamilton rating scale (74), which have high interrater reliability (75) to assess the intensity of depression and follow change in symptomatology. These widely utilized scales allow objective measures of clinical outcome and assume international relevance. This is important as 74% of the patients represented in Table 4 are from studies originating outside the United States.

The inclusion of a placebo is necessary to exclude spontaneous responders who would otherwise obscure the plasma concentration effect correlation. The same is true for non-responders, and exclusion criteria in the present study extended to patients who had depression of more than 12 months duration. These patients would be less likely to respond at any plasma concentration. It should be kept in mind that a major goal of plasma concentration effect correlation studies is to define the concentration range at which patients who will respond, do respond.

Reisby and Gram also excluded some patients with delusions and hallucinations. Patients with these depressive characteristics may define a group of depressed patients who are appropriately treated with electroconvulsive therapy and are less likely than others to respond to tricyclics (76). As psychiatric research becomes more sophisticated in terms of identifying subgroups of drug responding patients, correlations of plasma concentration to response should become better defined.

Other considerations in study design include maintaining patients drug-free except for the tricyclic, and controlling dosage. A constant dosage is necessary to help define the therapeutic window, i.e., to have a broad range of plasma concentrations over which to evaluate response. This range becomes constricted if dosage is adjusted during therapy (77).

Appropriate timing and handling of blood samples are necessary for reproducibility of results. Only at steady-state, i.e., when drug has accumulated in the body where elimination equals daily intake, does a plasma concentration reflect equilibrium between free drug in plasma and at the site of action. The time to reach approximate steady-state on a constant dosage is four to five half-lives, or a minimum of one week. For research, this time is extended to two weeks to insure inclusion of possible slow eliminators. This recommendation holds for all tricyclics except protriptyline, which with its longer half-life could continue to accumulate in the body for 3 to 4 weeks or longer. Sampling should be performed during the elimination phase of the drug, which is a minimum of 8 hours after the last dose. The most convenient time is in the morning hours before the first dose of the day. Plasma concentrations determined at this time are comparable between patients on a once-a-day or three times-a-day dosage schedule (78,79). All samples should be analyzed in the same laboratory, especially for the results of a multicenter study to be meaningful. The assay should be sensitive, specific, and measure all active metabolites of interest.

The development of the full antidepressant effects of tricyclics is often preceded by a lag period lasting up to several weeks. Thus, a minimum of 3 to 4 weeks should be allowed for patients to respond before correlating plasma concentration to effect. In the Reisby and Gram study, correlations were made at 5 and 6 weeks.

## Clinical Response in Adults

When the data from this Danish study were analyzed, a linear correlation was found between improvement in depression and total plasma concentration of imipramine plus desipramine. Critical lower limits for antidepressant response were determined to be 45 ng/ml or greater for imipramine plus 75 ng/ml or greater for desipramine. A combined plasma concentration of 240 ng/ml differentiated well between responders and non-responders, and there was no indication of an upper concentration limit for the antidepressant effect.

Glassman and Perel et al (80) studied 60 patients receiving 3.5 mg/kg/day of imipramine and reported a median plasma concentration of 180 ng/ml of combined imipramine plus desipramine. The best response was associated with a combined concentration greater than

TABLE 4. STUDIES OF TRICYCLIC PLASMA CONCENTRATION AND CLINICAL RESPONSE

| Drug | Indication | Total Studies | Total Pts Studied | Relationship Yes | Relationship No | Usual Range of doses (mg/day)[d] | Probable ng/ml Therapeutic Range[a] |
|---|---|---|---|---|---|---|---|
| Imipramine | Adult Depressive Illness | 10 | 232 | 9 | 1 | 75–300 | > 180[b] |
| Nortriptyline | Adult Depressive Illness | 12 | 397 | 7 | 5 | 30–100 | 50–150 |
| Amitriptyline | Adult Depressive Illness | 11 | 321 | 7 | 4 | 75–300 | 120–250[b] |
| Desipramine | Adult Depressive Illness | 3 | 56 | 2 | 1 | 75–300 | 75–160 |
| Doxepin | Adult Depressive Illness | 3 | 42 | 2 | 1 | 75–300 | > 110[b] |
| Protriptyline | Adult Depressive Illness | 2 | 49 | 2 | —— | 15–60 | 70–240 |
| Imipramine | Prepubertal Depressive Illness | 1 | 30 | 1 | —— | 1.5–5.0 mg/kg/day | 150–250[b] |
| Imipramine/[c] Desipramine | Childhood Enuresis | 1 | 40 | 1 | —— | 25–75 | > 150 |

[a] Tentative, most require confirmation except imipramine and nortriptyline in adults
[b] Parent drug plus secondary amine metabolite
[c] Desipramine was found effective but is unapproved for this use
[d] Manufacturer's suggested doses for adults

562

225 ng/ml. Poor response was associated with total concentrations below 150 ng/ml. Their data indicated that an additional 24% of patients improved when plasma concentrations exceeded 200 ng/ml in the non-responders at the conclusion of the study. These two studies provide strong evidence for improving patient care through monitoring plasma concentrations and support a linear therapeutic plasma concentration range for imipramine.

For nortriptyline, the plasma concentration response relationship appears to be curvilinear. The observation that patients classified as suffering from endogenous depression showed the best antidepressant effect with an intermediate plasma concentration range of 50 to 139 ng/ml (81) has been confirmed by additional studies (82–84). The poor antidepressant response to high plasma concentrations was shown in a study where plasma concentrations were specifically manipulated to be within the range of 50 to 150 ng/ml or above this presumed therapeutic window (85). Patients with plasma concentrations greater than 180 ng/ml improved when plasma concentrations were lowered below 150 ng/ml.

From the studies of amitriptyline plasma concentration and response, it can be concluded that a positive relationship exists. Whether this relationship is linear or curvilinear is unclear. Combining the results of studies supporting a linear response (86–88), the concentration for most responders will fall between 80 and 220 ng/ml for combined amitriptyline and nortriptyline with a lower limit of approximately 80 to 120 ng/ml and no diminution in response above 220 ng/ml. The studies supporting a curvilinear response (89–91) would limit the upper range to 220 to 250 ng/ml. The two largest amitriptyline studies (38,92) found no useful relationship of concentration to effect. As only one-third of patients in the World Health Organization trial (92) responded, this study may have included a high proportion of tricyclic non-responders and has been criticized on that basis (93). The trial reported by Robinson et al (38) found only a weak positive correlation between tricyclic concentration and improvement.

Protriptyline, doxepin, and desipramine have not been thoroughly studied. For protriptyline, the study of Biggs and Ziegler (94) supports a plasma concentration range of greater than 70 ng/ml. One additional protriptyline study found a curvilinear response with a range of 165 to 240 ng/ml for responders (95). For doxepin, Friedel and Raskind (96) reported that improvement was related to a plasma concentration of greater than 110 ng/ml from an uncontrolled study of 15 patients. Kline et al (97) reported a correlation between improvement and desmethyldoxepin concentration and not with doxepin in a study of

12 outpatients. Desipramine concentrations have been reported in relation to clinical response in three studies but steady-state conditions were not assured in any of these (98–100). Twenty-six outpatients were studied in the largest desipramine study, and improvement was related to concentrations up to 160 ng/ml. The data suggest that the therapeutic response declines at plasma concentrations above 160 ng/ml (100).

An important consideration of plasma concentration monitoring relates to the concentration necessary during maintenance therapy to prevent recurrences of depression. The majority of concentration-effect studies have been of short duration (4 to 6 weeks) yet tricyclics are useful to maintain some patients in remission for years (101). It is currently recommended that tricyclics be continued for 6 to 8 months after a depressive episode has been successfully treated (102). There is controversy whether maintenance therapy should be continued at the same dosage, and hence, plasma concentration as used during an active illness, or be reduced. Coppen and Ghose et al (103) have shown the value of maintaining plasma concentrations in the range of 190 to 240 ng/ml when maintenance doses of amitriptyline are used, as 42% of patients in a sample of 32 who were non-compliant or received placebo relapsed within one year compared to none who continued treatment. Kragh-Sorensen found relapses in depression in 3 of 22 patients on maintenance therapy associated with low plasma concentrations of nortriptyline (104). When plasma concentrations were adjusted back to their previous concentration, depression remitted. The decision to maintain a patient on tricyclics after immediate recovery will depend largely on the history of that patient's previous depressive episodes.

In summary, the most evidence for a defined therapeutic range exists for imipramine and nortriptyline. A therapeutic range for amitriptyline probably exists and difficulty in defining its limits may relate to the heterogenity of the patients studied. Therapeutic ranges for protriptyline, doxepin, and desipramine await confirmation. Two published studies indicate that plasma concentrations should be maintained in the same range for continuation therapy as for treatment of active depression. A summary of current knowledge regarding presumed therapeutic plasma concentrations of tricyclics along with the manufacturers suggested doses is provided in Table 4. The combinations of amitriptyline with either chlordiazepoxide or perphenazine are commonly prescribed, but there are no published studies reporting tricyclic plasma concentrations in relation to antidepressant effects involving these products.

## Clinical Response in Pediatrics

For indications other than depression in adults, little plasma concentration-response data exist. Pugh-Antich et al (105) have examined the relationship between clinical response and plasma concentration of imipramine in prepubertal major depressive disorder. In nondelusional subjects, aged 6 to 12 years, a total plasma concentration of imipramine plus desipramine of 146 ng/ml separated responders from non-responders. Eleven of the 13 patients were treated as outpatients, but good evidence for steady-state was produced by weekly blood sampling for 4 consecutive weeks. The optimal response mirrored the plasma concentration range for response of endogenous depression in adults and was correlated to a total plasma concentration above 220 ng/ml of imipramine plus desipramine.

In a study of childhood enuresis where either imipramine or desipramine was administered, clinical improvement was associated with a total imipramine plus desipramine, or desipramine concentration alone, of 150 ng/ml or greater (106). As with studies of depression in adults, overlap was present in plasma concentrations of responders and non-responders. As non-responders were present with relatively high plasma concentrations and no antienuretic effect, apparently a high plasma concentration alone is not a sufficient condition for efficacy. Nevertheless, there may be good reason to monitor plasma tricyclic concentrations in enuretic children. These patients may be more susceptible to side effects from higher plasma concentrations of free drug than when a similar total plasma concentration exists in adults. This is because tricyclics are less avidly bound to plasma proteins in children (107).

Linnoila et al (108) treated six hyperactive children with 25 to 100 mg/day of imipramine and observed therapeutic response to be rapid and satisfactory in all patients. Plasma concentrations of imipramine plus desipramine were relatively low (mean = 56 ± 40 ng/ml) indicating the plasma concentration associated with therapeutic response in depressed adults does not apply for this use of imipramine in children.

## Correlations with Toxicity

A number of studies have correlated side effects with tricyclic plasma concentration. Asberg et al (109) found a weak positive correlation between common subjective side effects scored on a rating scale and plasma concentration of nortriptyline. Ziegler et al (110) identified increased perspiration and dry mouth as correlating to nortriptyline plasma concentration; however, these are of no practical value, as many subjective effects of tricyclics are also symptoms of depression. Objective measures such as change in visual accommodation (111) or reduction in salivary flow (112) are correlated to plasma concentration, but are impractical to measure.

Tricyclics may produce unwanted effects on the cardiovascular system when plasma concentrations are in the therapeutic range. Unfortunately, the chronotropic response (113) and orthostatic changes in blood pressure (114) which commonly occur with therapy do not correlate well with steady-state plasma concentrations. Fortunately, in situations of overdosage, plasma concentrations are of value. Tricyclic plasma concentrations of 1,000 ng/ml or greater have been used to define a serious overdosage and are associated with greater frequency of need for respiratory support, development of unconsciousness, seizures, and cardiac arrhythmias (115). The most reliable sign for evaluating the seriousness of overdosage was found to be a QRS duration of 0.1 second or greater on the ECG. Measurement of plasma concentration following an overdose may be valuable as the correlation between amount of drug ingested by history and plasma concentration is significant, but weak.

Knowledge of the plasma tricyclic concentration may be helpful to avoid incipient toxicity as well as define overdosage. An occasional patient taking usual doses of imipramine will have plasma concentrations of imipramine plus desipramine at steady-state between 600 and 900 ng/ml (unpublished observations). Surprisingly, these patients may voice no complaint of bothersome side effects or show symptoms of toxicity. There are no data which support any beneficial antidepressant effect from increasing plasma concentrations to this magnitude, but data exist demonstrating conduction defects with plasma concentrations not far above the therapeutic range for nortriptyline (116). It would thus be judicious to lower the dosage in any patient found to have plasma concentrations greater than the presumed therapeutic range.

## Additional Considerations

As early as 1965, Kuhn (117) suggested that a hydroxylated metabolite of imipramine contributed to its antidepressant effect. There is now accumulating evidence that this is actually the case. The 2-hydroxylated metabolites of imipramine and desipramine block the reuptake of neurotransmitters (118,119) are present in cerebrospinal fluid (120), and behave like antidepressants in classical animal screening tests (119). Until recently (121,122), no analytical method was readily available to quantitate these compounds in plasma. Prospective studies correlating clinical response to measurement of these hydroxylated compounds, along with imipramine and/or desipramine, are needed. Whether their measurement will improve concentration response correlations or not, it may be useful to measure these hydroxy compounds since they are cardiotoxic (123) and occasionally accumulate to plasma concentrations greater than their parent compounds (120).

The antidepressant response of the tertiary amine tricyclics (imipramine, amitriptyline, doxepin) appears to be linear, while that of the secondary amines (desipramine, nortriptyline, protriptyline) appears to be curvilinear. This relationship is complicated by the fact that desipramine and nortriptyline are metabolites of imipramine and amitriptyline, respectively. A question arises of whether the pharmacodynamics may change and a curvilinear response become predominant when the concentration of a secondary amine metabolite rises above a certain limit. It is equally possible that the presence of the tertiary amine parent drug may alter the response of its secondary amine metabolite to maintain a linear relationship. Support for this contention may be found in the work of Linnoila et al (14) who found that nortriptyline concentrations within erythrocytes (and presumably across other membrane barriers as well) were influenced by the presence of amitriptyline.

The relative potency of the tricyclics is also of concern. Is is appropriate to simply sum the plasma concentrations of imipramine or amitriptyline with their secondary amine metabolites, or should a proportion of one be added to the other? The critical limits of 45 ng/ml plus 75 ng/ml for imipramine and desipramine, respectively (50,71), suggest unequal potencies for their antidepressant effect. Gram also found that orthostatic blood pressure changes correlated better with plasma concentration when using two times the measured imipramine concentration plus the desipramine concentration than when the imipramine plus desipramine concentration was used alone (124). Using isobolographic analysis (125), Perel has analyzed the results from his studies and determined that imipramine may be two to three times as potent in its antidepressant effect as desipramine (36). At the present time, there is no choice but to simply sum the concentrations of the tertiary tricyclics with their active secondary amine metabolites.

As most evidence for defined therapeutic ranges applies to patients classified as having endogenous depression, it may be questionable to extrapolate to other types of depression, such as neurotic or delusional, which have different symptoms (126), neuroendocrine characteristics (127,128), and possibly plasma concentration-response relationships.

There is an additional problem posed by the introduction of the third edition of the diagnostic and statistics manual of the American Psychiatric Association (DSM-III). This manual, which is widely used to classify psychiatric patients, has dropped from its nomenclature terms such as endogenous and neurotic depression, which were formerly used for classifying patients in many plasma concentration-effect studies. Some difficulty may arise in applying presumed therapeutic plasma concentration ranges determined in patients classified in one manner to those now classified differently. This issue and the others above may be resolved with additional research.

## CLINICAL APPLICATION OF PHARMACOKINETIC DATA

Pharmacokinetic data can be applied to predict dosing regimens to achieve targeted steady-state plasma concentrations in individual patients. At least three approaches are possible: [1] empirically adjusting dosage based on random plasma concentrations, [2] dosing based on total body clearance determined from a single dose study, and [3] dosing based on a single plasma concentration obtained after the first dose.

### Dosing from Random Plasma Concentrations

The conventional technique of adjusting dosages involves a delay of two weeks or longer until steady-state conditions are assumed and plasma concentration can be determined. For example, consider a patient taking 150 mg of oral imipramine/day, who at the end of two weeks of continuous treatment achieves a combined imipramine plus desipramine plasma concentration of 90 ng/ml. An upward dosage adjustment is desirable, either immediately or after 4 weeks if the patient remains non-responsive, to increase the steady-state to within the presumed therapeutic range of > 180 ng/ml. To calculate a new daily dosage, clearance is first determined from its inverse relationship to steady-state plasma concentration (Cpss):

$$\text{Cpss} = \frac{\text{F·D}}{\text{Cl}_T \cdot \tau}$$

(Eq. 1)

where "F" is the fraction of the daily dose absorbed, assumed to be constant and equal to unity, "D" is the daily dose, "$\text{Cl}_T$" is the total body clearance, and "$\tau$" is the dosage interval, equal to one day for ease of calculation. After solving for $\text{Cl}_T$, substitution of the new desired steady-state, 180 ng/ml, into Equation 1 allows calculation of the required daily dose, 300 mg. It is easily seen that these calculations are equivalent to dividing the steady-state concentration, 90 ng/ml, by the daily dosage, 150 mg, to determine the ng/ml plasma concentrations produced by each mg of drug administered per day, and dividing this quotient into any desired Cpss to determine dosage. Inherent in basing dosage changes in this simple manner are the following assumptions:

a. the systemic availability remains constant,
b. enzyme stimulation or inhibition does not occur between the first Cpss and subsequent determinations, and
c. metabolism remains linear over the dosage range employed.

The above assumptions cannot usually be validated. Some deviation from the predicted steady-state often occurs, but the magnitude is usually inconsequential. This method remains the simplest pharmacokinetic approach to adjustment of dosing without making additional assumptions of individual pharmacokinetic parameters based on population means. For the tricyclics, this would be a tenuous generalization given their variable metabolism.

For this example patient, rather than immediately doubling the daily dosage to 300 mg, the Food and Drug Administration approved limit for imipramine, a cautious posture is preferred with a gradual increase in dose, especially if the patient already reports side effects which might increase in severity and jeopardize treatment adherence if dosage is too rapidly increased.

### Dosing from Single Dose Body Clearance

A pharmacokinetic approach to predict dosage at the outset of therapy is to determine the total body clearance from a single dose. This involves precisely timed, multiple blood samples obtained during the concentration time course of a single dose for 48 to 72 hours or longer. Many useful pharmacokinetic parameters can be determined from these data and the principle of superposition can be applied to predict the dose necessary to result in a targeted steady-state (129). This approach has been successfully used by investigators working with imipramine (43), nortriptyline (58), and desipramine (130). A Swedish study found that the pharmacokinetics of nortriptyline allowed accurate prediction of desipramine plasma concentrations in the same subjects. In the United States, Ziegler et al (8,131) found that the pharmacokinetics of doxepin and protriptyline were not correlated in the same subjects. This inconsistency in findings may be related to the metabolism of the individual drugs or to the study subjects, but implies a warning if concentrations of one tricyclic are predicted on the basis of the pharmacokinetics of another. Metabolism among different tricyclics given to the same patient may be strikingly different, thus tolerance and/or therapeutic benefit with one tricyclic may not occur with another.

A disadvantage of determining clearance from a single dose is the 3 to 5 days required for study. Also, such pharmacokinetic work-ups are expensive, usually require institutionalization, and may delay initiation of treatment. Under certain conditions the determination of clearance in this manner will be valuable. As depression tends to be a recurring illness, the information gained should allow efficient dosing for years to come. However, by determining plasma concentration at steady-state, and calculating clearance from Equation 1, the knowledge gained from a protracted single dose study is obviated for future use.

## Dosing from First Dose Trough Concentration

A third approach to pharmacokinetic dosing has been reported for nortriptyline by Cooper and Simpson (42) and Montgomery et al (40), and for imipramine and desipramine by Brunswick et al (41).

These investigators administered a single oral dose of tricyclic, determined several plasma concentrations before a second dose was given, and correlated these values to steady-state after a constant maintenance dose. The concentration at 24 hours correlated well with the steady-state value in all reports and was utilized in formulating dosage tables to predict maintenance doses from a single plasma concentration following a test dose. The original references should be consulted for these recommendations, but one should be cognizant of certain limitations when predicting dosage in this manner.

The extent to which a drug will accumulate during multiple dosing can be determined by comparing the minimum plasma concentration at steady-state ($C_{min}^{ss}$) with that after the first dose ($C_{min}^1$). For the tricyclics, which demonstrate pharmacokinetics best described by the common two-compartment open model with first-order absorption, the equation which describes this relationship is termed the accumulation ratio, R (129):

$$R = \frac{C_{min}^{ss}}{C_{min}^1} = \frac{1}{1 - e^{-\beta\tau}} \tag{Eq. 2}$$

where $\beta$ is the terminal rate for drug elimination from the body. If dosage is held constant and the pharmacokinetic parameters that determine elimination do not change between the first dose and steady-state, then the $C_{min}^1$ to $C_{min}^{ss}$ relationship should be suitable for predictive purposes if it is either linear or reproducible among patients.

Figure 4 shows experimental and theoretical data which demonstrate the $C_{min}^1$ to $C_{min}^{ss}$ relationship for imipramine. Test doses of 50 mg followed in 24 hours by a constant maintenance dose of either 25 or 100 mg per day produced linearity over a limited range of $C_{min}^1$ values. Pharmacokinetic simulations predict that a disproportionate and pronounced degree of drug accumulation, more than has been experimentally demonstrated, may occur in patients with the relatively slower rates of elimination and higher $C_{min}^1$ values. The lack of agreement between the theoretical and experimental data indicate the need for caution in employing suggested doses of tricyclics based on published serum concentration data. Dosage predictions outside the range experimentally tested should not be made, and warrant testing at each clinical and analytical site to confirm their practical utility for the intended patient population.

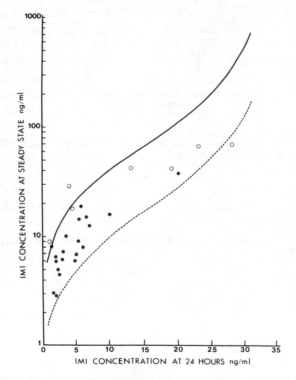

FIGURE 4. Theoretical relationship between the 24-hour serum concentration of imipramine following a 50 mg test dose ($C_{min}^1$) and steady-state serum concentration ($C_{min}^{ss}$) during a regimen of 25 mg/day (dashed line) and 100 mg/day (solid line). Solid circles are experimental data from Brunswick et al[41] and open circles are from DeVane, Wolin, and Jusko (to be published).

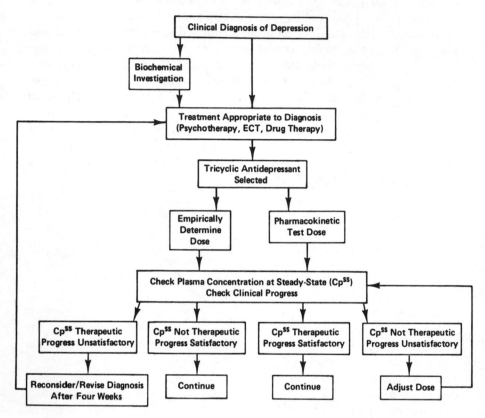

FIGURE 5. Pharmacokinetic approach to the treatment of depression.

**Treatment of Depression**

The schematic diagram in Figure 5, adapted from the approach of Sjoqvist (132) illustrates how to apply tricyclic plasma concentration data in the treatment of depression. Once the clinical diagnosis of depression is made, appropriate treatment may include tricyclics. The value of supportive psychotherapy should not be underestimated. Future research developments in the biochemical classification of depression may determine which tricyclic is specific for an individual patient. Dosage may be selected empirically, using the information in Table 4 and beginning with a small dose to minimize initial side effects, or with use of a pharmacokinetic test dose followed by stepwise increments to a maintenance dose determined by one of the prediction methods discussed above. Whether or not a tricyclic is selected for which a defined therapeutic range exists, measurement of plasma concentration at the expected steady-state (four to five half-lives, Table 1) is useful to assess absorption and compliance and to identify individuals who achieve excessive plasma concentrations. The latter should be especially avoided in the elderly and those with pre-existing cardiac disease.

When patient progress is satisfactory, including absence of unacceptable side effects, no adjustment in dose is necessary unless plasma concentrations are excessive. When patient progress is unsatisfactory, a dosage adjustment may be necessary to increase or decrease the plasma concentration to within the therapeutic range. This can be accomplished with the use of Equation 1. When presumed therapeutic concentrations exist, at least 4 weeks should elapse with continuous dosing to allow for the usual lag in full efficacy before reconsidering diagnosis or changing therapy. If a switch to another tricyclic is made, dosage should be titrated in the same manner as before. One should be mindful of the factors in Table 3 when continuing patients on maintenance therapy and recheck plasma concentration when recrudescence of symptoms or unexpected side effects occur. With this approach, the variability in plasma concentrations, which may undermine therapeutic success, can be minimized.

## ASSAY METHODS

Clinicians must realize that laboratory workers may not produce simple objective measurements of tricyclic plasma concentrations that are comparable between laboratories. There are technical difficulties in estimating the nanogram concentrations involved, and meticulous attention is required for assay reproducibility. There have been very few comparisons between different methods, and the clinician is advised to inquire about internal quality control and cross-check laboratory results when routinely ordering assays.

Many analytical techniques have been applied in the assay of tricyclics. These have been recently reviewed (133) and the most common methods are summarized in Table 5. The selection of a particular method will depend on such factors as cost, ease of operation, and applicability to research as well as clinical monitoring. No single assay is best for both purposes; however, some general guidelines can be stated for laboratories beginning measurement of tricyclics.

For identification of compounds in research, the combination of a mass spectrometer with gas chromatography (GC-MS) is unsurpassed. This method is highly reliable, but requires access and time on very expensive equipment. Regarded as the standard by which other methods should be compared for specificity, it is doubtful whether its use in community hospitals is feasible.

Gas chromatography (GC) has been the most popular chromatographic technique in clinical chemistry, and several different detection systems can be used in conjunction for quantitation of tricyclics. An alkali flame ionization detector (AFIP), sometimes called a nitrogen detector, has the selectivity and sensitivity for research use and is not as difficult to operate as GC-MS. Electron-capture (GC-EC) is another detection system for GC and is more sensitive than AFIP; however, its operation requires more technical skill, and poor specificity is a drawback.

High performance liquid chromatography (HPLC) is an increasingly popular analytical technique offering tremendous separation capability but has not yet been applied to measurements of all the available tricyclics. When coupled with a fluorescence detector, it is a highly sensitive and specific assay. While moderately expensive, HPLC is a good compromise for research and clinical monitoring due to its ease of operation.

A promising method is radioimmunoassay (RIA), which has high sensitivity, requires only a small quantity of sample, and does not involve the extensive sample preparation inherent in most other methods. Specificity, however, may be a problem due to cross reaction of antibodies with metabolites and compounds of similar structure. Ultimately, this method may become widely used in hospitals which presently own a scintillation counter owing to its ease of operation and low cost after initial set-up.

An important consideration is the proper collection of samples. While use of vacuum stoppered glass tubes has greatly simplified collection of blood in clinical chemistry, use of Vacutainers (Becton-

TABLE 5. ANALYTICAL METHODOLOGIES FOR TRICYCLIC ANTIDEPRESSANT PLASMA CONCENTRATIONS

| Method[a] | Sample[c] Requirement | Speed | Sensitivity | Specificity | Difficulty of Operation | Cost | References |
|---|---|---|---|---|---|---|---|
| GC-MS | 1–4 ml | 15 samples/hr | 1.0 ng/ml | Excellent | High | High | 148–150 |
| GC-AFIP | 1–2 ml | 6–8 samples/hr | 5 ng/ml | Good | Moderate | Moderate | 151–153 |
| GC-EC | 1–3 ml | 6–8 samples/hr | 5–10 ng/ml | Moderate[b] | Moderate | Moderate | 159–160 |
| HPLC | 1 ml | 4–6 samples/hr | 1 ng/ml | Good | Low | Moderate | 121,154–155 |
| RIA | < 1.0 ml | > 10 samples/hr | < 1 ng/ml | Poor[b] | Low | Initially high then low | 156–158 |

[a] For abbreviations see text
[b] Assays may not distinguish between parent compound and metabolites
[c] Serum or plasma

Dickinson) introduces a laboratory error into the measurement of tricyclics (134). Spurious reductions in measured plasma concentrations result from interference of a plasticizer contained within the rubber stoppers, which displaces basic drugs from their plasma protein binding sites (135). This causes a re-equilibration with red cells and thus a lowering of measurable concentration when plasma is separated. Venoject tubes (Kimble-Terumo, Inc.) have been shown to be free from this interference (136). Alternate methods of blood collection include the use of all glass systems or transfer of blood from a glass syringe to unstoppered tubes. If blood must be collected with Vacutainers, discarding the stopper immediately after collection will minimize the interference (137). Plasma samples of imipramine and desipramine stored in tightly capped polypropylene or glass tubes and frozen at $-15$ degrees centigrade remain stable for at least six months (unpublished observations).

## PROSPECTUS

The diagnostic entities of depression will become more precisely defined by biologic criteria in the future. The largely empiric basis for selection among tricyclics can be improved when consideration of their inhibitory properties for serotonin and norepinephrine reuptake clearly become useful. Drugs affecting other neurotransmitters, such as those acting on histamine, may become useful adjuncts in the future treatment of depression. Already, mianserin and iprindole, which do not share all the central actions of the conventional tricyclics, yet are antidepressant, are being tested abroad. There is a well deserved and renewed interest in research with monoamine oxidase inhibitors.

For the present, tricyclics are generally the most useful drugs in the pharmacologic management of depression. With advances in assay methodology has come research demonstrating their pharmacokinetic profile of pre-systemic elimination, extensive distribution, and prolonged clearance through hepatic metabolism. The slowness of onset of the tricyclics' antidepressant effects seems to be unrelated to their pharmacokinetics. The antidepressant response does not parallel either the accumulation of drug in plasma to steady-state or the onset of pharmacologic blockade of neurotransmitter reuptake. Rather, it relates more likely to other neurochemical events such as the increase in norepinephrine release which occurs after development of presynaptic alpha receptor subsensitivity (138). Thus, research with loading doses or parenteral therapy, which could be hazardous due to production of high peak concentrations, cannot be justified on a pharmacokinetic basis.

The application of pharmacokinetic data appears to be most useful in assuring compliance, avoiding incipient toxicity, and in adjustment of doses to produce presumed therapeutic plasma concentrations. Research in this latter area should continue, as these concentration ranges require further definition. The promise of predicting accurate maintenance doses from a first dose concentration may decrease the number of dosage adjustments necessary for many patients and represents a therapeutic advance in clinical drug therapy.

## ACKNOWLEDGMENTS

Supported in part by Grant No. 20852 from the National Institutes of General Medical Sciences, National Institutes of Health.

## REFERENCES

1. Akiskal HS and McKinney WT: Overview of recent research in depression. Arch Gen Psychiatry 1975; 32:285–305.
2. Morris JB and Beck AT: The efficacy of antidepressant drugs. Arch Gen Psychiatry 1974; 30:667–674.
3. Hammer W and Sjoqvist F: Plasma levels of monomethylated tricyclic antidepressants during treatment with imipramine like compounds. Life Sciences 1967; 6:1895–1903.
4. Moody JP, Tait AC and Todrick A: Plasma levels of imipramine and desmethylimipramine during therapy. Br J Psychiatry 1967; 113:183–193.
5. Schildkraut JJ: Current status of the catecholamine hypothesis of affective disorders. In: Lipton M, DiMascio A and Killam KF (eds): *Psychopharmacology: A Generation of Progress.* Raven Press, New York; 1978:1223–1234.
6. Murphey DL, Campbell I and Costa JL: Current status of the indoleamine hypothesis of the affective disorders. In: Lipton M, DiMascio A and Killam KF (eds): *Psychopharmacology: A Generation of Progress.* Raven Press, New York; 1978:1235–1247.
7. Maxwell RA and White HL: Tricyclic and monoamine oxidase inhibitor antidepressants: structure-activity relationships. In: Iverson LL, Iverson SD and Snyder SH (eds): *Handbook of Psychopharmacology, Vol. 14.* Plenum Press, New York; 1978:83–155.
8. Ziegler VE, Biggs JT and Wylie LT et al: Protriptyline kinetics. Clin Pharmacol Ther 1978; 23:580–584.
9. Alexanderson B, Borga O and Alvan G: The availability of orally administered nortriptyline. Europ J Clin Pharmacol 1973; 5:181–185.
10. Gram LF and Overo KF: First-pass metabolism of nortriptyline in man. Clin Pharmacol Ther 1975; 18:305–314.
11. Gram LF and Christiansen J: First-pass metabolism of imipramine in man. Clin Pharmacol Ther 1975; 17:555–563.

12. Charalampous KD and Johnson PC: Studies of C[14]-protriptyline in man: plasma levels and excretion. J Clin Pharmacol 1967; 7:93–96.
13. Routledge PA and Shand DG: Presystemic drug elimination. Ann Rev Pharmacol Toxicol 1979; 19:447–468.
14. Linnoila M, Dorrity F and Jobson K: Plasma and erythrocyte levels of tricyclic antidepressants in depressed patients. Am J Psychiatry 1978; 135:557–561.
15. Souner R and Orsulak PJ: Excretion of imipramine and desipramine in human breast milk. Am J Psychiatry 1979; 136:451–452.
16. Gram LF, Kofod B, Christiansen J and Rafaelsen OJ: Imipramine metabolism: pH-dependent distribution and urinary excretion. Clin Pharmacol Ther 1970; 12:239–244.
17. Elonen E, Linniola M, Lukkari I and Mattila MJ: Concentrations of tricyclic antidepressants in plasma, heart and skeletal muscle after their intravenous infusion to anaesthetized rabbits. Acta Pharmacol et Toxicol 1975; 37:274–281.
18. Hobbs DC: Distribution and metabolism of doxepin. Biochem Pharmacol 1969; 18:1941–1954.
19. Christiansen J and Gram LF: Imipramine and its metabolites in human brain. J Pharm Pharmacol 1973; 25:604–608.
20. Borga O, Azarnoff DL, Forshell GP and Sjoqvist F: Plasma protein binding of tricyclic antidepressants in man. Biochem Pharmacol 1969; 18:2135–2143.
21. Piafsky KM and Borga O: Plasma protein binding of basic drugs II. Importance of $\alpha_1$-acid glycoprotein for interindividual variation. Clin Pharmacol Ther 1977; 22:545–549.
22. Bickel MH: Binding of chlorpromazine and imipramine to red cells, albumin, lipoproteins and other blood components. J Pharm Pharmacol 1975; 27:733–738.
23. Danon A and Chen Z: Binding of imipramine to plasma proteins: effect of hyper-lipoproteinemia. Clin Pharmacol Ther 1979; 25:316–321.
24. Schmid K: $\alpha_1$-acid glycoprotein. In: Putnam FW (ed): *The Plasma Proteins, Vol. I*, Academic Press, Inc. 1975:184–228.
25. Piafsky KM, Borga O, Odar-Cederlof I, Johansson C and Sjoqvist F: Increased plasma protein binding of propranolol and chlorpromazine mediated by disease-induced elevations of plasma $\alpha_1$-acid glycoprotein. N Engl J Med 1978; 299:1435–1439.
26. Glassman AH, Hurwic MJ and Perel JM: Plasma binding of imipramine and clinical outcome. Am J Psychiatry 1973; 130:1367–1369.
27. Potter WZ, Muscettola G and Goodwin FK: Binding of imipramine to plasma protein and to brain tissue: relationship to CSF tricyclic levels in man. Psychopharmacology 1979; 63:187–192.
28. Bertilsson L, Braithwaite R, Tybring G, Garle M and Borga O: Techniques for plasma protein binding of demethylchlorimipramine. Clin Pharmacol Ther 1979; 26:265–271.
29. Gram LF: Metabolism of tricyclic antidepressants: A review. Dan Med Bull 1974; 21:218–228.
30. Sjoqvist F, Berglund F, Borga O, Hammer W, Andersson S and Thorstrand C: The pH-dependent excretion of monomethylated tricyclic antidepressants in dog and man. Clin Pharmacol Ther 1969; 10:826–833.
31. Alexanderson B and Borga O: Urinary excretion of nortriptyline and five of its metabolites in man after single and multiple oral doses. Europ J Clin Pharmacol 1973; 5:174–180.

32. Minder R, Schnetzer F and Bickel MH: Hepatic and extrahepatic metabolism of the psychoactive drugs, chlorpromazine, imipramine and imipramine-N-oxide. Naunyn-Schmiedebergs Arch Pharmacol 1971; 268:334–347.
33. Dencker H, Dencker SJ, Green A and Nagy A: Intestinal absorption, demethylation, and enterohepatic circulation of imipramine. Clin Pharmacol Ther 1976; 19:584–586.
34. Von Bahr C and Orrenius S: Spectral studies on the interaction of imipramine and some of its oxidised metabolites with rat liver microsomes. Xenobiotica 1971; 1:69–78.
35. Perel JM, O'Brien L, Black NB, Bellward GD and Dayton DG: Imipramine and chlorpromazine in hepatic microsomal systems. In: Forrest IS, Carr CJ and Usdin E (eds): *The Phenothiazines and Structurally Related Drugs,* Raven Press, New York. 1974:201–212.
36. Perel JM, Stiller RL and Glassman AH: Studies on plasma level/effect relationships in imipramine therapy. Comm in Psychopharmacology 1978; 2:429–439.
37. Gram LF, Sondergaard I, Christiansen J et al: Steady-state kinetics of imipramine in patients. Psychopharmacology 1977; 54:255–261.
38. Robinson DS, Cooper TB, Ravaris CL et al: Plasma tricyclic drug levels in amitriptyline-treated depressed patients. Psychopharmacology 1979; 63:223–231.
39. Maas JW: Biogenic amines and depression. Arch Gen Psychiatry 1975; 32:1357–1361.
40. Montgomery SA, McAuley R, Montgomery DB, Braithwaite RA and Dawling S: Dosage adjustment from simple nortriptyline spot level predictor tests in depressed patients. Clin Pharmacokinetics 1979; 4:129–136.
41. Brunswick DJ, Amsterdam JD, Mendels J and Stern SL: Prediction of steady-state imipramine and desmethylimipramine plasma concentrations from single-dose data. Clin Pharmacol Ther 1979; 25:605–610.
42. Cooper TB and Simpson GM: Prediction of individual dosage of nortriptyline. Am J Psychiatry 1978; 135:333–335.
43. Potter WZ, Zavadil AP and Goodwin FK: Prediction of steady-state plasma concentration of imipramine. Psychopharmacol Bull 1978; 14:29–33.
44. Beaubien AR and Pakuts AP: Influence of dose on first-pass kinetics of $^{14}$C-imipramine in the isolated perfused rat liver. Drug Metabolism Disposition 1979; 7:34–39.
45. Amsterdam J, Brunswick DJ and Mendels J: High dose desipramine, plasma drug levels, and clinical response. J Clin Psychiatry 1979; 40:141–143.
46. Alexanderson B: Prediction of steady-state plasma levels of nortriptyline from single oral dose kinetics: A study in twins. Europ J Clin Pharmacol 1973; 6:44–53.
47. Nies A, Robinson DS, Friedman MJ et al: Relationship between age and tricyclic antidepressant plasma levels. Am J Psychiatry 1977; 134:790–793.
48. Ziegler VE and Biggs JT: Tricyclic plasma levels—effect of age, race, sex, and smoking. JAMA 1977; 238:2167–2169.
49. Musa MN: Imipramine: relationship of age to steady-state plasma level in endogenous depression. Res Comm Psychol Psychiat Behavior 1979; 4:205–208.
50. Gram LF, Reisby N, Ibsen I et al: Plasma levels and antidepressant effect of imipramine. Clin Pharmacol Ther 1976; 19:318–324.
51. Raskin A: Age-sex differences in response to antidepressant drugs. J Nervous Mental Disease 1974; 159:120–130.

52. Raskin A and Crook TH: Antidepressants in black and white inpatients. Arch Gen Psychiatry 1975; 32:643–649.
53. Wheatley D: Potentiation of amitriptyline by thyroid hormone. Arch Gen Psychiatry 1972; 26:229–233.
54. Perel JM, Shostak M, Gann E, Kantor SJ and Glassman AH: Pharmacodynamics of imipramine and clinical outcome in depressed patients. In: Gottschalk L and Merlis S (eds): *Pharmacokinetics of Psychoactive Drugs: Blood Levels and Clinical Response,* Spectrum-John Wiley, New York. 1976:229–241.
55. Norman TR, Burrows GD, Maguire KP, Rubinstein G, Scoggins BA and Davies B: Cigarette smoking and plasma nortriptyline levels. Clin Pharmacol Ther 1977; 21:453–456.
56. Jusko WJ: Influence of cigarette smoking on drug metabolism in man. Drug Metabolism Rev 1979; 9:221–236.
57. Braithwaite R, Montgomery S and Dawling S: Nortriptyline in depressed patients with high plasma levels. II. Clin Pharmacol Ther 1978; 23:303–308.
58. Alexanderson B: Pharmacokinetics of nortriptyline in man after single and multiple oral doses: the predictability of steady-state plasma concentrations from single-dose plasma level data. Europ J Clin Pharmacol 1972; 4:82–91.
59. Gram LF and Overo KF: Drug interaction: inhibitory effect of neuroleptics on metabolism of tricyclic antidepressants in man. Br Med J 1972; 1:463–465.
60. Wharton RN, Perel JM, Dayton PG and Malitz S: A potential clinical use for methylphenidate with tricyclic antidepressants. Am J Psychiatry 1971; 127:1619–1625.
61. Gram LF, Overo KF and Kirk L: Influence of neuroleptics and benzodiazepines on metabolism of tricyclic antidepressants in man. Am J Psychiatry 1974; 131:863–866.
62. Kuhn R: The treatment of depressive states with G-22355 (imipramine hydrochloride). Am J Psychiatry 1958; 115:459–464.
63. Prange AJ, Wilson IC, Rabon AM and Lipton MA: Enhancement of imipramine antidepressant activity by thyroid hormone. Am J Psychiatry 1969; 126:457–469.
64. Saraf K and Klein DF: The safety of a single daily dose schedule for imipramine. Am J Psychiatry 1971; 128:483–484.
65. Mendels J and Digiacomo J: The treatment of depression with a single daily dose of imipramine pamoate. Am J Psychiatry 1973; 130:1022–1024.
66. Schuckit MA and Feighner JP: Safety of high-dose tricyclic antidepressant therapy. Am J Psychiatry 1972; 128:1456–1459.
67. Bloomingdale LM and Bressler B: Rapid intramuscular administration of tricyclic antidepressants. Am J Psychiatry 1979; 136:1092–1093.
68. Gram LF: Plasma level monitoring of tricyclic antidepressant therapy. Clin Pharmacokinetics 1977; 2:237–251.
69. Glassman AH and Perel JM: Tricyclic blood levels and clinical outcome: A review of the art. In: Lipton M, DiMascio A and Killam KF (eds): *Psychopharmacology: A Generation of Progress,* Raven Press, New York. 1978:917–922.
70. Risch SC, Huey LY and Janowsky DS: Plasma levels of tricyclic antidepressants and clinical efficacy: Review of the literature—Parts I and II. J Clin Psychiatry 1979; 40:4–16; 53–69.
71. Reisby N, Gram JF, Beck P et al: Imipramine: Clinical effects and pharmacokinetic variability. Psychopharmacology 1977; 54:263–273.
72. Spitzer RL and Fleiss JL: A re-analysis of the reliability of psychiatric diagnosis. Br J Psychiatry 1974; 125:341–347.

73. Beck AT, Ward CH, Mendelson M, Mock J and Erbaugh J: An inventory for measuring depression. Arch Gen Psychiatry 1961; 4:561–571.
74. Hamilton M: A rating scale for depression. J Neurol Neurosurg Psychiatry 1960; 23:56–62.
75. Beck P, Gram LF, Dein E, Jacobsen O, Vitger J and Bolwig TG: Quantitative rating of depressive states. Acta Psychiat Scand 1975; 51:161–170.
76. Kantor SJ and Glassman AH: Delusional depressions: Natural history and response to treatment. Br J Psychiatry 1977; 131:351–360.
77. Davis JM, Erickson S and Dekirmenjian H: Plasma levels of antipsychotic drugs and clinical response. In: Lipton M, DiMascio A and Killam KF (eds): *Psychopharmacology: A Generation of Progress,* Raven Press, New York; 1978:905–915.
78. Ziegler VE, Knesevich JW, Wylie LT and Biggs JT: Sampling time, dosage schedule, and nortriptyline plasma levels. Arch Gen Psychiatry 1977; 34:613–615.
79. Ziegler VE, Biggs JT, Rosen SH, Meyer DA and Preskorn SH: Imipramine and desipramine plasma levels: relationship to dosage schedule and sampling time. J Clin Psychiatry 1978; 39:660–663.
80. Glassman AH, Perel JM, Shostak M, Kantor SJ and Fleiss JL: Clinical implications of imipramine plasma levels for depressive illness. Arch Gen Psychiatry 1977; 34:197–204.
81. Asberg M, Cronholm B, Sjoqvist F and Tuck D: Relationship between plasma level and therapeutic effect of nortriptyline. Br Med J 1971; 3:331–334.
82. Kragh-Sorensen P, Eggert-Hansen C and Asberg M: Plasma nortriptyline levels in endogenous depression. Lancet 1973; 1:113–115.
83. Montgomery S, Braithwaite R, Dawling S and McAuley R: High plasma nortriptyline levels in the treatment of depression. I. Clin Pharmacol Ther 1978; 23:309–314.
84. Ziegler VE, Clayton PJ, Taylor JR, Co BT and Biggs JT: Nortriptyline levels and clinical response. Clin Pharmacol Ther 1976; 20:458–463.
85. Kragh-Sorensen P, Eggert Hansen C, Baastrup PC and Hvidberg EF: Self-inhibiting action of nortriptyline's antidepressant effect at high plasma levels. Psychopharmacologia 1976; 45:305–312.
86. Kupfer DJ, Hanin I, Spiker DG, Grau T and Coble P: Amitriptyline plasma levels and clinical response in primary depression. Clin Pharmacol Ther 1977; 22:904–911.
87. Ziegler VE, Co BT, Taylor JR, Clayton PJ and Biggs JT: Amitriptyline plasma levels and therapeutic response. Clin Pharmacol Ther 1976; 19:795–801.
88. Ziegler VE, Clayton PJ and Biggs JT: A comparison study of amitriptyline and nortriptyline with plasma levels. Arch Gen Psychiatry 1977; 34:607–612.
89. Montgomery SA, McAuley R, Rani SJ, Montgomery DB, Braithwaite R and Dawling S: Amitriptyline plasma concentration and clinical response. Br Med J 1979; 1:230–231.
90. Braithwaite RA, Goulding R, Theano G, Bailey J and Coopen A: Plasma concentration of amitriptyline and clinical response. Lancet 1972; 1:1297–1300.
91. Vandel S, Vandel B, Sandoz M, Allers G, Bechtel P and Volmat R: Clinical response and plasma concentration of amitriptyline and its metabolite nortriptyline. Europ J Clin Pharmacol 1978; 14:185–190.
92. Coopen A, Montgomery S, Ghose K, Rama Rao VA and Bailey J: Amitriptyline plasma concentration and clinical effect—A World Health Organization collaborative study. Lancet 1978; 1:63–66.

93. Potter WZ and Goodwin FK: Antidepressant drug levels and clinical response. Lancet 1978; 1:1049–1050.

94. Biggs JT and Ziegler VE: Protriptyline plasma levels and antidepressant response. Clin Pharmacol Ther 1977; 22:269–273.

95. Whyte SF, Macdonald AJ, Naylor GL and Moody JP: Plasma concentrations of protriptyline and clinical effects in depressed women. Br J Psychiatry 1976; 128:384–390.

96. Friedel RO and Raskind MA: Relationship of blood levels of Sinequan® to clinical effects in the treatment of depression in aged patients. In: *Sinequan® (doxepin HC1): A Monograph of Recent Clinical Studies,* Excerpta Medica, 1975:51–53.

97. Kline NS, Cooper TB and Johnson B: Doxepin and desmethyldoxepin serum levels and clinical response. In: Gottschalk LA and Merlis S (eds): *Pharmacokinetics of Psychoactive Drugs—Blood Levels and Clinical Response,* Spectrum, New York; 1976:221–228.

98. Amin MM, Cooper R, Khalid R and Lehmann HE: A comparison of desipramine and amitriptyline plasma levels and therapeutic response. Psychopharmacology Bull 1978; 14:45–46.

99. Khalid R, Amin MM and Ban TA: Desipramine plasma levels and therapeutic response. Psychopharmacology Bull 1978; 14:43–44.

100. Friedel RO, Veith RC, Bloom V and Bielski RJ: Desipramine plasma levels and clinical response in depressed outpatients. Comm Psychopharmacology 1979; 3:81–87.

101. Prien RF, Klett J and Caffey EM: Lithium carbonate and imipramine in prevention of affective disorders. Arch Gen Psychiatry 1973; 29:420–425.

102. Gelenberg AJ and Klerman GL: Antidepressants: Their use in clinical practice. Rational Drug Therapy 1978; 12(4):1–7.

103. Coopen A, Ghose K, Montgomery S, Rama Rae VA, Bailey J and Jorgensen A: Continuation therapy with amitriptyline in depression. Br J Psychiatry 1978; 133:28–33.

104. Kragh-Sorensen P, Eggert Hansen C, Larson N-E, Naestoff J and Hvidberg EF: Long-term treatment of endogenous depression with nortriptyline with control of plasma levels. Psycholog Med 1974; 4:174–180.

105. Puig-Antich J, Perel JM, Luptakin W et al: Plasma levels of imipramine and desmethylimipramine and clinical response in prepubertal major depressive disorder. J Am Acad Child Psychiatry (in press).

106. Rapoport JL, Mikkelsen EJ, Zavadil AP et al: Childhood enuresis II. Psychopathology, plasma tricyclic concentration and antienuretic effect. Arch Gen Psychiatry (in press).

107. Winsberg BG, Perel JM, Hurwic MJ and Klutch A: Imipramine protein binding and pharmacokinetics in children. In: Forrest IS, Carr CJ and Usdin E (eds): *The Phenothiazines and Structurally Related Drugs,* Raven Press, New York; 1974:425–431.

108. Linnoila M, Gualtieri T, Jobson K and Staye J: Characteristics of the therapeutic response to imipramine in hyperactive children. Am J Psychiatry 1979; 136:1201–1203.

109. Asberg M, Cronholm B, Sjoqvist F and Tuck D: Correlation of subjective side effects with plasma concentrations of nortriptyline. Br Med J 1970; 4:18–21.

110. Ziegler VE, Taylor JR, Wetzel RD and Biggs JT: Nortriptyline plasma levels and subjective side effects. Br J Psychiatry 1978; 132:55–60.

111. Asberg M and Germanis M: Ophthalomological effects of nortriptyline—relationship to plasma level. Pharmacology 1972; 7:349–356.

112. Bertram U, Kragh-Sorensen P, Rafaelsen OJ and Larson N-E: Saliva secretion following long-term antidepressant treatment with nortriptyline controlled by plasma levels. Scand J Dent Res 1979; 87:58–64.
113. Freyschuss U, Sjoqvist F, Tuck D and Asberg M: Circulatory effects in man of nortriptyline, a tricyclic antidepressant drug. Pharmacologia Clinica 1970; 2:68–71.
114. Glassman AH, Bigger JT, Giardina EV, Kantor SJ, Perel JM and Davis M: Clinical characteristics of imipramine-induced orthostatic hypotension. Lancet 1979; 1:468–472.
115. Petit JM, Spiker DG, Ruwitch JF, Ziegler VE, Weiss AN and Biggs JT: Tricyclic antidepressant plasma levels and adverse effects after overdose. Clin Pharmacol Ther 1977; 21:47–51.
116. Vohra J, Burrows GP and Sloman G: Assessment of cardiovascular side effects of therapeutic doses of tricyclic antidepressant drugs. Aust NZ J Med 1975; 5:7–11.
117. Kuhn R: Untersuchungen uber mogliche zusammenhange zwischen metaboliten-ausscheidung und krankheitsverlauf depressive zustande unter imipramin-medikation. Psychopharmacologia 1965; 8:201–222.
118. Javaid JI, Perel JM and Davis JM: Inhibition of biogenic amines uptake by imipramine, desipramine, 2-OH-imipramine and 2-OH-desipramine in rat brain. Life Sci 1979; 24:21–28.
119. Potter WZ, Calil HM, Manian AA, Zavadil AP and Goodwin FK: Hydroxylated metabolites of tricyclic antidepressants: preclinical assessment of activity. Biological Psychiatry 1979; 14:601–613.
120. Potter WZ, Calil HM, Zavadil AP et al: Steady-state concentrations of hydroxylated metabolites of tricyclic antidepressants in patients: relationship to effect. Psychopharmacology Bull (in press).
121. Sutfin TA and Jusko WJ: High performance liquid chromatographic assay for imipramine, desipramine, and their 2-hydroxylated metabolites. J Pharm Sci 1979; 68:703–705.
122. Stiller RL and Perel JM: Simultaneous determinations of imipramine, desmethylimipramine and their 2-hydroxy metabolites in plasma by nitrogen selective detection gas chromatography. J Pharm Sci (in press).
123. Jandhyala BS, Steenberg ML, Perel JM, Manian AA and Buckley JP: Effects of several tricyclic antidepressants on the hemodynamics and myocardial contractility of the anesthetized dogs. Europ J Pharmacol 1977; 42:403–410.
124. Gram LF, Beck P, Reisby N, Nagy A and Christiansen J: Factors influencing pharmacokinetics and clinical effects of tricyclic antidepressants. In: Garattini S (ed): *Depressive Disorders,* Schattauer Verlag, New York; 1978:337–346.
125. Gessner PK: The isobolographic method applied to drug interactions. In: Morselli PL, Cohen SN and Garattini S (eds): *Drug Interactions,* New York; 1974:349–362.
126. Kiloh LG and Garside RF: The independence of neurotic depression and endogenous depression. Br J Psychiatry 1963; 109:451–463.
127. Sweeney D, Nelson C, Bowers M, Maas J and Heninger G: Delusional versus non-delusional depression: neurochemical differences. Lancet 1978; 2:100–101.
128. Schlesser MA, Winokur G and Sherman BM: Genetic subtypes of unipolar primary depressive illness distinguished by hypothalamic-pituitary-adrenal axis activity. Lancet 1979; 1:739–741.
129. Gibaldi M and Perrier D: *Pharmacokinetics,* Marcel Dekker, New York; 1975.
130. Alexanderson B: Pharmacokinetics of desmethylimipramine and nortriptyline in man after single and multiple oral doses—a cross-over study. Europ J Clin Pharmacol 1972; 5:1–10.

131. Ziegler VE, Biggs JT, Wylie LT, Rosen SH, Hawf DJ and Coryell WH: Doxepin kinetics. Clin Pharmacol Ther 1978; 23:573–579.
132. Sjoqvist F: A pharmacokinetic approach to the treatment of depression. Int Pharmacopsychiat 1971; 6:147–169.
133. Gupta R and Molnar G: Measurement of therapeutic concentrations of tricyclic antidepressants in serum. Drug Metabolism Rev 1979; 9:79–97.
134. Brunswick DJ and Mendels J: Reduced levels of tricyclic antidepressants in plasma from Vacutainers. Comm Psychopharmacology 1977; 1:131–134.
135. Borga O, Piafsky KM and Nilson OG: Plasma protein binding of basic drugs I. Selective displacement from $\alpha_1$-acid glycoprotein by tris(2-butoxyethyl) phosphate. Clin Pharmacol Ther 1977; 22:539–544.
136. Veith RC, Raisys VA and Perera C: The clinical impact of blood collection methods on tricyclic antidepressants as measured by GC/MC-SIM. Comm Psychopharmacology 1978; 2:491–494.
137. Cochran E, Carl J and Hanin I: Effect of Vacutainer stoppers on plasma tricyclic levels: A reevaluation. Comm Psychopharmacology 1978; 2:495–503.
138. Crews FT and Smith CB: Presynaptic alpha receptor subsensitivity after long-term antidepressant treatment. Science 1978; 202:322–324.
139. Brinkschulte M and Breyer-Pfaff U: Binding of tricyclic antidepressants and perazine to human plasma. Naunyn-Schmiedeberg's Arch Pharmacol 1979; 380:1–7.
140. Campbell IC and Todrick A: Plasma protein binding of tricyclic antidepressant drugs. J Pharm Pharmacol 1970; 22:226–227.
141. Ziegler VE, Biggs JT, Ardekani AB and Rosen SH: Contribution to the pharmacokinetics of amitriptyline. J Clin Pharmacol 1978; 18:462–467.
142. Jorgensen A and Hanson V: Pharmacokinetics of amitriptyline infused intravenously in man. Europ J Clin Pharmacol 1976; 10:337–341.
143. Rogers HJ, Morrison PJ and Bradbrook ID: The half-life of amitriptyline. Br J Clin Pharmacol 1978; 6:181–183.
144. Overo KF, Gram LF and Hansen V: Kinetics of nortriptyline in man according to a two compartment model. Europ J Clin Pharmacol 1975; 8:343–347.
145. Gram LF and Overo KF: First-pass metabolism of nortriptyline in man. Clin Pharmacol Ther 1975; 18:305–314.
146. Alvan G, Borga O and Lind M: First-pass hydroxylation of nortriptyline: concentrations of parent drug and major metabolites in plasma. Europ J Clin Pharmacol 1977; 11:219–224.
147. Moody JP, Whyte SF, MacDonald AJ and Naylor GP: Pharmacokinetic aspects of protriptyline plasma levels. Europ J Clin Pharmacol 1977; 11:51–56.
148. Biggs JT, Holland WH, Chang S, Hipps PP and Sherman WR: Electron beam ionization mass fragmentographic analysis of tricyclic antidepressants in human plasma. J Pharm Sci 1976; 65:261–268.
149. Jenkins RG and Friedel RO: Analysis of tricyclic antidepressants in human plasma by GLC-chemical-ionization mass spectrometry with selected ion monitoring. J Pharm Sci 1978; 67:17–23.
150. Claeys M, Muscettola G and Markey SP: Simultaneous measurement of imipramine and desipramine by selected ion recording with deuterated internal standards. Biomed Mass Spectrom 1976; 3:110–116.
151. Dorrity F, Linnoila M and Habig RL: Therapeutic monitoring of tricyclic antidepressants in plasma by gas chromatography. Clin Chem 1977; 23:1326–1328.
152. Bailey DN and Jatlow PI: Gas-chromatography analysis for therapeutic concentrations of imipramine and desipramine in plasma, with use of a nitrogen detector. Clin Chem 1976; 22:1697–1701.

153. Cooper TB, Allen D and Simpson GM: A sensitive method for the determination of amitriptyline and nortriptyline in human plasma. Psychopharmacology Comm 1976; 2:105–116.
154. Van Den Berg JHM, DeRuwe HJJM and Deelder RS: Column liquid chromatography of tricyclic antidepressants. J Chromatography 1977; 138:431–436.
155. Watson ID and Stuart MJ: Quantitative determination of amitriptyline and nortriptyline in plasma by high-performance liquid chromatography. J Chromatography 1977; 132:155–159.
156. Brunswick DJ, Needleman B and Mendels J: Specific radioimmunoassay of amitriptyline and nortriptyline. Br J Clin Pharmacol 1979; 7:343–348.
157. Brunswick DJ, Needleman B and Mendels J: Radioimmunoassay of imipramine and desmethylimipramine. Life Sci 1978; 22:137–146.
158. Midha KK, Loo JCK, Charette C, Rowe ML, Hubbard JW and McGilveray IJ: Monitoring of therapeutic concentrations of psychotropic drugs in plasma by radioimmunoassays. J Anal Toxicol 1978; 2:185–192.
159. Borga O and Garle M: Application of isotope derivative technique to assay of secondary amines: estimation of desipramine by acetylation with [$^3$H]-acetic anhydride. J Chromatography 1972; 68:77–88.
160. Wallace JE, Hamilton HE, Goggin LK and Blum K: Determination of amitriptyline at nanogram levels in serum by electron capture gas liquid chromatography. Anal Chem 1975; 47:1516–1519.
161. Gram LF, Anderson PB, Overo KF and Christiansen J: Comparison of single dose kinetics of imipramine, nortriptyline and antipyrine in man. Psychopharmacology 1976; 50:21–27.

# 18

# Lithium

Amdi Amdisen, M.D.

## INTRODUCTION/BACKGROUND

The application of pharmacokinetics to therapy with the lithium ion, $Li^+$ (in the following simply called "lithium"), is still an obscure issue for many clinicians. The prime difficulty is probably the after-effects of the precarious situation which was created in the mid-fifties, when adjustment of the lithium dosage according to its serum concentrations was introduced on a basis which, in retrospect, is unsatisfactory.

In 1950 Talbott (1) proposed that the plasma lithium concentration should never exceed 1.00 mmol/l during maintenance therapy, or toxicity would result. However, neither Noack and Trautner (2) nor Schou et al (3) were able to demonstrate any correlation between serum lithium concentrations and either therapeutic or toxic effects. In both these studies, there were patients with serum lithium concentrations close to 3.00 mmol/l without symptoms of intoxication. There was also a patient who suffered severe intoxication in spite of a serum concentration as low as 0.60 mmol/l (3). Since most patients in the study by Schou et al (3) showed serum lithium concentrations within a range of 0.50 to 2.00 mmol/l, they recommended this as the therapeutic range (4,5,6).

These procedures and recommendations were not well based on lithium pharmacokinetics and did not consider the influence of dosing or formulation on the blood concentration time course over the day (Figures 1 and 2). The toxicity of lithium was becoming more apparent, and there was an urgent need for new methods if the drug was to be used safely (7,8,9,10,11,12). Further need for close monitoring was apparent after the first systematic trial of lithium for long-term "prophylactic" treatment of frequently relapsing psychotic patients (9).

In terms of the usual *twelve-hour standardized serum lithium concentration (12h-stSLi)*, (13) a value above 1.50 mmol/l may cause acute

586

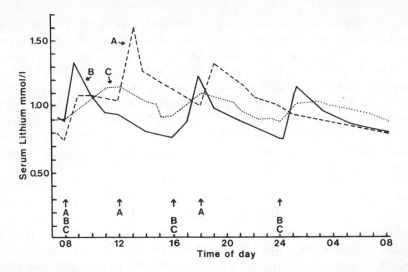

FIGURE 1. Fluctuations of the serum lithium concentration during steady-state. A, B and C all illustrate a 43-year-old man weighing 82 kg and given 12 mmol of lithium t.i.d. A: Conventional time regimen and conventional lithium carbonate tablets. B: Exactly 8 hours between intake of conventional lithium carbonate tablets. C: Exactly 8 hours between intake of sustained-release tablets with a controlled dissolution (Lithionit® Durettes®). (From Amdisen and Sjögren (67): Acta Pharmaceutica Suecica 1968; 5:465–472, with permission).

or subacute renal impairment, and thereby a corresponding reduction in lithium elimination. If treatment continues without dose reduction, a vicious circle leading to intoxication may easily be started (14,15). This consequence of an *acute* renal toxicity of lithium at modest concentrations (10,11) explains why any therapeutic dosage should be regarded as near-toxic (2). This acute kidney impairment at only slightly elevated lithium levels is a likely precursor to most intoxications (11), which later progress further because the decline in renal function renders the maintenance dosage too high (10,11,16).

Gershon and Trautner were the first to study the pharmacokinetic properties of lithium in man (9). These investigators made three remarkable recommendations: (a) therapeutic ranges of either 0.80 to 1.00 or 1.30 to 1.50 mmol Li$^+$/l in plasma; (b) employ monthly plasma concentration measurements, and, if these ranges could not be maintained, (c) abandon the lithium treatment because of its dangerousness without these safeguards. Figures 1, 2 and 9 show that using conventional lithium tablets, it would be difficult to maintain most patients within these narrow ranges unless the time interval between blood drawing and the last dose, and the number of doses per day had been standardized. In retrospect, the explanation for the success of the narrow ranges of Gershon and Trautner may have been that all their patients had four-times-a-day lithium doses in a fixed regimen, and blood was drawn at a fixed time point more than 8 to 10 hours after the last dose. Such standardized procedures might have occurred as part of hospital routine. Unfortunately, this standardization was overlooked by subsequent investigators and these recommendations were almost immediately forgotten.

Plasma concentrations of lithium must be interpreted within the context of time of blood sampling, dosage schedule employed and lithium preparation given. For example, a value of 2.00 mmol/l in serum or plasma could be without concern if blood had been taken at the peak time after intake of conventional tablets (see Figures 1, 2 and 9). On the other hand, the same serum lithium concentration could also indicate progressing toxicity if the sample were obtained prior to the morning dose (11).

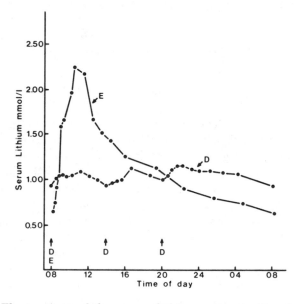

FIGURE 2.   Fluctuations of the serum lithium concentration during steady-state. D illustrates a 52-year-old woman weighing 57 kg and E a 27-year-old woman weighing 53 kg. D: t.i.d.-regimen adapted to the patient's private life during use of sustained-release tablets with a controlled dissolution (Litrarex®). E: Single-dose regimen of conventional lithium carbonate tablets. (From Amdisen: Lithiumbehandling. Copenhagen: Dumex, 1975, with permission.)

The observation of rapidly fluctuating serum concentrations during the day led to routine blood drawing early in the morning before the first lithium dose of the day (20) or, alternatively, 6 to 8 hours after either the morning or the mid-day dose. Then, in 1974, attention was drawn to the importance of the dosing regimen (Figure 9) (14,15). During the following years, a sampling interval of twelve hours was gradually introduced (22) and the level of the interindividual therapeutic range was lowered correspondingly (see below). It is surprising that scientific papers dealing with lithium still cite lithium concentration values without providing any information about such essential variables as dosage regimen and its relation to blood sampling and dissolution properties of the lithium preparation used. This omission almost always results in making a stated lithium concentration useless, and often directly misleading.

It should be stressed that patients may be pushed directly into intoxication if one fails to recognize that each dosing regimen demands a specific standardization of safety limits. For example, a dangerous situation would emerge if a single daily dosing regimen with conventional lithium tablets were combined with blood drawing just before the dose (cf. Figure 2) and concentrations were adjusted to the 12h-stSLi therapeutic value.

The last two decades have witnessed a rapid expansion of pharmacokinetic knowledge and techniques. Regrettably, a general application of these techniques to lithium therapy has been hampered by misunderstandings resulting from premature introduction of the lithium concentration as a monitoring device, before its proper use was appreciated. Because lithium monitoring was characterized as a rather unreliable tool to be used only as a supplement to symptom-oriented monitoring of lithium treatment (27), the implications of this warning were not appreciated by most clinicians and research workers.

A chronic toxic effect of lithium on the kidneys and the thyroid gland has long been appreciated (28,29,30). It was, however, thought that only when patients became symptomatic with tremor, polyuria and weight gain would these side effects be of more than a minor importance. During the last few years, it has become evident that myxedema (31) and impaired renal concentrating ability (11,16,32,33,34,35,36,37) often occur with a severity and frequency that make them clinically serious.

In rats, the chronic renal toxicity of lithium is dose- and duration-dependent (38,39). Therefore, the individual *minimum* effective concentration level in man should be continually sought.

Ideally, we should start all over again and carry out prospective investigations assessing the benefits of acute antimanic lithium treatment and long-term prophylactic effects of $Li^+$ in diminishing relapse rates. Such investigations would be ethically unacceptable; these patients are suffering from a socially disabling and potentially life-threatening disorder. Furthermore, Cade in 1949 (8) and Noack and Trautner in 1951 (2), provide an instruction for lithium therapy by thorough and continuous symptom supervision. Finally, early studies on monitoring serum concentrations have strongly indicated that a lithium dosage producing 12h-stSLi values below 0.30 mmol/l would be without therapeutic effect, and that values above 1.30 mmol/l would give no further improvement in antimanic treatment (41), but would expose patients to acute intoxication (10,11,15).

In 1973 Frazer et al (42,43) showed that lithium concentrations in the brain of rats were better correlated with erythrocyte concentrations than with serum concentrations. In man, however, the brain concentration may be 50 to 100% higher than the comparable serum concentration (18) while that of erythrocytes is only about 40 to 50% (44) (i.e. about one-fourth of the concentration in the brain). The lithium concentration of erythrocytes and the erythrocyte-plasma ratio have attracted much interest during recent years, both as potential control measures and potential predictors of outcome. The results are still inconclusive and contradictory (44,45,46,47,48) and therefore have only limited utility in applied pharmacokinetics. The same holds true for saliva lithium concentrations, primarily because of poor reproducibility of the concentration course, and interindividual differences greater than those found with serum lithium (49,50).

## Absorption

When lithium is used as a pharmacological agent, it is always administered orally. The usual dosage forms may be either conventional or sustained-release tablets (51). Parenteral administration has only rarely been tried (52) because of fear of serious adverse reactions produced by the high peak concentration immediately following the injection. Injectable depot lithium preparations have never been marketed, and the manufacture of such products may have proven impossible. Administration per rectum would not be feasible because of painful diarrheas caused by the local irritating effect of lithium (53).

If a fasting person takes lithium in the form of a dilute solution (i.e., lithium chloride), absorption is rapid. This rapid absorption is reflected by a steeply rising serum lithium concentration. In normal volunteers, the absorption half-time ranges from 6 to 17 minutes (54). The peak concentration is usually reached after about 15 to 45 minutes, and serum concentrations then decline in two phases (Figure 3). Experiments with delayed release preparations, and experiments with rectal administration have shown that lithium is readily absorbed

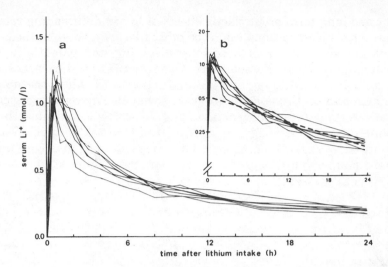

FIGURE 3.   24-hour course of serum lithium concentrations of seven volunteers after intake of a single dose of 24 mmol of lithium as the chloride in
300 ml of water. (a) Conventional diagram. (b) Semilog diagram. (From Amdisen (15): Danish Medical Bulletin 1975; *22*:277–291, with permission).

throughout the gastrointestinal tract (53). Urinary recovery during
steady-state is essentially 100% after intake of a dilute lithium chloride solution, indicating that absorption from aqueous solutions is
essentially complete.

Thus, disintegration and dissolution properties of lithium tablets
usually influence both course and completeness of the absorption
(15,55,56). Figure 4 shows that conventional tablets produce an erratic
and often unpredictable serum concentration-time course. While absorption may be almost as rapid as after intake of a lithium chloride
solution, at other times it may occur even slower than after the sustained-release preparations. It is also noteworthy that the two sustained-release preparations are released both slowly and consistently.
However, when a sustained-release preparation is not consistently
released, it may produce serum concentrations much more erratic
than those of conventional tablets (57) and the loss through feces may
be much greater and much more variable (15). Even when high quality
tablets are used, as much as about 15% of the lithium may not be
absorbed (15,58,59).

During the first 6 to 10 hours after a dose, fluctuations in dissolution
of the drug preparation and in the absorption course will be reflected
as variability in serum concentration. Therefore, blood sampling
should be more than 10 hours after the last dose.

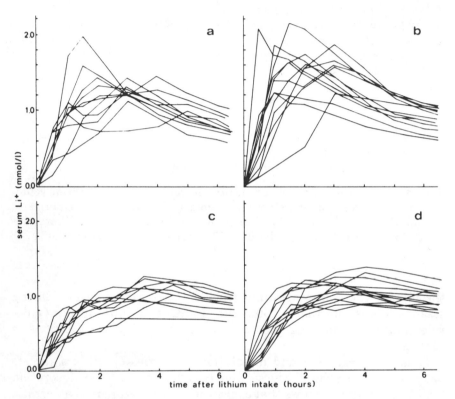

FIGURE 4. Courses of the serum lithium concentration during the first six hours after intake of a single dose of conventional tablets (a and b), and sustained-release tablets (c and d). a and c, about 0.7 mmol Li⁺/kg body weight; b and d, about 0.85 mmol Li⁺/kg body weight. a = conventional lithium carbonate tablets. b = conventional lithium citrate tablets. c = sustained-release tablets, Lithionit® Duretter®. d = sustained-release tablets, Litarex®. (From Amdisen (14): Nordisk Psykiatrisk Tidsskrift 1974; 28:407–430, with permission).

## Distribution

After absorption, lithium is unevenly distributed among a multitude of compartments (3,18,60,61,62,63). For example, a concentration of less than half of the corresponding serum concentration is encountered in erythrocytes (44), spinal fluid (cf. Fig. 12) (11,64) and liver, whereas the thyroid gland, bone and brain have concentrations more than 50% above the serum concentration. In muscle, heart, lung and kidney, the concentration is almost equal to that in serum.

The decline in serum concentrations is biphasic and can be described by a two-compartment model. Initial lithium distribution is into a central distribution space of 24 to 38% of the body weight, and the final distribution space averages 50 to 100% of body weight (15,54). The central space is larger than the extracellular space, and the steady-state distribution space is larger than total body water. Both observations indicate that lithium is also bound somewhere in the body, although no protein-binding in plasma has been demonstrated (65).

There seems to be a strong trend towards a smaller final distribution volume in elderly persons, on average about 90% of the body weight compared to about 120% in younger people (66). This implies that geriatric patients will require a smaller dosage to achieve therapeutic steady-state serum concentrations. This must be considered when instituting therapy in a patient over 55 years old (66).

## Excretion

Lithium is not metabolized. Wherever it is present, it is most likely to be fully biologically active, which means that it is potentially toxic if concentrations are elevated. Although this may be of concern for the distal nephron, no evidence has appeared to raise a corresponding degree of concern for the epithelium of the renal pelvises, ureters, bladder and urethra. After intake of a dilute solution of lithium chloride, urinary recovery is about 100% (15). In this experimental situation, the unavoidable loss of lithium through feces and sweat is negligible. However, when a lithium preparation with poor bioavailability is used, substantial amounts of non-absorbed lithium may be lost through feces (15,53,55,57,67). In the case of protracted watery stools or profuse sweating, the possibility of an extraordinary loss of lithium has not yet been investigated.

The lithium ion readily passes the glomerular membrane, but since renal plasma clearance (15,17,65,68,69,70,71) is about 20% of the glomerular filtration rate, about 80% of the lithium filtered through the glomeruli must be reabsorbed by the renal tubules. It is possible that this takes place exclusively in the proximal convoluted tubules, with roughly the same absorption ratio as sodium and water (72). The result is a renal lithium clearance of plasma which varies interindividually from about 8 to about 40 ml/min (15,71).

The renal clearance of lithium may be influenced by several variables. Reductions in the renal clearance of lithium are seen with any type of kidney impairment; these reductions develop very slowly with increasing age (37), rapidly during occurrence of chronic or subchronic renal diseases, and more rapidly in connection with acute kidney disorders. The sensitivity of lithium clearance to slowly developing kidney impairments is a principal reason for using lithium serum concentrations for routine monitoring of treatment. The problem of drug default (non-compliance) might be another important reason (45). However, if the lithium concentration is to be regarded as a reliable monitoring tool, patient non-compliance must be eliminated by thorough information and training of the patients and their close relatives.

Of more importance, however, may be that most long-term lithium-treated patients have an increased diuresis (11,37,73). The reasons are probably a lithium-produced impaired renal response to antidiuretic hormone (35,74,75) and an impaired renal concentrating ability caused by chronic interstitial nephropathy (11,16,33,34). The former is a consequence of a subchronic nephrotoxic effect, the latter of a *chronic* nephrotoxic effect of lithium, in both cases at therapeutic concentration levels. The occurrence of one or both of these impairments makes the lithium patient especially vulnerable to dehydration in risk situations such as fever diseases, watery stools and/or vomiting for a prolonged period, loss of appetite (note this possibility during a depressive relapse) and hot weather (e.g., travel in countries with a hot climate). Even frequent sauna bathing may represent a definite risk of dehydration with fatal consequences (76). Dehydration, regardless of its origin, results in a negative sodium balance. The kidney attempts to save sodium by increasing proximal reabsorption. Since Li and Na are handled similarly in the proximal tubules, the reabsorption of Li is increased and thereby a reduced renal lithium clearance results (11,16).

Treatment with natriuretic diuretics rapidly induces a pronounced reduction of renal lithium clearance (77), as does treatment with indomethacin (78). In addition, the excretion fraction of lithium may be reduced by about 50% when the urinary sodium excretion falls below 2 mmol per day (70). For patients taking lithium, such concurrent treatment creates a complicated situation which demands careful supervision of diuretic drug treatment so that the total amount of lithium in the body is kept at a safe level.

Negative sodium balance quickly leads to sodium depletion in the lithium-treated rat, while in man the development is presumably slower (69,70). Most non-medical slimming diets are short of sodium, and they share with salt-poor diets the same difficult monitoring problems that arise during diuretic therapy.

Aminophylline may enhance renal lithium elimination (79), but it has not been demonstrated to have any substantial importance in the treatment of lithium poisoning. One might speculate that consumption of varying amounts of coffee (caffeine) might cause a worsening of intraindividual reproducibility of serum lithium concentrations.

A 50% enhancement of human renal lithium elimination has been observed with intake of extreme amounts of sodium (70). Sodium loading was efficient in the treatment of intoxicated rats (69,80,81) and overloading with sodium has been recommended for the treatment of lithium intoxication in man (82,83). However, this procedure has not only proven clinically unsatisfactory because of a too weak and short-lasting effect (11), but also dangerous because in some patients it produced severe hyperosmolarity (11,84).

During the later part of pregnancy, both creatinine clearance and lithium clearance often increase, subsequently decreasing to pre-pregnancy values shortly after delivery. This change in renal function may create difficulties in monitoring lithium treatment during pregnancy and delivery (85).

Finally, both lithium clearance and creatinine clearance show a circadian rhythm, with higher values during daytime. The practical implications of this observation are difficult to evaluate at present, because the day-night difference was only observed in three healthy volunteers and also was found to be very small (86).

The amount of lithium excreted per unit time through the kidneys varies proportionally with the lithium concentration in plasma. Otherwise stated, the net lithium elimination is governed by linear first-order processes. As a simplified illustrative example, assume that: (a) the lithium concentrations in plasma and glomerular filtrate are equal; (b) the glomerular filtrate amounts to 150 liters and the diuresis to 1000 ml during the 24 hours of the day; (c) the 1000 ml of urine are produced with a constant velocity; and (d) the lithium excretion is 20% of the amount filtered by the glomeruli. In this hypothetical case, the lithium concentration in urine will be 30 times the simultaneous concentration in plasma. For the single-dose regimen shown in Figure 2 this would mean a variation of urinary lithium from about 25 mmol/l to about 75 mmol/l.

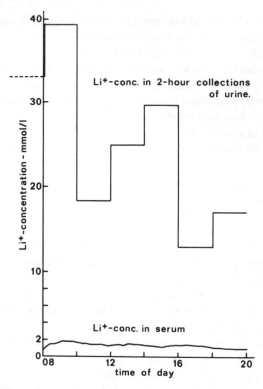

FIGURE 5. Concomitant fluctuations during daytime of the lithium concentration in serum and urine. Female patient on long-term treatment taking 24.3 mmol of lithium twice daily (8 a.m. and 8 p.m.) in the form of conventional lithium carbonate tablets. The urine volume of the 12 hours shown was within the high normal range, 1196 ml. (From Amdisen (88): Johnson FN, ed. *A Handbook of Lithium Therapy.* MTP, Lancaster 1979, with permission.)

In reality, the renal water excretion is not constant; it varies considerably during the day, producing both maximally high and extremely low urinary concentrations. It is not only early in the morning that maximally concentrated urine is normally produced but also occasionally during the day (87). Furthermore, most lithium patients already suffer from their lithium-induced increase of the urine volume (16,37). Many patients also suffer from an impaired ability to concentrate maximally (16,35,37), so that they presumably do not experience the very high urinary lithium concentrations. Nevertheless, a lithium concentration in urine of about 15 mmol/l is common (16,37). This value is still potentially toxic to almost all tissues. Figure 5 shows that in spite of a diuresis of almost 2½ liters per day, rather high urinary lithium concentrations may still appear. High concentrations are reached not only in the early morning hours, but also incidentally during the day.

Because lithium is not metabolized and is eliminated exclusively through the kidneys, both the renal clearance and elimination half-life are expressions of the wash-out rate from the central distribution space, of which plasma is a minor part. Thus, the dosage required to reach a certain concentration is in ratio to renal clearance directly, and elimination half-life inversely.

Since steady-state will essentially be reached after four to six elimination half-lives, it is of practical importance to assess the half-life of lithium during the elimination phase (beta-phase). If lithium were always ingested as a dilute solution of lithium chloride, where the absorption half-time is 6 to 17 minutes (54), and this is added to the distribution half-time of 40 to 90 minutes, it would be possible to determine elimination half-life by using a few blood samples drawn during an adequate period of time starting about twelve hours after intake of a suitable test dose. When lithium tablets are used, the absorption half-time may comprise more than one hour. In this situation, it is necessary to postpone the drawing of the first blood sample until 15 to 20 hours after the lithium dose. Unfortunately, the last blood sample will very often show a lithium concentration too low to be determined with satisfactory accuracy.

Because of this, the elimination half-life has been estimated by determining serial concentrations after a lithium dose and fitting the data to a two-compartment model. In this situation, lithium elimination half-life varies between 14 and 33 hours (15,54,89,90). It should be noted, however, that all the subjects studied were healthy, and for the most part normal volunteers. A cautious conclusion may be that steady-state is reached within eight days after initiation of treatment.

It might be useful to remember the general rule that the dosage required to produce a specified concentration level, for example the mean, is related to the elimination-rate constant ($K_{el}$). As a crude approximation, it may be said that a lower dosage requirement implies a slow elimination rate constant, and these patients would need a longer period of time to reach steady-state.

**Circadian variation of elimination half-life.** Preliminary data strongly indicate that some patients show a comparatively great variation of elimination half-life between daytime and nighttime, amounting to a night-to-day ratio of about 2.5 (15). In the choice of specifications for standardization, this has been a contributory reason for placing the blood drawing for treatment control in the morning instead of allowing a free choice between morning or late evening.

## CONCENTRATION VERSUS RESPONSE AND TOXICITY

### Therapeutic Concentrations

The therapeutic concentration range refers to those limits between which the lithium-responding patients are distributed according to the mean level of their individual control concentrations during steady-state. Some patients respond on a low concentration, many others require a medium level, while others require a higher concentration (10).

As regards the twelve-hour serum lithium, the range was estimated to be 0.30 to 1.30 mmol/l (40). This range was supported by analyzing 84 lithium responders (15) comprising the patient material of Baastrup et al (91) and by studying directly the 12h-stSLi in about 80 lithium responders (10).

Prien and Caffey (92) found a less satisfactory treatment efficacy among periodically depressive patients with concentration means between 0.50 and 0.80 mmol/l and more satisfactory above 0.80 mmol/l. They also found that manic patients needed 0.90 to 1.40 mmol/l to achieve antimanic effect (41). In Prien's studies, however, the blood was drawn after an interval of less than twelve hours, i.e. *8 to 12 hours.* The concentration range would have been roughly 20 to 25% lower if all blood samples had been drawn at an interval of twelve hours.

In the study by Jerram and McDonald (93) the relapse-repressive effect was found to be equally good at concentrations between 0.50 and 0.69 mmol/l and at concentrations just above and just below this range, but in this study the blood was drawn *12 to 16 hours* after the last dose. This means that the ranges would probably have been roughly 15 to 20% higher for the 12-hour samples.

In conclusion, when the individual velocities of the concentration fall during the period 8 to 16 hours after the last dose are considered, there seems to be no real disagreement among all the authors just mentioned—even the clinical impression of Gershon and Trautner from 1956 (9) seems to be in accordance.

Stokes et al (52) found the treatment efficacy for mania to increase with increasing serum lithium from 0.20 to 2.00 mmol/l. However, they had too few treatment periods with concentrations above 1.40 mmol/l to either prove or refute the proposed decline in improvement rate suggested by Prien et al (41). The concentrations cited by Stokes et al (52) are also somewhat difficult to interpret. Although the concentrations used are admittedly steady-state values, the drug preparation was a lithium chloride solution given in four doses per day, and the blood was drawn in the morning before the first dose of the day; no information was given about the exact points in time for the four dose administrations during the day, especially the last one, or about the blood sampling time in the morning. The overall concentration profile is therefore insufficiently known, and the information loses credibility.

All things considered, the therapeutic range of Figure 6 is probably an acceptable guideline when one exception is taken into consideration: according to Prien et al (41) and supported by Stokes et al (52), a satisfactory acute antimanic effect can hardly be expected below a mean 12h-stSLi of about 0.80 mmol/l.

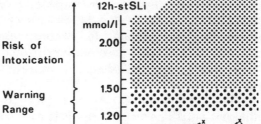

FIGURE 6. The curve of the figure demonstrates the check values of 12h-stSLi in a 42-year-old man during start and follow-up of lithium treatment. The first three controls were made on three consecutive weekdays after intake during the preceding week of one Litarex® tablet (6 mmol Li⁺) at 8 a.m. and 8 p.m. According to the values found, the dosage was then increased to three Litarex® tablets twice daily. The following four controls of 12h-stSLi correspond to once every week, the next five to once every month, and the rest to one every second to third month. (From Amdisen (13): Journal of Analytical Toxicology 1978; 2:193–202. Preston Publ., Inc., with permission.)

## Toxic concentrations of 12h-stSLi

Our entire present knowledge about the relation between lithium concentration and lithium poisoning is based on clinical experience. For most patients, 12h-stSLi concentrations even as high as 1.50 to 2.50 mmol/l are not in themselves life-threatening and such patients may avoid passing into a fatal state of poisoning in spite of having experienced the symptoms of slight intoxication: apathy and sluggishness, drowsiness, lethargy, sleepiness, speech difficulty, varying coarse and irregular tremor, smaller myoclonic twitchings, muscular weakness and ataxia. But in patients whose renal resistance towards lithium is in the lower range, and whose kidneys therefore react by impaired functioning and a reduced lithium elimination, the above conditions may easily progress to a fatal poisoning unless the daily lithium dose is reduced or the treatment stopped (10,11).

As it is not possible to isolate in advance the less vulnerable patients, a 12h-stSLi of 1.50 mmol/l should *always* be regarded as serious until repeated controls of the serum lithium level have shown whether the patient is actually suffering from an impending lithium intoxication or if other and more innocent explanations of the high 12h-stSLi can be found. It is not unusual, for example, for a patient to forget to omit the morning lithium dose before the blood sampling.

A 12h-stSLi of 2.50 to 3.50 mmol/l demands immediate and urgent action. A 12h-stSLi concentration above 3.50 mmol/l should be regarded as highly life-threatening (11). In both cases the treatment of choice is hemodialysis—with peritoneal dialysis as a less satisfactory alternative. Treatment should be instituted irrespective of the presence of intoxication symptoms, because in some patients the symptoms are delayed for a period of up to two or three days (11,18,19).

When the serum lithium concentration is below 2.50 mmol/l and the time interval from the last intake of lithium is 12 hours or more, serum lithium should be determined every third hour and the values plotted on a semilog scale versus time. Extrapolation backwards in time may disclose that 12 hours after the last dose the concentration had been 2.50 mmol/l or more, and the patient belongs to one of the two serious categories above. Furthermore, since renal function may have been progressively impaired before the examination, the 12-h value estimated by backward extrapolation should be regarded as a minimum value.

When the 12h-stSLi concentration is estimated below 2.50 mmol/l, but the semilog diagram shows that the concentration is falling at a slower rate than 10% per 3 hours, a progression towards acute anuria is possible. Such a patient should also be treated with hemodialysis.

Conservative treatment with special concern for water and electrolyte balance should only be employed for patients with a lithium excretion rate greater than 10% per 3 hours.

## Exceptions

A few patients, whose sensitivity to the toxicity of lithium was apparently exceptionally pronounced, developed severe symptoms within the therapeutic range of 12h-stSLi, thus making treatment impracticable (41,94,95). Combined treatment with lithium and neuroleptic drugs may be employed (31), but some react to this combination with a state of confusion (9,25,94,96). None of these reported cases is quite satisfactorily elucidated, especially not with respect to pharmacokinetic data. However, since severe toxic reactions do occur at 12h-stSLi levels below 1.30 mmol/l, such patients should be admitted to hospital for close supervision.

Since resistance to toxic agents usually decreases with increasing age, elderly patients should be dosed to 12h-stSLi values above 0.70 mmol/l with caution (97).

## CLINICAL APPLICATION OF PHARMACOKINETIC DATA

**Serum lithium course from early morning to late afternoon on a day off lithium.** Figure 7 shows that when the last lithium dose has been given at 6 p.m. the concentration falls during the period 8 a.m. to 3 p.m. on the following day showing "half-lives" of from 5 to 35 hours, with most subjects placed between 8 and 20 hours. Figure 8 is a constructed illustration of three representative "patients" with the same mean serum lithium during treatment before the day off lithium. The data show that if the standardized time interval is longer than twelve hours, the comparability between serum concentrations of virtually comparable patients is lost. The choice of twelve hours is not optimal, but shortening of the time interval would impose other disadvantages relating to absorption and distribution overlap with elimination.

**Dosage.** Some patients need only to be placed within the lower part of the therapeutic *concentration* range and have only a low lithium clearance; such patients require very low dosages. Other patients need high concentrations and have high lithium clearances, and they need very high daily dosages. The therapeutic dosage range for lithium patients as a group is therefore very wide, from about 4 mmol (150 mg Li carbonate) of lithium per day (98) up to about 80 to 100 mmol (3500 mg Li carbonate) per day (10). Because of the low therapeutic

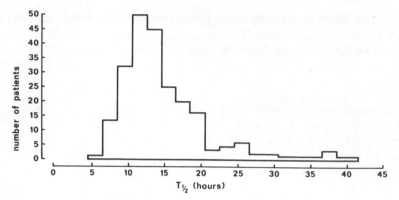

FIGURE 7. Distribution of 226 persons according to their lithium half-life, T½, during daytime. Drawing of blood samples for determination of the serum lithium concentration took place at 8 a.m. and about 3 p.m. Note the "T½" is used as an estimate of the velocity of the fall from morning to evening on a day off lithium during steady-state, although the determination in most cases was made after a single dose. (From Amdisen (14): Nordisk Psykiatrisk Tidsskrift 1974; 28:407–430, with permission.)

index of lithium, the dosage of one particular patient may be highly dangerous to another, even after only a few days' intake, making pharmacokinetic monitoring of patients taking lithium an integral part of therapy.

The mean dosage from larger studies has been about 30 mmol of lithium per day (16,37). The amount is of the same order of magnitude as the total amount of lithium present in the body during lithium treatment (54).

**Dose regimen.** The influence of the dosage regimen on the fundamental 24-hour profile of the plasma lithium concentration is illustrated by Figure 9. In this figure, the curves are constructed on the basis of a two-compartment model to give an impression of the profiles corresponding to a "patient" with a shorter elimination half-life and taking a fast-releasing tablet. The mean concentrations are equal for all four dose regimens in this particular "patient". The one-dose-per-day regimen deviates in every essential respect from the other three dose regimens. It is especially worth noting that the multiple-dose regimens show almost equal values twelve hours after the last dose.

**Specifications for the twelve-hour standardized serum lithium (12h-stSLi) concentration for monitoring of the therapeutic dosage.**

(a) Blood obtained in the morning before the first lithium dose, exactly (± 30 minutes) twelve hours after the evening dose.

(b) The daily dosage separated into two or more doses - (preferably t.i.d.)

(c) The dosage regimen, both number of doses and points in time of intake, carefully observed at least the day before taking the blood sample.

(d) Steady-state conditions.

(e) (If available and practically feasible for the patient, only lithium preparations with a controlled release should be used.)

In case of urgency where blood may be drawn irrespective of standardized conditions, the best estimate of the corresponding 12h-stSLi should be made on the basis of knowledge about both the time and the magnitude of the last lithium intake, the dosage regimen (both number of doses and points of time of intake) and properties of the lithium preparation used.

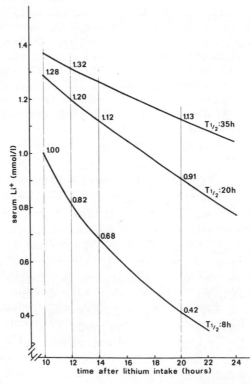

FIGURE 8. Computer constructed curves based on steady-state, dose administration every 12 hours, and similar mean concentrations previous to the time interval shown. The three curves illustrate fast-normal excretors (T½ 8 hours), slow-normal excretors (T½ 20 hours) and abnormal slow excretors (T½ 35 hours), respectively (cf. Fig. 7). (From Amdisen (15): Danish Medical Bulletin 1975; 22:277–291, with permission.)

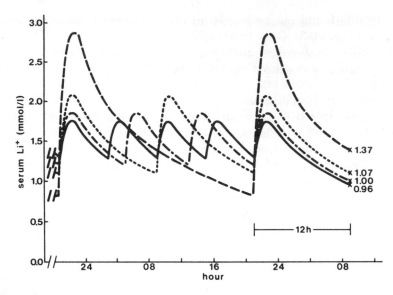

FIGURE 9. The fundamental importance of the dose regimen for fluctuations of the serum lithium concentration and 12h-stSLi. Computer constructed curves according to a two-compartment model of a "patient" with a short elimination-T½ (13 hours) and taking fast-release tablets with a controlled dissolution. (From Amdisen (14): Nordisk Psykiatrisk Tidsskrift 1974; 18:407–430, with permission.)

The primary aim of adapting pharmacokinetics to lithium therapy has been exploitation of the possibility of continual monitoring of the individual patient. None of the hallmarks of the concentration profile during the day (for example the maximum value, the minimum value, or perhaps the overall shape of the total 24-hour concentration course) seems to be of special importance with lithium use. Thus, standardizing the time factor for blood sampling has been considered of prime importance in achieving intraindividual reproducibility. The consideration of first and foremost importance is maintaining an adequate distance from the greater and more unpredictable concentration fluctuations during the absorption and distribution phase. The 12h-stSLi has been adopted from considerations of both the convenience for daily life and the possibility of establishing general guidelines for safe treatment. As a consequence, the choice of 12 hours for the time interval has been regarded as the optimal compromise.

Figures 10 and 11 illustrate the intraindividual reproducibility of 12h-stSLi which is achievable in practice, and they also reveal that a 12h-stSLi should not be judged in isolation but in consideration of previous values (45). Only pronounced deviations should lead to direct action, while smaller deviations should lead to repetition of 12h-stSLi, repeatedly if necessary, for clarification of apparent fluctuations.

Table 1 enumerates ten factors which may disturb the reliability of 12h-stSLi. Numbers 1 through 4 and number 10 should be controlled by repeated instruction of the patient. A non-cooperative patient should be put on long-term lithium treatment very reluctantly because of the risk of non-adherence to the drug treatment. Factor numbers 4 through 7 may be brought under the physician's control through inquiries, and proper choice of laboratory and lithium preparation.

**Practical use of the 12h-stSLi.** There is no therapeutic reference range for the one-dose-per-day regimen. Figure 6 is valid for multiple dose regimens only. It is my personal opinion that three doses per day should be preferred, although the tablet intake should be integrated with the patient's lifestyle.

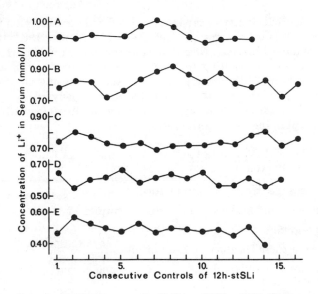

FIGURE 10.   Intraindividual reproducibility of 12h-stSLi. Twice weekly check values in 5 persons taking conventional lithium carbonate tablets (8.1 mmol Li$^+$ per tablet). A: 2 tablets at 8 a.m., 1 tablet at 2 p.m. and 2 tablets at 9 p.m. B: 2 tablets at 8 a.m., 2 p.m. and 9 p.m. C: 1 tablet at 8 a.m., 2 p.m. and 9 p.m. D: 1 tablet at 8 a.m., 2 p.m. and 9 p.m. E: 1 tablet at 8 a.m. and 9 p.m. (From Amdisen (13): Journal of Analytical Toxicology 1978; 2: 193–202. Preston Publ., Inc., with permission.)

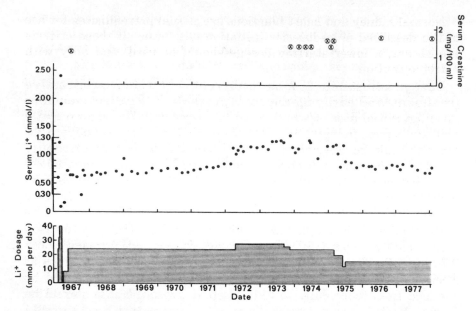

FIGURE 11. Reproducibility of the standardized SLi control value in a male patient (born 1931) of consummate treatment compliance. 1967–1970: 15h-stSLi; 1971 to date: 12h-stSLi. Notice (a) that the patient was started in 1967 on too high a dosage resulting in a slight lithium intoxication and a few weeks' interruption of lithium treatment; (b) the decreasing dosage requirement concomitant with decreasing renal function (slowly rising serum creatinine). (From Amdisen (13): Journal of Analytical Toxicology 1978; 2:193–202. Preston Publ., Inc., with permission.)

TABLE 1. VARIABLE FACTORS OF POTENTIALLY CRUCIAL
IMPORTANCE FOR THE RELIABILITY OF 12h-stSLi*

1. Lithium dosage (treatment compliance).
2. Time interval in blood sampling (deviation from 12 hours).
3. Dosage regimen.
4. Accuracy of the laboratory determination.
5. Lithium content of the drug preparation and variation within and between batches.
6. Dissolution properties of the drug preparation.
7. Bioavailability of the drug preparation.
8. Alimentary intake of sodium and extrarenal loss of sodium.
9. Coffee drinking?
10. Natriuretic and other drugs influencing renal elimination.

*Listed in the order of estimated practical importance.

606

Normal kidney and heart functions are crucial prerequisites for use of the described procedure for initiation of lithium. If these criteria are absent, a lower starting dosage should be used, and only with extreme caution.

**Dosage adjustment in long-term treatment (relapse-repressive treatment) and easily managed hypomania.** The patient should be given an initial dose of 4 to 6 mmol $Li^+$ twice daily, for example at 9 a.m. and 9 p.m., for eight days. On the following three weekdays, 12h-stSLi's should be determined. According to the direct proportionality (15) the maintenance dosage is now adjusted, showing a mean 12h-stSLi between only 0.80 and 1.00 mmol/l. A mean of 1.10 to 1.30 mmol/l would produce troublesome and sometimes unbearable toxic side effects.

Depending on the magnitude of dosage increment required to reach a 12h-stSLi of about 0.90 mmol/l (in elderly patients primarily only 0.70 mmol/l), the daily dosage is then increased by smaller steps at weekly intervals. At the same time the dosage regimen should be changed from twice daily to t.i.d. Each stepwise increase should be preceded with a serum level estimation, to ensure that the 12h-stSLi has reached the expected value. When the desired serum lithium level has been reached, 12h-stSLi should be measured every week for four weeks, and thereafter every month for five to six months, and then continually every other month. Gershon and Trautner (9) and Baldessarini and Lipinski (26) have recommended serum level determination at monthly intervals, which may prove to be safer.

If the treatment efficacy is unsatisfactory, the dosage should be increased to produce a 12h-stSLi mean between 1.10 and 1.30 mmol/l. Serum lithium should be maintained at this level long enough to find out whether the patient is a virtual non-responder, or eventually will respond to higher concentrations. When a patient maintained at a mean 12h-stSLi level of 0.80 to 1.00 mmol/l has been a responder, a continual search for the minimum effective 12h-stSLi should be started.

**Dosage adjustment in acute antimanic treatment. Mania treated with difficulty.** The following procedure should only be carried out during hospitalization, where serum lithium concentrations are available within 1 to 2 hours after blood drawing. It should not be used in patients with kidney or heart disease, abnormal serum creatinine and/or abnormal electrocardiogram. The patients should be under constant supervision for symptoms of lithium intoxication.

The patient should be given about 30 mmol $Li^+$ per day in three divided doses. 12h-stSLi must be measured daily from the first morning after start of treatment, and the dosage continually adjusted. In manic patients, each dose intake should be carefully supervised; in cases of noncompliance, the use of 12h-stSLi can be of more danger than advantage.

After the desired mean 12h-stSLi at steady-state has been reached, the concentration monitoring should be continued according to the same guidelines as given for long-term treatment.

**Concentration monitoring during use of diuretic drugs and other drugs influencing renal function, salt-free, salt-poor and slimming diets, and during pregnancy.** 12h-stSLi should be determined every other week.

**Pregnancy and Delivery.** Lithium treatment should be terminated about a week before delivery and then started again cautiously. Because of changes in renal function after delivery, daily measurement should be employed early, with regular monitoring until stable.

**Breastfeeding.** Lithium passes into the mother's milk and may even intoxicate the child (104). No recommendations have been given about control of the infant's lithium concentration during nursing. In my opinion, one should refrain from breastfeeding.

**Intercurrent disorders causing risk of dehydration.** If a patient is unable to counteract loss of water and sodium through adequate extra intake, and it is impossible to interrupt lithium treatment until the risk of dehydration no longer exists, 12h-stSLi should be measured daily.

**Lithium poisoning.** The active treatment of poisoning should be monitored by following the serum concentrations: (a) The efficacy of the hemodialysis should be determined by measurement of serum lithium at the start of dialysis and again at finish. A rebound should be anticipated. (b) If the serum lithium 6 to 8 hours after hemodialysis is greater than 1.00 mmol/l, the dialysis should be repeated (Figure 12). (c) The more slowly working peritoneal dialysis (Figure 13) presents no rebound and should be carried out until serum lithium concentrations are below 1.00 mmol/l.

**A single pretest for dosage adjustment?** There is direct proportionality between renal lithium clearance and the dosage required to achieve a certain level. This situation might be exploited by the use of a single-dose pretest. However, most internists distrust clearance methods based on quantitative urine collection unless at least three independent determinations are made. Furthermore, the pretest tends to overestimate the dosage requirement in patients who need a lithium dosage above 20 to 30 mmol Li$^+$ per day (71) and may increase the risk of intoxication. Therefore this pretest is not recommended.

The plasma concentration profile of each patient can be adapted to a mathematical equation which fits both the single-dose curve and

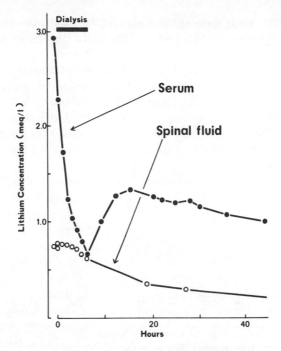

FIGURE 12. The effect of hemodialysis on the lithium concentration in serum and spinal fluid. Note the "rebound phenomenon" of serum lithium after finish of the dialysis. In the author's opinion the hemodialysis should have been repeated in this patient who never regained normal creatinine clearance. The patient was a 48-year-old severely lithium-intoxicated man with acute renal failure almost reaching anuria just before treatment with hemodialysis. (From Amdisen and Skjoldborg (64): The Lancet 1969; 2:213, with permission.)

the steady-state curve (15,54,89,99). In this manner, the single-dose can be used for a computer calculation of the maintenance dosage. This is obviously not convenient for daily practice, but the principle has been simplified to a single dose of 16 mmol of lithium, estimation of the 24-hour serum lithium value and reading the maintenance dosage from a table (100,101). Use of this procedure may be dangerous, because it assumes that a lithium preparation with both controlled release and adequate bioavailability is used. The procedure only secures a steady-state within the broad total therapeutic range, instead of placing the initial level around 0.90 mmol/l. The reliability of the recommendation over time is crucially dependent on the trustworthiness of the drug manufacturer. Furthermore, inspection of the table

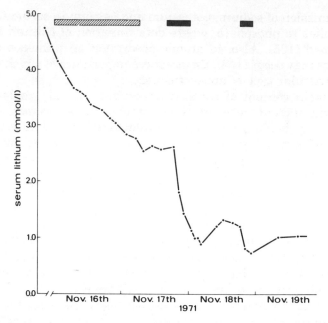

FIGURE 13. Li⁺-concentration in serum before, during and after dialysis in a 45-year-old, severely intoxicated woman.

▨▨▨▨ : Peritoneal dialysis, ████ : Hemodialysis.

(From Hansen and Amdisen (11): Quarterly Journal of Medicine 1978; 47:123–144, with permission.)

of Cooper et al (100,101) as well as the scatter within the diagram of Seifert et al (102) discloses the possibility of reaching a maintenance dosage which may be 50% too high. Thus, although the method has been acceptable for a certain limited period of time in the hands of experts (102,103), it should only be used where a highly reliable laboratory is available to clinicians with much experience with lithium.

## ASSAY METHODS

The only feasible principle for the laboratory determination of lithium is flame photometry, either by an emission flame photometer or an atomic absorption flame photometer. The methods are fundamentally equal for determination of lithium. The emission method has special demands, as it is absolutely necessary to correct for the background emission of sodium, potassium and calcium in serum (20). The same applies to phosphate, where determination of lithium in urine is concerned (105). Also, in atomic absorption an influence of these substances may occur (105), the practical importance of which depends on the particular type of apparatus used.

The protein content of serum represents a special problem, as it disturbs the suction and atomizing system of the apparatus. This can be avoided by using a sufficient dilution similar to that applied for determination of sodium and potassium in serum, but the influence of protein may still necessitate a correction. This problem can be solved by spiking the standard solution used for adjustment of the apparatus adequately with lithium-free serum or dextran (106), glucose, detergens, etc.

For a duplicate determination, 2 to 3 ml of serum are generally required, but some types of apparatus permit micromethods (see, for example, 106). When adequate precautions are taken, (i.e., by avoiding the use of tubes which contain lithium themselves) the serum can be stored directly for an unlimited period of time.

It would not be useful to give detailed instructions for the lithium determination, because technical details vary with the type of apparatus, and even from one particular instrument to another within the same type (20,107). The crucial point is that flame photometers exist which are not sufficiently accurate for lithium treatment. A reasonable coefficient of variation must be 1.5 to 2.0%, and such accuracy should be maintained by frequent controls.

## CONCLUSION

Although concentration monitoring of lithium therapy is admittedly indispensable, it is only supplementary to continuous symptom supervision. Severe intoxication may readily develop within the time interval between two serum concentration controls, even when the interval is as short as two weeks (10,11). The patient and the doctor responsible for the treatment must therefore meet several times during the initial phase of treatment (i.e. the first two or three months), so that both the patient and the close relatives are trained to become competent supervisors for poisoning symptoms. The repeated laboratory measurements are consequently also an aid in keeping in touch with the patient. Written instructions are valuable, but far from sufficient; in my opinion it is necessary to have the instructions repeated verbally at least once a year during long-term treatment.

However, applied pharmacokinetics in lithium therapy is still a young discipline and there is a continuous flow of new ideas, hypotheses and investigations. For example, Plenge (108) suggests that lithium administration every second day may be feasible. All these efforts will most certainly increase our knowledge and thereby our possibilities of offering patients a still safer and more efficient treatment.

## ACKNOWLEDGMENT

I am indebted to Mrs. Jytte Hildebrandt for invaluable assistance in preparation of the manuscript.

## REFERENCES

1. Talbott JH: Use of lithium salts as a substitute for sodium chloride. Arch Intern Med 1950; 85:1–10.
2. Noack CH and Trautner EM: The lithium treatment of maniacal psychosis. Med J Aust 1951; 38:219–22.
3. Schou M, Juel-Nielsen N, Strömgren E and Voldby H: The treatment of manic psychoses by the administration of lithium salts. J Neurol Neurosurg Psychiatry 1954; 17:250–60.
4. Schou M: Lithiumterapi ved mani. Praktiske retningslinier. (Treatment of mania with lithium salts. Practical considerations.—English summary.) Nord Med 1956; 55:790–4.
5. Schou M: Lithium in psychiatric therapy. Stock-taking after ten years. Psychopharmacology 1959; 1:65–78.
6. Gershon S and Yuwiler A: Lithium ion: A specific psychopharmacological approach to the treatment of mania. J Neuropsychiatry 1960; 1:229–41.
7. Amdisen A: Variation of serum lithium concentration during the day in relation to treatment control, absorptive side effects and the use of slow-release tablets. Acta Psychiat Scand 1969; Suppl. 207:55–7.
8. Cade JFJ: Lithium salts in the treatment of psychotic excitement. Med J Aust 1949; 3:349–52.
9. Gershon S and Trautner EM: The treatment of shock-dependency by pharmacological agents. Med J Aust 1956; 43:783–7.
10. Amdisen A: Serum level monitoring and clinical pharmacokinetics of lithium. Clin Pharmacokin 1977; 2:73–92.
11. Hansen HE and Amdisen A: Lithium intoxication. (Report of 23 cases and review of 100 cases from the literature.) Quart J Med, New Ser 1978; 47:123–44.
12. Grau K: Lithiumforgiftning. Et iatrogent fænomen i fremgang? (Lithium poisoning. An increasingly frequent iatrogenic phenomenon?—English summary.) Ugeskr Læg 1978; 140:720–1.
13. Amdisen A: Clinical and serum-level monitoring in lithium therapy and lithium intoxication. J Anal Toxicol 1978; 2:193–202.
14. Amdisen A: Farmakokinetikens praktiske konsekvenser belyst ved lithiumbehandlingens styrings- og kontrolproblemer. (The practical consequences of pharmacokinetics illustrated by monitoring and control problems in the lithium treatment.) Nord Psykiat Tidsskr 1974; 28:407–30.
15. Amdisen A: Monitoring of lithium treatment through determination of lithium concentration. Dan Med Bull 1975; 22:277–91.
16. Hansen HE, Hestbech J, Sørensen JL, Nørgaard K, Heilskov J and Amdisen A: Chronic interstitial nephropathy in patients on long-term lithium treatment. Quart J Med, New Ser 1979; 48:577–91.

17. Trautner EM, Morris R, Noack CH and Gershon S: The excretion and retention of ingested lithium and its effect on the ionic balance of man. Med J Aust 1955; 42:280–91.
18. Amdisen, A, Gottfries CG, Jacobsson L and Winblad B: Grave lithium intoxication with fatal outcome. Acta Psychiat Scand 1974; Suppl. 255:25–33.
19. Achong MR, Fernandez PG and McLeod PJ: Fatal self-poisoning with lithium carbonate. Can Med Ass J 1975; 112:868–70.
20. Amdisen A: Serum lithium determinations for clinical use. Scand J Clin Lab Invest 1967; 20:104–8.
21. Baastrup PC: Lithium in prophylaxis. Curr Psychiat Ther 1969; 9:125–31.
22. Amdisen A: Serum lithium estimations. Br Med J 1973; 2:240.
23. Goodman LS and Gilman A, eds. *The Pharmacological Basis of Therapeutics.* 5th ed. MacMillan Publ. Co., Inc., New York 1975.
24. Spring G, Schweid D, Gray C, Steinberg J and Horwitz M: A double-blind comparison of lithium and chlorpromazine in the treatment of manic states. Am J Psychiatry 1970; 126:1306–10.
25. Shopsin B and Gershon S: Pharmacology—toxicology of the lithium ion. In: Gershon S and Shopsin B, eds. *Lithium: Its Role in Psychiatric Research and Treatment.* Plenum Press, New York, London 1973.
26. Baldessarini RJ and Lipinski JF: Lithium salts. In: Klein DF and Gittelman-Klein R, eds. *Progress in Psychiatric Drug Treatment,* vol 2. Brunner/Mazel, New York 1976.
27. Strömgren E and Schou M: Lithium treatment of manic states. Postgrad Med 1964; 35:83–6.
28. Radomski JL, Fuyat HN, Nelson AA and Smith PK: The toxic effects, excretion and distribution of lithium chloride. J Pharmacol Exp Ther 1950; 100:429–44.
29. Sedvall G, Jönsson J, Pettersson U and Levin K: Effects of lithium salts on plasma protein bound iodine and uptake of I$^{131}$ in thyroid gland of man and rat. Life Sci 1968; 7:1257–64.
30. Amdisen A, Eskjær Jensen S, Olsen T and Schou M: Forekomst af struma under lithiumbehandling. (Development of goitre during lithium treatment.—English summary.) Ugeskr Læg 1968; 130:1515–18.
31. Amdisen A and Schou, M: Lithium. In: Dukes MNG, ed. *Side Effects of Drugs Annual* 2. Amsterdam, Oxford: Excerpta Medica 1978.
32. Simon NM, Garber E and Arief AJ: Persistent nephrogenic diabetes insipidus after lithium carbonate. Ann Intern Med 1977; 86:446–7.
33. Hansen HE, Hestbech J, Olsen S and Amdisen A: Renal function and renal pathology in patients with lithium-induced impairment of renal concentrating ability. In: Robinson BHB, Hawkins JB and Vereerstraeten P, eds. *Dialysis, Transplantation, Nephrology.* Proceedings of the European Dialysis and Transplant Association, vol 14. Pitman, Tunbridge Wells 1977.
34. Hestbech J, Hansen HE, Amdisen A and Olsen S: Chronic renal lesions following long-term treatment with lithium. Kidney Int 1977; 12:205–13.
35. Bucht G and Wahlin A: Impairment of renal concentrating capacity by lithium. Lancet 1978; 1:778–9.
36. Burrows GD, Davies B and Kincaid-Smith P: Unique tubular lesion after lithium. Lancet 1978; 1:1310.
37. Vestergaard P, Amdisen A, Hansen HE and Schou M: Lithium treatment and kidney function. A survey of 237 patients in long-term treatment. Acta Psychiat Scand 1979; 60:504–20.
38. Evan AP and Ollerich DA: The effect of lithium carbonate on the structure of the rat kidney. Am J Anat 1972; 134:97–106.

39. Yavorskii AN, Goryanov OA, Rychko AV and Samoilov NN: Role of the kidneys in the pathogenesis of lithium poisoning. Bull Exp Biol Med 1976; 82:1780–2.

40. Schou M, Amdisen A and Baastrup PC: The practical management of lithium treatment. Br J Hosp Med 1971; 6:53–60.

41. Prien RF, Caffey EM Jr and Klett CJ: Relationship between serum lithium level and clinical response in acute mania treated with lithium. Br J Psychiatry 1972; 120:409–14.

42. Frazer A, Mendels J, Secunda SK, Cochrane CM and Bianchi CP: The prediction of brain lithium concentrations from plasma or erythrocyte measures. J Psychiat Res 1973; 10:1–7.

43. Mendels J and Frazer A: Intracellular lithium concentration and clinical response: Towards a membrane theory of depression. J Psychiat Res 1973; 10:9–18.

44. Pandey GN, Dorus E, Davis JM and Tosteson DC: Lithium transport in human red blood cells. Arch Gen Psychiatry 1979; 36:902–8.

45. Müller-Oerlinghausen B: 10 Jahre Lithium-Katamnese. Nervenarzt 1977; 48:483–93.

46. Andrews S and Chiu E: The intracellular lithium level: Is it of any use? In: Johnson FN and Johnson S, eds. *Lithium in Medical Practice*. MTP, Lancaster 1978.

47. Greil W and Eisenried F: Lithium uptake by erythrocytes of lithium-treated patients: Interindividual differences. In: Johnson FN and Johnson S, eds. *Lithium in Medical Practice*. MTP, Lancaster 1978.

48. Cooper TB and Simpson GM: Kinetics of lithium and clinical response. In: Lipton MA, DiMascio A and Killam KF, eds. *Psychopharmacology: A Generation of Progress*. Raven Press, New York 1978.

49. Sims A, White AC and Garvey K: Problems associated with the analysis and interpretation of saliva lithium. Br J Psychiatry 1978; 132:152–4.

50. Sims A: Monitoring lithium dose levels: Estimation of lithium in saliva. In: Johnson FN, ed. *A Handbook of Lithium Therapy*. MTP, Lancaster (in press).

51. Schou M: Lithium preparations currently available. In: Johnson FN, ed. *A Handbook of Lithium Therapy*. MTP, Lancaster 1980.

52. Stokes PE, Kocsis JH and Arcuni OJ: Relationship of lithium chloride dose to treatment response in acute mania. Arch Gen Psychiatry 1976; 33:1080–4.

53. Amdisen A: Sustained release preparations of lithium. In: Johnson FN, ed. *Lithium Research and Therapy*. Academic Press, London, New York, San Francisco 1975.

54. Nielsen-Kudsk F and Amdisen A: An analysis of the pharmacokinetics of lithium in healthy volunteers. Eur J Clin Pharmacol 1979; 16:271–7.

55. Sugita ET, Stokes JW, Frazer A et al: Lithium carbonate absorption in humans. J Clin Pharmacol 1973; 13:264–70.

56. Poust RJ, Mallinger AG, Mallinger J, Himmelhoch JM, Neil JF and Hanin I: Absolute availability of lithium. J Pharm Sci 1977; 66:609–10.

57. Coppen A, Bailey JE and White SG: Slow-release lithium carbonate. J Clin Pharmacol 1969; May–June:160–2.

58. Tyrer S, Hullin RP, Birch NJ and Goodwin JC: Absorption of lithium following administration of slow-release and conventional preparations. Psychol Med 1976; 6:51–8.

59. Tyrer S: The choice of lithium preparation and how to give it. In: Johnson FN and Johnson S, eds. *Lithium in Medical Practice*. MTP, Lancaster 1978.

60. Schou M: Lithium studies. 3. Distribution between serum and tissues. Acta Pharmacol Toxicol 1958; 15:115–24.

61. Schou M, Amdisen A and Trap-Jensen J: Lithium poisoning. Am J Psychiatry 1968; 125:112–19.
62. Wraae O: The pharmacokinetics of lithium in the brain, cerebrospinal fluid and serum of the rat. Br J Pharmacol 1978; 64:273–9.
63. Nelson SC, Herman MM, Bensch KG, Sher R and Barchas JD: Localization and quantitation of lithium in rat tissue following intraperitoneal injections of lithium chloride. I. Thyroid, thymus, heart, kidney, adrenal, and testis. Exp Molec Pathol 1976; 25:38–48.
64. Amdisen A and Skjoldborg H: Hæmodialysis for lithium poisoning. Lancet 1969; 2:213.
65. Foulks J, Mudge GH and Gilman A: Renal excretion in the dog during infusion of isotonic solutions of lithium chloride. Am J Physiol 1952; 168:642–9.
66. Lehmann K and Merten K: Die Elimination von Lithium in Abhängigkeit vom Lebensalter bei Gesunden und Niereninsuffizienten. Int J Clin Pharmacol 1974; 10:292–8.
67. Amdisen A and Sjögren J: Lithium absorption from sustained-release tablets (Duretter®). Acta Pharmaceut Suec 1968; 5:465–72.
68. Schou M: Lithium studies. 2. Renal elimination. Acta Pharmacol Toxicol 1958; 15:85–98.
69. Thomsen K: The effect of sodium chloride on kidney function in rats with lithium intoxication. Acta Pharmacol Toxicol 1973; 33:92–102.
70. Thomsen K and Schou M: Renal lithium excretion in man. Am J Physiol 1968; 215:823–7.
71. Baastrup PC: Practical problems concerning lithium maintenance therapy. In: Vinar O, Votava Z and Bradley PB, eds. *Advances in Neuro-Psychopharmacology.* North-Holland Publ. Co., Amsterdam 1971.
72. Thomsen K: Renal handling of lithium at non-toxic and toxic serum lithium levels. Dan Med Bull 1978; 25:106–15.
73. Robak OH and Sætermo R: Behandling av litiumindusert polyuri. (Treatment of lithium-induced polyuria.) T Norske Lægeforen 1975; 95:436–9.
74. Forrest JN Jr, Cohen AD, Torretti J, Himmelhoch JM and Epstein FH: On the mechanism of lithium-induced diabetes insipidus in man and the rat. J Clin Invest 1974; 53:1115–23.
75. Asplund K, Wahlin A and Rapp W: D.D.A.V.P test in assessment of renal function during lithium therapy. Lancet 1979; 1:491.
76. Tonks CM: Lithium intoxication induced by dieting and saunas. Br Med J 1977; 2:1396–7.
77. Poust RI, Mallinger AG, Mallinger J, Himmelhoch JM, Neil JF and Hanin I: Effect of chlorothiazide on the pharmacokinetics of lithium in plasma and erythrocytes. Psychopharmacol Commun 1976; 2(3):273–84.
78. Leftwich RB, Oates JA and Frolich JC: Indomethacin decreases urinary lithium excretion and increases plasma lithium levels. Clin Res 1978; 26:14A.
79. Thomsen K and Olesen OV: Precipitating factors and renal mechanisms in lithium intoxication. Gen Pharmacol 1978; 9:85–9.
80. Thomsen K, Olesen OV, Jensen J and Schou M: Mechanism of gradually developing lithium intoxication in rats. In: Essman WB and Valzelli L, eds. *Current Developments in Psychopharmacology,* vol. 3. Spectrum Publ., Inc., New York 1976.
81. Thomsen K and Olesen OV: Lithium-induced acute renal failure in the rat. Toxicol Appl Pharmacol 1978; 45:155–61.
82. Schou M: Heutiger Stand der Lithium-Rezidivprophylaxe bei endogenen affektiven Erkrankungen. Nervenarzt 1974; 45:397–418.

83. Thomsen K and Schou M: The treatment of lithium poisoning. In: Johnson FN, ed. *Lithium Research and Therapy*. Academic Press, London, New York, San Francisco 1975.

84. Mann J, Branton LJ and Larkins RG: Hyperosmolality complicating recovery from lithium toxicity. Br Med J 1978; 2:1522–3.

85. Schou M, Amdisen A and Steenstrup OR: Lithium and pregnancy—II, Hazards to women given lithium during pregnancy and delivery. Br Med J 1973; 2:137–8.

86. Groth U, Prellwitz W and Jähnchen E: Estimation of pharmacokinetic parameters of lithium from saliva and urine. Clin Pharmacol Ther 1974; 16:490–8.

87. Curtis JR and Donovan BA: Assessment of renal concentrating ability. Br Med J 1979; 1:304–5.

88. Amdisen A: Monitoring lithium dose levels: Estimation of lithium in urine. In: Johnson FN, ed. *A Handbook of Lithium Therapy*. MTP, Lancaster (in press).

89. Caldwell HC, Westlake WJ, Connor SM and Flanagan T: A pharmacokinetic analysis of lithium carbonate absorption from several formulations in man. J Clin Pharmacol 1971; 11:349–56.

90. Poust RI, Mallinger AG, Mallinger J, Himmelhoch JM and Hanin I: Pharmacokinetics of lithium in human plasma and erythrocytes. Psychopharmacol Commun 1976; 2(3):91–103.

91. Baastrup PC, Poulsen JC, Schou M, Thomsen K and Amdisen A: Prophylactic lithium: Double-blind discontinuation in manic-depressive and recurrent-depressive disorders. Lancet 1970; 2:326–30.

92. Prien RF and Caffey EM Jr. Relationship between dosage and response to lithium prophylaxis in recurrent depression. Am J Psychiatry 1976; 133:567–70.

93. Jerram TC and McDonald R: Plasma lithium control with particular reference to minimum effective levels. In: Johnson FN and Johnson S, eds. *Lithium in Medical Practice*. MTP, Lancaster 1978.

94. Vinarova E, Uhlir O, Stika L and Vinar O: Side effects of lithium administration. Activ Nerv Sup (Praha) 1972; 14:105–7.

95. Strayhorn JM Jr and Nash JL: Severe neurotoxicity despite "therapeutic" serum lithium levels. Dis Nerv Syst 1977; 38:107–11.

96. Speirs J and Hirsch SR: Severe lithium toxicity with "normal" serum concentrations. Br Med J 1978; 2:815–6.

97. Velde CD van der: Toxicity of lithium carbonate in elderly patients. Am J Psychiatry 1971; 127:1075–7.

98. Cooper TB and Simpson GM: Plasma/blood level monitoring techniques in psychiatry. In: Gottschalk LA and Merlis S. eds. *Pharmacokinetics of Psychoactive Drugs*. Spectrum Publ., Inc., New York 1976.

99. Bergner P-EE, Berniker K, Cooper TB, Gradijan JR and Simpson GM: Lithium kinetics in man: effect of variation in dosage pattern. Br J Pharmacol 1973; 49:329–39.

100. Cooper TB, Bergner P-EE and Simpson GM: The 24-hour serum lithium level as a prognosticator of dosage requirements. Am J Psychiatry 1973; 130:601–3.

101. Cooper TB, Bergner P-PE and Simpson GM: The 24-hour serum lithium level as a prognosticator of dosage requirements. In: Klein DF and Gittelman-Klein R, eds. *Progress in Psychiatric Drug Treatment*, vol 2. Brunner/Mazel, New York 1976.

102. Seifert R, Bremkamp H and Junge C: Vereinfachte Lithiumeinstellung durch Belastungstest. Psychopharmacology 1975; 43:285–6.

103. Cooper TB and Simpson GM: The 24-hour lithium level as a prognosticator of dosage requirements: A 2-year follow-up study. Am J Psychiatry 1976; 133:440–3.

104. Skausig OB and Schou M: Diegivning under lithiumbehandling. (Breastfeeding during lithium treatment.—English summary.) Ugeskr Lag 1977; 139:400–1.
105. Amdisen A: The estimation of lithium in urine. In: Johnson FN, ed. *Lithium Research and Therapy.* Academic Press, London, New York, San Francisco 1975.
106. Cooper TB, Simpson GM and Allen D: Rapid direct micro method for determination of plasma lithium. Atom Absorpt Newslett 1974; 13:119–20.
107. Doerr P and Stamm D: Flammenphotometrische Lithiumbestimmung im Serum. Z Klin Chem Klin Biochem 1968; 6:178–82.
108. Plenge P: Lithium effects on rat brain glucose metabolism in long-term lithium-treated rats studied in vivo. Psychopharmacology 1978; 58:317–22.

# 19

# Heparin

Kim L. Kelly, Pharm.D.

## INTRODUCTION/BACKGROUND

The anticoagulant properties of heparin have been appreciated for nearly half a century since its isolation by McLean in 1916 (1). Despite the availability of heparin commercially for over 40 years, there continues to be controversy concerning its pharmacologic effects, the dosage necessary for certain of its properties, and methods to measure its effectiveness and standardize its potency.

Part of the reason for the difficulty in accurately assessing heparin's effects is that the compound is a polydisperse polysaccharide. When heparin is extracted from biological sources and subjected to separation by now standard methods, up to twenty-one separate components can be identified (2,3,4). In the native state, heparin probably occurs as a macromolecular complex with protein and/or a polysaccharide core (5,6).

Heparin is one of a group of sulfated glycosaminoglycans and is similar in some ways to the other members of that group, dermatan sulfate, heparan sulfate, and chondroitin sulfate, to name a few (5). Heparin is derived from biologic sources of which the two most important are porcine intestinal mucosa and beef lung. The majority of heparin utilized in the United States is from the porcine source, and only two of the thirty suppliers in the United States supply heparin from beef lung.

The basic structural unit of heparin appears to be a hexasaccharide containing two disaccharides of 2-sulfoiduronic acid-2-sulfoglucosamine and one disaccharide of glucuronic acid-2-sulfoglucosamine in an alpha-1,4 linkage (Figure 1). These units repeat in an unbroken fashion to construct units of varying chain length with molecular weights from 6000 to 30,000 daltons (7).

The anticoagulant activity of commercial heparin seems to reside in about one-third of the variable molecular weight components. Po-

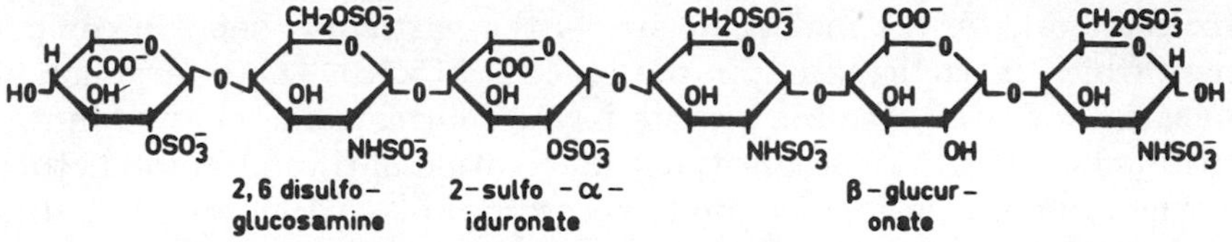
CH2OSO3
COO-
CH2OSO3
COO-
CH2OSO3
H
COO-
OH
HO
OSO3
NHSO3
OSO3
NHSO3
OH
NHSO3
2,6 disulfo-
glucosamine
2-sulfo -α-
iduronate
β-glucur-
onate

FIGURE 1 Heparin Structure.

tencies of the various molecular weight components varies, and the whole commercial preparations vary in potency depending on biologic source and the assay method (US Pharmacopoeia or British Pharmacopoeia) utilized to standardize the preparation (8).

The heterogeneity of heparin preparations and their assay methods are noted here so as to indicate the difficulty of measuring the "drug" itself versus measuring the effect of the preparation, which is more easily accomplished.

Physiologically, heparin has two functions which are well known (9). It enhances the release and possibly the activity of lipoprotein lipase, which is responsible for clearing the plasma of circulating lipids (10). While it is effective in this regard, it is not utilized to any major extent for this property. Heparin also has anticoagulant activity by interfering with coagulation factors (9,11). The anticoagulant effect of heparin appears not to involve an effect on platelets, although controversy exists in this area (12). The major effect of heparin seems to reside in its ability to augment the effects of the endogenously produced anticoagulant substance antithrombin III (13). During the sequence of activation of the various factors in the coagulation cascade, the factors are "activated" by being cleaved to fragments which are active serine proteases. The proteases then cleave other coagulation factors to eventually generate active thrombin, which is responsible for a protease activity on fibrinogen. This, in turn, generates units that subsequently polymerize to form fibrin. The coagulation sequence is adequately reviewed elsewhere (14).

The mechanism of action and relationship of heparin and antithrombin have been studied utilizing a number of different activated factors. The most commonly utilized model to study the interaction of the components is the reaction of thrombin with antithrombin III and heparin. In studying the interaction model, it has been noted that heparin binds to antithrombin III, to thrombin, and to the antithrombin-thrombin complex. The kinetics and affinities of these reactions depend in large part on the degree of N-sulfation of the heparin molecule and on the molecular size of the particular heparin component which is participating in the reaction (15,16). The interaction of heparin and antithrombin results in a conformational change in antithrombin III which enhances its inactivation of thrombin (and other serine proteases of the coagulation cascade) 50 to 100 fold (17). It is important to emphasize that the effect of heparin is only through enhancement of the activity of circulating antithrombin III, and it appears to have no anticoagulant activity other than by this mechanism.

Antithrombin III appears to be the major circulating inhibitor of coagulation. The amount of thrombin potentially available in only 10 ml of blood would be sufficient to clot all the fibrinogen in the body were it not for the rapid neutralization by antithrombin III. Antithrombin III deficiency has been noted in several kindred by various authors. In most reports of this deficiency [such as that of Marciniak (18)], the deficiency appears to be quantitative. The antithrombin III deficiency in these patients is not total, but rather levels 26 to 49% were noted in the above mentioned report, which is representative of other reports. One report of a qualitative alteration in antithrombin III exists where immunologic antithrombin III was present but activity was decreased (19). In patients who are deficient in antithrombin III, one would expect a tendency to thrombosis (which is indeed present) and also a decrease in the effectiveness of heparin therapy. In the study of Marciniak, while a decrease in the *in vitro* activity of heparin was noted, this defect was not parallel with the decrease in antithrombin III and the effect on heparin activity did not correlate with the profundity of the deficiency.

It is thus important to note that many factors affect the pharmacologic activity of heparin which are not related to the amount or type of heparin utilized. This variability and the interaction between heparin and antithrombin III has been recently reviewed (20).

As previously mentioned, heparin prepared commercially is from either porcine intestinal mucosa or bovine lung. Procedures utilized for the commerical purification and fractionation have been summarized by Rodén (21).

Certain *in vitro* differences in anticoagulant properties between porcine and bovine heparin do exist (22,23). These differences relate to potency against the active forms of the different coagulation factors, degree of sulfation, molecular size dispersion, and several other properties. Despite these *in vitro* differences (many of them noted with "research grade" and not commercial heparin), the effect upon human coagulation is not different between the two animal sources of heparin

(24,25,26). Since heparin is a strong organic acid, it is available as the sodium or calcium salt. Studies suggest that both *in vitro* and *in vivo* the potencies of either salt are equivalent (27,28), and that equivalence exists among the various sodium salts (25,26,29) which are the only salt forms available in the United States.

## Absorption

Heparin is administered clinically by the injectable route either subcutaneously, intramuscularly, or intravenously. Recently, the intrapulmonary administration of large doses of heparin by nebulization has been shown to produce anticoagulant activity in the blood for many days, but this technique is still experimental (30). Intravenous injection is clinically applied either by intermittent bolus administration or continuous infusions. Thus, in the clinical use of heparin, absorption from intramuscular or subcutaneous sites appears to be the only significant "absorptive" mechanism for heparin.

While no literature exists where the absorption rate has been specifically studied, several articles involving subcutaneous administration present enough data on anticoagulant activity (which is representative of blood levels) with time that statements concerning absorption can be made (24,28,31).

Heparin is absorbed slowly from subcutaneous sites. Absorption of the drug is so slow that a clear elimination phase is not discernible (assuming elimination to occur with the same half-life of approximately 90 minutes seen with intravenous heparin). Thus, anticoagulant effect over time subsequent to subcutaneous administration is in essence like "sustained-release" forms of medication, where absorption is a rate-limiting step. Subcutaneous administration of 10,000 units will generally provide anticoagulant effect (prolongation of appropriate test 1½ to 3 times) from after the first to the sixth hour of therapy (25), or may produce prolongation of coagulation but not into the therapeutic range (24). Dosages of 15,000 units subcutaneously may produce therapeutic levels from after the first through the tenth hour of therapy (26,28). In a study by Engelberg (31) subcutaneous administration of approximately 20,000 units led to therapeutic anticoagulant activity from the first through the 24th hour of therapy in the majority of patients, and up to 40 hours of therapy in a few patients. Unfortunately, studies of subcutaneous administration are few, they are all single-dose studies, and factors such as patient weight, site of injection, and concentration of the heparin product used, are not noted in most cases.

Thus, it would appear that subcutaneous heparin provides rapid therapeutic effect, with sustained activity which persists longer the larger the dose. For any individual patient, multiple doses and/or prolonged therapy should be closely monitored due to lack of data available in this area.

## Distribution

The distribution of heparin in the body is a complex process whereby injected heparin appears to quickly distribute to rapidly perfused tissues, and then distribute from those tissues back into the blood. This distribution process involves the reticuloendothelial systems within the liver, spleen, and lung primarily, which rapidly desulfate the drug (32). The apparent bimodality of distribution/catabolism during the first 30 minutes of heparin administration is only apparent with low doses of heparin by intravenous bolus administration. With doses above 5000 units, the decrease in active heparin in the blood appears unimodal, suggesting that uptake (and/or a certain portion of early catabolism) is saturated so that the decrease in active heparin in the blood appears linear or log-linear with time. Glimelius and coworkers have shown that heparin can bind reversibly to cultured human endothelial cells, suggesting that at least part of this bimodality may be the redistribution of the active compound (33). The volume of distribution of heparin is variable depending on dose of heparin, age of the patient, disease state, and perhaps actual body weight (if significantly greater than ideal body weight) (34,35,36,37,38). The volume of distribution will be designated $V_c$, since in most studies it is calculated by back extrapolation of the disappearance or pharmacologic effect curves, and since more than one compartment may be needed to describe its pharmacodynamics. Values for the volume of distribution from the literature are shown in Table 1. The majority of the values exceed the plasma volume and in some cases the blood volume (in ml/kg) (38,39); however, they are close enough that many authors have assumed a volume of distribution equivalent to blood volume in dosage calculations (40,41). Table 1 contains a list of volumes of distribution from data presented in several studies.

## Metabolism

Heparin activity in the plasma decreases with time by the processes of metabolism and excretion. Metabolism in large part is responsible for the loss of plasma heparin activity. Heparin is distributed to the reticuloendothelial system where it appears to undergo metabolism by N-desulfation (primarily) and O-desulfation. The metabolites found

TABLE 1. VOLUME OF DISTRIBUTION OF HEPARIN

| $V_c$ (estimate) ml/kg* | Author and Reference | Heparin Measurement Technique | Remarks |
|---|---|---|---|
| 57 ± 1 | Estes (34) | APTT Lee White (WBCT) | Mean value of 19 studies surveyed |
| 70 ± 28 | Simon (35) | Anti Xa Assay | 17 normal subjects |
| 62 ± 41 | Simon (35) | Anti Xa Assay | 14 patients— thrombophlebitis |
| 68 ± 49 | Simon (35) | Anti Xa Assay | 11 patients— pulmonary embolism |
| 78 ± 31 | Simon (35) | Anti Xa Assay | 7 patients—"liver disease" |
| 71 ± 41 | Simon (35) | Anti Xa Assay | 12 patients—"renal disease" |
| 127 ± 63 | Hirsch (36) | Protamine Titration | 16 patients—deep vein thrombosis and 4 patients— pulmonary embolism |
| 44 ± 4 | McAvoy (37) | Equation developed No new data | Re-analysis by two separate models of the data of Olsson (46) |
| 42 ± 6 | Goodman (38) | APTT | Value calculated from data presented in article |

* Values are mean ± standard deviation where information available

in blood have the same apparent molecular weight but lack sulfate substituents and biologic activity. The primary organs where this process takes place appear to be liver and spleen. There appears to be a secondary site of metabolism in the kidneys where cleavage of the polysaccharide chain occurs so that the majority of isotopically labeled heparin in the urine has a molecular weight of <1000 daltons (32).

## Excretion

Excretion of heparin in the urine appears to occur in several forms. Heparin in the urine may be as the unchanged drug, the partially desulfated (bioinactive) drug of the same molecular weight as the parent compound [which has been labeled uroheparin by McAllister and Demis (42)], and lower molecular weight breakdown products with variable activity. Urinary excretion of the unchanged drug appears to be a minor process, but the amount of unchanged drug, its desulfated metabolite, and their subsequent low molecular weight metabolites appears controversial (11,32,42).

## Elimination Kinetics

Perhaps the largest literature base on heparin kinetics involves studies of the disappearance of its effect over time. The average half-life (t½) of heparin effect has been reported to be about 90 minutes in normal individuals, but values from 30 to 360 minutes have been observed (43). Heparin elimination has been described almost exclusively from studies of bolus administration of single doses. The elimination t½ appears to be dose-dependent, and to be dependent upon disease states present in the patient, and upon the assay methodology utilized in determining the disappearance of heparin and/or its effects. Table 2 contains the results of several studies on the elimination of heparin, and while not exhaustive, it is representative of the complexity of the factors affecting heparin t½, diversity of dosages utilized for study, and the methods of measuring heparin or its pharmacologic effect. Assay methods utilized will be discussed in a subsequent section.

The decrease in heparin effect appears to have several points where there is agreement in the literature despite the noted complexity of the problem.

In a critical analysis of several papers, McAvoy (48) has noted that apparently large differences between half-lives noted in studies can be resolved when the data are analyzed by the same parameter (for example, extension of the WBPTT versus actual WBPTT). Half-lives should be specified by including the method of assessment, which falls into one of three basic categories: t½ of bioassayed heparin, t½ of extension of clotting time, and t½ of clotting time, which in the literature gives t½ in the neighborhood of 90 minutes with commonly recommended therapeutic doses (50,51). The measures of heparin effect and measurements of biologically active heparin levels in patients appear to be correlated to a significant degree; however, the variability in the correlations is also significant (36,38). This should not be surprising due to the large number of factors previously mentioned which affect heparin activity (52). Thus, extension of clotting time is not directly predictable from the knowledge of blood levels of heparin.

Heparin t½ appears to be related to its dose in many studies. Most studies suggest that in larger population samples there is significant variability in t½ related to dose (46,48,53). This variability in many instances still falls within the range of the noted 10-fold intraindividual variability in patients receiving approximately the same dose on a body-weight basis (38).

Kinetics of heparin tend to vary with disease state. While in cirrhosis there may be a modest increase in volume of distribution, generally this variable is relatively resistant to change associated with disease state. Half-life of heparin does vary with disease state, as noted by Hirsch (36), Simon (35), and others (44,54). Heparin t½ appears to decrease in patients with pulmonary embolism to approximately half its average value. This does not hold true for deep vein thrombosis. This change in heparin t½ with pulmonary embolism appears not to relate to release of platelet factor 4, as has been assumed from work with this antiheparin factor (55,79). Heparin t½ may be prolonged in liver disease, up to 50% longer than its average value (35,54).

## CONCENTRATION VERSUS RESPONSE AND TOXICITY

Blood levels of heparin are utilized primarily in pharmacokinetic studies, and not routinely in clinical practice. Certainly, blood levels vary with dose, and measurements of heparin effect on clotting are associated with blood levels of heparin within a given range.

Without any exogenous heparin administration, blood levels of heparin have been shown to be in the range of 0.15 to 0.18 units/ml (9). It has also been shown that at levels of 0.15 units/ml, heparin prevents the formation of intrinsic plasma thromboplastin and enhances neutralization of activated factor X. Despite this evidence, the presence of heparin in normal plasma and any physiologic function of heparin as an anticoagulant remain controversial (78). On bolus injection of 75 units/kg to normal volunteers, heparin concentrations varied from 1.0 unit/ml to 0.2 units/ml over 3 hours (35). In patients undergoing open heart operations and receiving bolus doses of 300 units/kg, initial plasma levels of heparin were 7.1 ± 0.77 (mean ± SD) units/ml, and during the study the authors noted that clotting times (WBCT) that were two to three times control were associated with plasma heparin levels of 0.43 to 0.85 units/ml respectively (38). Hirsch et al (36) noted that after bolus administration of 70 units/kg, heparin levels by protamine titration fell from 0.6 to 0.2 units/ml of plasma during the 90 minutes following heparin administration, and this was correlated with a fall in APTT from 105 to 65 seconds (control 40 seconds). The correlation coefficient between heparin level and APTT was only $r = 0.48$, and the variability increased with increasing plasma heparin concentrations.

TABLE 2. HALF-LIVES OF HEPARIN

| Half-Life (minutes)* | Intravenous Bolus Dosage (Units) | Author and Reference | Assay or Measurement Technique | Remarks |
|---|---|---|---|---|
| 87 ± 31 | Not mentioned | Estes (34) | Various—including WBCT, APTT | 19 studies summarized |
| 37 ± 5 | 2400–5000 U | Perry (41) | ACT | Dosages based on blood volume estimates dosed to approximate 0.6 U/ml blood level |
| 23 ± 4 | 1200–2500 U | Perry (41) | ACT | As above except doses given to approximate blood level of 0.3 U/ml |
| 107 ± 70 | 75 U/kg | Simon (35) | Anti Xa Assay | 17 normal subjects |
| 106 ± 104 | 75 U/kg | Simon (35) | Anti Xa Assay | 14 patients—Thrombophlebitis |
| 80 ± 63 | 75 U/kg | Simon (35) | Anti Xa Assay | 11 patients—Pulmonary Embolism |
| 80 ± 55 | 75 U/kg | Simon (35) | Anti Xa Assay | 7 patients—"Liver Disease" |
| 110 ± 62 | 75 U/kg | Simon (35) | Anti Xa Assay | 12 patients—"Renal Disease" |
| 93 ± 77 | 70 U/kg | Hirsch (36) | APTT | 15 patients—Deep Vein Thrombosis |
| 70 ± 16 | 70 U/kg | Hirsch (36) | Protamine Titration | Same 15 patients as above. Simultaneous measurements. |
| 53 ± 30 | 70 U/kg | Hirsch (36) | APTT | 4 patients with Pulmonary Embolism |
| 38 ± 2 | 70 U/kg | Hirsch (36) | Protamine Titration | Same 4 patients as above. Simultaneous measurements. |

| Value | Reference | Test | Dose | Notes |
|---|---|---|---|---|
| 119 ± 81 | Goodman (38) | APTT | 300 U/kg + 2400 U—pump | 24 patients undergoing open heart surgery. Large doses plus "pump primer" dose. |
| 75 ± 8 | Teien (44) | Polybrene Titration | 100 U/kg | 6 normal subjects |
| 64 ± 2 | Teien (44) | Thrombin Clotting Time | | Same 6 subjects as above. Simultaneous measurements. |
| 108 ± 19 | Teien (44) | Polybrene Titration | | 11 subjects with renal failure (5 of whom were nephrectomized) |
| 69 ± 14 | Teien (44) | Thrombin Clotting Time | | Same 11 subjects as above. Simultaneous measurements. |
| 97 ± 4 | Estes (45) | WBCT | 49–138 U/kg | 17 normal subjects |
| 103 ± 6 | Estes (45) | WBAPTT | 49–138 U/kg | 17 normal subjects |
| 80 ± 6 | Estes (45) | APTT | 49–138 U/kg | 17 normal subjects |
| 79 ± 4 | Estes (45) | PTT | 49–138 U/kg | 17 normal subjects |
| 56 ± 4 | Olsson (46) | TCT | 100 U/kg | 13 normal subjects |
| 96 ± 5 | Olsson (46) | TCT | 200 U/kg | 13 normal subjects |
| 152 ± 5 | Olsson (46) | TCT | 400 U/kg | 13 normal subjects |
| 89 | Estes (47) | WBAPTT | 40–150 U/kg | Relative dose to give blood level of 0.3 U/ml [McAvoy (48)] |
| 95 | Estes (47) | WBAPTT | 40–150 U/kg | Relative dose to give blood level of 0.6 U/ml [McAvoy (48)] |
| 102 | Perry (49) | ACT | 1200–2500 U | Relative dose to give blood level of 0.3 U/ml [McAvoy (48)] |
| 120 | Perry (49) | ACT | 2400–5000 U | Relative dose to give blood level of 0.6 U/ml [McAvoy (48)] |

* Values are mean ± standard deviation where information available

627

Hemorrhage is one of the major complications associated with heparin therapy. Logic would suggest that the more anticoagulated a patient is, the greater the chances of bleeding. While this may be true for excessively large doses, the correlation is difficult to make for dosages (and associated lengthening of clotting times) that are only 1 to 3 times higher than normally recommended dosages. Hemorrhage with heparin is not uncommon, and heparin therapy has resulted in "minor" hemorrhagic complications in 22 to 48% of patients in several studies, whereas "major" hemorrhage has been noted in from 1 to 33% of the patients, although it is generally less than 4% (56). Bleeding with heparin seems not to correlate well with clotting times in excess of the "therapeutic range" (57,58,59). This should not be surprising in view of the multiplicity of factors associated with bleeding during heparin therapy, which include drug interactions (60), age, sex, and intermittent bolus method of administration (57,58). Patients with preexisting hemostatic defects or thrombocytopenia secondary to heparin therapy (43,61) may have a higher incidence of bleeding.

## CLINICAL APPLICATIONS OF PHARMACOKINETIC DATA

### Dosing

Dosing heparin has for years been a matter of empiricism. The discovery that lower or "mini" doses of heparin have prophylactic efficacy has led to a more rational approach to dosing heparin based on the reason for administering the drug.

**Prophylactic Use of Small Doses.** Many conditions involving relative immobilization and potential activation of coagulation, such as surgery, stroke, myocardial infarction, and others, are associated with an increased incidence of venous thrombosis. In these patients several authors have demonstrated that low-dose subcutaneous heparin can decrease the incidence of lower extremity thrombosis as measured by $I^{125}$-fibrinogen scanning and other methods (56,61,62). This does not, however, appear to substantially change the mortality or morbidity from myocardial infarction since pulmonary embolism is an uncommon complication. A review of 27 studies of the use of low-dose heparin subcutaneously indicates that the incidence of deep vein thrombosis and pulmonary embolism have been substantially reduced in patients undergoing surgery. Patients with femoral neck fractures and total hip replacements are less likely to benefit. While surgical blood loss and transfusions have been noted to increase in some studies, the number of transfusions necessary for patients given low-dose heparin prior to surgery appears not to be significantly increased (64).

Most studies have utilized 5000 units subcutaneously every 8 or every 12 hours as prophylactic therapy, and for surgery patients the first dose is generally administered 2 hours prior to surgery. There has not been evidence to suggest that every 8 hour subcutaneous heparin is more effective than every 12 hour dosing. Assessment is complicated by the fact that studies of every 12 hour dosing were done primarily in the United States, where heparin potency is at least 10% greater than in Europe, where the majority of the every 8 hour dosing studies were done (65).

For prevention of thrombosis and possible embolism, heparin 5000 units subcutaneously every 12 hours is recommended, and where surgery is to be an inciting factor for thrombosis, the dosing should begin at least 2 hours prior to surgery. It is to be noted, however, that many cases of deep vein thrombosis occur days before surgery is accomplished in surgical candidates. Additionally, the blood levels of heparin and anticoagulant effect in patients receiving the low-dose regimen are quite variable, and no one yet knows what levels are optimal (66). In patients with myocardial infarction, the use of low-dose heparin is still controversial. The incidence of deep vein thrombosis, pulmonary embolus, and death from embolism is so low as to raise questions as to the cost effectiveness of utilization of subcutaneous heparin for all patients with myocardial infarction (67).

**Therapeutic Use.** The use of heparin in "full," "standard," "therapeutic," or "high" doses is the more time-honored method of heparin administration. Dosage regimens developed for heparin have been empirically chosen to keep coagulation studies prolonged anywhere from 1½ to 3 times their control values. This range can be most likely attributed to early work in dogs by Wessler and Morris (68).

If the correctness of this goal of therapy is accepted, then dosage regimens to achieve this desired effect are myriad. In general, therapeutic heparin is used to prevent extension of deep vein thrombosis and pulmonary embolism, and in existing pulmonary embolism, to prevent worsening of the situation, which might occur if clot formation instead of dissolution were a dominant process. Wessler and Gitel (43) have arbitrarily divided heparin dosing regimens into low, medium, and high, as shown in Table 3.

The division between medium (which represents the commonly utilized range for therapeutic doses) and high dosages centers around the evidence that the t½ of heparin is substantially shortened in pulmonary embolism. A larger dose seems justified in view of the data by Hirsch (36) indicating that following a standard bolus of 70 units/kg in patients with pulmonary embolism, the majority of APTT values were not in the "therapeutic range" of 60 to 80 seconds.

TABLE 3. HEPARIN DOSING REGIMENS

| Dosage (USP units/24 hr) | | Route | Clinical Indications |
|---|---|---|---|
| Low: | 10,000–15,000 | Subcutaneous, intravenous | 1. Elective abdominothoracic surgery<br>2. Acute myocardial infarction |
| Medium: | 20,000–60,000 | Intravenous (continuous or intermittent) | 1. Active venous thromboembolism<br>2. Disseminated intravascular coagulation |
| High: | 60,000–100,000 | Intravenous (continuous) | 1. Massive pulmonary embolism with shock |

Modified from Wessler S, Gitel SN. Blood 53:525, 1979.

In patients who have deep vein thrombosis and not pulmonary embolism, the dosages recommended to prevent progression of pulmonary embolism are those which have been shown to produce concentrations in the range of 0.3 to 1.0 units/ml of plasma, which have generally been shown to prolong most measures of coagulation to 1½ to 3 times their control values. It should be recognized and will be discussed later that the degree of prolongation does not correlate between coagulation measures (for example, 2 times control WBCT does not necessarily correspond to an APTT of 2 times control).

Many dosage recommendations are based on several assumptions.

1. Heparin t½ is approximately 90 minutes for the blood levels achieved by standard regimens (34,43).
2. The decrease in heparin effect with time can be adequately described by a one-compartment model (11,34,41).
3. Heparin is distributed in a volume that is approximated by volumes from plasma volume (44 ml/kg) to blood volume (55 to 75 ml/kg dependent on height) (34,35,38,39).
4. Heparin concentrations associated with "therapeutic" prolongation of clotting times range from 0.3 to 1.0 units/ml of blood or plasma (36,41,44).

To utilize some of these variables in a sample problem assuming first-order kinetics, the equation below is utilized to determine the infusion rate necessary to achieve an average plasma concentration of 0.5 units/ml for a volume of distribution of 60 ml/kg in a 70 kg man.

Assuming a t½ of 90 minutes (1.5 hr),

$$K_0 = (C) (V) (K)$$
$$K_0 = (0.5\ U/ml)\ [(60\ ml/kg)(70\ kg)]\ (0.462\ hr^{-1})$$
$$K_0 = 970\ units/hr$$
$$= 23{,}300\ units/24\ hr$$

It can be seen from the above equation that infusion dosages derived in this way come close to literature recommendations of 400 U/kg/24 hr as the dosage likely to anticoagulate the patient to an appropriate level (1½ to 3 times control) (36,39). Once the total dose per 24 hours is determined, it can be administered either via bolus injections at various time intervals, or as a continuous infusion. Several studies comparing intermittent to continuous infusions have reached conflicting results on the incidence of rethrombosis, hemorrhagic complications, doses, and dosage intervals necessary (57,58,70,71). The weight of evidence thus far suggests that continuous infusion is associated with less risk of hemorrhage than intermittent administration.

With the evidence of decreased t½ of heparin in pulmonary embolism, several authors have recommended dosages of 60,000 to 120,000 units/day. Currently there are no clinical trials bearing directly upon the necessity for or efficacy of these large doses, nor any that indicate the risk of hemorrhage from this dosage. Prudence would indicate that if the patient is moribund and high-dose therapy is contemplated, 60,000 units/24 hr for the first 24 hours may be acceptable, since the risk of bleeding in the first 24 hours seems, from other studies, to be low. Subsequently, doses should be reduced to the more commonly utilized range (72). Pharmacokinetic calculations of dosages and dosage regimens are still only approximations based on studies with wide variances. Kinetic approaches utilizing blood volume as the volume of distribution have aimed for effective blood concentrations which were derived from plasma (and not blood) measurements. Despite this, the dosages calculated still fall into the therapeutic range for anticoagulation the majority of the time (36,40). This is, no doubt, due to the magnitude of the therapeutic range, but may also be correlated with the high variability in the values one chooses for a given kinetic parameter. Certainly more work needs to be done to more accurately identify the appropriate pharmacokinetic parameters for heparin.

## Assessment of Heparin Effect

Blood levels of heparin are not generally available, nor are they particularly valuable in the clinical setting. Since there is only a modest correlation between levels of heparin in the blood and its effect

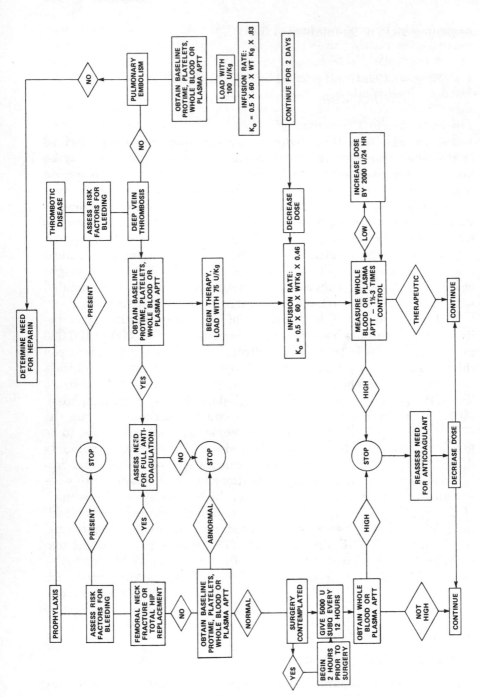

FIGURE 2  Algorithm for Clinical Use of Heparin.

as measured by prolongation of clotting times, it is better to directly measure the clotting time to assess heparin effect. Since hemorrhage is not convincingly related to the clotting time in standard dosing regimens, and since rethrombosis or thrombus extension may be related to inadequate prolongation of clotting time, it is prudent to direct one's effort to assuring that the anticoagulant effect does not fall below 1½ to 2 times control values. To this end, the use of bolus injections at short intervals (every 3 hours) or administration by continuous infusion seems most appropriate. When bolus administration is utilized, clotting time should be assessed at the time when plasma levels of heparin (or most commonly their effect on coagulation tests) are at their lowest, which is just before the next bolus dose. For continuous infusion, any time of sampling is appropriate. Clotting times should be assessed several times after any dosing adjustment, and at least daily during heparin therapy.

## ASSAY METHODS

Table 4 has been modified from that of Wessler and Gitel (43) as a partial list of methods utilized to regulate heparin dosage and to assay heparin concentration. Currently the only clinically utilized tests are those for regulating dosage. The current literature suggests that there is no single test of choice for monitoring heparin therapy. The original recommendations for "therapeutic" anticoagulation were done utilizing the whole blood clotting time of Lee and White (WBCT). Despite the only modest correlation of this test with newer, more rapidly performed tests, the therapeutic range of anticoagulation of 1½ to 3 times control has been applied to these tests also. Some support for this comes from the correlation of whole blood activated partial thromboplastin time (WBAPTT) with WBCT, the activated partial thromboplastin time (APTT) with the WBAPTT, and the activated clotting time (ACT) with APTT (45,73,74).

Generally the more recently introduced tests are preferred over the whole blood clotting time of Lee and White. This is because most of the newer tests are rapid (less than 3 minutes to complete) and reproducible. All the clinically utilized tests are measures of heparin's effect in blood (or plasma) which is *ex vivo* at the time of assay. The relevance of these measures to inhibition of thrombus formation or progression is only anecdotal based on cases of failure of patients to respond to the level of heparin which shows the proper effect in the *in vitro* tests. There are currently two tests which can be utilized to assess the anticoagulant effects *in vivo*, the $I^{125}$-fibrinogen t½ and the measurement of fibrinopeptide A. Neither of these is clinically utilized to any great extent at this time (75,76).

The utility of measuring anticoagulant effect has been questioned due to the fact that in many studies nearly 50% of the results of these tests are outside commonly accepted limits (57,58). It is, however, also important to note that recurrence or progression of thrombosis was most often (although not always) associated with anticoagulant effect that was lower than the clinically desired level (59). Controversy exists at the upper limit of coagulation prolongation as to whether there is a correlation of bleeding with excessive anticoagulation, but with so many factors associated with bleeding, it would be impossible to resolve the controversy until patients stratified according to these factors were studied (59,77).

TABLE 4.     HEPARIN MEASUREMENT TECHNIQUES

**Assays for Regulation of Dosage**

Activated clotting time (ACT)
Activated partial thromboplastin time (APTT)
Capillary tube clotting time
Partial thromboplastin time (PTT)
Thrombin time
Whole-blood clotting time (WBCT)
Whole-blood recalcification time

**Quantitative Assays for Heparin Concentration**

Activated partial thromboplastin time (APTT)
Whole-blood activated recalcification time (BART)
Anti-activated factor X (one-stage assay)
Anti-activated factor X (two-stage assay)
British Pharmacopoeia assay
Colorimetric assays
Polybrene titration assays
Protamine titration assays
Thrombin time
Thrombin generation and neutralization test (TNGT)
United States Pharmacopoeia assay
Whole-blood partial thromboplastin time (WBPTT)
Whole-blood activated partial thromboplastin time (WBAPTT)

**Assays for Effect on Thrombosis**

$I^{125}$-fibrinogen kinetics
Fibrinopeptide A

Modified from Wessler S, Gitel SN. Blood 53:525, 1979.

It is accepted practice to monitor heparin therapy with some measure of its anticoagulant effect. It is therefore recommended that patients receiving heparin by *any* method receive at least one control measurement and one measurement of clotting during therapy. For those patients receiving "therapeutic" doses of heparin, these tests should be repeated several times during the first few days of therapy and at least daily as long as therapy is continued.

There is no current evidence that any coagulation test is "better" than any other. Three tests which are quick, easily done and reproducible are: whole blood activated partial thromboplastin time (WBAPTT), activated clotting time (ACT), and the activated partial thromboplastin time (APTT). The first two utilize whole blood and can be done at the bedside. The last test is done in most clinical laboratories, but requires that the specimen be processed quickly so as to avoid any effect from platelet factor 4 which may be released while the specimen is being held in the collection container.

## SUMMARY

In summary, the factors affecting heparin therapy are many, from biochemical differences in commercial products, to interpatient variance, to the myriad of available monitoring tests. To stay within clinically established guidelines for dosage and administration of heparin seems prudent until more concrete information on heparin pharmacokinetics is available. Patients receiving heparin should be monitored with tests of coagulation that are simple and reproducible. These tests should be done to establish that the level of anticoagulation is within clinically accepted guidelines.

## REFERENCES

1. McLean J: The thromboplastic action of cephalin. Am J Physiol 1916; 41:250–257.
2. Jaques LB, Kavanaugh LW, Lavalle A: A comparison of biological activities and chemical analyses for various heparin preparations. Arzneimittel Forschung 1967; 17:744–778.
3. Jaques LB: What is "heparin"? In: Bradshaw RA, Wessler S (eds). Heparin: Structure, function, and implications. Adv Exp Biol Med 1975; 52:139–147.
4. McDuffie NM, Dietrich CP, Nader HB: Electrofocusing of heparin: Fractionation of heparin into 21 components distinguishable from other acidic mucopolysaccharides. Biopolymers 1975; 14:1473–1486.
5. Laurent TC: Interaction between proteins and glycosaminoglycans. Fed Proc 1977; 36:24–27.
6. Horner AA: The concept of macromolecular heparin and its physiologic significance. Fed Proc 1977; 36:35–39.
7. Silvan ME, Dietrich CP: Structure of heparin. J Biol Chem 1975; 250:6841–6846.

8. Walton PL, Rickets CR, Baugham DR: Heterogeneity of heparins. Brit J Haematol 1966; 12:310–326.
9. Engelberg H: Probable physiologic functions of heparin. Fed Proc 1977; 36:70–72.
10. Olivecrona T, Bengtsson G, Marklund SE, Lindahl U, Höök M: Heparin-lipoprotein lipase interactions. Fed Proc 1977; 36:60–64.
11. Coon WW: Some recent developments in the pharmacology of heparin. J Clin Pharmacol 1979; 19:337–349.
12. Zucker MB: Heparin and platelet function. Fed Proc 1977; 36:47–49.
13. Rosenberg RD: Actions and interactions of heparin and antithrombin III. N Engl J Med 1975; 292:146–150.
14. Davie EW, Fujikawa K: Basic mechanisms in blood coagulation. Ann Rev Biochem 1975; 44:799–829.
15. Feinman RD, Eddy HH: Interaction of heparin with thrombin and antithrombin III. Fed Proc 1977; 36:51–55.
16. Riesenfeld J, Höök M, Björk I, Lindahl U, Ajaxon B: Structural requirements for the interaction of heparin with antithrombin III. Fed Proc 1977; 36:39–43.
17. Waugh DF, Fitzgerald MA: Quantitative aspects of antithrombin and heparin in plasma. Am J Physiol 1956; 184:627–629.
18. Marciniak E, Farley CH, DeSimone PA: Familial thrombosis due to antithrombin III deficiency. Blood 1974; 43:219–230.
19. Sas G, Blasko G, Banhegyi D, Jako J, Palos LA: Abnormal antithrombin III (antithrombin III "Budapest") as a cause of familial thrombophilia. Thromb Diath Hemorrh 1974; 32:105–115.
20. Barrowcliffe TW, Johnson EA, Thomas D: Antithrombin III and heparin. Brit Med Bull 1978; 38:143–150.
21. Rodén L, Baker JR, Cifonelli A, Mathews MB: Isolation and characterization of connective tissue polysaccharides. Methods Enzymol 1972; 28:73–140.
22. Baugham DR, Woodward PM: A collaborative study of heparins from different sources. Bull Wld Hlth Org 1970; 43:129–149.
23. Barrowcliffe TW, Johnson EA, Eggleton CA, Thomas DP: Anticoagulant activities of lung and mucous heparins. Thromb Res 1977; 12:27–36.
24. Gomez-Perez F: Anticoagulant activity of two commercially available heparin preparations. J Clin Pharmacol 1972; 12:413–416.
25. Baltes BJ, Diamond S, D'Agostino RJ: Comparison of anticoagulant activity of two preparations of purified heparin. Clin Pharmacol Ther 1973; 14:287–290.
26. McMahon FG, Jain AK, Ryan JR, Lefton TE: Anticoagulant potency of mucosal lung heparin. Clin Pharmacol Ther 1975; 17:79–82.
27. Detrie P, Frileux C, Dreux C, Vairel EG, Leger L: Calcium heparinate: Properties and indications. La Presse Medicale 1962; 78:627–628.
28. Bender F, Aronson BS, Hougie C, Moser K: Bioequivalence of subcutaneous calcium and sodium heparins. Clin Pharmacol Ther 1980; 27:224–229.
29. Jain AK, McMahon FG, Ryan JR, Lefton TE: Comparison of anticoagulant activity of three preparations of heparin. Curr Ther Res 1974; 22:427–432.
30. Jaques LB, Mahadoo JR, Kavanaugh LW: Intrapulmonary heparin: A new procedure for anticoagulant therapy. Lancet 1976; 2:1157–1161.
31. Engleberg H: Prolonged anticoagulant therapy with subcutaneously administered concentrated aqueous heparin. Surgery 1954; 36:762–769.
32. Dawes J, Pepper DS: Catabolism of low dose heparin in man. Thromb Res 1979; 14:845–860.
33. Glimelius B, Bush C, Hook M: Binding of heparin on the surface of cultured human endothelial cells. Thromb Res 1978; 12:773–782.

34. Estes JW, Pelikan EW, Krüger-Thiemer E: A retrospective study of the pharmaco-kinetics of heparin. Clin Pharmacol Ther 1969; 10:329–337.
35. Simon TL, Hyers TM, Gaston JP, Harker LA: Heparin pharmacokinetics: Increased requirements in pulmonary embolism. Brit J Haematol 1978; 39:111–120.
36. Hirsch J, van Aken WG, Gallus AS, Dollery CT, Cade JF, Yung WL: Heparin kinetics in venous thrombosis and pulmonary embolism. Circulation 1976; 53:691–695.
37. McAvoy TJ: Pharmacokinetic modeling of heparin and its clinical implications. J Pharmacokinet Biopharm 1979; 7:331–354.
38. Goodman TL, Todd ME, Goldsmith EI: Laboratory observations and clinical impli-cations of monitoring the effect of heparin by bioassay. Surg Gynec Obstet 1976; 142:673–685.
39. Nadler SB, Hildago JU, Bloch T: Prediction of blood volume in human adults. Surgery 1962; 51:224–232.
40. Chenella FC, Gill AM, Kern JW, Floyd RA, McGehee WG: Improved methods for estimating initial heparin infusion rates. Am J Hosp Pharm 1979; 36:782–784.
41. Perry PJ, Herron GR, King JC: Heparin half-life in normal and impaired renal function. Clin Pharmacol Ther 1974; 16:514–519.
42. McAllister BM, Demis DJ: Heparin metabolism: Isolation and characterization of uroheparin. Nature 1966; 215:293–294.
43. Wessler S, Gitel SN: Heparin: New concepts relevant to clinical use. Blood 1979; 53:525–544.
44. Teien AN, Bjornson J: Heparin elimination in uraemic patients on dialysis. Scand J Haematol 1976; 17:29–35.
45. Estes JW: Kinetics of the anticoagulant effect of heparin. JAMA 1970; 212:1492–1495.
46. Olsson P, Lagergren H, Ek S: The elimination from plasma of intravenous heparin. Acta Med Scand 1963; 173:619–630.
47. Estes JW: The kinetics of heparin. Ann NY Acad Sci 1971; 179:187–204.
48. McAvoy TJ: The biologic half-life of heparin. Clin Pharmacol Ther 1979; 25:372–379.
49. Perry PJ: Anticoagulant half-life of heparin in human subjects with normal and impaired renal function. Ph.D. Dissertation. Stockton, Calif: University of the Pacific, 1973.
50. Genton E: Guidelines for heparin therapy. Ann Int Med 1974; 80:77–82.
51. Estes JW: The fate of heparin in the body. Curr Ther Res 1975; 18:45–57.
52. Estes JW: The heterogeneity of the anticoagulant response to heparin. J Clin Pathol 1972; 25:45–48.
53. Nyman D, Thunherr N, Duckert F: Heparin dosage in extracorporeal circulation and its neutralization. Thromb Diath Hemorrh 1975; 33:102–104.
54. Teien AN: Heparin elimination in patients with liver cirrhosis. Thromb Haemost 1977; 38:701–706.
55. Chiu HM, van Aken WG, Hirsch J, Regoeczi E, Horner AA: Increased heparin clearance in experimental pulmonary embolism. J Lab Clin Med 1977; 90:204–215.
56. Gallus A, Engel G: Heparin. Society of Hospital Pharmacists of Australia: Educa-tional Monographs, Woden A.C.T., 1978.
57. Mant MJ, Thong KL, Birthwhistle RV, O'Brien DB, Hammond GW, Grace MG: Hemorrhagic complications of heparin therapy. Lancet 1977; 1:1133–1135.
58. Salzman EW, Deykin D, Shapiro RM, Rosenberg R: Management of heparin ther-apy—controlled prospective trial. N Engl J Med 1975; 292:1046–1050.

59. Basu D, Gallus A, Hirsch J, Cade J: A prospective study of the value of monitoring heparin treatment with the activated partial thromboplastin time. N Engl J Med 1972; 287:324–327.

60. Colburn WA: Pharmacologic implications of heparin interactions with other drugs. Drug Metab Rev 1976; 5:281–293.

62. Wessler S, Yin ET: Theory and practice of minidose heparin in surgical patients. Circulation 1973; 47:671–676.

63. Gallus AS, Hirsch J, Tuttle RJ, et al: Small subcutaneous doses of heparin in prevention of venous thrombosis. N Engl J Med 1973; 288:545–550.

64. Kakkar VV: The current status of low-dose heparin in prophylaxis of thrombophlebitis and pulmonary embolism. World J Surg 1978; 2:3–18.

65. Council on Thrombosis of the American Heart Association: Prevention of venous thromboembolism in surgical patients by low-dose heparin. Circulation 1977; 55:423A–426A.

66. Brozovic M, Stirling Y, Klenerman L, Lowe L: Subcutaneous heparin and postoperative thromboembolism. Lancet 1974; 2:99–100.

67. Frishman WH, Ribner HS: Anticoagulation in myocardial infarction: Modern approach to an old problem. Am J Cardiol 1979; 43:1207–1213.

68. Wessler S, Morris LE: Studies in intravascular coagulation IV: The effect of heparin and dicoumarol on serum-induced venous thrombosis. Circulation 1955; 12:553–556.

69. Swanson M, Cacade L: Heparin therapy by continuous intravenous infusion. Am J Hosp Pharm 1971; 28:792–795.

70. Glazier RL, Crowell EB: Randomized prospective trial of continuous versus intermittent heparin therapy. JAMA 1976; 236:1365–1367.

71. Chiu HM, Hirsch J, Yung WL, Rogoeczi E, Gent M: Relationship between the anticoagulant and antithrombotic effects of heparin in experimental venous thrombosis. Blood 1977; 49:171–184.

72. Sutton GC: The management of pulmonary embolism. In: Nicolaides AN (ed): *Thromboembolism: Aetiology, Advances in Prevention and Management.* Medical and Technical Publishing, Lancaster, England 1975.

73. Blakely JA: A rapid bedside method for control of heparin therapy. Can Med Assoc J 1968; 99:1072–1076.

74. Mollitt DL, Gartner DJ, Madura JA: Bedside monitoring of heparin therapy. Am J Surg 1978; 135:801–803.

75. Blaisdell FW, Graziano CJ, Effeney DJ: In vivo assessment of anticoagulation. Surgery 1977; 82:821–837.

76. Yudelman IM, Nossel HL, Kaplan KL, Hirsch J: Plasma fibrinopeptide A levels in symptomatic venous thromboembolism. Blood 1978; 51:1189–1195.

77. Pitney WR, Pettit JE, Armstrong L: Control of heparin therapy. Brit Med J 1970; 4:139–141.

78. Goodman LS, Gilman A: *The Pharmacological Basis of Therapeutics.* 5th Ed. Macmillan Company, New York 1975.

79. Handin RI: Purification and properties of platelet factor 4. Fed Proc 1977; 36:50.

# 20

# Guidelines for Collection and Pharmacokinetic Analysis of Drug Disposition Data

William J. Jusko, Ph.D.

Many recent developments and efforts in both theoretical and applied pharmacokinetics have emphasized the principles of *physiological pharmacokinetics* and the use of *model-independent* approaches to analysis of drug disposition data. Physiological pharmacokinetics involves the deployment of pharmacokinetic models and equations based on anatomical constructions and functions such as tissue spaces, blood flow, organ metabolism and clearance, drug input sites, and mechanisms of partitioning, binding, and transport. While the complete application of physiologic systems analysis may require the extensive models proposed by Bischoff and Dedrick (1,2), even the simplest of pharmacokinetic treatments should have a physiologic basis for interpretation. Coupled with efforts to discern the physiologic elements of any set of data is the use of model-independent techniques in pharmacokinetics. This term applies to methods of data treatment and resultant parameters which either do not require a specific model in the analysis or yield the physiological elements of pharmacokinetics such as systemic clearance ($Cl_s$) or steady-state volume of distribution ($V_D^{ss}$) which apply regardless of the model used for calculation.

This chapter is intended to blend the natural components of both approaches to applied pharmacokinetics. A summary is provided of the most relevant concepts, models, equations, and caveats which may be useful in the design, analysis, and interpretation of pharmacokinetic experiments. References are provided for more complete details of the assumptions, derivations, and applications of these guidelines and relationships. This material may be helpful as a checklist in designing animal and human experiments in pharmacokinetics, in

639

reviewing drug disposition reports and, in fully expanded format, has served as a basis for a graduate course in physiological pharmacokinetics.

## Context of Pharmacokinetics

A pharmacokinetic analysis must be made in context of, be consistent with, and explain the array of basic data regarding the properties and disposition characteristics of the drug.

The tasks of model and equation selection and interpretation of data require a fundamental appreciation of and integration of principles of physiology, pharmacology, biochemistry, physicochemistry, analytical methodology, mathematics, and statistics. Pharmacokinetics is a distillation of many disciplines, and the relevant portions of these areas must be considered in reaching any conclusions regarding a particular set of data. The physicochemical properties of a drug such as chemical form (salt, ester, complex), stability, partition coefficient, pKa, and molecular weight can affect drug absorption, distribution, and clearance. A drug disposition profile must be correlated with studies of toxicity, structure-activity, disposition in alternative species, perfused organs, tissue or microsomal metabolism, tissue drug residues, and disease state effects. For example, a much larger $LD_{50}$ for oral doses of a drug compared with parenteral administration may be indicative of either poor gastrointestinal absorption (low aqueous solubility?) or a substantial first-pass effect. Drug metabolism data may be difficult to fully extrapolate between species, but the biotransformation rate ($V_{max}$ and $K_m$) of microsomes, homogenates, or perfused organs can often be applied directly to whole body disposition rates in the same species (1–3).

In general, the pharmacokinetic model and analysis should either conform to or account for the known properties and accumulated data related to the drug. One set of disposition data may misrepresent the characteristics of the drug because of any one or combination of reasons. Experienced judgment may be required to serve in the final interpretation and acceptance of any experimental findings and analysis.

## Array of Basic Data

Pharmacokinetic studies often serve to answer specific questions about the properties of a drug. For example, a limited experimental protocol can easily resolve the question of how renal impairment affects the systemic clearance of an antibiotic. In the total design and implementation of pharmacokinetic studies, an *ideal* and *complete* array of experimental data should include a number of considerations:

A. The dosage form should be pre-analyzed. All calculations stem from knowledge of the exact dose given (e.g., Clearance = Dose/AUC, where AUC is the area under the plasma concentration versus time curve). Most commercial dosage forms are inexact. Vials or ampules of injectables typically contain some overage and require analysis or aliquoting for administration of a precise dose. Solid dosage forms are required to yield an average of the stated quantity of drug with limited variability, but both may be inaccurate for pharmacokinetic purposes. Manninen and Koriionen (4) provided an excellent example of both the variability and lack of stated quantity of digoxin in many commercial tablets of this product. One product contained a range of 39 to 189% of the stated 0.25 mg dose of digoxin, while the most uniform product, Lanoxin® (Burroughs-Wellcome), exhibited a range of about 95 to 106% for one batch of drug. To evaluate the potential uncertainty of the dose of drug used in disposition studies, it may be necessary to collect and analyze replicate doses of the product used. Low dose and poorly soluble drugs may be most susceptible to erratic formulation.

B. Accuracy in administration of the dose should be confirmed. All doses should be timed exactly for starting time and duration of administration. Pharmacokinetic equations are available to correct data from short-term infusion studies to the intercepts expected after bolus injection for ease in subsequent calculations. The duration of multiple-dosing in relation to the terminal half-life is crucial for ascertaining whether steady-state conditions obtain. Materials used in drug administration may cause loss of drug. As one of the most dramatic examples, MacKichan et al (5) found immediate loss of about 50% of a dose of intravenous diazepam by adsorption during passage through the plastic tubing of an infusion set.

C. Attention to methods and sites of blood collection is needed. Blood samples should either be collected by direct venipuncture in clean glass tubes without anticoagulant and centrifuged while maintained at 37°C or assessment of possible artifacts from alternative procedures should be made. Maintenance of a heparin trap can result in increased free fatty acid concentrations in blood causing altered drug-protein binding (6). The type of plastic, commercial tube, or anticoagulant may be a factor

(7). Changes in temperature may alter red cell distribution of some compounds (8). These problems primarily pertain to weak bases such as propranolol and imipramine where plasma protein binding is extensive and displacement alters plasma-red cell drug distribution (7). Platelets accumulate marked concentrations of pyroxamidin which can be released during blood clotting, producing a 5-fold increase in plasma concentrations of this compound (9).

One of the major assumptions employed in most pharmacokinetic studies is that venous blood collected from one site adequately reflects circulating arterial blood concentrations. For practical purposes, most drug disposition studies use venous blood samples. This may require that the pharmacokinetic analysis be somewhat qualified. Arterial and capillary blood concentrations may differ markedly from venous blood concentrations of many drugs (10). The AUC of arterial versus venous blood is expected to be identical for a non-clearing organ and thus the principal difference expected is in distribution volumes. Physiologically, organ uptake of drugs occurs, of course, from the arterial blood. The clearance models described subsequently are based on arterial-venous extraction.

D.  Plasma (or blood) concentration data following intravenous injection provide partial characterization of drug disposition properties. Accurate assessment of volumes of distribution, distribution clearance ($Cl_D$), and systemic clearance ($Cl_s$) can only be attained with intravenous washout data. The kinetic relationships will be presented in greater detail in a later section. Three dosage levels should be administered to span the usual therapeutic range of the drug to permit assessment of possible dose-dependence (nonlinearity).

E.  Plasma (or blood) concentration data following oral doses of the drug in solution add additional pharmacokinetic parameters related to absorption and intrinsic clearance. The doses (or resultant plasma or blood concentrations of drug) should be comparable to those from the intravenous doses. These data permit assessment of linearity of either oral clearance ($Cl_{oral}$) or availability (FF*), and the minimum transit time for absorption ($\bar{t}_a$). If relevant, additional study of other dosage forms and routes of administration should be made. For these, the FDA guidelines for bioavailability studies should be consulted (11).

F.  Plasma protein binding and red cell partitioning should be measured over the expected range of plasma drug concentrations. Both rate and degree of binding and uptake are important.

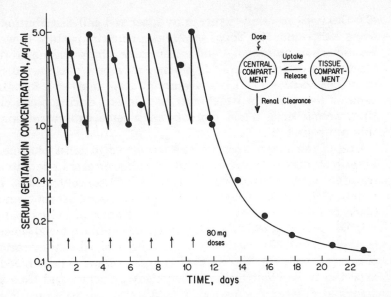

FIGURE 1. Plasma concentration versus time profile for gentamicin disposition during multiple dosing in a patient showing the prolonged terminal phase caused by strong tissue binding. This type of data was characterized with a two-compartment model (insert) which included prediction of drug remaining in body at time of death of patients. Data from Reference 14.

These data should be obtained at 37°C. This information may be needed for interpretation or normalization of clearances and nonlinear disposition patterns.

G. Urinary excretion rates of drug (as a function of time, dose and route of administration) should be measured to accompany the above studies. This is often a major route of drug elimination and analyses permit quantitation of renal clearance ($Cl_R$). Additional analyses of other excreta or body fluids (feces, milk, bile, saliva) if feasible and relevant may permit determination of other elimination or distribution clearances.

H. Many drug metabolites are either pharmacologically active or otherwise of pharmacokinetic interest. Oxidation products such as hydroxylated or demethylated metabolites are most commonly either active or toxic (12). Their measurement will allow evaluation of AUC and transit time and perhaps permit quantitation of metabolite formation and disposition clearances.

I. Multiple-dose and steady-state experiments are necessary if this is the mode of therapeutic use of the drug. Comparative single-

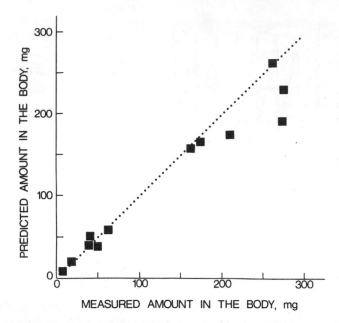

FIGURE 2.  Correlation of gentamicin accumulation in the body determined by pharmacokinetic analysis of serum concentration data (see Figure 1) and by direct analysis of body tissues obtained at autopsy from the same patients who were evaluated pharmacokinetically prior to death. Dotted line indicates perfect correlation. Data from References 14 and 15.

and multiple-dose studies may permit further assessment of linearity and/or allow determination of chronic drug effects such as enzyme induction (13), unusual accumulation (14), or self-induced alterations in disposition. For example, aminoglycoside uptake into tissues is extremely slow and was difficult to assess from single-dose studies. Multiple-dose washout measurements (Figure 1) led to observation of a slow disposition phase which was the result of tissue accumulation (14).

J.  Body tissue analyses add reality and specificity to drug distribution characteristics. Comprehensive studies in animals permit detection of unusual tissue affinity while generating partition coefficients ($K_{pi}$) for individual tissues ($V_{ti}$). This can lead to complete physiologic models for the drug in each species studied (1,2). Autopsy or biopsy studies in man may extend or complement pharmacokinetic expectations. This approach was found to be extremely helpful (see Figure 2) in confirming the strong tissue binding of aminoglycosides in man which was anticipated on the basis of serum concentration profiles (Figure 1, Ref. 15).

K. Comparable or partial drug disposition studies in patients with various diseases form the basis of clinical pharmacokinetics. Perturbations in organ function, blood flow, or response will often alter drug disposition which may warrant quantitative characterization. General principles may not always apply and each drug needs individualized study. For example, while hepatic dysfunction may diminish the rate of oxidation of many drugs such as most benzodiazepines, some compounds such as lorazepam are predominantly metabolized by glucuronide formation, a process largely unaffected by liver diseases such as cirrhosis (16). Each disease state may require evaluation of direct effects on pharmacokinetic processes such as changes in renal drug clearance caused by renal disease. However, indirect changes also require attention, such as the effects on both distribution and clearance caused by altered plasma protein binding (17).

This list is meant to be comprehensive. Many drug disposition questions may be resolved from selected, limited studies and alternative types of information may permit some experimental procedures to be omitted and validate various assumptions. However, it is the investigator's obligation to adequately assess the literature, to make no unwarranted assumptions, and to satisfy the demands of rigorous and precise experimentation.

## Drug Assays

There are several common concerns in the employment of various drug analysis techniques. Certainty in measurement of drugs or metabolites is a major *sine qua non* in pharmacokinetics and deserves considerable attention. To start, it is obvious that the assay method must be specific, sufficiently sensitive, and precise for the intended range of drug concentrations, especially in the presence of metabolites, secondary drugs, and in the occurrence of a disease state. Microbiological assays are notoriously unreliable in many of these regards. Other antibiotics often interfere in detection of the main drug. Active metabolites such as the desacetyl form of some cephalosporins (18) may be included in the measurements unless prior separation is made of the two active compounds. Limited microbiological sensitivity initially prevented adequate characterization of gentamicin in single-dose studies (14). An extreme case of metabolite inclusion is in use of radioisotopic tracers; total radioisotope counts generally yield total drug and metabolite activity and provide minimal pharmacokinetic data. Separation of parent drug and individual metabolites is required for pharmacokinetic specificity. Microbiologic, enzymatic, and radioimmunoassays may require preparation of standards in each patient's blank plasma for accurate pharmacokinetic data.

Coupled with assay reliability is concern for the stability of drug in biological specimens, even in the frozen state. An unusual case is ampicillin which is less stable frozen than when refrigerated (19). Some drug esters such as hetacillin (a prodrug of ampicillin), continue hydrolyzing in blood and during the bioassay, and imprudent handling of the blood specimens can confound the true disposition profiles of both prodrug and drug (20). Measurement of drug stability in blood will complement the pharmacokinetic profiling of a drug in discerning whether drug clearance can occur directly from blood or whether exposure to other body organs is required.

## Sample Timing

Appropriate pharmacokinetic evaluation requires properly timed specimens. The simplest and least ambiguous experiment is the determination of systemic plasma clearance at steady-state:

$$Cl_s = k_0/C_p^{ss} \qquad \text{(Eq. 1)}$$

where $k_0$ is the infusion rate and $C_p^{ss}$ is the steady-state plasma concentration. For this equation to apply, the infusion period must be sufficiently long to allow steady-state to be attained.

A specific compartmental type of analysis requires multiple blood samples to be collected during each phase of drug disposition. More frequent samples are needed for more rapid exponential phases. A pilot study or other preliminary data is usually necessary to aid in design of more extensive studies.

A common and severe problem in applied pharmacokinetics is the inadequate or incomplete measurement of drug washout from the system. This is often caused either by premature termination of sample collection or by analytical limitations. The 'true' terminal disposition phase must be examined in order for most aspects of the pharmacokinetic treatment and interpretation to be accurate. For example, the early distributive phase of aminoglycoside disposition had long been accepted as the only phase, yet more sensitive radioimmunoassays, lengthier studies, and evaluation of multiple-dose washout revealed the slower phase of prolonged drug release from tissues (see Figure 1).

The two principal model-independent, physiologic parameters in pharmacokinetics, systemic clearance and steady-state volume of distribution, are calculated by use of the area under the plasma concentration versus time curve (AUC) and the area under the moment curve (AUMC). Both area values require extrapolation of plasma concentrations to time infinity, and the AUMC is, in particular, prone to error from an inaccurate terminal slope. If analytical or ethical constraints limit blood sample collection and assays, saliva concentration monitoring and extended urine collection may aid in defining the terminal disposition slope while adding one or two other pharmacokinetic parameters to the analysis.

The "midpoint" $(\overline{C})$ is generally the most desirable time to collect blood samples to match an excretion interval to assess a time-dependent clearance process:

$$\text{Clearance} = \frac{\text{Excretion Rate}}{\overline{C}} = \frac{\text{Amount Excreted}}{\text{AUC}} \qquad \text{(Eq. 2)}$$

The arithmetic mean time is acceptable for slow processes but errors will be incurred if the kinetic process produces rapid changes in plasma concentrations. The mean transit time $(\overline{t})$ of the excretion interval provides a true time at which the blood sample should be collected to yield an accurate $\overline{C}$ and time-average clearance (21,22) for exponential processes:

$$\text{AUMC} = \text{AUC} \cdot \overline{t} = \overline{C} \cdot \overline{t}^2 \qquad \text{(Eq. 3)}$$

This requires foreknowledge of the shape of the plasma concentration versus time curve over the excretion interval in order to estimate the time of occurrence of $\overline{t}$. Curve-fitting may permit this to be done retrospectively.

It is common that an early exponential phase of drug disposition is missed because of infrequent blood sampling. For a polynomial curve with intercepts, $C_i$, and slopes, $\lambda_i$, the total AUC is:

$$\text{AUC} = \Sigma(C_i/\lambda_i) \qquad \text{(Eq. 4)}$$

If the initial distributive phase is missing $(C_1/\lambda_1)$, then the error incurred in calculation of a clearance parameter (Clearance = Dose/AUC) is:

$$\% \text{ of Cl Error} = 100 \times (C_1/\lambda_1)/\text{AUC} \qquad \text{(Eq. 5)}$$

Different degrees of error will be produced in the values of the volumes of distribution and distribution clearance as can be discerned by analogous inspection of later equations.

## Basic Physiologic Models

The evolution of complete physiologic models (1–3) and clearance concepts applied to perfused organ systems (23,24) with the restrictions incurred by the limited visibility of most blood or plasma drug disposition profiles has led to the employment of partial physiologic models for description of pharmacokinetic data. One such model is shown in Figure 3. Its construction and use should be viewed with some conceptual flexibility. The concepts described in this section will apply to linear or first-order processes unless otherwise stated.

**Volumes.** The drug in blood or plasma ($C_p$) is considered to be part of the central compartment ($V_c$). The minimum value of $V_c$ is plasma volume ($V_p$), but because drug either diffuses rapidly out of plasma or the number of early time data are limited, a $V_c$ larger than plasma volume is frequently observed.

Drug which is located outside of $V_p$ or $V_c$ is, of course, present in tissues. The apparent volume of the tissue compartment ($V_T$) has two basic determinants: physiologic weight or volume of each tissue ($V_{ti}$) and partition/distribution factors ($K_{pi}$). In analysis of plasma concentration versus time profiles, tissues must commonly be merged together (including the clearing organs); thus:

$$V_T = \Sigma(K_{pi} \cdot V_{ti}) \tag{Eq. 6}$$

This leads to definition of one of the primary model-independent, physiologic parameters, volume of distribution at steady-state ($V_D^{ss}$):

$$V_D^{ss} = V_c + V_T \tag{Eq. 7}$$

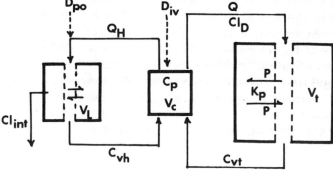

FIGURE 3. Basic physiologic pharmacokinetic model for drug distribution and elimination. Symbols are defined in the text. The clearance organ is pharmacokinetically perceived as separate from other compartments for drugs with high intrinsic clearances ($Cl_{int}$) allowing characterization of the first-pass input. Low clearance drugs may not exhibit separate distribution and clearance properties for the clearance organ (see Figure 1).

TABLE 1.  PHYSIOLOGICAL DETERMINANTS OF DRUG PARTITION OR
DISTRIBUTION RATIOS BETWEEN TISSUES AND PLASMA

Active Transport
Donnan Ion Effect
pH Differences
Plasma Protein Binding
Tissue Binding
Lipid Partitioning

If plasma ($f_{up}$) and tissue ($f_{ut}$) binding are the sole determinants of nonhomogeneous distribution of drug in the body, then one definition of $V_D^{ss}$ is:

$$V_D^{ss} = V_p + \frac{f_{ut}}{f_{up}} \cdot V_t \qquad \text{(Eq. 8)}$$

as proposed by Gillette (25) where $f_u$ is the fraction of drug unbound, and $V_t$ is the volume or the weight of all tissues except plasma. Other factors may also contribute to the partition coefficient of drugs between tissues and plasma (Table 1). Since by definition $V_p$ and $V_t$ comprise total body weight (TBWt):

$$\text{TBWt} = V_p + V_t \qquad \text{(Eq. 9)}$$

then the quotient of:

$$K_D = V_D^{ss}/\text{TBWt} \qquad \text{(Eq. 10)}$$

defines the distribution coefficient ($K_D$), a physicochemical/physiological measure of the average partition coefficient of the drug throughout the body. Approximate values of $K_D$ and the primary rationalization of the size of $K_D$ are provided in Table 2 for various common drugs.

One qualification of $V_D^{ss}$ is needed. Drug equilibration between plasma and tissue of a clearing organ also encompasses the blood flow ($Q_H$) and intrinsic clearance ($Cl_{int}$) (26). For hepatic tissue this yields the following relationship between the true partition coefficient ($K_{ph}$) and the apparent value which would be measured at steady-state ($K_{ph}^{ss}$):

$$K_{ph} = K_{ph}^{ss} \cdot (1 + \frac{Cl_{int}}{Q_H}) \qquad \text{(Eq. 11)}$$

**Distribution Clearance.** The least developed and appreciated element of the basic pharmacokinetic properties of drugs is the distribution clearance ($Cl_D$) or intercompartmental clearance. This term reflects the flow/transfer property of drugs, representing movement in

TABLE 2.  DISTRIBUTION COEFFICIENTS ($K_D$) FOR VARIOUS DRUGS
AND PROBABLE PHYSIOLOGIC/PHYSICOCHEMICAL CAUSE

| Drug | $K_D = \dfrac{V_D^{ss}}{TBWt}$ | Explanation/Indication |
|---|---|---|
| Indocyanine Green | 0.06 | Strong binding to plasma proteins and limited extravascular permeability. |
| Inulin | 0.25 | Limited distribution into plasma and interstitial fluid owing to large molecular weight (5500) and lack of lipid solubility. |
| Ampicillin | 0.25 | Limited intracellular distribution owing to poor lipid solubility. |
| Theophylline | 0.5 | Distribution primarily into total body water. |
| Antipyrine | 0.6 | Fairly equal distribution into total body water. |
| Gentamicin | 1.1 | Strong tissue binding common to aminoglycosides. |
| Tetracycline | 1.6 | Strong tissue binding to calcium in bone. |
| Diazepam | 1.7 | Appreciable lipid partitioning. |
| Digoxin | 8.0 | Strong binding to Na/K Transport ATPase in cell membranes. |
| Imipramine | 10.0 | Strong tissue binding common to many basic amines. |

and out of physiological spaces. The simplest assumption made in constructing a generalized model is that distribution clearance is equal in both directions; that is, clearance in equals clearance out of tissues.

Renkin has characterized distribution clearance in terms of transcapillary movement of small molecular weight substances (27). The model he proposed is depicted in Figure 4. Drug transfer from blood to tissues is represented by flow down a cylindrical tube (Q) with permeability (P) determined by diffusion across the capillary. Distribution clearance is thus defined by flow and permeability according to the relationship:

$$Cl_D = Q(1 - e^{-P/Q})$$ (Eq. 12)

Compounds with high tissue permeability will exhibit a limiting $Cl_D$ of Q:

$$\lim_{P \to \infty} Cl_D = Q$$ (Eq. 12a)

while those with low permeability are limited by P:

$$\lim_{P \to 0} Cl_D = P$$ (Eq. 12b)

One of the determinants of the capillary permeability of drug is molecular weight, as indicated in Table 3 (28). This description of distribution clearance, while based on capillary transfer, demonstrates its physiological and physicochemical basis. Other processes may be rate-limiting for specific drugs where the tissue barriers are cell membranes rather than blood vessel walls (29).

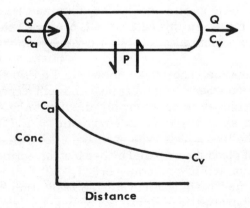

FIGURE 4. Model for distribution clearance where blood flow (Q) along the cylindrical tube and capillary permeability (P) are the primary determinants of drug loss from arterial blood ($C_a$). Drug concentration in the tube will decline monoexponentially according to distance (length) along the tube emerging at the venous concentration ($C_v$).

TABLE 3.   PERMEABILITY OF MUSCLE CAPILLARIES TO WATER-
SOLUBLE MOLECULES

| | Molecular Weight | Radius of Equivalent Sphere (Å) | Diffusion Coefficient | |
|---|---|---|---|---|
| | | | In water, D (cm$^2$/sec) $\times 10^5$ | Across Capillary, P (cm$^3$/sec. 100g) |
| Water | 18 | | 3.20 | 3.7 |
| Urea | 60 | 1.6 | 1.95 | 1.83 |
| Glucose | 180 | 3.6 | 0.91 | 0.64 |
| Sucrose | 342 | 4.4 | 0.74 | 0.35 |
| Raffinose | 594 | 5.6 | 0.56 | 0.24 |
| Inulin | 5,500 | 15.2 | 0.21 | 0.036 |
| Myoglobin | 17,000 | 19 | 0.15 | 0.005 |
| Hemoglobin | 69,000 | 31 | 0.094 | 0.001 |
| Serum Albumin | 69,000 | | 0.085 | <0.001 |

From Reference 28.

The $Cl_D$ can be perceived as a model-independent, physiologic parameter when summed for all distribution processes:

$$Cl_D = Cl_{d12} + Cl_{d13} + \ldots + Cl_{di} \qquad \text{(Eq. 13)}$$

Thus, apparent three-compartment ($Cl_{d12}, Cl_{d13}$) distribution can be
blended with two-compartment $Cl_D$ by combining $Cl_{d12}$ and $Cl_{d13}$ values
for the former model. In this context, $Cl_D$ becomes the total transcapillary distribution clearance (30) with cardiac output as the limiting
value (Q).

**Organ Clearance.** The model shown in Figure 3 represents the
common situation where drug must pass through a specific organ such
as the liver or kidney in order for elimination to be effected. It does
not apply in a situation such as enzymatic hydrolysis of the drug
occurring in the blood. This type of model allows characterization of
the dual role of blood flow (Q) and either biotransformation ($V_{max}$, $K_m$)
or renal filtration (GFR) and transport ($T_{max}$, $T_m$) on removal of drug
from the body and permits accurate representation of the effects of
route of administration (e.g., first-pass effects) on drug disposition.

Two types of clearing organ models have been proposed for hepatic
elimination: the "Jar" Model (1–3,23) (Figure 5) and the "Tube" Model
(31,32) (Figure 6). Both include blood flow for systemic drug access to
the organ and, as shown in the figures, currently assume that free or
unbound drug ($C_f$) in plasma equilibrates with free drug in the tissue

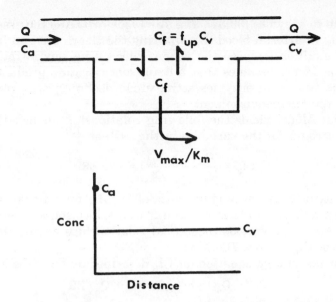

FIGURE 5.   The "well-stirred" or "jar" model for hepatic uptake and metabolism ($V_{max}/K_m$) of drug where instantaneous venous and hepatic equilibration of unbound ($C_f$) drug is assumed. Inflow and outflow (Q) are assumed to be identical.

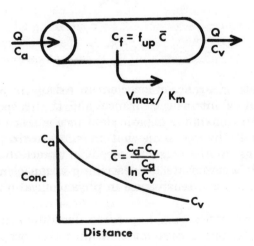

FIGURE 6.   The "tube" or "parallel tube" model for hepatic uptake and metabolism ($V_{max}/K_m$) of drug where venous concentrations ($C_v$) decline monoexponentially as flow (Q) carries drug past homogenously distributed sites of biotransformation. The log-mean concentration ($\bar{C}$) in the tube is indicated.

available to enzymes (33,34). The Jar Model involves the assumption that drug in arterial blood ($C_a$) entering the clearing organ instantaneously equilibrates with the venous blood drug concentration ($C_v$). The Tube Model assumes that a drug concentration gradient exists down the tube with enzymes acting upon declining drug concentrations in the microenvironment.

The Jar Model yields the following relationship for hepatic clearance to account for the variables in the system:

$$Cl_H = \frac{Q_H \cdot f_{up} \cdot Cl_{int}}{Q_H + f_{up} \cdot Cl_{int}} = Q_H \cdot ER \qquad \text{(Eq. 14)}$$

where intrinsic clearance is the ratio of $V_{max}/K_m$ for a linear biotransformation and ER is the Extraction Ratio. Wilkinson and Shand (24) have depicted the various theoretical relationships among the determinants of $Cl_H$ (Figure 7).

The corresponding equation for $Cl_H$ described by the Tube Model is:

$$Cl_H = Q_H(1 - e^{-f_{up} \cdot Cl_{int}/Q_H}) = Q_H \cdot ER \qquad \text{(Eq. 15)}$$

Pang and Rowland (35a) have compared the two hepatic models in terms of the effects of $Q_H$ and $Cl_{int}$ on $Cl_H$ and ER. Both models predict a lower limit of:

$$\lim_{Cl_{int} \to 0} Cl_H = f_{up} \cdot Cl_{int} \qquad \text{(Eq. 15a)}$$

and upper value of:

$$\lim_{Cl_{int} \to \infty} Cl_H = Q_H \qquad \text{(Eq. 15b)}$$

Thus the hepatic clearance of low clearance drugs is essentially equal to the product of intrinsic clearance and the fraction unbound in plasma (33). The maximum hepatic clearance will be organ blood flow. The two models diverge somewhat in characterizing intermediate clearance drugs. At the present time, it is uncertain which model is most generally appropriate for describing organ clearance. The Jar Model has had most extensive use in physiological pharmacokinetics (1–3).

The organ clearance models provide definitions for two types of general clearance terms. *Systemic clearance* ($Cl_s$) reflects any situation where drug is administered without its initially passing through the clearing organ. Intravenous, intramuscular, buccal, and subcutaneous injection of drugs yields plasma concentration versus time data governed by systemic clearance, e.g.:

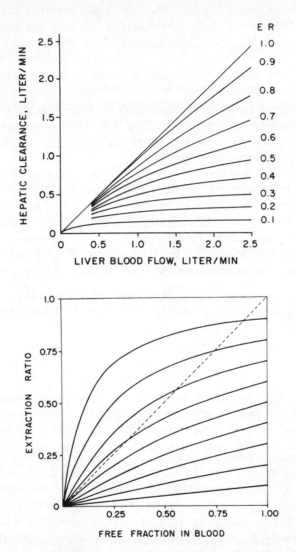

FIGURE 7. Top portion depicts the relationship between hepatic clearance ($Cl_H$) and liver blood flow ($Q_H$) drugs with low (ER = 0.1) to very high (ER = 1.0) values of intrinsic clearance. The bottom figure shows the expected effect of plasma protein binding on Extraction Ratio ($Cl_H = Q_H \cdot ER$) for drugs with increasing values of intrinsic clearance (low to high in sequential order). Both graphs portray the role of the variables controlling hepatic clearance in Equation 14. Taken from Reference 24; reproduced by permission of the author and the C.V. Mosby Co.

$$Cl_s = \frac{D_{IV}}{AUC_{IV}} = Q \cdot ER \qquad (Eq.\ 16)$$

The systemic clearance is equal to the sum of all organ clearance processes:

$$Cl_s = Cl_H + Cl_R + Cl_{other} \qquad (Eq.\ 17)$$

where the upper limit in removal of drug from the body can be perceived as the sum of each organ blood flow. For drugs subject to enzymatic degradation in blood, the upper limit of $Cl_s$ is, of course, $V_{max}/K_m$ for this biotransformation process.

The *intrinsic clearance* is a related, complementary term which reflects the maximum metabolic or transport capability of the clearing organ. It can be measured by directly introducing the drug into the circulation feeding the clearing organ. Oral, intraperitoneal, and rectal (in part) doses place the drug directly into the liver via the mesenteric vein. If the drug is fully absorbed ($F = 1$) and undergoes biotransformation entirely by the liver, then:

$$\frac{F \cdot D_{po}}{AUC_{po}} = Cl_{oral} \qquad (Eq.\ 18)$$

and:

$$\frac{F \cdot D_{po}}{f_{up} \cdot AUC_{po}} = Cl_{int} = \frac{V_{max}}{K_m} \qquad (Eq.\ 19)$$

where $Cl_{oral}$, or oral dose clearance, provides the intrinsic clearance uncorrected for protein binding ($f_{up}$) (33,34). Shand et al (34) have demonstrated that $V_{max}/K_m$ values from *in vitro* drug metabolizing systems can be used to predict reasonable values of ER for perfused organ disposition of various drugs where (from Equation 14):

$$ER = \frac{C_a - C_v}{C_a} = \frac{f_{up} \cdot Cl_{int}}{Q_H + f_{up} \cdot Cl_{int}} \qquad (Eq.\ 20)$$

These data are presented in Table 4.

If hepatic biotransformation causes removal of essentially the entire dose of drug, then the model shown in Figure 3 will often apply. A second clearing process can be added to the scheme to represent renal clearance (which is always one mechanism of systemic clearance in whole body disposition studies). One relationship which defines many of the common factors affecting renal clearance ($Cl_R$) is:

$$Cl_R = Q_{RP} \cdot ER = \left( f_{up} \cdot GFR + \frac{Q_{RP} \cdot f_{up} \cdot Cl_{int}^R}{Q_{RP} + f_{up} \cdot Cl_{int}^R} \right) (1 - f_R) \qquad (Eq.\ 21)$$

TABLE 4. COMPARISON OF DRUG EXTRACTION RATIOS PREDICTED FROM IN VITRO DRUG METABOLISM DATA AND OBSERVED IN LIVER PERFUSION STUDIES*

| Drug | In Vitro $V_{max}/K_m$ ml/(min)(g liver) | Extraction Ratio Predicted | Observed |
|---|---|---|---|
| Alprenolol | 23.5 | 0.92 | >0.90 |
| Propranolol | 10.0 | 0.83 | >0.90 |
| Lidocaine | 8.21 | 0.80 | >0.90 |
| Phenytoin | 1.99 | 0.50 | 0.53 |
| Hexobarbital | 1.60 | 0.44 | 0.33 |
| Carbamazepine | 0.11 | 0.05 | 0.04 |
| Antipyrine | 0.08 | 0.04 | 0.01 |

*From Reference 34.

where $Q_{RP}$ is the effective renal plasma flow, GFR is the glomerular filtration rate, $f_R$ is the fraction of drug reabsorbed in the tubules, and $Cl_{int}^R$ is the intrinsic renal transport, which under linear conditions is governed by the $T_{max}/T_m$ for the active transport process (35b).

Thus at least two model-independent, physiological elimination clearances can be generated from typical drug disposition data. Parenteral drug doses yield the total systemic blood/plasma clearance, while oral drug doses yield oral blood/plasma clearance (confounded with F, the bioavailability and by the presence of secondary presystemic clearance processes). The $Cl_{oral}$ can be used to generate the intrinsic clearance if F and plasma protein binding ($f_{up}$) are determined and drug elimination occurs entirely by hepatic biotransformation.

**Absorption.** Two properties of drugs exhibiting an absorption profile can be considered as model-independent, physiological parameters. These are the systemic availability (FF*) and the mean transit time for absorption ($\bar{t}_a$). The systemic availability represents the net fraction of the dose reaching the blood/plasma following possible losses from incomplete release from the dosage form or destruction in the gastrointestinal tract (F) and losses caused by first-pass metabolism during distribution from gut to liver to systemic circulation (F*):

$$F^* = 1 - \frac{f_{up} \cdot Cl_{int}}{Q_H} \qquad \text{(Eq. 22)}$$

The oral : IV AUC ratio indicates systemic availability:

$$FF^* = AUC_{po}/AUC_{IV} \qquad \text{(Eq. 23)}$$

A relatively new concept for characterizing drug absorption rate is the $\overline{t}_a$ (30,36). As indicated by its name, this parameter represents the average duration of time that drug molecules persist in the dosage form and GI tract (Figure 8). Drug absorption rate constants are usually the least secure of conventionally calculated pharmacokinetic parameters because of the complications incurred by incomplete release from the dosage form, irregular absorption, lag times ($\overline{t}_{lag}$), mixed zero-order and other dissolution rates, effects of changing GI motility and contents, GI blood flow effects, first-pass, blurred exponential terms in equations, and inadequate blood sampling (37). The $\overline{t}_a$ provides a quantitative parameter which basically summarizes how long, on average, drug molecules remain unabsorbed. It is calculated as follows for a low clearance drug:

$$\overline{t}_a = \overline{t}_{oral} - \overline{t}_{IV} - \overline{t}_{lag} \qquad \text{(Eq. 24)}$$

where the transit times of oral and IV doses of drugs can be obtained from their AUMC/AUC ratios (Figures 8 and 9) and $\overline{t}_{lag}$ is the lag time before absorption begins. The calculation is more complicated for high clearance drugs (see Equations 35–36).

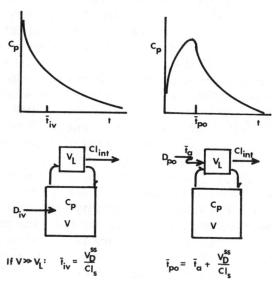

FIGURE 8.   Representations of the mean transit time for drugs administered by intravenous ($\overline{t}_{IV}$) and oral ($\overline{t}_{po}$) routes of administration. On the graph, the $\overline{t}$ reflects the average duration of time drug molecules persist in the body and can be visualized at the time point where the AUC is equal on both sides of the $\overline{t}$. In the models, the $\overline{t}$ is equal to the input $\overline{t}$ ($\overline{t}_a$) plus the ratio of $V_D^{ss} \div Cl_s$, if it can be assumed that $V >> V_L$.

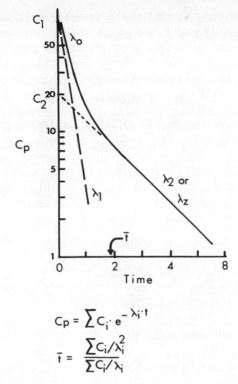

$$C_p = \sum C_i \cdot e^{-\lambda_i \cdot t}$$

$$\bar{t} = \frac{\sum C_i / \lambda_i^2}{\sum C_i / \lambda_i}$$

FIGURE 9. Log-linear intravenous drug disposition curve showing the biexponential decline in plasma concentrations ($C_p$) as a function of time (t). The SHAM properties include Slopes ($\lambda_0$, $\lambda_1$, and $\lambda_2$ or $\lambda_z$), Heights ($C_1$ and $C_2$), Area ($\sum C_i / \lambda_i$) and Moment ($\sum C_i / \lambda_i^2$).

## Time Average Parameters

The initial goal of any drug disposition study and minimum requirement in the pharmacokinetic analysis is the generation of four to six basic model-independent, physiologic parameters. The starting point in the analysis should involve curve-fitting the data as polyexponentials to characterize the SHAM properties (30,38):

S: Slopes     ($\lambda_i$: $\lambda_1$, $\lambda_2$...$\lambda_z$)
H: Heights    ($C_i$: $C_1$, $C_2$...$C_z$) (Intercepts)
A: Area       (AUC = $\sum C_i / \lambda_i$)
M: Moment   (AUMC = $\sum C_i / \lambda_i^2$)

(See Figure 9 for a depiction of these characteristics)

From these values, the data following intravenous doses of drug yield:
Systemic plasma or blood clearance:

$$Cl_s = D_{IV}/AUC \qquad \text{(Eq. 25)}$$

Volume of distribution at steady-state (29,39):

$$V_D^{ss} = D_{IV} \cdot AUMC/AUC^2 = Cl_s \cdot \overline{t}_{IV} \qquad \text{(Eq. 26)}$$

The mean transit time $(\overline{t}_{IV})$ of an IV bolus dose is determined by:

$$\overline{t}_{IV} = V_D^{ss}/Cl_s \qquad \text{(Eq. 27)}$$

The mean transit time of a function can also be viewed (Figures 8–10) as the time point where the AUC is equal on both sides. If the decline in plasma concentrations is multi-exponential, at least two additional parameters can be calculated:

The volume of the central compartment $(V_c)$:

$$V_c = D_{IV}/C_p^\circ = D_{IV}/\Sigma C_i \qquad \text{(Eq. 28)}$$

Distribution clearance:

$$Cl_D = V_c \cdot \lambda_o - Cl_s \qquad \text{(Eq. 29)}$$

where $\lambda_o$ is the slope or tangent of the initial distributive phase[1] (30,38) (see Figure 9).

The addition of drug disposition data $(AUC_{po})$ following oral doses $(D_{po})$ yields:

Apparent oral clearance:

$$Cl_{oral} = F \cdot D_{po}/AUC_{po} \qquad \text{(Eq. 30)}$$

Systemic availability:

$$FF^* = AUC_{po}/AUC_{IV} \qquad \text{(Eq. 31)}$$

Mean transit time for absorption:

$$\overline{t}_a = \overline{t}_{po} - \overline{t}_{IV} \qquad \text{(Eq. 32)}$$

---

[1]It may be inaccurate to calculate $\lambda_o$ in this fashion (see Reference 30). $Cl_D$ can be generated more precisely by constructing a specific model and solving for the individual clearance and volume terms including $Cl_{di}$. When multiple compartments exist, then $Cl_D = \Sigma Cl_{di}$ for the individual distribution clearances (Equation 13). For a biexponential curve, $Cl_D$ can be obtained from:

$$Cl_D = (\frac{C_1 \cdot \lambda_2 + C_2 \cdot \lambda_1}{C_1 + C_2})(V_D^{ss} - V_C) \qquad \text{(Eq. 29a)}$$

The AUC and AUMC can be generated by numerical integration to facilitate data analysis when the shape of the plasma concentration versus time curve is irregular (Figure 10):

$$AUC = \int_0^T C_p \cdot dt + \frac{C_p{}^*}{\lambda_z} \qquad \text{(Eq. 33)}$$

and

$$AUMC = \int_0^T t \cdot C_p \cdot dt + \frac{T \cdot C_p^*}{\lambda_z} + \frac{C_p{}^*}{\lambda_z{}^2} \qquad \text{(Eq. 34)}$$

where $\lambda_z$ is the terminal slope of the curve and $C_p{}^*$ and T are the last measured $C_p$ and time values. The quotient terms provide extrapolations of each function to time infinity. Numerical integration can be carried out by various methods to generate both the AUC and AUMC values (40). The ratio of AUMC/AUC provides the $\bar{t}$ for the particular function.

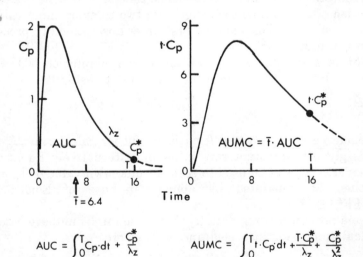

$$AUC = \int_0^T C_p \cdot dt + \frac{C_p^*}{\lambda_z} \qquad AUMC = \int_0^T t \cdot C_p \cdot dt + \frac{T \cdot C_p^*}{\lambda_z} + \frac{C_p^*}{\lambda_z^2}$$

FIGURE 10. Graphical depiction of the Area (AUC) and Moment (AUMC) properties of a pharmacokinetic disposition (Cp vs. t) curve. The last measured plasma concentration $(C_p^*)$ at $t = T$ is extrapolated to time infinity using the terminal slope $(\lambda_z)$ of the log-linear disposition curve. The mean transit time $(\bar{t})$ is indicated on the AUC curve and in relation to the AUMC. Note the larger portion of the AUMC curve requiring extrapolation compared to the AUC curve.

The transit time approach must be somewhat qualified when a clearance organ accounts for removal of drug from the plasma (C.L. DeVane and W.J. Jusko, to be published). For the type of model depicted in Figure 8, the exact definition of $\bar{t}$ for a bolus dose of drug introduced *either* into V or $V_L$ is:

$$\bar{t} = \frac{V(Q + Cl_{int}) + Q \cdot V_L}{Q \cdot Cl_{int}} \qquad \text{(Eq. 35)}$$

(where protein binding is not considered). If it can be assumed that V (or actually $V_D^{ss}$) is appreciably greater than $V_L$, then the second term in the numerator can be neglected and, with a substitution from Equation 14, this equation reduces to:

$$\bar{t} = \frac{V(Q + Cl_{int})}{Q \cdot Cl_{int}} = \frac{V_D^{ss}}{Cl_s} \qquad \text{(Eq. 36)}$$

This relationship forms the basis of calculation of the transit time for absorption from Equation 24 and 32. It should be noted that, while $\bar{t}_a$ is a reflection of the mean persistence time of drug molecules at the absorption site, it can be converted into two common input rate processes if applicable. For a simple first-order absorption ($k_a$) process, $\bar{t}_a$ is identical to $k_a^{-1}$ (36).

In the case of either zero-order absorption or infusion ($k_0$) of drug for a time duration of $T_I$, the transit-time relationship is:

$$\bar{t} = \frac{V_D^{ss}}{Cl_s} + \tfrac{1}{2}T_I \qquad \text{(Eq. 37)}$$

This equation in rearranged form is useful for calculating $V_D^{ss}$ when drug is given by constant rate infusion. Alternatively Equation 37 together with $\bar{t}_{IV}$ can be used to seek an unknown value of $T_I$, and $k_0$ can then be generated by appropriate use of Equation 31 ($k_0 = FF^* \cdot D_0/T_I$).

Plasma protein binding data ($f_{up}$ = fraction unbound) are essential for calculation of intrinsic clearance (33) where:

$$Cl_{int} = \frac{V_{max}}{K_m} = \frac{F \cdot D_{po}}{f_{up} \cdot AUC_{po}} \qquad \text{(Eq. 38)}$$

This equation applies when complete hepatic biotransformation of the drug occurs. The value of $f_{up}$ can also be introduced into the equation for hepatic clearance (Equation 14). Similar use of $f_{up}$ can be found in the equation for renal clearance (Equation 21).

Other time-average clearance terms can be calculated if drug excretion by specific pathways is measured:

$$Cl_{excretory} = \frac{\text{Amount Excreted}}{\text{AUC}} \qquad \text{(Eq. 39)}$$

This relationship is most often applied to renal clearance calculations (see Equation 21).

Wagner (41) has developed a useful array of general equations which can be employed along with the SHAM parameters for calculating the time-course of drug amount in the body and other properties of polyexponentials. These are listed in Table 5.

One relationship which can be added to Wagner's array is Vaughan's equation for estimating the first-order rate constant for drug absorption (42):

$$k_a = \cfrac{\lambda_z}{1 - \cfrac{(C_z)_{IV}}{F \cdot (C_z)_{po}} \cdot \cfrac{D_{po}}{D_{IV}}} \qquad \text{(Eq. 40)}$$

where $C_z$ and $\lambda_z$ are the intercept and slope of the terminal phase of disposition. This equation applies only to low clearance drugs and is most helpful for estimating $k_a$ for further application of specific models and curve-fitting procedures.

Deconvolution methods form an alternative model-independent approach to assessing both the type and rate of drug input to the systemic circulation (43). They are not appropriate, however, for high clearance drugs, because the use of an IV disposition curve for characterizing the output function does not reflect the intrinsic clearance of the drug which effects removal of part or all of an oral dose of drug.

For linear pharmacokinetic systems, the time-average parameters can be extrapolated to steady-state situations. Steady-state plasma concentrations ($C_p^{ss}$) are determined by four factors (44):

$$C_p^{ss} = \frac{F \cdot D_o}{Cl \cdot \tau} \qquad \text{(Eq. 41)}$$

where $D_o$ is either the oral or intravenous dose, Cl applies as the respective oral or systemic clearance, and $\tau$ is the dosing interval. Distribution parameters obviously do not influence steady-state conditions, although $V_D^{ss}$ affects the time required to attain steady-state during continuous dosing. As a rule of thumb, it requires more than four durations of $\lambda_z$ to attain $C_p^{ss}$; the minimum value of $\lambda_z$ is:

$$\lim_{Cl_{int} \to 0} \lambda_z = Cl_s / V_D^{ss} \qquad \text{(Eq. 42)}$$

TABLE 5. CALCULATION OF PHARMACOKINETIC PARAMETERS AND FUNCTIONS BASED ON POLYEXPONENTIAL EQUATIONS FOR BOLUS INTRAVENOUS INJECTION

General disposition equation:

$$C_p = \Sigma C_i \cdot e^{-\lambda_i \cdot t}$$

SHAM Properties:

$$\lambda_i = \text{Slopes}$$
$$H_o = \Sigma C_i \quad \text{(Height)}$$
$$A = \Sigma C_i/\lambda_i \quad \text{(Area)}$$
$$M = \Sigma C_i/\lambda_i^2 \quad \text{(Moment)}$$

Physiologic Parameters:

$$Cl_s = D_{IV}/A$$
$$V_c = D_{IV}/H_o$$
$$V_D^{ss} = D_{IV} \cdot M/A^2$$

$Cl_D$ (biexponential only):

$$Cl_D = (\frac{C_1 \cdot \lambda_2 + C_2 \cdot \lambda_1}{H_o}) \, (V_D^{ss} - V_c)$$

Others:

$$\lambda_z = \text{Terminal slope}$$
$$t_{1/2\,z} = 0.693/\lambda_z$$
$$V_{D\beta} = D_{IV}/A \cdot \lambda_z$$

$A_E$ (Amount Eliminated to time t):

$$A_E = D_{IV} \cdot A_o^t/A_o^\infty$$

$A_B$ (Amount in Body at time t):

$$A_B = D_{IV} - A_E$$

Partly from References 38, 39, and 41.

## Pharmacokinetic Models

Deployment of specific compartmental or physiologic models should be with sound biopharmaceutical and physiologic justification for their construction. The number of exponential terms in decline of plasma drug concentrations is not a direct indication of a specific model (46). Drug disposition usually occurs with each portion of a curve comprised of mixed absorption, distributive, mixing, volume, clearance, and recycling elements which can vary among subjects and with dose and time (45,46). The visibility of an exponential phase usually depends on the route and speed of drug administration and the intensity of blood sampling. Thus bolus doses are usually preferred in pharmacokinetics because they improve determination of the distributive phase of disposition. Slopes and intercepts of any curves are seldom unique.

On the other hand, if a model is justified, there would be loss of information about the drug disposition system if the pharmacokinetic analysis was limited to the time-average parameters. The use of a specific model is most often justified when characterizing time or concentration dependent processes and for assessing drug input rates. Recognition of the different behavior of high clearance drugs when administered by oral and parenteral routes implies the functioning of the first-pass organ clearance model (Figure 3) rather than an ordinary two-compartment model with clearance from either $V_c$ or $V_T$.

The development and solution of specific models requires an extensive array of physiologic and mathematical considerations which have been addressed in many monographs (48) and textbooks (30,43,47,49). Only some general principles are presented here.

The number of parameters (NP) which can be calculated for a given compartmental/physiologic model is dependent on:

EX, the number of exponentials visible in the plasma or blood concentration versus time pattern;

PE, the number of elimination or excretory pathways suitably measured;

TS, the number of tissue spaces or binding proteins analyzed;

NL, the number of visible nonlinear features in the data;

according to:

$$NP = 2EX + PE + 2TS + NL \qquad \text{(Eq. 43)}$$

providing that accurate and sufficient data are obtained. The 2EX segment is neglected if *all* tissues and fluid spaces of the body are analyzed in a full physiological assessment.

Examples of application of Equation 43 can be given. The biexponential decline in plasma drug concentrations (EX = 2) after intravenous drug injection together with urinary excretion data (PE = 1) yields NP = 5 (i.e., $V_c$, $Cl_D$, $Cl_s$, $V_D^{ss}$ or $V_T$, and $Cl_R$) (48). Tissue analyses allow calculation of $Cl_{di}$ and $K_{pi}$ for each specific tissue space. Each nonlinear condition may permit calculation of one additional parameter (both $V_{max}$ and $K_m$ instead of their ratio of $V_{max}/K_m$ or $Cl_{int}$).

In construction and characterization of models, the volume and clearance terms are preferable in quantitation of the fundamental properties of drugs rather than rate constants, because of their physiologic and physicochemical bases. Rate constants are *ratio* terms. Most commonly, for example, for a two-compartment systemic clearance model (Figure 1) they are:

TABLE 6. EFFECT OF CHANGING SYSTEMIC CLEARANCE
ON VALUES OF $V_{D\beta}$ AND $V_D^{ss}$

Parameters maintained constant:

$$V_c = 12 \text{ L.}$$
$$V_T = 8 \text{ L.}$$
$$Cl_D = 12 \text{ L/hr.}$$

| $Cl_s$ (L/hr.) | $V_{D\beta}$ (L.) | $V_D^{ss}$ (L.) | $\lambda_z$ (hr.$^{-1}$) |
|---|---|---|---|
| 0.12 | 20.0 | 20.0 | 0.006 |
| 1.2 | 20.3 | 20.0 | 0.059 |
| 12.0 | 24.0 | 20.0 | 0.500 |
| 120.0 | 89.2 | 20.0 | 1.345 |

Adapted from Reference 50.

$$k_{el} = Cl_s/V_c \qquad \text{(Eq. 44)}$$

$$k_{12} = Cl_D/V_c \qquad \text{(Eq. 45)}$$

$$k_{21} = Cl_D/V_T \qquad \text{(Eq. 46)}$$

Rate constants, therefore, do not quantitate individual processes. Similarly, slope values ($\lambda_i$) and half-lives ($t_{1/2z}$) are complex functions of distribution and clearance and may not adequately reflect the individual elements of a system. Again, for the two-compartment systemic clearance model, the multiple determinants of $\lambda_i$ slopes can be assessed from:

$$\lambda_1^+, \lambda_2^- = -b \pm \sqrt{b^2 - 4c} \qquad \text{(Eq. 47)}$$

where

$$-b = \frac{Cl_s}{V_c} + \frac{Cl_D}{V_c} + \frac{Cl_D}{V_T} \qquad \text{(Eq. 47a)}$$

$$c = Cl_s \cdot Cl_D/V_c \cdot V_T \qquad \text{(Eq. 47b)}$$

As pointed out above, $\lambda_z$ approaches a limiting value of $Cl_s/V_D^{ss}$ for low clearance drugs (Equation 42 and Table 6).

The employment of models has also led to introduction of a time- and clearance-dependent volume of distribution parameter, $V_{D\beta}$ or $V_D^{area}$. This parameter is calculated from:

$$V_{D\beta} = F \cdot D_o/AUC \cdot \lambda_z \qquad \text{(Eq. 48)}$$

and represents a proportionality factor between plasma concentrations and amount of drug in the body during the terminal or $\lambda_z$ phase of disposition. As shown in Table 6, it is affected by elimination and changes as clearance is altered (50). A slower clearance allows more time for drug equilibration into tissues and creates a smaller $V_{D\beta}$. It can be noted that:

$$\lim_{Cl_s \longrightarrow 0} V_{D\beta} = V_D^{ss} \qquad \text{(Eq. 48a)}$$

and thus $V_{D\beta}$ is often used to represent $V_D^{ss}$ for low clearance drugs.

## Sundry Observations

In the absence of adequate information to calculate either the time-average pharmacokinetic parameters or to evolve a specific model, at least two summary characteristics of the drug or metabolite can be used to describe the data. These are the AUC and the $\bar{t}$. The AUC is a fundamental characteristic of each compound which is determined by:

$$AUC = \frac{\text{Amount (Absorbed or Formed)}}{\text{Total Clearance (Systemic or Oral)}} \qquad \text{(Eq. 49)}$$

It may not be possible to fully define the numerator or denominator of the equation, but the net effect of these pharmacokinetic determinants can be described as the AUC. Similarly, the $\bar{t}$ is a mixed function of total volume of distribution, systemic clearance, and input rate (Equation 24) and can be used to summarize an important time element of the system. This approach may be most helpful for characterizing drug metabolites where, in many cases, neither the amount formed or the clearance mechanism may be ascertained (51,52). In both cases, calculation of AUC and $\bar{t}$ requires extrapolation of $C_p$ versus time data to time infinity, and the $\lambda_z$ should be measured as accurately as possible.

Blood clearance, rather than plasma clearance, may be the most relevant measure of drug elimination rate if the drug partitions/diffuses rapidly between red cells and plasma (35,53–55). Clearance is a proportionality constant between the removal or transfer rate (dx/dt) and substrate concentration (S):

$$\frac{dx}{dt} = Cl \cdot S, \text{ or Velocity} = \frac{V_{max}}{K_m} \cdot S \qquad \text{(Eq. 50)}$$

The inappropriate use of plasma rather than blood concentration may yield a clearance value which does not represent the true output from the system. Some drugs do not enter red cells or their efflux is so slow (e.g., PAH, Reference 54) that plasma concentrations serve as the

TABLE 7. RELATIONSHIP BETWEEN PHYSIOLOGIC PROPERTIES AND BODY WEIGHT AMONG MAMMALS: PROPERTY = (BODY WEIGHT)$^{Exponent}$

| Property | Exponent |
|---|---|
| Creatinine Clearance | 0.69 |
| Inulin Clearance | 0.77 |
| PAH Clearance | 0.80 |
| Basal $O_2$ Consumption | 0.73 |
| Endogenous N output | 0.72 |
| $O_2$ Consumption by liver slices | 0.77 |
| Kidneys Weight | 0.85 |
| Heart Weight | 0.98 |
| Liver Weight | 0.87 |
| Stomach and Intestines Weight | 0.94 |
| Blood Weight | 0.99 |

Data from Reference 57.

clearance substrate and the maximum systemic (renal) clearance is plasma flow rather than blood flow. The rate of red cell efflux of drug must be sufficiently rapid in comparison with the organ transit time of RBC for drug removal/equilibration to be of quantitative importance (55,56). Similar considerations pertain to the role of plasma protein binding in organ drug uptake. The current clearance models assume that drug equilibration between plasma proteins and tissue water is relatively rapid compared with transit through the organ. This accounts for experimental observations with drugs such as propranolol (34) where extraction ratios approach unity in spite of greater than 90% binding of this drug to plasma proteins. Further definition and evaluation of organ clearance rates for drugs with slow binding or red cell partition rates will require measurements of the rates of drug uptake and release from both plasma proteins and red blood cells.

Pharmacokinetic parameters related to volume or clearance should be normalized to standard body size. Most physiologic flow and clearance functions can be correlated among species in parallel with body surface area (Table 7) and the most logical expression of clearance appears to be liters/hr/1.73m$^2$. Adolph's data (57) suggest that organ sizes and body space sizes are more proportional to total body weight. Thus volumes expressed as liters/kg seem appropriate and thereby directly yield the distribution coefficient ($K_D$, Equation 10, Table 2). The question of whether to normalize pharmacokinetic parameters according to surface area or body weight is difficult to resolve in man alone. Humans show greatest changes or differences in body size at neonatal and infant ages; at this time developmental effects complicate this type of correlation. Normalization is most important for averaging data from individuals of markedly different sizes.

## Nonlinear Pharmacokinetics

The SHAM analysis yields pharmacokinetic parameters which are dose- and time-average values. In this fashion they may adequately represent the properties of the drug in a general sense, but will have limited application to drug disposition either at other doses, as a function of time, or as a function of plasma or blood concentrations. A similar effect may result from use of a specific model or equation where linear functions fit the data but are used inappropriately. Kinetic analysis allowing parameters to vary as a function of time or plasma concentrations may sometimes be feasible to evaluate whether nonlinearity exists. For example, serial renal clearances can be assessed as a function of free or total plasma concentrations to determine whether saturable tubular secretion or reabsorption of drug occurs (Equation 21).

The Michaelis-Menten function (58):

$$\text{Velocity} = \frac{V_{max} \cdot C_p}{K_m + C_p} \text{ or } \frac{T_{max} \cdot C_p}{T_m + C_p} \tag{Eq. 51}$$

is generally useful to characterize active biotransformation or transport of drugs where limited enzyme capacity exists. Other sources of dose-dependence (rather than dose-proportionality) which may produce other types of nonlinear curves include zero-order (or other) release from drug dosage forms, saturable plasma or tissue protein binding, and product (metabolite) inhibition of metabolism (59).

The presence of nonlinear kinetics in some aspect of drug disposition may be determined in several ways. It is generally most useful to assess pharmacokinetic parameters over several dosage levels. While the Michaelis-Menten decline in phenytoin or salicylate plasma concentrations readily reveals a characteristic nonlinearity at sufficiently high doses, either lower doses or the presence of mixed absorptive, distributive, and elimination exponentials may obfuscate the occurrence of nonlinearity (59,60).

Techniques for discerning nonlinearity include the following:

A.  Lack of superposition (dividing all $C_p$ values by Dose) indicates some type of dose-dependence, but further evaluation of the basic pharmacokinetic parameters is needed to determine the type of nonlinearity.

B. The AUC disproportionate to dose indicates that either FF* or clearance (systemic or oral) is nonlinear.

C. The AUMC or $\bar{t}$ change with dose indicates that either absorption rate, $V_D^{ss}$, or clearance ($Cl_s$ or $Cl_{oral}$) is nonlinear.

D. Further calculation of $Cl_s$, $Cl_{oral}$, $V_c$, $V_D^{ss}$, $Cl_D$, FF*, and $\bar{t}_a$ is needed to evaluate whether nonlinearity exists in one or more of these parameters. Significant and consistent changes must occur in relation to dose and thus three dose levels are helpful. For a Michaelis-Menten process, these doses should produce maximum $C_p$ values which are below and in excess of the $K_m$ value if possible.

E. Nonlinearity may or may not alter either $\lambda_z$, the fractional excretory composition of drug metabolites, or amount excreted unchanged in urine. However, changes in one or more of these parameters usually indicates the presence of nonlinearity.

F. The input rate will alter the AUC and other parameters derived from the AUC of a nonlinear drug. The calculation of FF* = $AUC_{po}/AUC_{IV}$ is distorted for drugs with nonlinear elimination clearance (60).

## Curve Fitting

Both the SHAM analysis and data characterization with a specific pharmacokinetic model share the basic need of adequate curve-fitting of experimental data to appropriate equations. The slopes and intercepts which underlie the SHAM approach and the specific parameters which can be generated when using a formulated model will depend on the number and placement of experimental points, the quality of the assay, the completeness of data collection, and other aspects already described.

Several curve-fitting programs are in frequent use with NONLIN as the most common (61). All of these share a common mechanism of being iterative procedures based on approximation of nonlinear mathematic functions with partial linear Taylor series estimates. Each program must be used extensively with diverse equations and types of data for the user to gain familiarity and experience with the reliability and range of application. However, some general guidelines can be recommended for appropriate use of nonlinear least-squares regression computer programs:

A. Multiple functions (plasma concentrations, urinary excretion rates) for each dosage level and sampled compartment should be employed simultaneously to allow all measured data to influence the analysis and to generate parameters common to all disposition data for the drug (see Figure 11; from Reference 20).

B. Weighting functions are usually necessary to offset the non-Gaussian distribution of error in pharmacokinetic data, thereby preventing large numbers from predominating in the least squares criteria (62). For example, the data in Figure 11 show a 100,000-fold range of values and the weighting function used was essentially $1/Y_i$.

C. Reasonable initial parameter estimates can be obtained either using SHAM analysis, curve stripping, or preliminary evaluation of the data. The initial estimates may bias the fitting and can be designed to do so if justified by additional information about the system. For example, the NONLIN program permits assignment of minimum and maximum parameter values. Factors such as plasma volume for $V_c$ and cardiac output or organ blood flow for distribution clearance or systemic clearance may be used to physiologically limit the parameter range.

D. The absence of systematic deviations between the measured data and fitted curves is one of the most important criteria for a suitable least-squares fit (63). This pertains to all functions; such deviations in one or more functions may be indicative of nonlinearity, an inappropriate predictor equation, or an improper least-squares fitting. Inspection of graphs of all measured and fitted pharmacokinetic data is most useful (see Figure 11) in this regard.

E. Coefficients of determination ($r^2$) or correlation (r) are usually very high even for unsuitable curve fittings. This alone is not a good criterion.

F. Small, reasonable, or explainable (lack of data) standard deviations should be expected for the individual fitted parameters.

G. The iterative procedure should attain satisfactory convergency rather than reaching a specified upper limit in number of iterations.

H. The predictor equations, when possible, should incorporate corrections such as lag-time for absorption, duration of short-term drug infusion, and other adjustments for perturbations from ordinary or bolus dose disposition patterns.

In general, the most important use of curve-fitting techniques is to obtain parameters for an accurate AUC according to Equation 4 ($\Sigma C_i/\lambda_i$). Alternative methods for calculating the AUC such as La-Grange Polynomials, Spline, and Log-Trapezoidal (in part) offer im-

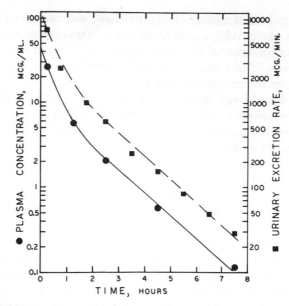

FIGURE 11.   Plasma concentrations ($C_p$) and urinary excretion rates (dXu/dt) of ampicillin as a function of time. The data were fitted with two functions simultaneously ($C_p = C_1 \cdot e^{-\lambda_1 t} + C_2 \cdot e^{-\lambda_2 t}$) and dXu/dt $= Cl_R(C_1 \cdot e^{-\lambda_1 t} + C_2 \cdot e^{-\lambda_2 t})$ yielding five basic parameters (20).

proved curve resolution over the common Trapezoidal Rule when a specific function cannot be discerned from the data pattern (40) or for providing initial estimates of parameters such as clearance.

## Statistical Considerations

The design, analysis, and interpretation of pharmacokinetic data require many logical uses of statistics to assure a lack of bias in the arrangement of studies, in curve fitting, and to employ standard tests to assess possible significant differences between treatments. Several important points can be noted specially in consideration of pharmacokinetic data.

Prior to an experiment, the number of subjects or animals needed to discern an effect or lack thereof can be estimated using an appropriate statistical method of "determination of the power of the test" (64). For, say, a bioavailability study, this method usually predicts the need for far more subjects than most investigators are willing to include. Pharmacokinetic studies of this nature involve intensive human and analytical work, and multiple blood sampling points form the basis of each AUC value. Thus 10 to 18 subjects has become an unofficial compromise norm for many types of cross-over drug disposition studies. This compromise was based on extensive experience and ethical concerns and limitations.

Multiple dose levels and routes of drug administration in groups of subjects or animals should entail use of a balanced cross-over design to randomize or equalize drug or sequence effects on the subjects (64). A well planned study facilitates the later statistical analysis considerably.

Averaging data often distorts pharmacokinetic parameters. The arithmetic mean can be used when averaging normally distributed data. This has the advantage of yielding interpretable standard deviations and facilitating subsequent statistical tests. Unfortunately, pharmacokinetic data often follow a log-normal distribution for which the geometric mean yields the best measure of the central tendency of the data. The geometric mean is awkward or impossible to employ in statistical tests.

Correlation and least-squares regression analyses are often performed to assess interrelationships between pharmacokinetic parameters. A frequent problem arises when both variables contain experimental error, for example, when assessing drug excretion or clearance versus creatinine clearance (see Figure 12). This does not affect a correlation analysis, but the ordinary least-square regression entails the requirement that one variable (the abscissa value) contains no error. Appropriate techniques exist for "fitting straight lines when both variables are subject to error". Riggs et al (65) indicate that no one method is universally appropriate; however, the writer prefers the "weighted perpendicular method" as a reasonable first-choice procedure for many types of pharmacokinetic data where the error is reasonably proportional to the variance of parameters in each dimension. This method is easily programmed on small computers.

## Ethical Factors

Part of any study design includes a clear and reasonably detailed protocol to standardize all elements of the investigation and to make certain that all collaborators and assistants follow proper directions. These protocols usually serve a dual purpose in grant applications and for submission to Committees on Human Research.

Guidelines exist for use of both animals and human subjects in pharmacological experimentation. Common sense must usually pre-

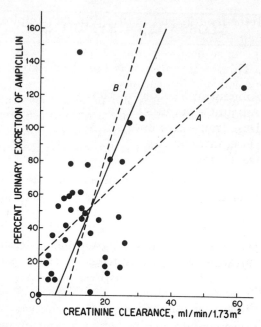

FIGURE 12.  Relationship between percent urinary excretion of ampicillin (Y) and normalized creatinine clearance (X) in a group of infants. Data are from Kaplan et al (66). Lines A and B show the results of regressing variable Y on X and X on Y, respectively, while the solid line shows the results of the perpendicular least-squares regression method (65). The last method comes nearest to depicting the true relationship which, physiologically, should have a zero-intercept and the same mean as the other lines.

vail. Well planned experiments and expert use of pharmacokinetic methods can aid considerably in minimizing the amount of risk to which patients or volunteers need be exposed. Further evolution of principles of physiological pharmacokinetics and "animal scale-up" methods will add greater meaningfulness to *in vitro* and animal studies which may eventually lead to the need for only confirmatory experiments in man.

## ACKNOWLEDGMENTS

The skilled secretarial assistance of Ms. Tracey McCarthy is appreciated.

Supported in part by Grant 20852 from the National Institute of General Medical Sciences, NIH.

# GLOSSARY OF SYMBOLS

## Amounts

| | |
|---|---|
| $A_B$ | Amount in the body at time t |
| $A_E$ | Amount eliminated up to time t |
| $D_o$ | Dose (route variable) |
| $D_{IV}$ | Dose, intravenous |
| $D_{po}$ | Dose, oral |

## Times

| | |
|---|---|
| t | Variable time |
| T | A specific time |
| $\bar{t}$ | Mean transit time |
| $\bar{t}_a$ | Mean transit time for absorption |
| $\tau$ | Duration of dosing interval |

## Concentrations

| | |
|---|---|
| $C_p$ | Plasma concentration |
| $C_b$ | Blood concentration |
| $C_p^{ss}$ | Steady-state plasma concentration |
| $C_p^*$ | Last measured plasma concentration |
| $\bar{C}$ | Time-average concentration |
| $C_f$ | Unbound or free concentration |
| $C_a$ | Arterial plasma or blood concentration |
| $C_v$ | Venous plasma or blood concentration |
| $C_i$, $C_z$, $H_O$ | Intercepts of plasma concentration versus time curve |
| $K_m$, $T_m$ | Michaelis-Menten constant (metabolism, renal transport) |

## Clearances

| | |
|---|---|
| Cl | Clearance, mechanism variable |
| $Cl_s$ | Systemic clearance resulting from a non-first pass dose |
| $Cl_{oral}$ | Oral clearance where drug first enters the circulation passing initially through the liver |
| $Cl_{int}$ | Intrinsic metabolic clearance = $V_{max}/K_m$ for biotransformation |
| $Cl_{int}^R$ | Intrinsic renal clearance = $T_{max}/T_m$ for transport |
| $Cl_R$ | Renal clearance |
| $Cl_M$ | Metabolic clearance |
| $Cl_H$ | Hepatic clearance |

P          Transcapillary permeability

$Cl_D$       Total distribution clearance

$Cl_{di}$       Distribution clearance to/from specific sites or compartments

## Volumes, Weights

$V_p$       Volume of plasma compartment

$V_c$       Volume of central compartment

$V_T$       Apparent volume of tissue compartment ($\Sigma K_{pi} \cdot V_{ti}$)

$V_D^{ss}$       Steady-state volume of distribution

$V_{D\beta}$       Apparent volume of distribution during $\lambda_z$ or terminal phase

$V_L$       Volume or weight of liver

TBWt     Total body weight

## Fractions

$f_{up}$       Fraction unbound in plasma

$f_{ut}$       Fraction unbound in tissue

$f_R$       Fraction reabsorbed in kidney tubules

F          Fraction of dose available from dosage form

F*        Fraction available following first-pass metabolism

FF*       Systemic availability

ER        Extraction Ratio: $(C_a - C_v)/C_a$

## Flows

Q          Blood or plasma flow

$Q_H$       Hepatic blood flow

$Q_{RP}$     Effective renal plasma flow

## Ratios

$K_p$, $K_{pi}$    Tissue:Plasma partition coefficient

$K_D$       Body:Plasma distribution ratio ($V_D^{ss}$/TBWt)

## Areas

A, AUC    Area under plasma (or blood) concentration versus time curve

M, AUMC   Area under moment curve

## Rate Constants, Slopes

$k_a$       Absorption rate constant

$k_o$       Zero-order infusion rate

$\lambda_i$, $\lambda_z$      Slopes of plasma concentration versus time curve

$k_{el}$       Elimination rate constant ($Cl_s/V_c$)

$k_{12}$          Distribution rate constant from plasma to tissues $(Cl_D/V_c)$

$k_{21}$          Distribution rate constant from tissues to plasma $(Cl_D/V_T)$

**Rates**

$V_{max}$          Maximum velocity of metabolism

$T_{max}$          Maximum velocity of transport

$dXu/dt$        Urinary excretion rate

# REFERENCES

1. Bischoff KB and Dedrick RL: Thiopental pharmacokinetics. J Pharm Sci 1968; 57:1346–51.
2. Dedrick RL: Animal scale-up. J Pharmacokin Biopharm 1973; 1:435–61.
3. Rane A, Wilkinson GR, and Shand DG: Prediction of hepatic extraction rate from *in vitro* measurement of intrinsic clearance. J Pharmacol Exp Ther 1977; 200:420–24.
4. Manninen V and Koriionen A: Inequal digoxin tablets. Lancet 1973; 2:1268.
5. MacKichan J, Duffner PK, and Cohen ME: Adsorption of diazepam to plastic tubing. N Engl J Med 1979; 301:332–3.
6. Wood M, Shand DG, and Wood AJJ: Altered drug binding due to the use of indwelling heparinized cannulas (heparin lock) for sampling. Clin Pharmacol Ther 1979; 25:103–7.
7. Cotham RH and Shand D: Spuriously low plasma propranolol concentrations resulting from blood collection methods. Clin Pharmacol Ther 1975; 18:535–8.
8. Chavarri M, Luetscher JA, Dowdy AJ and Ganguly A: The effects of temperature and plasma cortisol on distribution of aldosterone between plasma and red blood cells: Influence on metabolic clearance rate and on hepatic and renal extraction of aldosterone. J Clin Endocrinol Metab 1977; 44:752–9.
9. Garbe A, Steiner K, and Nowak H: The accumulation of pyroxamidin—a new antihypertensive—in platelets and its significance in blood level determinations. Naunym-Schiedberg's Arch Pharmacol 1980; 311:in press.
10. Chou W: Arterial blood clearance approach for the rapid derivations of general equations for calculating commonly needed pharmacokinetic parameters of drugs involving hepatic, renal and/or pulmonary elimination—Limitations of multi-compartmental model analyses. Academy of Pharmaceutical Sciences, Washington DC, May 1980.
11. Food and Drug Administration: Bioequivalence requirements and *in vivo* bioavailability procedures. Federal Register 1977; 42:1623–53.
12. Tognoni G, Latini R, and Jusko WJ: *Frontiers in Therapeutic Drug Monitoring.* New York, NY: Raven Press, 1980.
13. Levy RH and Dumain M: Time-dependent kinetics VI: Direct relationship between equations for drug levels during induction and those involving constant clearance. J Pharm Sci 1979; 68:934–6.
14. Schentag JJ, Jusko WJ, Plaut ME, Cumbo TJ, Vance JW, and Abrutyn E: Tissue persistence of gentamicin in man. JAMA 1977; 238:327–9.

15. Schentag JJ, Jusko WJ, Vance JW, Cumbo TJ, Abrutyn E, DeLatre M, and Gerbracht LM: Gentamicin disposition and tissue accumulation on multiple dosing. J Pharmacokin Biopharm 1977; 5:559–77.
16. Kraus JW, Desmond PV, Marshall JP, Johnson RF, Schenker S, and Wilkinson GR: Effects of aging and liver disease on disposition of lorazepam. Clin Pharmacol Ther 1978; 24:411–9.
17. Jusko WJ and Gretch M: Plasma and tissue protein binding of drugs in pharmacokinetics. Drug Met Rev 1976; 5:43–140.
18. Cabana BE, Van Harken DR, and Hottendorf GH: Comparative pharmacokinetics and metabolism of cephapirin in laboratory animals and humans. Antimicrob Ag Chemother 1976; 10:307–17.
19. Savello DR and Shangraw RF: Stability of sodium ampicillin solutions in the frozen and liquid states. Am J Hosp Pharm 1971; 28:754–9.
20. Jusko WJ and Lewis GP: Comparison of ampicillin and hetacillin pharmacokinetics in man. J Pharm Sci 1973; 62:69–76.
21. Oppenheimer JH, Schwartz HL, and Surks MI: Determination of common parameters of iodothyronine metabolism and distribution in man by noncompartmental analysis. J Clin Endocrinol Metab 1975; 41:319–24, 1172–3.
22. Larson KB and Snyder KL: Measurement of relative blood flow, transit-time distributions and transport-model parameters by residue detection when radiotracer recirculates. J Theor Biol 1972; 37:503–29.
23. Rowland M, Benet LZ, and Graham G: Clearance concepts in pharmacokinetics. J Pharmacokin Biopharm 1973; 1:123–36.
24. Wilkinson GR and Shand DG: A physiologic approach to hepatic drug clearance. Clin Pharmacol Ther 1975; 18:377–90.
25. Gillette JR: Factors affecting drug metabolism. Ann N Y Acad Sci 1971; 179:43–66.
26. Chen H-SG and Gross JF: Estimation of tissue-to-plasma partition coefficients used in physiological pharmacokinetic models. J Pharmacokin Biopharm 1979; 7:117–25.
27. Renkin EM: Effects of blood flow on diffusion kinetics in isolated, perfused hindlegs of cats: A double circulation hypothesis. Amer J Physiol 1955; 183:125–36.
28. Pappenheimer JR: Passage of molecules through capillary walls. Physiol Rev 1953; 33:387–423.
29. Schultz JS and Armstrong W: Permeability of interstitial space of muscle (rat diaphragm) to solutes of different molecular weights. J Pharm Sci 1978; 67:696–700.
30. Lassen NA and Perl W: *Tracer Kinetic Methods in Medical Physiology.* New York, NY: Raven Press, 1979.
31. Nagashima R and Levy G: Effect of perfusion rate and distribution factors on drug elimination kinetics in a perfused organ system. J Pharm Sci 1968; 57:1991–3.
32. Bass L: Current models of hepatic elimination. Gastroenterology 1979; 76:1504–5.
33. Levy G and Yacobi A: Effect of plasma protein binding on elimination of warfarin. J Pharm Sci 1974; 63:805–6.
34. Shand DG, Cotham RH, and Wilkinson GR: Perfusion-limited effects of plasma drug binding on hepatic drug extraction. Life Sci 1976; 19:125–9.
35a. Pang KS and Rowland M: Hepatic clearance of drugs. I. Theoretical considerations of a "well-stirred" model and a "parallel tube" model. Influence of hepatic blood flow, plasma and blood cell binding, and the hepatocellular enzymatic activity on hepatic drug clearance. J Pharmacokin Biopharm 1977; 5:625-53.
35b. Levy G: Effect of plasma protein binding on renal clearance of drugs. J Pharm Sci 1980; 69:483.

36. Yamaska K, Nakawaga T, and Uno T: Statistical moments in pharmacokinetics. J Pharmacokin Biopharm 1978; 6:547–58.
37. Perrier D and Gibaldi M: Calculation of absorption rate constants for drugs with incomplete availability. J Pharm Sci 1973; 62:225.
38. Caprani O, Sveinsdottir E, and Lassen N: SHAM, a method for biexponential curve resolution using initial slope, height, area, and moment of the experimental decay type curve. J Theor Biol 1975; 52:299–315.
39. Benet LZ and Galeazzi RL: Noncompartmental determination of the steady-state volume of distribution. J Pharm Sci 1979; 68:1071–4.
40. Yeh KC and Kwan KC: A comparison of numerical integrating algorithms by trapezoidal, LaGrange, and Spline approximation. J Pharmacokin Biopharm 1978; 6:79–98.
41. Wagner JG: Linear pharmacokinetic equations allowing direct calculation of many needed pharmacokinetic parameters from the coefficients and exponents of polyexponential equations which have been fitted to the data. J Pharmacokin Biopharm 1976; 4:443–67.
42. Vaughan DP, Mallard DJH, and Mitchard M: A general method of determining the first order input rate constant of a drug that is directly absorbed into the central compartment. J Pharm Pharmacol 1974; 26:508.
43. Simon W: *Mathematical Techniques for Biology and Medicine.* Cambridge, MA: The MIT Press, 1977.
44. Wagner JG, Northam JI, Alway CD, and Carpenter OS: Blood levels of drug at the equilibrium state after multiple dosing. Nature 1965; 207:1301–2.
45. Chiou W: Potential pitfalls in the conventional pharmacokinetic studies: Effects of the initial mixing of drug in blood and the pulmonary first-pass elimination. J Pharmacokin Biopharm 1979; 7:527–36.
46. Wagner JG: Linear pharmacokinetic models and vanishing exponential terms: Implications in pharmacokinetics. J Pharmacokin Biopharm 1976; 4:395–425.
47. Gibaldi M and Perrier D: *Pharmacokinetics.* New York, NY: Marcel Dekker, 1975.
48. Benet LZ: General treatment of linear mammillary models with elimination from any compartment as used in pharmacokinetics. J Pharm Sci 1972; 61:536–41.
49. Wagner JG: *Fundamentals of Clinical Pharmacokinetics.* Hamilton, IL: Drug Intelligence Publications, 1975.
50. Jusko WJ and Gibaldi M: Effects of change in elimination on various parameters of the two-compartment open model. J Pharm Sci 1972; 61:1270–3.
51. DeVane CL and Jusko WJ: Pharmacokinetics of high clearance drugs and their metabolites. In: Usdin E, Dahl SG, Gram L, Lingjaerde O, eds. *Clinical Pharmacology in Psychiatry.* London: MacMillan and Co., 1980:in press.
52. Pang KS and Gillette JR: A theoretical examination of the effects of gut wall metabolism, hepatic elimination, and enterohepatic recycling on estimates of bioavailability and of hepatic blood flow. J Pharmacokin Biopharm 1978; 6:355–67.
53. Wilkinson GR: Pharmacokinetics of drug disposition: Hemodynamic considerations. Ann Rev Pharmacol 1975; 15:11–27.
54. Phillips RA, Dole VP, Hamilton PB, Emerson K, Archibald RM, and Van Slyke DD: Effects of acute hemorrhage and traumatic shock on renal function of dogs. Am J Physiol 1945; 145:314–36.
55. Goresky CA, Bach GB, and Nadeau BE: Red cell carriage of label. Its limiting effect on the exchange of materials in the liver. Circ Res 1975; 36:328–51.
56. Perl W: Red cell permeability effect on the mean transit time of an indicator transported through an organ by red cells and plasma. Circ Res 1975; 36:352–7.

57. Aldoph EF: Quantitative relations in the physiological constitutions of mammals. Science 1949; 109:579–85.
58. Michaelis L and Menten ML: Die kinetik der invertinwirkung. Biochem Z 1913; 49:333–69.
59. Levy G: Dose dependent effects in pharmacokinetics. In: Tedeschi DH and Tedeschi RE, eds. *Importance of Fundamental Principles in Drug Evaluation*. New York, NY: Raven Press, 1968.
60. Jusko WJ, Koup JR, and Alvan G: Nonlinear assessment of phenytoin bioavailability. J Pharmacokin Biopharm 1976; 4:327–36.
61. Metzler CM, Elfring GL, and McEwen AJ: A users manual for NONLIN and associated programs. Research Biostatistics, The Upjohn Co., Kalamazoo, MI, 1974.
62. Daniel C and Wood FS: *Fitting Equations to Data*. Wiley-Interscience, New York, 1971.
63. Boxenbaum HG, Riegelman S, and Elashoff RM: Statistical estimations in pharmacokinetics. J Pharmacokin Biopharm 1974; 2:123–48.
64. Westlake WJ: The design and analysis of comparative blood-level trials. In: Swarbrick J, ed. *Dosage Form Design and Bioavailability*. Philadelphia: Lea and Febiger, 1973; 149–79.
65. Riggs DS, Guarnieri JA, and Addelman S: Fitting straight lines when both variables are subject to error. Life Sci 1978; 22:1305–60.
66. Kaplan JM, McCracken GH, Horton LJ, Thomas ML, and Davis M: Pharmacologic studies in neonates given large doses of ampicillin. J Ped 1974; 84:571–7.

# Index

Troleandomycin *(Contd.)*
  And Theophylline Clearance 107
Tube Model 651
Tuberculosis
  Streptomycin In 175
  Transport Maximum 87-88
    Of PAH 88

## U

Urea
  Diet 34
  GI Bleed 34
  Hemoperfusion Of 52
  Hypercatabolic States 34
  Production 34
  Serum Concentration 34
Urine pH Effects
  On Lidocaine Excretion 356
  On Procainamide Excretion 411
  On Quinidine Excretion 441
  On Salicylate Excretion 491-492
  On Tricyclic Antidepressants 558-559

## V

Valproic Acid
  Distribution In Cirrhosis
  Phenytoin Interaction 296,315

Vancomycin
  Consult Service 27
  In Renal Failure 36
Velosef(Tm)
  See Cephradine
Vincristine
  In Renal Failure 36
  Methotrexate Interaction 522
  Pharmacokinetic Parameters 522
Vitamin E
  Also See Alpha Tocopherol
  In Premature Infants 80
Volume Of Distribution
  Also See Specific Drug
  Steady-State 647

## W

Warfarin
  Consult Service 28
  In Renal Failure 36
  In Viral Hepatitis 61

## Z

Zollinger-Ellison Syndrome
  Digoxin Metabolism 325

## ACKNOWLEDGEMENT

The Editors graciously thank Mr. Larry F. Barker who developed the computer program which indexed this book.

*Publisher's Note:* The computer tape of the index subsequently provided direct data input for typesetting.

75767